PRACTICAL HANDBOOK OF

Human Biologic Age Determination

PRACTICAL HANDBOOK OF

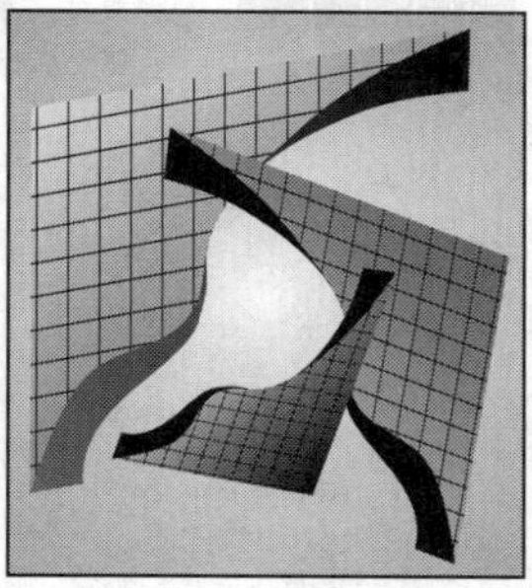

Human Biologic Age Determination

Edited by

Arthur K. Balin, M.D., Ph.D., F.A.C.P

Executive Director

American Aging Association

President

Longevity Research, Inc.

Private Practice

Dermatology

Chester, Pennsylvania

CRC Press

Boca Raton Ann Arbor London Tokyo

Library of Congress Cataloging-in-Publication Data

Practical handbook of human biologic age determination / edited by
Arthur K. Balin.
p. cm.
Includes bibliographical references and index.
ISBN 0-8493-0129-7
1. Man—Age determination. 2. Aging. I. Balin, Arthur K.
QP86.P695 1994
612.6—dc20 93-43792
CIP

International Standard Book Number 0-8493-0129-7
Library of Congress Card Number 93-43792
Printed in the United States of America 1 2 3 4 5 6 7 8 9 0
Printed on acid-free paper

PREFACE

Although functional decline appears to be an inevitable and inescapable consequence of aging, there are often considerable differences between individuals with respect to the rate and extent of this decline. Individuals may be young or old in relation to their number of years. As a result, age-related disease or age-related death may occur at different chronological ages. It follows that the true or practically relevant age of an individual is not adequately defined by the time that has elapsed since birth, but by a figure reflecting the individual's progressive inability to respond adaptively to an environmental stress that leads to a decreased viability and increased vulnerability to death. The degree of age-related vulnerability is defined as "biological age".

There has been a great surge of interest in techniques or treatments that might delay the process of human aging. Transferring information, obtained in the basic research laboratory or from studies with animals, to humans is hampered by the time it takes to ascertain whether a specific intervention will extend the mean and maximum human life span. Aging research will be markedly enhanced by techniques that measure the biologic age of an individual because these tests could be used to estimate the effectiveness of therapeutic interventions designed to retard the aging process and extend the length of healthy, productive life. In this volume we review scientific studies that have measured various parameters that change with chronologic age. Our objective is to explore these parameters and follow longitudinally those which will give the highest likelihood of reflecting biological age.

The molecular mechanisms of biologic aging have been under active investigation by a small number of investigators over the last 40 years, but a substantial increase in the quantity and quality of basic aging studies occurred in the mid 1970s, concomitant with the formation of the National Institute on Aging. Development of useful model systems to study aging, along with the advent of the revolution in molecular biology, is likely to greatly accelerate the rate of aging research and increase the likelihood that significant advances will be made in the foreseeable future. *We already have the technology to determine why we age.* It is only a matter of committing sufficient resources to this problem. Whether we will be able to modify the rate of aging in humans depends on the mechanisms that are responsible for the aging process. Therefore, it is possible that we will discover why we age, and perhaps we will then learn that there is nothing we can do to modify the process.

However, there are a number of clues that have developed that suggest that it might be possible to influence or modify the aging process in whole or in part. Studies have shown that it is possible to alter the basic rate of aging in a number of animal systems. In cold-blooded animals, such as the housefly, cooler temperatures and reduced activity will slow the rate of aging and extend the maximum life span of the longest-lived survivor by 400%. In warm-blooded animals, such as the mouse and the rat, caloric restriction will extend the life span of the longest lived survivor by 200%. Studies have shown, in these animal systems, that these manipulations also retard the appearance of many of the age-related diseases such as diabetes and cancer.

One of the problems with using animal systems to study the basic causes of aging is that many of the effects of a specific intervention or manipulation may be unrecognized when death is the end point of the study. Disease and disordered metabolism are difficult to diagnose in experimental animals because the base of knowledge about diseases in different animal species, the number of veterinarians and the intrinsic difficulty in early detection of disease in animals, and the quantity and quality of veterinary autopsies are inferior to what is available in human medicine. Knowledge of disease and the ability to diagnose early perturbations in the human body makes using the human system particularly appropriate when elucidating the basic mechanisms of human aging. There have been a number of treatments postulated, based on research that already exists, that propose modifying the aging process in humans in whole or in part. Many more are likely to come in future years as a result of the increasing interest and active research being done.

How are we going to tell whether any specific treatment can retard the aging process? At present, the only reliable way to do this would be to give a group of people the treatment and wait 40 or 50 or 60 years to see whether the treatment worked. Multiple studies would need to be done for every proposed treatment. This will take many lifetimes and enormous expense. In order to provide short cuts to this procedure, we wish to be able to measure the rate of aging in an individual. If we could reliably measure how old a person's body is, then we could give them any specific treatment and measure their biologic age again in a few years and be able to rapidly tell whether a specific intervention was useful in retarding the rate of aging.

A number of individuals have been attempting to develop ways to measure the rate of aging in people. Many of them have given this problem serious consideration for many years and have developed approaches that they believe will be useful. A large proportion of these individuals provide their thoughts and approaches to this problem in this volume.

When a test or battery of tests is developed to determine a human's biologic age, the initial validation of the predictive power of the test must be made by following a group of people serially for sufficient years until they have died and the reliability of the parameters chosen can be ascertained. It would be very discouraging to set up a large study, measure a number of parameters in people for 50 or 60 years, and then analyze the data and learn that no measured parameter predicted biologic age. To try to prevent this outcome, it is necessary to measure as many of the most likely predictive factors as possible. For that reason, it is particularly important to have the thoughts of virtually every investigator that has considered the problem collected in one volume. This handbook should provide the basis on which any investigator trying to set up a study to measure biologic age can draw upon existing expertise. This work will stand as a landmark in the development of our ability to measure human biologic age and therefore to ascertain what interventions can retard the aging process in humans.

Arthur K. Balin, M.D., Ph.D., F.A.C.P.
Chester, Pennsylvania

CONTRIBUTORS

Jozef Adam, M.D., Ph.D.
Department of Medical Chemistry and Biochemistry
Safárik University
Kosice, Slovakia

Bruce N. Ames, Ph.D.
Department of Biochemistry
University of California
Berkeley, California

Arthur K. Balin, M.D., Ph.D., F.A.C.P.
American Aging Association *and*
Longevity Research, Inc. *and*
Private Practice
Dermatology and Mohs Micrographic Surgery and Cutaneous Oncology
Chester, Pennsylvania

Douglas M. Bowden, M.D.
Department of Psychiatry and Behavioral Sciences
University of Washington
Seattle, Washington

Larry J. Brant, Ph.D.
Gerontology Research Center
National Institute on Aging
Francis Scott Key Medical Center
Baltimore, Maryland

Wojtek J. Chodzko-Zajko, Ph.D.
School of PERD
Kent State University
Kent, Ohio

Ward Dean, M.D.
The Center for Bio-Gerontology
Pensacola, Florida

Tamara L. Dubina, M.D., Ph.D.
Hadassah Medical School
The Hebrew University
Jerusalem, Israel

W. John Elder, M.D.
Transamerica Life Companies
Los Angeles, California

Myrvin H. Ellastad, M.D.
Memorial Heart Institute of Long Beach
Long Beach, California

Pertti Era, Ph.D.
Department of Health Sciences *and*
Gerontology Research Center
University of Jyväskylä
Jyväskylä, Finland

James L. Fozard, Ph.D.
Gerontology Research Center
National Institute on Aging
Francis Scott Key Medical Center
Baltimore, Maryland

Toshiyuki Furukawa, M.D., D.Med.Sci.
Osaka National Hospital
Osaka, Japan *and*
Research Center for Advanced Science and Technology
University of Tokyo
Tokyo, Japan

Eino Heikkinen, M.D., Ph.D.
Department of Health Sciences *and*
Gerontology Research Center
University of Jyväskylä
Jyväskylä, Finland

Daniel Hershey, Ph.D.
Department of Chemical and Nuclear Engineering
University of Cincinnati
Cincinnati, Ohio

Richard Hochschild
Hoch Company
Corona Del Mar, California

Gerhard Hofecker, D.V.M., Ph.D.
Austrian Society of Geriatrics and Gerontology *and* Institute of Physiology
University of Veterinary Medicine
Vienna, Austria

J. William Hollingsworth, M.D.
Medical Service
San Diego Veterans Administration Hospital
and Department of Medicine
University of California
San Diego, California

Edwin B. Hutchins, Ph.D.
The HEALTHIER PEOPLE NETWORK, Inc.
Decatur, Georgia

Stanley Kaplan, Ph.D.
Prickard, Lowe and Garrick
Newport Beach, California

Sankar N. Koyal, Ph.D.
Division of Pulmonary Medicine
UCLA-VA Medical Center
Los Angeles, California

William E. Lee, III, Ph.D.
Department of Chemical Engineering
University of South Florida
Tampa, Florida

Donald G. Lindsay, M.D.
University of Southern California
College of Medicine
Los Angeles, California *and*
Foundation for Research in Aging
Ventura, California

Frédéric C. Ludwig, M.D., D.Sc.
School of Medicine
University of California
Irvine, California

Anna-Liisa Lyyra, Ph.Lic.
Department of Statistics
University of Jyväskylä
Jyväskylä, Finland

Jonathan R. Matias
Orentreich Foundation for the Advancement of Science
Cold Spring on Hudson, New York

E. Jeffrey Metter, M.D.
Gerontology Research Center
National Institute on Aging
Francis Scott Key Medical Center
Baltimore, Maryland

Andrej Molnár, M.D., Ph.D.
Department of Social Medicine
Faculty of Medicine
Safárik University
Kosice, Slovakia

Vincent M. Monnier, M.D.
School of Medicine
Institute of Pathology
Case Western Reserve University
Cleveland, Ohio

Robert F. Morgan, Ph.D.
Division of Geropsychology
International Association of Applied Psychology *and*
Department of Psychology
Antioch University at Santa Barbara
Santa Barbara, California

Eitaro Nakamura, Ph.D.
Department of Environmental Sciences
Faculty of Integrated Human Studies
Kyoto University
Kyoto, Japan

Andrej Nicák, M.D., Ph.D.
Department of Pharmacology
Safárik University
Kosice, Slovakia

Hans Niedermüller, D.Sc., Ph.D.
Institute of Physiology
University of Veterinary Medicine
Vienna, Austria

David S. Orentreich, M.D.
Orentreich Foundation for the Advancement of Science
Cold Spring on Hudson, New York *and*
Department of Dermatology
Mount Sinai School of Medicine
New York, New York

Norman Orentreich, M.D.
Orentreich Foundation for the Advancement of Science
Cold Spring on Hudson, New York *and*
Department of Dermatology
New York University School of Medicine
New York, New York

William Regelson, M.D.
Department of Medicine
Medical College of Virginia
Virginia Commonwealth University
Richmond, Virginia

Werner Ries, M.D.
Department of Gerontology
University of Leipzig
Leipzig, Germany

Lewis C. Robbins, M.D. (Deceased)
Indianapolis, Indiana

Arthur B. Robinson, Ph.D.
Oregon Institute of Science and Medicine
Cave Junction, Oregon

Laurelee R. Robinson (Deceased)
Oregon Institute of Science and Medicine
Cave Junction, Oregon

A. Ruiz-Torres, M.D., Ph.D.
Institute for Gerontologic and Metabolic Research
Universidad Autónoma de Madrid
Division of Endocrinology and Nutrition
Hospital de la Princesa
Madrid, Spain

Silverio Santiago, M.D.
Division of Pulmonary Medicine
UCLA-VA Medical Center
Los Angeles, California

Donald Schwartz, M.D.
Memorial Medical Center of Long Beach
Long Beach, California

David R. Sell, Ph.D.
School of Medicine
Institute of Pathology
Case Western Reserve University
Cleveland, Ohio

Robert A. Short, Ph.D.
Washington State University
Spokane, Washington

Monika Skalicky, D.Sc.
Institute of Physiology
University of Veterinary Medicine
Vienna, Austria

Harri Suominen, Ph.D.
Department of Health Sciences *and*
Gerontology Research Center
University of Jyväskylä
Jyväskylä, Finland

Adrian J. Williams, M.D.
Division of Pulmonary Medicine
UCLA-VA Medical Center
Los Angeles, California

Darrell D. Williams, Ph.D.
Regional Primate Research Center
University of Washington
Seattle, Washington

Jay A. Zimmerman, Ph.D.
Department of Biological Sciences
St. John's University
Jamaica, New York

Dedicated To
Lewis C. Robbins, M.D.
1909–1990

This book is a tribute to the prescience that Dr. Lewis C. Robbins exhibited throughout a long and productive career. With a positive outlook, always encouraging fellow scientists who were creative in thought and young in spirit, Dr. Robbins anticipated the direction the health sciences would take a half century ahead of most of his colleagues. A career public health officer from 1941 to 1968, he participated in the preparation of the first surgeon general's report on the health hazards of tobacco. A staunch soldier in the battle against chronic diseases, his seminal work on the appraisal of health risks helped to arm health care providers and added untold years to the lives of thousands of people. The field of prospective medicine developed around this work. The concept that our knowledge of the natural history of disease can be employed to help ordinary people anticipate the consequences of their lifestyle habits and, in so doing, make changes to alter the course of events is central to this idea.

TABLE OF CONTENTS

OVERVIEW

RISK APPRAISAL

PHYSIOLOGIC ASSESSMENT

For a detailed description of the contents of this book, see the first page of each chapter.

PHYSIOLOGIC ASSESSMENT (CONTINUED)

METABOLIC PROFILES

ORGAN SYSTEM APPROACHES

For a detailed description of the contents of this book, see the first page of each chapter.

ORGAN SYSTEM APPROACHES (CONTINUED)

BIOCHEMICAL MEASUREMENTS

NONHUMAN MODEL STUDIES

STATISTICAL ANALYSIS

For a detailed description of the contents of this book, see the first page of each chapter.

STATISTICAL ANALYSIS (CONTINUED)

For a detailed description of the contents of this book, see the first page of each chapter.

OVERVIEW

CHAPTER 1

BIOLOGICAL AGING MEASUREMENT — ITS RATIONALE, HISTORY, AND CURRENT STATUS

WARD DEAN

TABLE OF CONTENTS

I. INTRODUCTION

Benjamin Franklin[29] coined the famous one liner, "all would live long, but none would be old". The purpose of aging research is clearly to gain an understanding of the aging process so that we can devise methods to slow it down, live longer, and it is hoped, ultimately reverse the aging process.

Denham Harman,[33] in creating the American Aging Association (AGE), clearly proclaimed that "the purpose of AGE is to help people live better longer, through the promotion of biomedical aging studies directed toward slowing down the aging process(es)".[33]

The growing scientific interest in aging retardation is evidenced by an increasing number of books on this subject written by physicians and scientists for physicians and scientists.[6,7,21,24,25,30,31,52,59]

Thousands of people around the world are currently engaged in self-experimentation with a variety of potential age-retarding regimens, whether approved by the majority of the gerontological community or not. These regimens range from moderate exercise and dietary modifications to caloric restriction, megadose vitamin therapy, and various forms of pharmacotherapeutic intervention.[64]

Currently, this vast human experiment is largely unmonitored. The only way to truly determine the efficacy (or lack thereof) of any of these gerontotherapeutic regimens is to wait 50 to 100 years or so, and evaluate the results retrospectively. This method is eminently impractical for those of us now living, however.

Clearly, it is necessary to develop a means to evaluate potential life-extending gerontotherapeutic regimens over a short period of time (2 to 5 years). Probably the best way to do this is to develop

0-8493-0129-7/94/$0.00+$.50

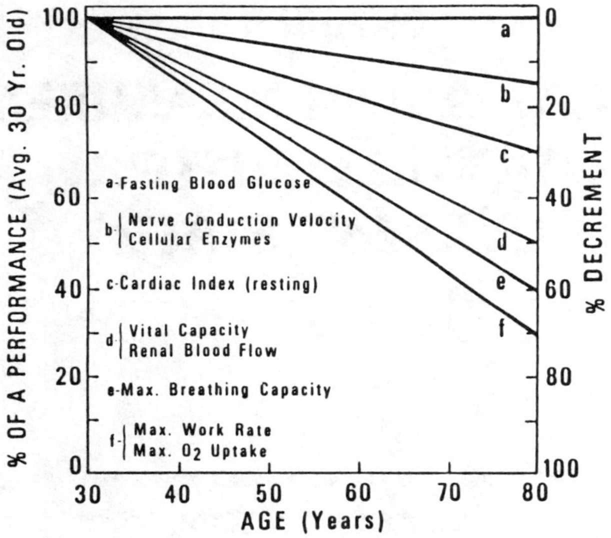

Figure 1 Schematic linear representation of the decline of various physiological functions with age.[67]

a system to measure biological age. Agents that cause a significant retardation in aging rate or reduction in biological age would clearly warrant intensified testing and evaluation.

II. WHAT IS AGING?

The definition of aging is surprisingly often not well agreed upon, even by many gerontologists. Bernard Strehler[69] has probably given the most useful definition of aging by proposing four criteria that a biological change must meet in order to qualify as aging:

1. Aging is universal. The changes occur in all older members of the species.
2. Aging is intrinsic. Aging does not result from modifiable, environmental variables, although environmental variables may accelerate aging.
3. Aging is progressive. Its onset is a gradual, cumulative occurrence.
4. Aging is deleterious. This is the most characteristic change that differentiates aging from development.

Thus, the often-heard statements that "aging begins at birth" or "aging begins at conception" are clearly wrong. Aging is, by definition, detrimental to the organism. As Richard Cutler of the National Institute on Aging (NIA) says, "Aging is bad. Growth and development are good." Growth and development processes are not "aging". Therefore, aging and its deleterious changes begin sometime in middle age, between 25 and 35.

III. AGING AS A DISEASE

Webster's Dictionary defines disease as "an alteration of a living organism that impairs its function". As we age, the functional capacity of nearly every organ and organ system is reduced (Figure 1). As chronological age increases, the morbidity and mortality from almost every disease also increases (Figure 2). Many scientists[21,24,39,41] now propose that the aging process itself may be viewed as a disease in its own right.

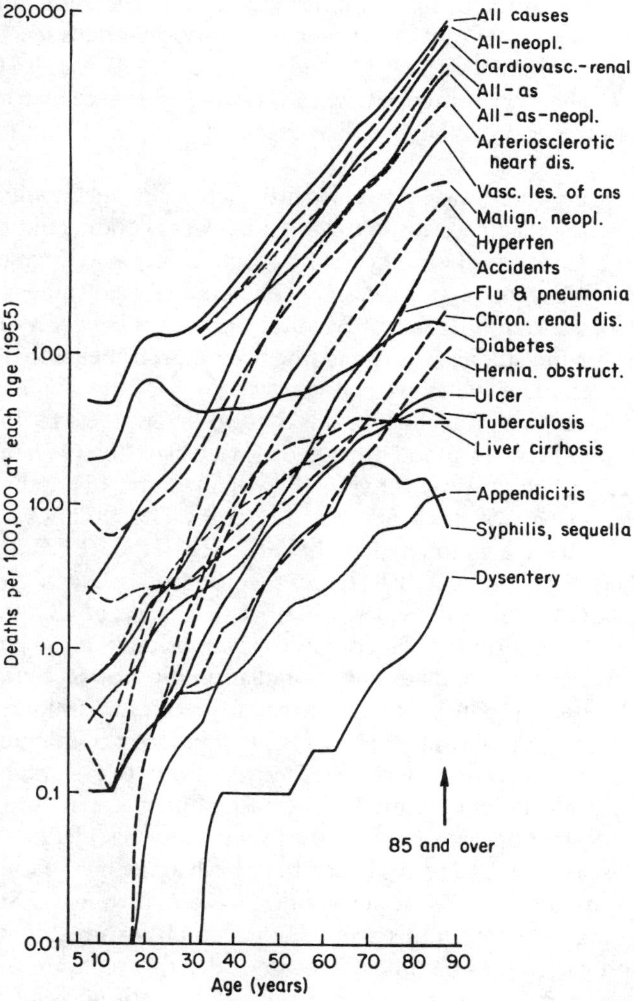

Figure 2 Increase in age-specific death rates from selected causes.[40]

IV. DIAGNOSING THE DISEASE

Biological age is an abstract concept commonly expressed by a comment that a person looks older or younger than his chronological age. In simple terms, biological age is a composite score based on how one's appearance, physiological, biochemical, and neuropsychological condition compares with the "average" for his chronological age. Longitudinal measurements of biological age can be used to calculate aging rates, and to monitor the progress of aging and efficacy of intervention.

V. MULTIPLE REGRESSION EQUATION-DERIVED AGING MEASUREMENT SYSTEMS

The first published study of aging measurement was written in 1951 by Dr. I. M. Murray[48] of the State University of New York College of Medicine. Reporting on research done at Dalhousie

University, Murray pioneered the technique of using multiple regression equations to calculate a biological age from a battery of physiological and anthropometric tests. His test battery was comprised of: (1) visual accommodation, (2) auditory acuity, (3) systolic blood pressure, (4) dark adaptation; and (5) hand grip strength. Murray noted, as did others who followed[26,27] that those who were older often scored younger than expected, and those who were younger scored older than expected.

For the next 10 years, there was apparently little activity in the aging measurement field. In the early 1960s, a series of aging measurement studies were conducted on Japanese survivors of the Hiroshima-Nagasaki atomic bomb blasts, by a joint U.S.-Japanese research team from the Atomic Bomb Casualty Commission (ABCC).[38] The studies were under the direction of J. William Hollingsworth (currently Chief of Medical Services, University of California at San Diego). The impetus for the studies was to test the then-current belief that radiation exposure was a cause or an accelerant of the aging process.[19]

Again, the multiple regression technique was used to determine a biological age from nine tests: (1) skin elasticity, (2) systolic blood pressure, (3) vital capacity, (4) hand grip strength, (5) light extinction time, (6) vibratory sensitivity, (7) visual acuity, (8) auditory acuity, and (9) serum cholesterol. An analysis of this work is presented by Dr. Hollingsworth in Chapter 2.

A series of studies followed, conducted by the successor to the ABCC, the Radiation Effects Research Foundation (RERF).[5] The RERF studies used only six of the original nine parameters: (1) hand grip strength, (2) skin elasticity, (3) vibratory sensitivity, (4) light extinction time, (5) auditory acuity, and (6) near vision. Their studies were reported in more detail, and concluded that contrary to popular belief among scientists, radiation did not accelerate aging.

Alex Comfort,[16] founding editor of the journal *Experimental Gerontology*, addressed the question in 1969 when he proposed a battery of tests to measure physiological age.[16] Nearly half of Comfort's comprehensive test battery was derived from the work of Hollingsworth.[38] However, Comfort did not describe a method of evaluating the mass of information that he proposed, nor did he follow up with further developments of his idea.

By the early 1970s, a number of teams began to publish aging measurement studies. A series of reports emerged from the Veterans Administration's Normative Aging Study in Boston, and were published together.[4,14,20,28,60] Of this group, only Damon's study[20] contained the complete details of his tests and calculation methods, allowing others to replicate his work.

In The Netherlands, scientists from The Netherlands Institute for Preventive Medicine, under the leadership of Professor J. M. Dirken,[26] published a detailed series of aging measurement test batteries designed to develop a functional age system that could be used as a criterion for retirement. Although the system was not formally adopted, the tests appear to have provided the foundation for the test battery on which Hochschild's[37] computerized H-SCAN are based.

Also of significance was Dirken's rediscovery of what Murray[48] had found, that the multiple regression technique caused a skewing of the regression line about the mean, i.e., those who were older scored younger, and those who were younger scored older than their chronological ages. Dirken devised a method to correct this anomaly.

The first of only three long-running continuing series of aging measurements was published in 1972 by Professor Werner Ries of Karl Marx University, Leipzig, Germany.[53-56] The studies by Ries and his colleagues are unique in that they were the first to utilize a specifically designed instrument, the Geromat, that combined a number of tests.[55] The Geromat did not of itself produce a composite score of biological age like that of Hochschild[37] (discussed later), but was used in conjunction with other standard tests.

Another long-running series was that of Professor Eino Heikkinen and co-workers at the University of Jyväskylä in Jyväskylä, Finland. In 1974, Heikkinen[34,35] published the first of a series of aging measurement studies. Heikkinen's first test battery was based on only three tests: (1) vital capacity, (2) vibratory sensitivity, and (3) auditory acuity. Numerous studies have been

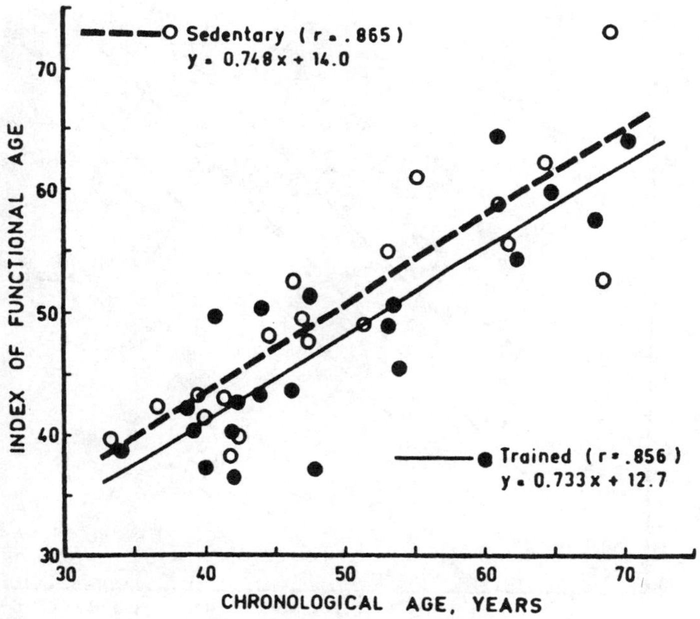

Figure 3 Biological ages of physically active subjects are generally younger than those who are sedentary. (From Suominen, H., in *Studies in Sport, Physical Education and Health II*, Komi, P.V., Ed., University of Jyväskylä, Jyväskylä, Finland. With permission.)

generated subsequently by scientists from Jyväskylä, using a variety of tests. One of Heikkinen's colleagues[70] found that physical fitness had a profound biological age-lowering effect, confirming a common belief that exercise may be the best antiaging "pill" currently available (Figure 3).

The third long-term series of aging measurement studies is the ongoing research of the Romanian National Institute of Gerontology and Geriatrics.[2,3] Their test battery is extensive, consisting of more than 40 tests. It is particularly interesting in that one of its objectives is to evaluate the controversial "Romanian youth drug" Gerovital, or GH3.

From the mid-1970s, aging measurement seemed to be developing into a hot topic among gerontologists, and a proliferation of studies were published from institutes around the world. In 1975 Dr. Toshiyuki Furukawa and associates[32] at Osaka University, Osaka, Japan, developed several aging measurement test batteries. One of the major contributions made by Furukawa was his comparison of hypertensives and diabetics with healthy controls. Not surprisingly, his results confirmed that the biological ages of the healthy subjects were younger (Figure 4). This appears to confirm the long-held belief that diabetes and hypertension actually cause accelerated aging.

A short time later, Webster and Logie[74] of the University of New South Wales, Kensington, Australia published a study based on the results of a routine health screen performed by a mobile testing laboratory. Years later, Webster[73] confirmed that the reason he did not pursue his studies was due to adverse pressure from his peers.

At about the same time Webster's paper appeared, Dr. Gary Borkan[8] was completing his Ph.D. thesis on aging measurement. Borkan then joined the team at the Boston Veterans Administration, where he continued the work begun earlier by Damon and associates and published a series of studies[9-11] before abandoning gerontology and aging humans to pursue a career with aging furniture as an antique dealer.

Dr. Eitaro Nakamura[49,50] at the University of Kyoto, Kyoto, Japan, has been continuing in the tradition established in that country by Hollingsworth and co-workers and Furukawa.

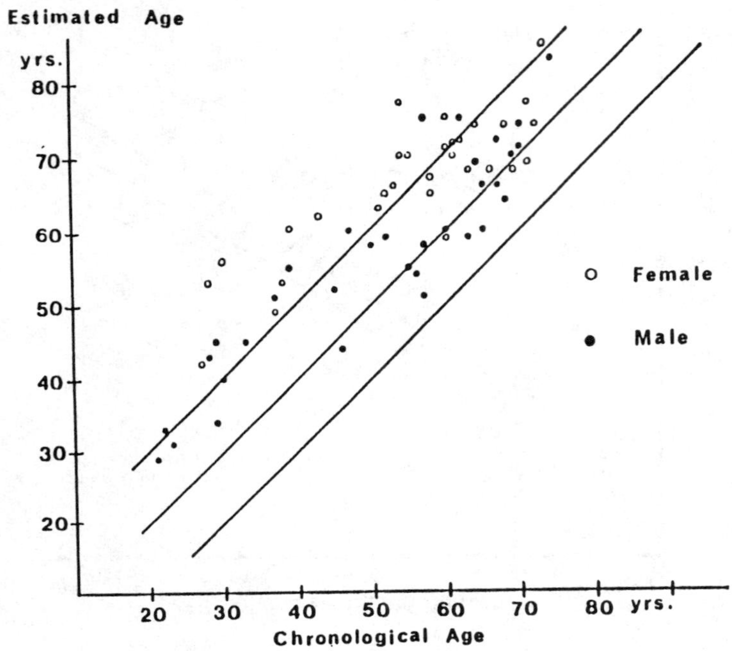

Figure 4 Biological ages of a group of hypertensive subjects (dots and circles) compared to the biological age ranges of a large group of normal subjects (lines). (From Furukawa, T. et al., *J. Gerontol.*, 30, 422, 1975. With permission.)

Nakamura's research is similar to that of Suominen in Finland in evaluating the effect of exercise and fitness on aging. Nakamura's results confirm those of Suominen — that exercise is an effective way to reduce biological age.

A great deal of work in this field is also being conducted in the former Soviet Union. Drs. T. L. Dubina and A. Ya. Mints performed studies on an exceptional population ranging in age from 60 to 100 years.[27,43] No other team has focused on subjects in such an advanced age bracket. Dubina's work is unique in several other ways, in that she independently discovered the artifactual skewing of the regression line about the mean, and calculated correction factors using a technique almost identical to Dirken's earlier work. She has also been conducting longitudinal measurements, indicating that it is possible to measure the rate of aging with sequential measurements (Figure 5). This should be of particular significance for evaluating interventionist therapies.

Another Russian team, headed by Professor Anatoli V. Tokar and Dr. Vladimir P. Voitenko evaluated the comparative aging rates of men and women[71] and found that women age faster in youth, but that men age faster in old age.

Although the cited studies confirm the feasibility of aging measurements, the measurements have not been validated by relating them to the individual's life span. Despite this, Dr. Hiroshi Shimokata and colleagues[66] at the University of Nagoya, Nagoya, Japan, have used a varied and comprehensive series of aging measurement tests to evaluate the progress of their subjects, and used the information to advise them of interventions to retain their youth and reduce their biological age.

Finally, Professor A. Ruiz-Torres at the Institute of Investigative Gerontology in Madrid, Spain, developed a simple six-parameter test battery for biological age based on his "Two-Compartment Model" of the aging process.[63] His aging measurement system is unique in that (1) the parameters measured are directly related to his theory of aging, (2) their normalization

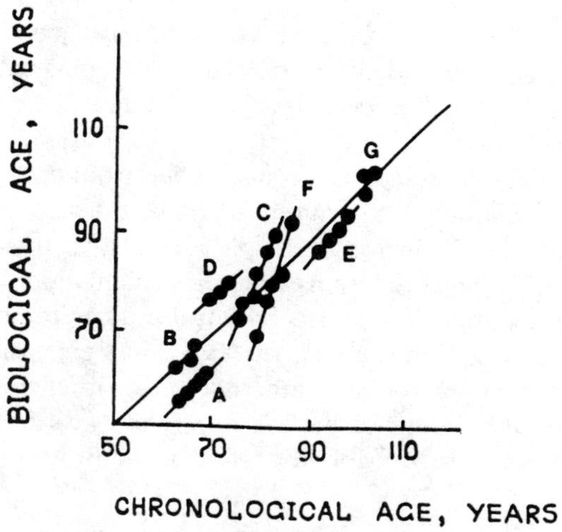

Figure 5 Longitudinal assessment of biological age in six subjects, showing differences in aging rates. (From Dubina, T.L. et al., *Exp. Gerontol.*, 19, 133, 1984. With permission.)

should have a beneficial effect with regard to reducing biological age, and (3) should lead to the development of effective gerontotherapeutic agents.

VI. OTHER APPROACHES TO AGING MEASUREMENT

Closely correlated with the concept of aging measurement is that of health risk appraisal, an approach originated by Drs. Lewis C. Robbins and Jack Hall.[57] The health risk appraisal identifies the leading cause of death at each age, an individual's risk factors for succumbing to these causes of mortality, and calculates an individual "risk age" based on these data.

This approach has now gained wide acceptance, as indicated by its adoption by the Centers for Disease Control,[13] and the formation of a professional society, The Society for Prospective Medicine, based on the principles originally espoused by Robbins and Hall.

Another true pioneer in aging measurement who has persisted with the same tenacity as Heikkinen, Ries, and the Romanians, is Dr. Robert Morgan, formerly Dean of Academic Affairs at the Pacific Graduate School of Psychology, Menlo Park, CA.[44-47] Morgan developed a simple test, the Adult Growth Examination, which uses three parameters to evaluate biological age. These tests (blood pressure, near vision, and auditory acuity) are given equal weight, the values are compared to population norms, and biological age is determined by the middle value. The simplicity of this test belies its accuracy and reproducibility. Morgan's system is one of the most widely tested aging measurement systems, and has been used by many scientists to evaluate interventionist therapies.[72]

Dr. Daniel Hershey, Professor of Chemical Engineering, Department of Chemical and Nuclear Engineering, University of Cincinnati, conceived the entropic theory of aging. He developed a method of deriving entropy production of living organisms from basal metabolic rates.[36] With his combined knowledge of gerontology, engineering, and thermodynamics, Hershey developed an office whole body calorimeter and computer program to determine basal metabolic rate (BMR) and to calculate entropy production. These calculations allowed Hershey to plot "life span tracks" for individuals and to attempt to predict their life expectancy.

Many scientists have noted the close correlation of maximal oxygen uptake with the aging process[58,61] and believe that it may be one of the most accurate parameters to assess biological age. Unfortunately, $VO_{2\,max}$ measurements are complex, expensive, require a motivated subject, and may not be accomplished by those who are disabled in some way. Dr. Wojtek J. Chodzko-Zajko[15] determined an index of physiological status (IPS) based on a battery of noninvasive tests that closely correlates with $VO_{2\,max}$. It appears that this IPS may be an excellent biomarker and indicator of biological age.

Dr. Richard Hochschild, an independent researcher from Corona Del Mar, CA, has developed a self-contained computerized aging measurement device which comprises a battery of 12 tests.[37] The tests used in his device are nearly identical to those of Dirken (previously described). Hochschild's approach is a dramatic improvement upon the labor-intensive test batteries employed by the majority of scientists who utilized the multiple regression equation technique. By completely automating the test, the test is less expensive, can be administered faster, and is less subject to the operator error inherent in the other test batteries. Hochschild's system is limited, however, as it does not include any tests of cardiovascular performance or clinical chemistry. This approach is probably the wave of the future, however.

VII. AGING MEASUREMENT CONFERENCES AND SYMPOSIA

At a satellite conference of the International Congress of Gerontology and Geriatrics in Kiev, Russia in 1963, it was resolved that a primary focus for gerontological research should be to determine a means to measure biological age. In addition to probably being the impetus for many of the earlier aging measurement studies, the major result of this declaration was a World Health Organization pamphlet by Francois Bourliere.[12]

In 1981 Dr. William Regelson's Foundation for Integrative Biological Research (FIBER) held a conference on biomarkers in Boston. The FIBER conference was followed shortly thereafter by a conference sponsored by the NIA, "Biological Markers of Aging", and by the published proceedings of that conference.[51] Surprisingly, none of the scientists who conducted aging measurements in humans were invited to present papers at the NIA conference. The speakers were restricted to NIA grant recipients. Regelson held a second, larger conference in 1982, widely regarded as the best conference ever held on aging measurement to that time.[52]

The International Congress of Gerontology and Geriatrics in New York in 1985 included a symposium on aging measurement, but it was largely confined to philosophical discussions about whether aging could be measured. Several presenters did describe aging measurement studies with insects and mice, but again, none of the scientists who conducted aging measurements in humans were invited to present, although many of these scientists were in the audience. That same year, a more productive, but less well publicized, conference organized by Professor A. Ruiz-Torres was held by the University Institute of Investigative Gerontology in Madrid.[61]

Another symposium was held at the 1987 Gerontological Society meeting. Although this was more comprehensive than most previous symposia, again, inexplicably, none of the scientists who conducted aging measurements in humans were invited, and the subject again revolved around studies on lower animals and discussions of whether age could be measured. The proceedings were published as a special issue of *Experimental Gerontology*.[68]

At the meeting of the Board of Directors of the AGE in 1987, a draft of my monograph on aging measurement was circulated.[21] Because the scientists who had conducted aging measurements in humans had never been brought together at one symposium, it was decided that the subject of the annual symposium at the next AGE meeting would be the measurement of human physiological age. All of the leading aging measurement scientists in the world were to be invited.

Organized and chaired by Dr. Arthur Balin, this conference was clearly a landmark in gerontology. The collected papers should stand as a significant advance in the science of aging measurement, as chapters were solicited from nearly every scientist in the world involved in human aging measurement. More recently, conferences have been held in Vienna, Austria[58] and Bologna, Italy,[42] and have focused on aging measurement and biomarkers, respectively.

VIII. CONTROVERSIES IN AGING MEASUREMENT

The major detractors to progress in aging measurement are the discouraging, but widely circulated negative appraisals of the concept by several scientists who have reviewed, but never personally conducted research in the field.[1,17,18] Briefly, the criticisms of Costa and McCrae stem from: (1) their lack of understanding of the purposes of aging measurement, (2) their contention that present techniques do not allow the accurate measurement of biological age (they believe that because biological age has not been as accurately measured as they would like, it can never be accurately measured), and (3) that current aging measurements are not measurements of the fundamental mechanisms of aging and are therefore of no value.

Costa and McCrae repetitively criticize the idea of using biological age as a replacement for chronological age. They totally overlook its more widely accepted use as a measurement of relative aging status, aging progression, and as a means of evaluating the efficacy of interventionist regimens.

Their second criticism is analogous to those of scientists who claimed in 1902 that powered flight was impossible because it had never been done before, or who proclaimed in 1959 that man would never set foot on the moon.

Their third criticism demonstrates conclusively that Costa and McCrae do not think in practical terms. It is not necessary to understand mechanisms of a biological process to measure and treat it. For example, although physicians may not fully understand the mechanisms regarding the etiology of hypertension, this does not prevent measuring high blood pressure, treating it, and reducing the accompanying morbidity and mortality. The same holds true for most diseases.

The other major detractor, Adelman, appeared to be more concerned about a potential diversion of funds into biomarker research and away from projects that he believes would provide more fundamental information regarding the etiology of the aging process. He does not have any conceptual difficulties with aging measurement. In fact, Adelman succinctly sums up the purposes and values of biomarkers and aging measurements. He states that biomarkers may be used as:

1. A means to measure the degree of functional age as opposed to chronological age
2. A means to ascertain a rate of aging
3. A standard by which to assess the effectiveness of therapeutic interventions
4. A means to document successful aging

All of the criticisms of Costa and McCrae and Adelman have been reviewed and answered in detail elsewhere.[21-23]

IX. SUMMARY

The development of a widely accepted system to measure biological age is of paramount importance for the advancement of clinical gerontology. The numerous studies cited in this chapter attest to the fact that biological age can be and is being measured by many teams around the world. Further research is needed to identify biomarkers more closely related to the fundamental cause(s) of aging. Such biomarkers will greatly enhance the development of more accurate and more sensitive systems of aging measurement, which should accelerate the development of effective gerontotherapeutic agents and regimens.

REFERENCES

1. Adelman, R.C., *Testing the Theories of Aging*, CRC Press, Boca Raton, FL, 1982.
2. Aslan, A., Dumitru, M., Vrabiescu A., Enachescu, G., and Jucovschi, V., Evaluation of the biological age, *Romanian J. Gerontol. Geriatr.*, 1, 143, 1980.
3. Aslan, A., Vrabiescu, A., Enachescu, G., Ionescu, T., and Mihailescu, V., Assessment criteria for the biological age and the effectiveness of the eutrophic therapy, *Romanian J. Gerontol. Geriatr.*, 1, 13, 1983.
4. Bell, B., Auditory functional age, *Aging Hum. Dev.*, 3, 183, 1972.
5. Belsky, J.L., Moriyama, I.M., Fujita, S., and Kawamoto, S., Aging Studies in Atomic Bomb Survivors, Tech. Rep., RERF TR 11-78, Radiation Effects Research Foundation.
6. Bjorksten, J., *Longevity, A Quest*, Bjorksten Research Foundation, Madison, WI, 1981.
7. Bjorksten, J., *Longevity 2. Past, Present, Future*, JAB Publishing, Charleston, SC, 1987.
8. Borkan, G.A., The Assessment of Biological Age during Adulthood, Ph.D. dissertation, University of Michigan, Ann Arbor, 1978, Dissertation Abstracts International, 39/06-A, 3682 (University Microfilms No 78228-61).
9. Borkan, G.A., Factors in clinical aging: variation in rates of aging, in *Intervention in the Aging Process, Part A, Quantitation, Epidemiology, and Clinical Research*, Regelson, W. and Sinex, F.M., Eds., Alan R. Liss, New York, 1983.
10. Borkan, G.A., Norris, A.H., Assessment of biological age using a profile of physical parameters, *J. Gerontol.*, 55, 177, 1980.
11. Borkan, G.A., and Norris, A.H., Biological age in adult-hood: comparison of active and inactive U.S. males, *Hum. Biol.*, 52, 787, 1980.
12. Bourliere, F., *The Assessment of Biological Age in Man*, World Health Organization, Geneva, 1970.
13. Breslow, L., Fielding, J., Afifi, A.A., Couldson, A., Kheifets, L., Valdiviezo, N., Goetz, A., McTyre, R., Peterson, K., and Dane, K., Risk Factor Update Project, U.S. Department of Health and Human Services, Centers for Disease Control, Center for Health Promotion and Education, Atlanta, 1985.
14. Burney, S.W., Laboratory functional age, *Aging Hum. Dev.*, 3, 189, 1972.
15. Chodzko-Zajko W.J. and Ringel, R.L., Physiological fitness measures and sensory and motor performance in aging, *Exp. Gerontol.*, 22, 317, 1987.
16. Comfort, A., Test battery to measure ageing rate in man, *Lancet*, December 27, 1411, 1969.
17. Costa, P.T. and McCrae, R.R., Functional age: a conceptual and empirical critique, in *Proc. 2nd Conf. Epidemiology of Aging*, Haynes, S.G. and Geinleib, M., Eds., National Institute on Aging, Bethesda, MD, 1977.
18. Costa, P.T. and McCrae, R.R., Concepts of functional or biological age, in *Principles of Geriatric Medicine*, Andres, R., Bierman, E.L., and Hazzard, W.R., Eds., McGraw Hill, New York, 1985.
19. Curtis, H.G., *Biological Mechanisms of Aging*; Charles C Thomas, Springfield, IL, 1966.
20. Damon, A., Predicting age from body measurements and observations, *Aging Hum. Dev.*, 3, 169, 1972.
21. Dean, W., *Biological Aging Measurement — Clinical Applications*, The Center for Bio-Gerontology, Pensacola, FL, 1988.
22. Dean, W., In defense of the concept of biological aging measurement — current status, *Arch. Gerontol. Geriatr.*, 7, 191, 1988.
23. Dean, W., Biomarkers of aging (letter), *Exp. Gerontol.*, 23, 139, 1988.
24. Dilman, V.M., *The Law of Deviation of Homeostasis and Diseases of Aging*, John Wright/PSG, Boston, 1981.

25. Dilman, V.M. and Dean, W., *The Neuroendocrine Theory of Aging and Degenerative Disease*, The Center for Bio-Gerontology, Pensacola, FL, 1992.
26. Dirken, J.M., *Functional Age of Industrial Workers*, Wolters-Noordhoff Publishing, Gröningen, Sweden, 1972.
27. Dubina, T.L, Mintz, A.Y., and Zhuk, E.V., Biological age and its estimation. III. Introduction of a correction to the multiple regression model of biological age and assessment of biological age in sectional and longitudinal studies, *Exp. Gerontol.*, 19, 133, 1984.
28. Fozard, J., Predicting age in the adult years from psychological assessments of abilities and personality, *Aging Hum. Dev.*, 3, 175, 1972.
29. Franklin, B., *Poor Richard's Almanac*, 1749.
30. Frolkis, V.V., *Aging and Life Prolonging Processes*, Springer-Verlag, New York, 1982.
31. Frolkis, V.V. and Muradian, K.K., *Life Span Prolongation*, CRC Press, Boca Raton, FL, 1992.
32. Furukawa, T., Inoue, M., Kajiya, F., Inada, H., Takasugi, S., Fukui. S., Takeda, H., Abe, H., Assessment of biological age by multiple regression analysis, *J. Gerontol.*, 30, 422, 1975.
33. Harman, D., Brochure, American Aging Association, Omaha, NE, 1979.
34. Heikkinen, E., Assessment of functional ageing, in *Lectures on Gerontology, Vol. 1: On Biology of Ageing, Part B*, Vidik, A., Ed., Academic Press, New York, 1982.
35. Heikkinen, E., Kiiskinen, A, Kayhty, B., Rimpela, M., Vuori, I., Assessment of biological age, *Gerontologia*, 20, 33, 1974.
36. Hershey, D., *A New Age Scale for Humans*, Lexington Books, Lexington, MA, 1980.
37. Hochschild, R., The H-SCAN — an instrument for the automatic measurement of physiological markers of aging, in *Intervention in the Aging Process, Part A*, Regelson, W. and Sinex, F.M., Ed., Alan R. Liss, New York, 1983.
38. Hollingsworth, J.W., personal communication.
39. Johnson, H.A., Is aging physiological or pathological?, in *Relations between Normal Aging and Disease*, Johnson, H.A., Ed., Raven Press, New York, 1985.
40. Kohn, R.R., *Principles of Mammalian Aging*, 2nd ed., Prentice Hall, Englewood Cliffs, NJ, 1978.
41. Kohn, R.R., Aging and age-related diseases: normal processes, in *Relations between Normal Aging and Disease*, Johnson, H.A., Ed., Raven Press, New York, 1985.
42. Licastro, F., Ed., *Proc. 1st Int. Congr. Biomarkers of Aging: Expression and Regulation*, Editrice, Bologna, Italy, 1992.
43. Mints, A.Y., Dubina, T.L., Lysenyk, V.P., Zhuk, E.V., Determination of individual biological age and evaluation of aging degree, *Physiol. Zh.*, 30, 39, 1989.
44. Morgan, R.F., The adult growth examination: preliminary comparisons of physical aging in adults by sex and race, *Perceptual Motor Skills*, 27, 595, 1968.
45. Morgan, R.F., *Conquest of Aging: Modern Measurement and Intervention*, Applied Gerontology Communications, Pueblo, CO, 1977.
46. Morgan, R.F., *Interventions in Applied Gerontology*, Kendall/Hunt Publishing, Toronto, 1981.
47. Morgan, R.F., The Adult Growth Examination Adult Body Age Test Manual. International Association of Applied Psychology, Division of Gerontological Psychology, Fresno, CA, 1986.
48. Murray, I.M., Assessment of physiologic age by combination of several criteria — vision, hearing, blood pressure and muscle force, *J. Gerontol.*, pp. 120, 1951.
49. Nakamura, E., The aged people and its physiological ages in relation to work capacity, *Kyoiku Igaku*, 28, 2, 1982.
50. Nakamura, E., The assessment of physiological age based upon a principal component analysis of various physiological variables, *J. Kyoto Pref. Univ. Med.*, 8, 757, 1985.
51. Reff, M.E. and Schneider, E.L., *Biological Markers of Aging*, U.S. Government Printing Office, Washington, D.C., 1982.
52. Regelson, W. and Sinex, F.M., *Intervention in the Aging Process, Parts a and b*, Alan R. Liss, New York, 1983.
53. Ries, W., Problems associated with biological age, in *Proc. 9th Int. Congr. Gerontology and Geriatrics*, Kiev, Russia, 1972.
54. Ries, W., Problems associated with biological age, *Exp. Gerontol.*, 9, 145, 1974.

55. Ries, W. and Poethig, D., Chronological and biological age, *Exp. Gerontol.*, 19, 211, 19??.
56. Ries, W. and Sauer, I., *Biologisches Alter — Problem und Bericht*, Akademie Verlag, Berlin, 1991.
57. Robbins, L. and Hall, J.H., *How to Practice Prospective Medicine*, Methodist Hospital of Indiana, Indianapolis, IN, 1970.
58. Robert, L. and Hofecker, G., *The Theoretical Basis of Aging Research* (Vienna Aging Series, Vol. 2), Facultas Universitatsverlag Wien, Vienna, 1990.
59. Roberts, J., Adelman, R.C., and Cristofalo, V.J., *Pharmacological Intervention in the Aging Process*, Plenum Press, New York, 1977.
60. Rose, C.L., The measurement of social age, *Aging Hum. Dev.*, 3, 153, 1972.
61. Ruiz-Torres, A., *Biological Age and Aging Risk Factors*, Tecnipublicaciones, Madrid, 1987.
62. Ruiz-Torres, A., Slagado, A., and Hollander, C.F., *Biological Age and Aging Risk Factors*, Instituto Universitario de Investigacion Gerontological y Metabolica, Madrid, 1985.
63. Ruiz-Torres, A., Agudo, A., Vicent, D., and Beier, W., Measuring human aging using a two-compartmental mathematical model and the vitality concept, *Arch. Gerontol. Geriatr.*, 10, 69, 1990.
64. Schneider, E.L. and Reed, J.D., Life extension, *N. Engl. J. Med.*, 312, 1159, 19??.
65. Shephard, R.J. and Kavanaugh, T., The effects of training on the aging process, *Phys. Sports Med.*, 6, 33, 1978.
66. Shimokata, H., Shibata, K., and Kuzuya, F., Assessment of biological aging status, *J. Jpn. Soc. Intern. Med.*, 74, 1344, 19??.
67. Shock, N.W., Systems integration, in *Handbook of the Biology of Aging*, Finch, C.E. and Hayflick, L., Eds., Van Nostrand Reinhold, New York, 1982.
68. Sprott, R.L. and Baker, G.T., III, Biomarkers of aging, *Exp. Gerontol.*, 23, 223, 1988.
69. Strehler, B.L., *Time, Cells, and Aging*, Academic Press, New York, 1977.
70. Suominen, H., Effects of physical training in middle-aged and elderly people, in *Studies in Sport, Physical Education and Health 11*, Komi, P.V., Ed., University of Jyväskylä, Jyväskylä, Finland, 1978.
71. Voitenko, V.P. and Tokar, A.V., The assessment of biological age and sex differences of human aging, *Exp. Aging Res.*, 9, 239, 1983.
72. Wallace, R.K., Dillbeck, M., Jacobe, E., and Harrington, B., The effects of the transcendental meditation and TM-SIDHI program on the aging process, *Int. J. Neurosci.*, 16, 53, 1982.
73. Webster, I.W., personal communication, 1984.
74. Webster, I.W., Logie, A.R., A relationship between functional age and health status in female subjects, *J. Gerontol.*, 31, 546, 1976.

CHAPTER 2

THE HIROSHIMA STUDIES OF PHYSIOLOGICAL AGE: A HISTORICAL NOTE*

J. WILLIAM HOLLINGSWORTH

Sputnik will almost certainly be considered, historically, as the most significant world event of the 1950s. Surprisingly the Hiroshima studies on aging were almost a direct offshoot from Sputnik. In 1957, the U.S. was the leader in world technology, confident and secure in its prowess. Russia seemed a big, uncouth nation, unsophisticated but earnest, a nation that might challenge our scientific and technical lead sometime in the future, perhaps late in the 20th century. On October 4, 1956, that complacency was shattered forever when Sputnik I, a 184-lb space capsule, pierced the atmosphere 584 mi above Earth and orbited the planet for more than 1 year. Sputnik generated an enormous outpouring of old-fashioned patriotism in the U.S. as we examined the fundamental social and educational structure of our society. Nobel laureates left their laboratories to help devise better ways to teach mathematics, and industries and educational institutions brought in high school students to teach them science. American science in general wanted to help.

In Japan from 1955 to 1957, the Atomic Bomb Casualty Commission (ABCC), operated jointly by the US-Japan National Academies of Science, was having trouble meeting its responsibility of determining the late effects of the atomic bombings on the citizens of Hiroshima and Nagasaki. The acute effects of radiation had been described, and an epidemic of acute leukemia was being effectively studied. In the 2 years before Sputnik, a committee of the U.S. National Research Council and its Japanese equivalent, headed by the famous epidemiologist, Thomas Francis of the University of Michigan, had devised a two-pronged long-term scientific strategy consisting of a large basic epidemiological study of the quarter million survivors of the bombings, and a clinical study of survivors, called the Adult Health Study. A sample of approximately 20,000 in Hiroshima and Nagasaki would be constituted in the Adult Health Study, consisting of three basic subsets based on bomb exposure history: (1) radiation exposed, within 2000 m of the bomb epicenters, a group in whom acute radiation symptoms had been prominent in 1945; (2) persons in the cities at the time of the bombings, but beyond the 2,000 meters range and thus not experiencing the acute radiation syndrome but fully participating in the physical and social upheaval that followed destruction of the sites; and (3) a control group of people who resettled the cities after the war. The Adult Health Study sample would be randomly brought to the clinics in Hiroshima and Nagasaki every 2 years for examination and studies. The findings of ABCC, later reorganized as Radiation Effects Research Foundation (RERF), have been derived since 1958 from the basic scientific structure envisaged in the Francis Report.

At the time of Sputnik in October 1957, Dr. R. Keith Cannan, a former Professor of Biochemistry at New York University and then head of the Biology and Medicine Section of the National Academy of Sciences, was trying to reorganize ABCC to carry out the basic strategy of the

* Dr. Stuart C. Finch, Director of Research, Radiation Effects Research Foundation, Hiroshima, greatly facilitated this review by searching the archives of ABCC/RERF. His interest and encouragement is appreciated.

0-8493-0129-7/94/$0.00+$.50

Francis Report. One major element had been established: the Academy's own statistical unit would take over the key Department of Statistics at ABCC, and Dr. Gilbert W. Beebe would assume that responsibility in the summer of 1958. In New Haven, CT, the Department of Internal Medicine at Yale University under the concerned leadership of Dr. Paul B. Beeson was meeting weekly in the post-Sputnik era to consider ways to improve our nation's scientific position, and Dr. Cannan in early 1958 addressed one of those weekly luncheons about ABCC and its need for continuity of leadership of the Medical Service by rotation of clinical scientists from a parent department in the U.S., i.e., Yale. Myself, Stuart Finch, and Larry Freeman were among the young faculty at that luncheon, and we provided in that order the first three Yale-nominated Chiefs of Medicine, each serving for 2 years. By March 1957, I was appointed as the first to serve in Japan.

The aging studies came about primarily as I pondered the logistics of the ABCC Adult Health Study, and how to involve young doctors productively in what essentially was a well-subject examination of a randomly selected population of all ages. Young American house staff-level doctors were to be inducted through the mechanism of the doctor draft, assigned to the Public Health Service and then sent to ABCC; young Japanese doctors were to be recruited from Japanese universities. Little was known about late sequelae of total body irradiation, but animal studies had detected life shortening following radiation exposure, mostly from induction of cancer but possibly because of somatic mutations leading to acceleration of the generalized aging process. I was quite skeptical of the hypothesis, but studying physiologic measures of aging in the radiation-exposed and control populations seemed a valid undertaking for ABCC, and a splendid way to get young physicians involved in clinical research.

Having decided to utilize the variably aged population of the Adult Health Study to assess physiologic measurements of age, I delved into the *Index Medicus* to find publications on aging, and began to contemplate more fully the feasibility and the desirability of measuring age biologically rather than chronologically. In deciding on the tests, we recognized that they had to be simple, nonthreatening to the subjects, easy to administer in a clinic setting, and readily reduced to numbers for computer storage. As we began to really uncover or devise usable tests, it became clear that not all tests could be performed on a single day, but with about 25 randomly selected subjects coming daily to the ABCC clinic, a sample for perhaps 2 to 3 months would yield a substantial number of tests in a highly representative group of the population under observation.

By the time we got to Japan in July 1958, I had about a dozen little projects on physiological age detailed in one or two typed pages and supported by photostats of key references. Most of the tests arranged themselves into organ systems and were variables which could be measured in each subject and which would yield a finite quantitation. A few tests related to conditions whose prevalence increased with age in a population but were only present in certain subjects; presence or absence of gastric achlorhydria or of bacteriuria are examples of this type of age-associated condition.

When we got to Hiroshima, we began to parcel out projects (and often expand them) with the young doctors who were there. The Americans were mostly from New York, having been recruited by Dr. Cannan through his New York connections. Sam Switzer from Albert Einstein University was interested in hypertension and cardiovascular disease, and he teamed up with one of our most experienced Japanese staff, Katsuhiko Yano, on several studies related to heart disease and hypertension. Quantitative bacteriuria was just being used in epidemiological research, and its study in Japanese women confirmed the findings elsewhere of increasing numbers of bacteriuric subjects with age.[1] The bacteriuric subjects had no excess hypertension, however, a finding which was at odds with existing dogma but which is now widely accepted.

Blood pressure levels were strongly associated with age in the nonatherosclerotic Japanese, similar to data from Europe and the U.S.[2]

Historically, both Drs. Switzer and Yano maintained their interest in cardiovascular disease and hypertension. Before his death in an automobile accident in the early 1960s, Switzer was Assistant

Professor of Medicine at Albert Einstein University. Dr. Yano stayed on in Hiroshima for a few years, obtained proper training in epidemiology in the U.S., and now directs the Honolulu Heart Study, a major geoepidemiology study center.

Emphysema of the lung was an accepted process in the elderly, thought to be related to loss of elasticity of the lung. We performed pulmonary function tests on the Hiroshima subjects, and reported the total vital capacity and 1-min forced expiratory time. It was useful to confirm fall in lung function related to age without lung irritants because the Japanese population of the late 1950s consisted mostly of nonsmokers. One sidelight of the lung tests was that nurses were worn out by testing 25 to 30 subjects daily. Each subject had to be taught the test and then exhorted by the nurse to make maximal respiratory effort. One nurse lost 10 lb as a result of this cheerleading-type activity.

The appearance of aging is reflected to a major extent by wrinkled skin and gray hair, and we measured these two obvious components of aging. Gray hair was an excellent parameter in the Japanese with their jet-black hair, except that the nurses who made the estimates became aware of a significant number of elderly women who, like their western counterparts, dyed their hair; the nurses became quite proficient at getting at the root of things, as some punster remarked. Wrinkles are the dermal reflection of the generalized loss of elastic tissue which occurs with age, and we found in the available literature a good paper on measurement of skin elasticity. Basically, a spring-type pincers was used to provide a standard pinch of the forearm, and we measured the time for the pinch to disappear as the elastin springs back. In young people, the pinch retracts immediately, while in the very old the time exceeds 3 min. Skin retraction time seemed an excellent representation of loss of elasticity with age, a process now well understood biochemically and one which may be fundamental to the aging process.[3]

Neuromuscular changes with age are obvious, manifested by decrease in strength and agility. Strength in the hands was readily measured with a commercially available dynamometer.[4] In the 1950s, loss of vibratory sensation and of light touch was well-recognized clinically as a concomitant of aging; we found a vibrometer which applied a standard stimulus, and the patient signaled when the vibration ceased. The test was reliable, and its strong association with age in the Japanese subjects helped support the loss of sensory nerve function as a feature of age, and not of peripheral vascular atherosclerosis.[4] Agility seems to involve both a central nervous system function (reaction time, or stimulus recognition) and peripheral action (response time). We were unable to sort out this complex parameter into its components, but Seymour Bogitch, the engineer at the ABCC, was fascinated with the problem, and he devised something we called the light extinction test. His gadget consisted of a row of ten light bulbs with a turn off switch below each bulb. When the apparatus was operating, lights switched on in irregular sequence and with irregular time intervals, much like a modern symphony or, in cliche, without rhyme or reason. The apparatus measured the total time that the lights were on. Agile people scored short times. This test seemed to yield good age discrimination.[4]

The special senses of sight, hearing, and taste become dysfunctional with age. Presbyopia, the far sightedness of the elderly, is thought to reflect, perhaps with skin elasticity, a change in the chemistry of the collagen of the lens tissue of the eye. Although many Japanese are myopic, we decided to use visual acuity as one of our tests of biologic age. Hearing is easily quantitated with an instrument (the audiogram) which measures the loss of high frequency hearing which is a regular feature of age, and we used the audiogram as a reliable age-related test.[5] Taste was simply too complex to measure.

Several conditions were studied in which incidence of the variable in the population was the age-related parameter. Turner and Hollingsworth showed that tuberculosis was more common in the aged, as predicted, but it was similar in irradiated and nonirradiated subjects. The study provided one indication that the irradiation of lymphoreticular tissue did not lead to reactivation of tuberculosis.[6] Knittle used a new commercially available test for achlorhydria, in which a blue dye was conjugated to a binding protein. The dye-protein complex was too large to be absorbed from the intestine, but if gastric pH was low the complex was cleaved and the blue dye was absorbed and then excreted in the urine; in order words, blue urine after the capsule indicated normal gastric acidity. The test seemed to work well for us in epidemiological surveys, although it never caught on as a clinical test for achlorhydria. As expected, the incidence of achlorhydria rose with age and was the same in irradiated and nonirradiated subjects.[7] About 10 years later Pastore et al.,[8] testing the hypothesis that gastric cancer was more likely in achlorhydrics, used the Knittle population to prove that point.[8]

It was known that certain types of so-called naturally occurring serum antibodies, mostly the macroglobulin antibodies to blood group substances, fell substantially with age. We proved this nicely in the Japanese sample,[9] and although the mechanism remains obscure, the test is a good variable in population surveys. When searching the literature for the blood group antibody date, we came across a German publication from the 1920s that basically said that it took more blood group antibody to agglutinate erythrocytes from the elderly than from young subjects. In other words, erythrocyte agglutinability declined with age. We found the same thing and reported it.[10] A few years later, back in New Haven, I was pondering this observation, which might imply that the erythrocyte membrane made by the elderly is different from that made by the young, since the average age of the erythrocyte in a blood sample is 60 d in both groups. Alternatively, some factor in the circulation of the elderly might affect the red cell membrane after the membrane was formed. I tried to repeat the Hiroshima experiments, in somewhat desultory fashion with months between experiments, but could not repeat them. Finally, I wrote to Japan to Dr. Howard Hamilton, collaborator and Chief of Laboratories at ABCC, and he failed to repeat the original observations. We both suspected a technical bias in the tests, but were never sure. More than 5 years had elapsed since the original report, and the report itself had elicited such little interest that I did not bother to retract the paper. I still wonder whether the change is real. A clearly defined defect in the red cell membrane in the elderly would prove a boon to our understanding of the aging process, and perhaps we should keep the red cell in mind as a readily sampled tissue of proven age.

By early 1960, all the studies of aging had been completed. Although none of the tests gave the slightest indication of a radiation effect, ABCC and particularly our statisticians understood the importance to the staff of having publications from their experience. Dr. Beebe and his staff performed the analyses, and Dr. Beebe really taught each of us how to report population epidemiology, and indeed how to write medical papers. By common consent, each of us determined to have at least a first draft manuscript with ABCC before we left in July 1960. Nonetheless, the basic series of publications was drawn out over almost a decade (see bibliography).

Mr. Seymour Jablon, who succeeded Dr. Beebe at ABCC from 1961 to 1964, was to work with me to try to put it all together as biologic age, in contradistinction to chronological age. Together we selected the tests to be analyzed, and Mr. Jablon was to give statistical weight in the assignment of a given biological age to an individual subject. The tests we used are shown in Table 1. They were selected mostly because of good statistical fit with age with acceptable variability, and for their uniform application within the sample. Some tests (i.e., blood group antibodies) were not being performed during the time interval of these other tests and thus were not available for comparison. Of the tests selected, several exhibited decreased statistical reliability because data from all ages were used to compute a statistical regression. For example, skin elasticity is a remarkably good variable between ages 40 and 75, but is not measurable below age 40; including the below-40 age group simply lowers the correlation coefficient value. Indeed, most of the tests diverged with age uniformly only after age 40, and the entire statistical manipulation would have been more pertinent if restricted to the over-40 age group. Of the sample of 437 subjects, however, only 238 are aged 40 or above. Thus, the power of this population sample to help define physiological age and compare that measurement with longevity is limited.

Fujita and his colleagues[11] in 1986 submitted an abstract to the meeting of the Japanese Society of Public Health, computing a physiological age for a sample studied at ABCC/RERF. They found no overall statistical excess of deaths over a 15-year period in the more physiological old half of the

Table 1 Tests used in computing physiological age, with their correlation coefficients with chronological age

		Sample size[a]	Correlation
1.	Skin elasticity	433	+0.604
2.	Systolic blood pressure	437	+0.519
3.	Total vital capacity	429	–0.402
4.	Hand grip strength	437	–0.323
5.	Light extinction test	435	+0.488
6.	Quantitative vibrometer	437	+0.537
7.	Visual acuity	433	–0.423
8.	Audiometry, 4000 cyc/s	436	+0.596
9.	Serum cholesterol	426	+0.234

[a] *A total of 437 subjects.*

sample. These investigators located a sample of 8153 subjects who participated in six different tests of aging and divided the sample into those whose estimated physiological age was higher or lower than the mean for their biological age. That abstract has not been expanded to a full publication, but the detailed analysis and perhaps the correlation of each individual test with the fact of death might be quite rewarding. In 1975 Finch and Beebe[12] reviewed all the data from ABCC/RERF on aging, including pathological studies and mortality, and failed to detect any radiation-related acceleration of the aging process.

I have recounted the genesis and the execution of the Hiroshima/Nagasaki studies on physiological aging. The work was primarily an assessment of the validity and value of individual tests of physiological variables with age. Although the concept was to attempt to define physiological age, we recognized that it might be more a statistical tour-de-force than an effective and useful biological tool, because the concept would have to be validated against the fact of death. After 30 years, the fact and cause of death of many subjects in that sample is now known and recorded in Hiroshima in the Radiation Effects Research Foundation's massive data bank. The question was then, and now, do the physiological young live longer than the physiological older, and if so, what parameters of age predict this most validly?

REFERENCES

1. Switzer, S., Bacteriuria in a health population and its relation to hypertension and pyelonephritis, *N. Engl. J. Med.*, 264, 7, 1961.
2. Switzer, S., Hypertension and ischemic heart disease in Hiroshima, Japan, *Circulation*, 28, 368, 1963.
3. Hollingsworth, J.W., Ishi, G., and Conard, R.A., Skin aging and hair aging in Hiroshima, *Geriatrics*, 16, 27, 1961.
4. Hollingsworth, D.R., Hollingsworth, J.W., Bogitch, S., and Keehn, R.J., Neuro-muscular tests of aging in Hiroshima subjects, *J. Gerontol.*, 24, 276, 1969.
5. Hollingsworth, J.W., Hashizume, A., and Jablon, S., Correlations between tests of aging in Hiroshima subjects — an attempt to define "physiologic age", *Yale J. Biol. Med.*, 38, 11, 1965.
6. Turner, R.W. and Hollingsworth, D.R., Tuberculosis in Hiroshima, *Yale J. Biol. Med.*, 36, 165, 1963.
7. Knittle, J.L., Achlorhydria in the ABCC-JNIH Adult Health Study Sample, Hiroshima 1959, ABCC Tech. Rep. 11-60, 1959.
8. Pastore, J.O., Kato, H., and Belsky, J.L., Serum pepsin and tubeless gastric analysis

as predictors of stomach cancer, *N. Engl. J. Med.*, 286, 279, 1972.
9. Hollingsworth, J.W., Hamilton, H.B., Beebe, G.W., and Yamasaki, M., Blood group antibody levels in Hiroshima, *Blood*, 17, 462, 1961.
10. Hollingsworth, J.W., Hamilton, H.B., and Ishii, G., Age-related changes in erythrocyte agglutinability in Hiroshima subjects, *J. Appl. Physiol.*, 16, 1093, 1961.
11. Fujita, S., Sasaki, H., Yoshimehi, O., Neriishi, K., Kato, H., and Hosoda, Y., *Abstr. Annu. Meet. Japanese Society of Public Health*, Sendai, 1986.
12. Finch, S.C. and Beebe, G.W., Biological effects of aging, *J. Rad. Res.*, 16, 108, 1975.

CHAPTER 3
ASPECTS OF QUANTITATION OF HUMAN AGING

William Regelson

TABLE OF CONTENTS

0-8493-0129-7/94/$0.00+$.50

I. INTRODUCTION

Because of the cost, time, and uncertainty involved, we cannot expect the effective entry of physicians or the pharmaceutical industry into the search for antiaging drugs unless bioquantitation establishes parameters of change that can be reasonably measured over short periods of time. This will enable antiaging drugs to become acceptable to the academic medical community, the patent office, and Food and Drug Administration (FDA) regulatory authorities.

Aging assessment is primarily concentrated on the elderly, but for it to become an adjunct to clinical intervention, assessment of physiologic age must be made periodically throughout adult life to enable us to act prophylactically to improve the quality of our survival as we age. Clinical evaluation of biochemical or physiological age must go beyond nutritional assessment or evaluation of the chronically ill, but must include quantitation of broad aspects of the developing aging syndromes in healthy individuals. The problems associated with this have been effectively discussed in texts on gerontology[23,63,173,185,186,235] and in reviews.[17,87,132,139,186,187,189]

As an example of a commercially available quantitative system, the H-SCAN (Hoch Company, Corona Del Mar, CA)[95,95a] has been used by insurance companies to evaluate physiologic performance in order to determine biologic age. As discussed in this volume by Hochschild, this instrument provides bioquantitation of forced vital capacity; hearing (highest audible pitch); vision (accommodation in diopters); touch sensitivity at fingertip; motor control (alternate button tapping); memory; longest chain, auditory, and visual reaction time, movement time; and decision reaction. The H-SCAN provides a computerized test system with a format that can be self-administered and that is economic as to cost, time, and space. The individual's data can be readily related to nutritional, biochemical, or socioeconomic factors as well as to chronologic age.

Bioquantitation of aging has been reviewed in the text *Intervention in the Aging Process*,[185,186] which presents a discussion of the range of methodology for age measurement that was in place or potentially useful up to 1983. The problem of translating physiologic measurement to age quantitation is hazardous as it is immediately associated with survival prediction, a controversial area when regression analysis is related to human populations. Reviews or texts that provide quantitative information are listed in Regelson and Sinex's previous work,[185,186] refer to the classic work of Shock,[214] and are updated. Currently, animal experimentation that searches for biomarkers aids in the selection of parameters that might be clinically useful.[87,215] Dean's[44] manual for biological aging measurement provides a broad compendium of available physiologic tests. This review, like its predecessor,[185,186] is meant to be both practical and speculative as to clinical application.

Of major future potential is the use of biopsy, tissue culture, or sampling techniques that will determine peptide, enzyme, DNA or RNA changes regarding DNA configuration, repair, or enzymatic change. Techniques that determine free radical formation, tissue antioxidant levels, or DNA physical state can provide information that is useful to the quantitation of mutational and radiation exposure as well as aging.[7,40,86]

It is not the purpose of this chapter to distinguish clearly intrinsic biologic clocks (factors related to changes in neuroendocrine, immune, biochemical or nucleochromatin status) from extrinsic factors (dietary, exercise, or psychosocial influences) that govern aging. Intervention in aging must combine an understanding of all these factors,[185,186] as the author contends that what is intrinsic today and resistant to change in the aging process will be modifiable tomorrow. In that regard, the author feels that aging is primarily a syndrome of defined biochemical and physiologic identity rather than merely the cumulative effect of individual chronic diseases. The concept of aging, as a biologic syndrome, is important if a more effective entry of academia and the pharmaceutical industry into this field is to be effective. We must mobilize resources for intervention to avoid age-related debility and dependency before it becomes clinically evident, for which bioquantitation is best suited.

II. BIOQUANTITATION: PHYSIOLOGIC PARAMETERS IMMEDIATELY AVAILABLE OR ADAPTABLE TO CLINICAL TESTING

A. RESPIRATORY: FORCED VITAL CAPACITY (FVC)

Currently the most important measurable index of aging that summates physical changes is the evaluation of forced vital capacity (FVC).[44,114,221] The importance of pulmonary changes with age has been demonstrated by the Framingham Heart Study, which showed in its 20-year mortality study that death related predictably to biennially measured vital capacity. Excess mortality at low vital capacity was noted in the elderly as well as the young in both sexes and in nonsmokers as well as smokers. This relationship was independent of disease states and vital capacity predicted for both long- and short-term mortality.

The differences between respiratory function in young and old may depend on age-related differences in central processing of inspiratory volume and elastic load. Scarpace et al.[207] have shown β-agonist affinity and adrenylate cyclase activity to be decreased in the lungs of senescent rats. Muscle force may be more important than lung volume changes in providing respiratory clues to older subjects.[226] In that regard, the maximal sniff test as an assessment of diaphragmatic function may be of value.[158]

B. MUSCLE FUNCTION: HAND GRIP STRENGTH

Age changes in respiratory capacity may be due to loss of muscle power or a stiffer, less compliant chest wall or diaphragm. A major correlate of FVC is decline in hand grip strength. This is not surprising as the effect of age on vital capacity is thought to relate to compliance or recoil factors in the chest wall,[44,161] although this is controversial because age changes in lung collagen have been reported.[9]

With regard to the above, vital capacity may be the respiratory equivalent of the senile gait with implications of a Parkinson equivalency. Supporting this claim, Sastry et al.[204] have reported a decline in response of the aging isolated rat hemidiaphragm to acetylcholine or electrical stimulation. Studies of vital capacity in Parkinson's disease and the senile gait in relation to prognosis and survival data are needed.

C. CARDIAC FUNCTION

This has been well reviewed by Walsh,[236] Lakatta,[130] and Rosenthal,[200] with discussions of vascular and autonomic functions. A fall in resting cardiac output with age has been known for many years,[19] and alterations in cardiac function with aging have been discussed by Lakatta[129,130] in animal models and by Gerstenblith[73] and Shephard[213] in their discussions of cardiovascular aging in man.

The influence of age on exercise hemodynamics has been reviewed by Ehrsam et al.[57] With age, right heart pressures, flow resistance, catecholamine response increases or changes,[149] and clinical aspects of this are pertinent to exercise as an intervention strategy.

Cardiac index and age are inversely related. In addition, renal blood flow decreases with age and a trend exists for an increase in systemic vascular resistance and mean blood pressure and a decrease in peripheral blood flow.[58]

Of possible clinical significance, Yin et al.[249] found that they could quantify cardiac hypertrophy as an age-related event in the rat with tibial strength, which was superior to body weight as a standard for chronologic comparison.

D. RENAL FUNCTION

The decline in clinical renal function, as seen in 24-h endogenous creatinine clearance studies, begins essentially in the middle of the fourth decade.[58,220] Progressive changes in the renal handling of creatinine or inulin have resulted in age-adjusted normative standards developed by the National Institute on Aging (NIA) Gerontology Research Center.[202] Functional changes correlate with glomerular sclerosis and the thickening of all capillary basement membranes in aging rats.[109] The pathogenesis of age-related renal changes has been reviewed by Goldstein et al.[75]

E. BONE LOSS

Bone loss is a significant problem leading to skeletal collapse and fracture and is a leading cause of disability in elderly women, with 200,000 hip fractures annually in the U.S.[50] Heaney[91] has discussed a variety of techniques that are clinically applicable to quantitate this problem, as have Smith et al.[218] in their excellent review.

Heaney[91] lists radiogrammetry, single or dual photon absorptiometry (photodensometry), total and partial body neutron activation analysis, computed tomography (CT), Compton-scanner, biopsy, and calcium balance as techniques to measure patterns of skeletal change with bone loss in the aged.

CT may be our best available tool for bone loss measurement, but it is an expensive procedure. Currently, bone densitometers designed for office use are available to provide screening technology at more reasonable cost.

In regard to factors affecting aging, there is a progressive increase in serum parathyroid hormone with age, with a change in total serum calcium.[31] After the sixth decade, 1,25-dihydroxy vitamin D (D_3) decreases in serum and calcium absorption decreases with age. In *in vitro* tissue culture sampling rabbit articular chondrocytes lose reproductive capacity with aging or serial passage.[52]

Susceptibility to osteoporosis can be identified by utilizing a short-term gonadotrophin-releasing hormone (GRH) antagonist which can identify, based on female Rhesus monkey studies, urinary calcium excretion.[1]

Most recently, antihormones have been discovered in women which antagonize follicle-stimulating hormone (FSH) action on ovarian granulosa cells.[41] The antihormones were induced by the administration of GRH in hypogonadal women, which resulted in immunoreactive FSH that was deglycosylated to produce an FSH inhibitor. The search for similar antihormones might explain the dynamics of menopause, osteoporosis, and other age-related changes.

F. FINGERNAIL GROWTH–WOUND HEALING

Orentreich's group[167] has developed a simple, inexpensive, noninvasive technology for measurement of nail growth. They have found that the rate of fingernail growth, measured over 1 year, can give quantifiable information when correlated with age. Linear nail growth decreases 50% over the life span of humans and dogs which relates to vascularization and techniques allow measurement as part of a simple outpatient clinical evaluation. Cutaneous wound healing provides an alternative technique that can be clinically standardized,[35] although patient acceptance would be a problem.

G. SENSORY AND NEUROLOGIC CHANGES

Sensory changes include measurement of auditory, visual, and neurologic changes, sleep disorders, stimulus response changes, and posture, balance, and cognitive changes that for the sake of space cannot be discussed here, but require a more extensive review.[185] Aspects of this are addressed in this volume, with particular reference to visual changes.

The reader is referred to Landfield's work[131,132] and recent commentary for a review of what is required in central nervous system (CNS) determinations. Of particular interest is Zbuzek and Wu's[250] report on age-related decline in vasopressin in rat plasma. This is pertinent not only to urinary output with aging, but has sensory significance in that vasopressin has a nonopioid pain-inhibiting role. However, Miller[159] has found an increase in vasopressin release in older rats.

Olfactory pathways show senile plaque formation and the loss of olfactory sensitivity occurs with aging and may be a harbinger for the development of Alzheimer's disease.[37] The author is skeptical of this except as being solely representative of a receptor deficiency problem, because odor distinction requires a long-term memory of reference substance. However, olfaction declines with age and olfactometers and taste sensitivity galvanic stimulation measurement techniques are available.[54]

Apart from nuclear magnetic resonance (NMR) and CT scanning and positron emission tomography (PET) brain scans, the development of neurometrics, utilizing computerized profiles of brain electrical activity (electroencephalography, EEG), can now be quantitated and localized for age-related appraisal of CNS function.[108]

H. ENDOCRINE

Finch and Landfield[64] reviewed both neuroendocrine and autonomic alterations which involve immunomodulation because of brainstem involvement in immune function.

While the level of glucocorticoids is a factor in aging and age-related response to stress,[64,131] the one adrenocortical hormone that clearly declines with age and constitutes a readily evaluable biomarker is dehydroepiandrosterone (DHEA) or DHEA-sulfate (DHEA-S).[157,168,188] This hormone, at age 80, declines to 10 to 20% of values seen at age 20 and is discussed in detail by Zimmerman in this volume. Of major importance, DHEA-S values in men aged 56 to 79 years were significantly lower in those with heart disease, and in contrast, in those with highest DHEA-S values there was a 36% reduction in mortality from any cause.[12] This has been addressed by Zimmerman in this volume and in the reviews by Regelson et al.[188,188a-c]

The decline in DHEA with advancing age has particular validity for resistance to infection as it has been shown that its oral and subcutaneous administration enhances resistance to lethal coxsackie B4, and herpes simplex type II in mice.[137] The DHEA values in patients with acquired immunodeficiency syndrome/human immunodeficiency virus (AIDS/HIV) infection are remarkably reduced.[154]

Most resistance to viral infection induced by DHEA is mediated via the immune system[137] and the buffering action of this hormone, which has antistress, anticarcinogenesis, antitumor, and antidiabetogenic action, makes its action particularly pertinent to aging.[188] DHEA is orally well tolerated clinically where mild androgenic effects have been seen in studies of advanced cancer and multiple sclerosis;[188] studies in senile dementia, depression, and AIDS are ongoing.

Another role for DHEA relates to its inhibition of glucose-6 phosphate dehydrogenase (G6PD), which governs nonspecific drug hydroxylases which affect carcinogenicity and lipid peroxidation involved in aging.[124]

In another area, the clinical decline in thyroid function with age and its significance to physiologic decline has been discussed in detail in the Regelson review, "The Evidence for Pituitary and Thyroid Control of Aging".[186] The role of the thyroid hormones in aging is supported by the joint action of thyroid and growth hormone during a postweaning 30-d period in Snell-Begg progeric dwarf mice, which resulted in doubling or tripling of life span.[60,61] More recently, Fabris et al.[62] have shown that thyroid function clinically modulates thymic endocrine activity through effects on thymulin, a zinc-dependent thymic hormone. This is not surprising in view of the classical work of Lurie,[140] who reported that resistance in rabbits to tuberculosis was governed by thyroid hormone activity which related to its stimulation and maintenance of immune and phagocytic function.

Evaluation of thyroid hormonal function with particular reference to the convenience of whole body calorimetry is discussed by Daniel Hershey in this volume. His technology will enable us to conveniently measure overall oxygen utilization as a function of aging, with reference to thyroid and hypophyseal activity.[49] This is pertinent to clinical evaluation of the concept of a so-called decreased oxygen consumption hormone (DECO) with aging as proposed by Denckla.[186] In another area, autoimmunity to the thyroid gland increases in incidence with age, and is present in euthyroid individuals possibly related to elevated cholesterol values.[46] Gonzalez and Quapri[76] have shown a delay in thyroid response to thyroid-releasing hormone (TRH) in aging dogs. A similar clinical decline in the aged is described by Jacques et al.[106] and Kaiser[111] regarding thyroid-stimulating hormone (TSH) and prolactin response.

The role of estrogen, GRH, and testosterone was discussed in many lengthy reviews.[184,186,188] It is sufficient to say that bioquantitation and clinical data indicate that estrogen replacement in menopausal women is a logical intervention program that should require clinical and biochemical quantitation.[184]

The changes in glucose metabolism, insulin and other related hormones deserve more specific review.[153,216] Because of our interest in hypophyseal control of aging and our interest in the action of DHEA,[188] and with the combined possibility of a thyroid-related effect on endocrine programmed age, we have reviewed these relationships.[186,188]

The rise in parathyroid hormone with age and the decline in 1,25-dihydrocalciferol can be bioquantitated in relation to osteoporosis, as well as immune and vascular responses.[245]

Another hormone or neuroendocrine modulator that declines clinically with age is melatonin.[142] This hormone plays a role in stimulating immune responsiveness, inducing sleep, and affecting circadian rhythms and sexual function.[116,187]

Somatotropin augments the activity of cytolytic T cells, natural killer cells, interleukin-2 (IL-2) production, and delayed type hypersensitivity mediated by T cells.[60,178,179] It governs response to T-dependent antigens and production of thymulin. The pituitary cells that secrete somatotropin and prolactin decrease with age.[179] Of interest to the free radical concept of aging, somatotropin is responsible for priming macrophages for the generation of superoxide.[56] Measurement of somatropin and prolactin produced by pituitary acidophilic cells could provide quantitative measures useful for age quantitation as evidence exists for age-related alterations in growth hormone[219] and prolactin production.[152]

Type II diabetes in the elderly is characteristic of aging, but its relationship to obesity and the fundamental process of aging is not clear. As a biomarker, glucose tolerance or insulin response requires elaborate testing to go beyond simple definition.[153]

Somatostatin, which can affect insulin levels, is remarkably increased in the elderly, providing another endocrine-related biomarker.[199]

III. IMMUNOLOGIC PARAMETERS

It has been shown in a variety of animal and clinical models that with age, immunologic response declines.[24,53,66,90,144,169,237] The evidence is presented in some detail in the author's previous paper on biomarkers.[185] More recently, Murasko et al.[163] have shown that aged negative responders to phytohemagglutinin (PHA), concanavalin A (Con A), or pokeweed mitogen (PWM) blastogenesis had twice the mortality of positive responders. Death was primarily due to cardiovascular disease, suggesting the lack of immune responsiveness is a signal for disease other than those attributed to immune resistance.

Long-term cultures of human T cells show age-related decreases in doubling capacity despite the presence of T cell growth factors.[77,104,183,237] There is a decline in the number of cells dividing *in vitro* for a second or third time from older donors when stimulated by PHA *in vitro*. Weksler et al.[237] indicate that cultures from old donors have only one fifth the number of lymphocytes dividing for a third time as did cultures from younger donors.[104] This may be due to a decline in nucleolar organizing regions which have been found to decline along with RNA synthesis in PHA-stimulated lymphocytes of the aged.[43]

Despite evidence for an age-related decline in *in vitro* mitotic capacity, colony forming capacity and PHA-stimulated kinetics may actually increase with age.[42,138]

deWeck's group[47] have shown changes in lymphocyte populations in the elderly as measured by cytofluorometric responses to lectin and leukokine mitogenic stimulation. This has been related in mice to an increase in null cells and a decrease in T lymphocytes. Singh et al.[217] have studied the immunologic deficiencies that are associated with Down syndrome and Alzheimer's disease, i.e., decrease in immunoglobulin M (IgM), decline in T_4 suppressor activity, and rise in autoantibodies to brain and cerebral amyloid.

Of pertinence to thymic function and aging, Fabris et al.[61] have described thymic functional deficiency in Down syndrome and aging which was improved by zinc on *in vitro* addition to plasma. As discussed previously, lymphocyte activation and aging show changes in seasonal and diurnal cyclicity in mice, suggesting the importance of a melatonin effect.[22,142]

Cinader et al.[34] have shown that suppressor immune activity increases with age in SJL mice which can be reversed by lipid-containing diets with a high ratio of unsaturated to saturated phospholipid. Rivnay et al.[192] and Schinitsky et al.[208] have shown that lymphocytic responses in the aging mouse can be enhanced by lecithin (AL721) administration but whether these membrane fluidizers can change surface lymphocyte properties[156] or reverse the age-related loss of antibacterial immunity requires more data.[171]

The role of neuroimmunomodulation, as it is affected by changes in environmental stimuli or emotional factors to which the aged are particularly vulnerable, was discussed by Kelley[118] in an excellent comparative physiologic review.

Bridge et al.[21] have shown that monoamine oxidase activity shows enhanced thermolability in older lymphocytes which might be pertinent to lymphocyte-related autonomic adrenergic responses. In another area, Horan and Fox[99] present evidence that increased endotoxin absorption from the gastrointestinal (GI) tract or, its declining detoxification, could be responsible for age-altered enhanced autoimmunity or hypoimmune response. Evidence exists of altered capacity to repair DNA injury in lymphocytes,[122] which may relate to the unwinding of the supercoiled state of DNA with age.[89]

There is a marked age-related decline in human sera IgG with a less marked decline in IgM[135] beginning at age 60. Of additional pertinence to aging quantitation is the evidence that old mice have difficulty generating a T cell response to lymphocytic choriomeningitis virus.[51] This implies that an age quantitative measure could be developed in relation to the measurement of vaccine response. Murasko et al.[163] suggests that immune responsiveness may be among the best biomarker for age prognostics.

IV. FACTORS REQUIRING VALIDATION AND LONG-TERM STUDY

A. AUTONOMIC FUNCTION

Autonomic function has been reviewed by Pfeiffer et al.,[176] Kulheimer,[127] Wollner and Spalding,[244] and Wagner et al.[234] who placed emphasis on temperature control.

Clinically, plasma noradrenaline levels are elevated in healthy elderly individuals with exaggerated responses to tilting.[231] Despite this, cardiovascular responses are attenuated in the elderly as compared to younger subjects.[175] In this regard, monoamine oxidase (MAO) elevation accompanies aging in a variety of circulating blood elements and clinical responses.[21,115]

Pfeiffer et al.[175] have attempted to assess the clinical role of the autonomic nervous system with aging. They found evidence of a decline in both sympathetic and parasympathetic responses as measured by pupillary and cardiac respiratory variation in heart rate. Both plasma norepinephrine and mean blood pressure increased with age, which may represent compensatory responses to functional autonomic decline, with particular reference to baroreceptor function.

Adrenergic receptor affinity data for β-adrenergic agonists and their receptor responses decline with aging in target tissue such as adipocytes, CNS, heart, lymphocytes, and lung.[128,207] This has been related to differences in cutaneous vascular responses in Alzheimer's disease and to iontophoretic administration of adrenergic and cholinergic drugs.[100] Platelet membranes that contain MAO show alterations in fluidity in Alzheimer's disease.[254]

In this category are pyrogenic responses to IL-1 or endotoxin, which decline with age in most species.[81,203] Additional studies showing changes in autonomic response with sleep may have value regarding age-related sleep responses.[252]

Of importance to intervention, strenuous acute exercise regimens reduce catecholamine levels in the heart of aged rats (27 months), but chronic exercise attenuates the decline.[149]

B. BIOCHEMICAL ASSAYS

The metabolism of certain drugs, i.e., aspirin, barbiturates, ethanol, coumadin, and morphine analgesic, alters with aging. With regard to drug metabolism, what are needed are standardized tests, independent of ongoing or previous drug administration, to establish the functional capacity of nonspecific drug hydrolases to metabolize a given agent. This is a measure of multiple metabolic factors including endoplasmic reticulum, protein and RNA synthesizing capacity, peroxisome, cytochrome levels, and hormonal metabolism, all of which influence the detoxification of drugs and should be able to provide a functional measure related to age.[107] Stadtman[223] has discussed the theoretical aspects of the possible role that mixed function oxidases (MFOs) play in the aging process.

Age influences hepatotoxicity in rats and in this regard, allyl alcohol injury was more severe with age.[190] With respect to intervention, age-related decreases in drug metabolism are associated with rises in δ-aminolevulinic synthetase activity which was restored when stimulated by testosterone administration.[14] Drug metabolism in aging has been reviewed by Van Bezooijen[230] as a potential measure of protein synthetic capacity, respiratory pigment response, and hormone production.

Although not studied in senescence, but pertinent to aging, Elcombe[59] has found that peroxisomal enzyme induction by clofibrate or phthalate, which induces hepatic catalase, fatty acid β-oxidases, and amino oxidases, is less actively synthesized in long-lived vs. short-lived species.

Age-related CNS responses to drugs[205] involve changes in the CNS as a function of endorphins or opiate binding.[11] This is seen in both pain and feeding studies.[80] Opioid sensitivity with aging is modulated by pineal function and the production of melatonin which decreases with aging.[116,187]

Pertinent to the above, β-endorphin immunoreactivity decreases in the cerebrospinal fluid (CSF) of Alzheimer's patients.[112] This is not surprising in view of the alterations in the molecular forms of endorphins found in the aging rat hypothalamus.[239] The response of the aging rat to the inhibition of feeding responses to opioid antagonists, i.e., naloxone, is distinct from that seen in younger animals, and this reflects on elevated endorphin levels in older animals.[80]

Burchinsky[26] has reviewed the role of neurotransmitter receptors and pharmacologic agents with aging, but has made no reference to the work of Papavasiliou et al.[170] who showed improved motor function and increased life span with L-dopa feeding in mice. This suggests the importance of basal ganglia functional changes.

C. VOLATILES IN EXPIRED AIR

The volatiles include clinical measurement of hydrocarbons, aldehydes, ketones, esters, ethers, nitrogen and sulfur compounds,[79,126] isoprene/acetone ratios,[68] and pentane and ethane formation related to exercise-mediated free radical formation in rats. The above is pertinent to the work of Robinson and co-workers whose data regarding urinary volatiles are presented in this volume.[195-197]

Respiratory excretory products, which can be measured in expired air as a function of age, can also provide a potential measure of capacity to cope with exercise and free radical generation, as well as diagnose diabetes and possibly lung cancer.

D. CENTRAL NERVOUS SYSTEM FUNCTION

As discussed previously, apart from measuring psychomotor function,[132] there are quantitative changes in brain volume and density that accompany aging. In support of this, deLeon et al.[45] reported cognitive defects that correlate with cortical atrophy on CT scan in senile dementia as have George et al.,[71] who found increases in ventricular volume in this population. Bioquantitative assays in this diagnostic sphere require their own review. Of interest, Chodzko-Zajko and Ringel[33] have found physiologic correlates, i.e., lens accommodation, two-point discrimination, acoustic analyses, and reaction time, to relate to declining motor performance with aging. Again, this was discussed in detail in Dean's text[44] and by Hochschild.[95,95a]

E. CHOLESTEROL, PHOSPHOLIPID RATIOS, MEMBRANE VISCOSITY, AND AGING

Aging is associated with a decrease of protein, cholesterol, and phospholipids in brain cell membranes which accompanies increased viscosity.[28] As mentioned previously, increased viscosity has also been reported by Rivnay et al.[192] as a function of increased cholesterol to phospholipid ratios in rat brains and lymphocytes which can be reversed by egg lecithin feeding of the proper phospholipid ratios (AL721). These effects are said to govern narcotic addiction and immune responsiveness.

Gershfeld[72] has described saturated to desaturated lecithin ratios as a predictive factor in coronary disease, and there are reports of increased arterial wall sphingomyelin with age.[201]

Murthy et al.[164] have reviewed fatty acid and triglyceride changes with aging and describe fatty acid elevations and uptake in the liver with enhanced triacylglycerol synthesis in aging rats which could be evaluated in clinical aging.

Cholesterol and low density lipoprotein (LDL) are indicative of coronary risk, but it might be more effective to study age-related differences in apolipoprotein E, which is involved not only in cholesterol transport, but in injury and tissue regeneration.[143]

F. MONOAMINE OXIDASE

We have discussed evidence for the elevation of this enzyme complex with progressive age.[21,115,151] Monoamine oxidase exists in two separate forms and in addition to its presence in readily sampled platelets is found in mitochondrial membranes and can be extracted from muscle and blood vessel walls. Levels rise in the myocardium of aging rats.[151]

G. XANTHINE OXIDASE

In congenic mice higher levels of this enzyme reflect on shorter survival,[124] which is of interest as regards its role in free radical formation.

H. AMINO ACID AND RELATED PATTERNS

Patterns of amines, amides, and amino acids change in urine and blood[67,194-197] as do bound to unbound amino acid patterns.[191] In another area, hyaluronic acid is elevated in the urine of the progeric Hutchinson-Gilford syndrome,[251] with only a modest age-related increase in controls. Similar effects have been seen in Werner's syndrome and hyaluronate changes could be a reflection of antiangiogenic activity. Based on this, refinements of assays for hyaluronate excretion might have value in age estimations.

Robinson et al.[198] have spoken of molecular profiles of aging and a symposium on this was held in 1984.[3] Pertinent to the "free radical concept" of aging, Brown's group[16] reported that valine, tyrosine, isoleucine, tryptophan, and other amino acids, in decreasing order of importance, protect *Escherichia coli* from hyperbaric oxygen toxicity. It would be interesting to see whether clinical amino acid profiling in aging correlates with amino acid differences that may relate to oxygen protection or lipofuscin formation.

I. ENZYME PROTEIN/PEPTIDE PATTERNS

The search for age-related enzyme differences which are not conveniently located in serum or plasma for evaluation requires sampling of blood elements or biopsy combined with tissue culture techniques for what will become applied cytogerontology. Aspects of this are found in Frolkis' text[65] on the physiology of cell aging.

The search for isozyme or enzyme or protein/peptide differences with two-phase gel electrophoresis makes assay techniques of this type feasible.[222,223] The Andersons[8] have been trying to develop peptide profiling as a major commercial venture in order to create a diagnostic laboratory for proteins and peptides in the study of disease. This requires the development of a library of serum and urine for computerized comparative scanning of serum- or tissue-derived gels. A library of this kind could be made available under the control of the Orentreich Foundation, which possesses over 30 years of vertical patient study material from the Kaiser-Permanente Foundation group practice.

Enzyme differences of proven laboratory potential include:

1. 5'-Nucleotidase in lymphocytes and cultured fibroblasts. Sun and Holland[225] have shown that 5'-nucleotidase rises in cell senescence and is absent in growing tumor cells. Along with changes in 5'-nucleotidase, another enzymatic age change involving nucleic acid synthesis has been described by Hards and Patterson,[84] who showed increases in glycinamide ribonucleotide synthetase during *in vitro* aging of human fibroblast cell lines.
2. Ribonucleotide reductase. This is another enzyme involved in replicative activity which decreases with age[48] in fibroblasts. In view of the iron dependency of this enzyme, this could reflect on the availability of iron-containing growth factors.
3. Another enzyme that may reflect on cellular aging is G6PD,[78,101] which is inhibited by DHEA.[188]
4. Glutamine synthetase activity increases by 25% in whole brain of old rats, but decreases in liver cells. Cao Danh et al.[29] feel that this could be an enzymatic change related to detoxifying ammonia. In this regard, ammonia, apart from its effects on pH and the CNS, has other physiological effects which include inhibition of interferon.[105]

5. Superoxide dismutase (SOD) and catalase. In a study of species-related life expectancy Cutler's group[228] has emphasized that levels of SOD relate to life span as a function of metabolic rate. The measurements were made on the basis of liver, heart, and brain sampling. It would be of interest to see if this assay could be applied to tissue culture or blood samples with correlates of metabolic rate related to Hershey's[92,93] clinical calorimetric metabolic measurement or if it would relate to tolerance to oxidative stress.[103]
6. α-Glycerophosphate dehydrogenase and malic enzyme. Age-related changes occur in hepatic and renal expressions of these enzymes which can be modulated by chronic administration of triiodothyronine.[206] This is particularly interesting because of the Denckla hypothesis that aging may reflect a declining sensitivity to thyroid hormone.[186]

J. LONG-TERM EFFORT; MISCELLANEOUS

Other measurements require much longer efforts for clinical application and validation. Some of them, i.e., measurement of sexual dysfunction or measurement of GI function require specialized attention or measurement techniques that could be inconvenient or expensive.[185]

Hollander and Dadufalza[98] have shown pancreatic protein and amylase secretion to decline in aging rats, although this has not been confirmed clinically.[82] The timing and sample size in human studies do not rule out the eventual clinical significance of observations regarding age-related exocrine enzyme secretion changes in the rat. In further support of Hollander and Dadufalza,[98] exocrine secretion of parotid amylase in rats decreases with age, suggesting that salivary gland secretion could be a more convenient clinical approach to measure exocrine function with age.[121]

Other measurements that may be of value, some of which have been discussed previously, include: steroid responses to stress, aldosterone assay, sex hormonal assays, growth hormone, thyroid stimulating or releasing hormones, thyroid hormone, the study of glucoregulatory hormones, prolactin, melatonin, vitamin D_3, parahormone, and vasopressin. Prolactin is particularly important in view of the reports that it has immunostimulatory, dopaminergic, and salt- and water-regulatory action.

All of these assays are influenced by circadian variation governing sampling techniques. In addition, it must be recognized that immunologic quantitation of hormone levels may not account for abnormalities in receptor affinities that are not revealed by the usual direct immunologic hormone assays.

Additional assays of immunologic response in lymphocytes could include evaluation of IL-2 induction and response, natural killer cell distribution, phosphokinase and cyclic nucleotide activity, and changes in purine nucleoside phosphorylase and other enzymes needed for DNA synthesis. Lymphocyte membrane fluidity, movement of surface markers, lactic acid dehydrogenase isozyme ratios, and measurement of adrenergic receptors, adrenocorticotropic hormone, and endorphin receptors which have been identified in lymphocytes.

In another area, thymosin fractions can now be quantitated and identified by immunologic technique. Autoantibodies change with age[94] as do colony-forming lymphocytes,[42] monocyte responses,[10] and sister chromatid exchange in lymphocytes to mutational agents.[165]

Other areas that require long-term study include red cell membrane sensitivity to perfringolysin or chymotrypsin,[150] changes in hemoglobin composition and glycosylation of red cell membranes (the latter has been used for diabetic monitoring),[30,162] measurement of osmotic fragility, sphericity index, Na,K-ATPase levels, acetylcholine esterase, polyamine oxidase and MAO levels, changes in lipid peroxidation[110,147] and charge density, and changes in electron spin resonance.[232] These all have potential utility in quantitative aging studies.[185]

Pertinent to study of changes in membrane response are observations that show an age-related decline in adrenocortical membrane potential to extracellular potassium concentration.[141] There are also studies indicating declines in mitochondrial membrane synthesis.[145]

Other studies that may have value include measurement of hemolytic sensitivity to oxidants, oxidized glutathione and phosphatidylethanolamine content, and glycoprotein changes.

One group of enzymes of possible significance to aging that have not been examined is glutathione S-transferases, important to sulfhydryl availability and leukotriene/prostaglandin E_2 metabolism.

Hair, fingernail, and skin scrapings have value in technologies that include cation or trace metal quantitation via secondary gamma emission and atomic absorption, but this area currently lacks serious clinical acceptance.

The platelet is another readily available blood element that shows functional alteration with aging.[115] Above age 59, platelets have shown enhanced aggregation to adenosine diphosphate and collagen, as well as increases in MAO activity.[20] Platelet membrane fluidity was shown to be increased in an Alzheimer familial cohort.[254]

Collagen or tendon biopsy, while uncomfortable, could provide information related to age change as collagen solubility alterations are age markers in rodents. Sorbitol concentration, and nonenzymatic browning could be quantitated in tissue of this type.[30,162] Similarly, in this tissue, lysyl oxidase, which rises in diabetic animals, also should be looked at as an age marker.[241]

Muscle biopsy provides another sampling alternative with regard to lipofuscin levels and changes in dehydroascorbic acid and glycoproteins, which have been reported to change in muscle with age in animal models.[185] Glucocorticoid receptors decrease in the muscle of mature rats.[212] These receptors have also been shown in hepatic cells,[113] and this may provide a marker for age-related changes.

With appropriate tissue sampling biochemical parameters could be examined. These include enzymes such as ornithine decarboxylase involved in polyamine metabolism, δ-amino levulinic acid synthetase (δ-ALA-S) involved in heme metabolism, and methionine sulfoxide dismutase, which are important to lens cataracts and lung emphysematous changes. Other enzymes of interest include δ-6-desaturase, lipoprotein lipase, SOD, and succinate dehydrogenase, CoQ reductase, aldehyde dehydrogenase, and glutathione S-transferase.[185]

The first enzyme of heme synthesis δ-ALA-S decreased 67% with age in both drug-induced and spontaneous controls in the liver of Fisher 344 rats. The decrease was present in mitochondria, and the hepatic mitochondrial content decreased with aging.[172,211] There is high activity for microsomal heme oxygenase and a low-level δ-ALA-S in livers of senescent female rats[172] and a decline in heart and brain cytochrome oxidase with age,[2] along with the decline in δ-ALA-S.[15]

Protein peptide patterns, measurement of racemization of proteins, measurement of protein deamidation and protease sensitivity, changes in isoenzyme patterns, and measurement of changes in transfer RNA methylation or acylation[148] may also be of value with more study.[185]

The author has discussed deamidation of protein as a potential biomarker in a previous review.[185] The concept of aging, as a function of altered proteins leading to enzymatic changes or protease vulnerability, has been reviewed by Stadtman,[223] several texts,[3,4] and reviews[246,246a,247] on nonenzymatic deamidation of asparaginyl and glutaminyl residues in peptides and proteins. The alteration of proteins includes prooxidation[238] and the action of MFOs and nonenzymatic browning (Maillard reaction),[30,162,166] as well as glycosylation, which may be responsible for tissue changes in diabetes and aging.

Pertinent to an age-related quantitation of protein changes are proteins that show deamidation which include adrenocorticotropic hormone, alcohol dehydrogenase, amylase, aspartate aminotransferase, calmodulin, carbonic anhydrase, growth hormone, hemoglobin, lysozyme, prolactin, ribonucleases, somatomammotropin, substance P, and triosephosphate isomerase.[246,246a]

There is evidence that the calcium-binding S100 protein found in the CNS may be pertinent to Down syndrome.[5] The genomic expression for a beta subunit of this protein is found on chromosome 21 and its expression should be examined as a function of age.

For biomarker purposes, what is missing in age-related studies of deamidation of protein is a targeted peptide or enzyme that can provide profiles of peptide change or protease sensitivity as a key biomarker. When two-phase gel electrophoresis and staining techniques such as have been applied by the Andersons[8] are finally routinized, these patterns will be determined and characterized for clinical automation.

Susceptibility to proteases is a function of age and liver cytosol proteins are more readily digested in young than in old animals, which may reflect on the prolonged survival of albumin in older rats.[238]

With regard to the above, age-related scrutiny are amino acid sequences that are rapidly degraded. This is the PEST amino acid sequence, so-called because it is rich in proline, glutamic acid, serine and threonine.[246] The PEST region and the role of ubiquitin, which affects protease or peptide degradation, as age-related biomarkers deserves scrutiny.

A possible way to develop a window into protein or peptide age changes is to examine changes that have been found in well-characterized tissue such as the lens of the eye.[96] The hope would be to find similar clinical changes in plasma and readily available cells such as lymphocytes or through skin biopsy and/or tissue culture. Importantly, Brunauer and Clark[25] found an age-dependent accumulation of D-aspartic acid in human erythrocytes. This should be searched for in other tissues.

Biodegradation of polyamines is enhanced in older cells. This may be due to the action of amine oxidase or aldehyde dehydrogenases.[32] Labeling of amino acids derived from putrescine and spermidine also has been found to increase in older cells.[210] Catabolic conversion of putrescine or spermidine to amino acids in old cells was eight-fold greater than in young cells, and circulating cells show a decrease in polyamines with increasing age.[32] One key factor in polyamine synthesis is *S*-adenosyl-L-methionine decarboxylase which decreases with age.

Trace metal analysis requires a more extensive review, but there is an increase with age in the ratios of copper to ceruloplasmin in human males.[147] Vistines et al.[232] have shown with electron spin resonance (ESR) that lipofuscin in CNS ceroid in dogs and man is associated with age-related metal binding of copper and iron. Dyundikova et al.[55] have shown a significant decline in rat aortic copper concentration with age which deserves clinical evaluation in readily obtained tissue. This is important to age-related collagen changes as copper deficiency is associated with the decline in lysyl oxidase.[241]

Electron spin resonance of *in vitro* neuronal lipopigments shows the presence of metal complexes that could be quantitated.[232] Again, this could be valuable in the exploration of biopsiable cells in culture or from blood sources.

Iron accumulates in organs with aging in mice[147,243] or with hypothyroidism, and it would be interesting to see whether total iron values of tissue biopsies or culture could reflect on clinical age in humans. This may be critical to the free radical concept of aging in view of its role in oxidation.

K. TISSUE CULTURE, BLOOD SAMPLE, OR BIOPSY ASSAY

There are similarities between *in vitro* and *in vivo* aspects of cellular aging.[155] The problems of donor age, which can define clonal differentiation or growth in tissue culture skin fibroblasts, have been frequently discussed.[119] Apart from the measurement of RNA, protein metabolism, or DNA repair, one technique to define differences between cells of young vs. old origin is to stress cells by defining *in vitro* sensitivity to radiation,[18] radiation repair,[88,248] or sensitivity to carcinogens or prooxidants such as dioxin.[134] Alternatively, baseline measurements can be obtained on age pigments by microspectrofluorometric techniques because these accumulate with age in nondividing cells.[123]

Regarding tissue culture, Cristofalo's group[39,102] have discussed the role of tissue culture as a technique to study age modulation as have others. Cells in tissue culture progressively lose responsiveness to mitogenic components in serum.[165,185] Cultures lose response to epidermal growth factor, insulin, and dexamethasone, although the concentrations that elicit the response remain the same, indicating that the portion of cells responding decline.[177] Morphologic changes of differentiation of fibroblasts can be useful in determining aging,[125] and as discussed previously, studies of lymphocytes provide an opportunity distinct from solid tissue biopsied cells in tissue culture. As examples, sister chromatid exchange to mitomycin declines in old donor lymphocytes.[165]

Our capacity to grow cells in culture and determine growth kinetics, enzyme, autocrine responses, and DNA repair alterations should make tissue culture techniques useful for quantitation of functional age. In this regard, nuclear area increases with senescence and progressive donor age,[133] as do changes in the nucleolus forming chromosomal regions in metaphase fibroblasts and lymphocytes.[27] The importance of this is seen in presentations by Stephens and Lipetz[224] and Williams[240] in which the physical state of DNA and DNA repair capacity ascertained from blood or biopsy samples may relate to chronologic age or to species survival capacity.

Yamamoto et al.[248] have presented data regarding DNA cross-linked material which increases with age in rabbit liver. Gensler[70] and Gensler and Bernstein[69] have looked at this in studies of cells from isolated hamster lung and kidney cells. Unscheduled DNA repair did not change until the animals had exceeded two thirds of their life span and related data has been presented by Plesko and Richardson.[182] Goldstein and Shmookler-Reis[74] have shown *in vitro* changes in lymphocytes from old donors related to extrachromosomal DNA species, and Piko et al.[188] have discussed changes in mitochondrial DNA with aging that could be ascertained with *in vitro* study. These changes are varied as there is an age-related decline in mitochondrial protein synthesis related to iron deficiency.[145] Torrelio et al.[229] have reported that senescent fibroblast cell lines can be identified by changes in phosphoribosylpyrophosphate (P-RIB-PP) levels. In view of the role P-RIB-PP plays in DNA synthesis and repair, its measurement in isolated biopsy material could constitute a potential biomarker for aged cells, as does the response of these cells to growth factors.[36]

Immortal cell lines maintain 5-methylcytosine residues in their DNA while senescent cells lose methylated DNA. The changes in DNA methylation may distinguish between embryonic and adult functional differences that could be critical to the aging process[242] and vital to organ and embryonic tissue transplantation.

Minkowitz et al.[160] have developed enzyme profiles from skin biopsies of dermal fibroblasts and found suggestive variation in five enzymes that could provide comparative information with age. As discussed previously, Sun and Holland's[225] work with 5'-nucleotidase can provide information as to senescence in tissue culture models and Pereira-Smith et al.[174] have found inhibitors of DNA synthesis in the membranes of senescent cells. The relationship of age-related changes to chromatin has been reviewed by Thakur,[227] but he has missed the interesting observations of Stephens and Lipetz[224] and Williams.[240]

Williamson and Kilo[241] have found lysyl oxidase levels to be abnormal in the connective tissue of diabetic animals. Berenson et al.,[13] in discussing the role of sulfated polysaccharides in atherosclerosis, have found age-related differences in blood vessel walls. The above is pertinent to the age-related predicting effect of hexosamine values in aging rat tissue[97] and glycosylation of protein which could be revealed by biopsy or tissue culture technique. These observations are also pertinent to the work of Kay[117] regarding Band 3 glycoproteins which appear with senescence in red blood cells and nucleated cells.

As discussed previously, in tissue culture one can measure responses to ultraviolet or free radical injury and repair and/or response to epidermal growth factor and other cytokines. Changes in MAO activity in skin fibroblasts can be quantitated for donor age. The latter shows a three- to tenfold increase in MAO with senescence of cell lines *in vitro*.[85] This may relate to catecholamine effects on keratinocytes, and be pertinent to plasma or platelet increases in MAO.[20,21]

Once tissue culture survival patterns are established, response to peptide or transferrin and other growth factors by *in vitro* aging cells can be ascertained in a fashion similar to that seen for lymphocyte response to lectins and leukokines.

In this regard, there is an inverse correlation between *in vitro* replicative capacity and age of the donor for a wide range of cells which may relate to explant outgrowth, onset of cell culture senescence, life span, doubling time, percent of replicating cells, and number of cells at confluence. Automated systems for monitoring these *in vitro* differences eventually will be needed. These were previously developed by the Nobelist, Don Glaser, at the University of California, Berkeley. Glaser's group[38] developed elaborate computerized TV monitored tissue culture systems that provided continuous three-dimensional monitoring of tissue culture growth patterns from biopsy or single cell clonal lines. Unfortunately, this expensive program was scuttled before it could be applied, but these techniques have been rediscovered by Schmidt-Ullrich et al.[209] In 1988 the capacity of DNA to unwind was associated with the initiation of DNA replication during the cell cycle.[193]

The above tissue culture methodology lends itself to studies of free radical toxicity as a function of aging. Hagihara et al.[83] claim that lipid peroxide levels were found in low density, low protein fractions in higher concentration in old than in younger individuals. The spin resonance technique may be useful in determining prooxidant/antioxidant age-related activity. Von Zglinicki and Bimmler[233] have described a decline in intracellular water with aging in hepatocytes and monocytes which they feel is of mitochondrial origin.

Additional areas of tissue culture change that can be measured include patterns of glycosaminoglycans, collagen, peroxidase effects, changes in energy mechanics and DNA and DNA polymerase, as well as histone changes, DNA template, protein synthesis and RNA synthetic activity; measurement of nucleolar organizing activity, microtubulin synthesis, or colchicine sensitivity; measurement of Na,K-ATPase and membrane changes; changes in autocrine regulatory responses, i.e., changes in receptor availability, production and response to IL_1, IL_2, IL_3, erythrocyte growth factor, transforming growth factor, interferons, somatostatin, insulin-related factors, and other cytokinase and regulatory peptides. It is essential in studies of this type to be aware that serum or plasma nutritional culture systems may contain inhibitory substances which contribute to senescence which could also be evaluated from donor sources for age evaluation.[136] In support of the differences in tissue culture media responses, Kihara et al.[119] has found S6 protein phosphorylation responses in senescence to be governed by serum factors.

V. DISCUSSION

The importance of biomarker determinations, while not necessarily providing immediate answers, provides the motivation to seek changes in what has been considered immutable: that the functional decline of aging, with the loss of quality of life, is an irreversible fact of man's fate. It is my feeling that if we quantitate age-related changes as an integrated profile for vertical study for each individual, we provide a challenge to each of us to intervene in an effort to alter our fate. For this to happen, it is important to motivate the policymakers of the health science community who can only be influenced by measurement of "before and after" treatment.

At a more basic level of biomarker study, cytogerontologic assays can help us understand the more fundamental changes of aging that affect cell cycle, DNA repair, protein synthetic, translational or membrane events. Thus, does 5'-nucleotidase enzyme activity, which increases with senescence, have fundamental significance along with Band-3 glycoprotein cell membrane changes or changes in nucleochromatin, DNA repair, or membrane fluidity? The techniques exist if biopsy and tissue culture methodology for aging studies should generate enthusiasm equal to the interest that developed for *in vitro* chemotherapy assays in cancer patients.

In this chapter, and in texts[185,186] the author has discussed what he considers to be among the most promising techniques to measure age-related physiology. Clinical groups with a strong interest in bioquantitation are those in cardiovascular rehabilitation, sports medicine, Alzheimer's disease study, orthopedics, rheumatoid disease and diabetic control where performance and/or pathophysiology are age-related. Bioquantitation and intervention are now in place as profitmaking ventures for cardiac rehabilitation and improvement of athletic performance.

Of recent importance to bioquantitation, Papaconstantinou[255] has found a decline in acute reactive proteins to stress. This age-related decline of the liver's response to injury provides a rapid assay for quantitation of age and its reversal.

Despite the problems of deciding on which measures of quantitation will have validity and the statistical hurdles related to "bottom-line" predictions of death and/or debility, we should be greatly encouraged by the work in Harrison and Archer's[87] laboratory, which shows that in a food-restricted mouse model, six physiologic tests predicted the value of dietary control. Despite caveats that a focus on bioquantitation would displace financial resources from basic aging research, centers of excellence that would quantitate physiologic age should be the primary goal for the National Institute on Aging[214] as well as the insurance industry.[185] With the above in place, rational intervention with single or multiple strategies becomes possible as we can ascertain youthful change or maintenance, which is the essential goal of intervention.

REFERENCES

1. Abbasi, R. and Hodgen, G.D., Predicting the predisposition to osteoporosis gonadotrophin-releasing hormone antagonist for acute estrogen deficiency test, *JAMA*, 255, 1600, 1986.
2. Abu-Erreish, G.M. and Sanadi, D.R., Age-related changes in cytochrome concentration of myocardial mitochondria, *Mech. Age. Dev.*, 7, 425, 1978.
3. Adelman, R.C. and Dekker, E.E., Eds., *Modification of Proteins During Aging*, Alan R. Liss, New York, 1984.
4. Adelman, R.C. and Roth, G.S., Eds., *Altered Proteins and Aging*, CRC Press, Boca Raton, FL, 1983.
5. Allore, R., O'Hanlon, P., and Price, R., Gene encoding the B subunit of S100 protein is on chromosome 21: implications for Down's syndrome, *Science*, 239, 1311, 1988.
6. Ambrecht, H.J., Changes in calcium and vitamin D metabolism with age, in *Nutritional Intervention in the Aging Process*, Ambrecht, H.J., Pendergast, J.M., and Coe, R.M., Eds., Springer-Verlag, New York, 1988, 69.
7. Ames, B., The assay of endogenous oxidative DNA damage as related to aging, in *Practical Handbook of Human Biologic Age Determination*, Balin, A.K., Ed., CRC Press, Boca Raton, FL, 1994, 397.
8. Anderson, N.G. and Anderson, N.L., The Human Protein Index: A Proposal for the Organization of Molecular Anatomy. A Report of the Human Protein Task Force, Molecular Anatomy Program, Argonne National Laboratories, Argonne, IL, 1981.
9. Androtti, C., Bussotti, A., Cammelli, D. et al., Connective tissue in aging lung, *Gerontology*, 29, 377, 1983.
10. Antonaci, S., Jirillo, E., Lucivero, G. et al., Humoral immune response in aged humans: suppressor effect of monocytes on spontaneous plaque forming cell generation, *Clin. Exp. Immunol.*, 52, 387, 1983.
11. Bardo, M. T., Bhatnagar, R.K., and Gebhart, G.F., Age-related differences in the effect of chronic administration of naloxone on opiate binding in rat brain, *Neuropharmacology*, 22, 453, 1983.

12. Barret-Conner, E., Khaw, K.-T., and Yen, S.S.C., A prospective study of dehydroepiandrosterone sulfate, mortality, and cardiovascular disease, *N. Engl. J. Med.*, 315, 1519, 1986.
13. Berenson, G.S., Radhakrishnamurthy, S.R., Srinivasan, S.R. et al., The extracellular matrix of atherosclerosis, in *Comparative Pathobiology of Major Age-Related Diseases. Current Status and Research Frontiers*, Migaki, G. and Scarpelli, D.G., Eds., Alan R. Liss, New York, 1984, 307.
14. Bitar, M. and Weiner, M., Modification of age-induced changes in heme and hemoproteins by testosterone in male rats, *Mech. Age. Dev.*, 23, 285, 1983.
15. Bitar, M.S. and Shapiro, G.H., Aberration of HEME and hemoprotein in aged female rats, *Mech. Age. Dev.*, 38, 189, 1987.
16. Boehme, D.E., Vincent, K., and Brown, O.R., Oxygen and toxicity inhibition of amino acid biosynthesis, *Nature*, 262: 418, 1976.
17. Borkan, G.A., Factors in clinical aging: variation in rates of aging, in *Intervention in the Aging Process*, Part A, Regelson, W. and Sinex, F.M., Alan R. Liss, New York, 1983, 99.
18. Bourgeois, C.A., Raynaud, N., and Diatloff-Zito, C., Effect of low dose rate ionizing radiation on the division potential of cells in vitro. III. Cytogenetic analysis of human fibroblasts, *Mech. Age. Dev.*, 17, 225, 1981.
19. Bradfonbrener, M., Landowne, M., and Shock, N.W., Changes in cardiac output with age, *Circulation*, 12, 557, 1955.
20. Bridge, T.P., Jeste, D.V., Wise, C.D. et al., Platelet monoamine oxidase in an aged general population and elderly schizophrenics, *Psychopharmacol. Bull.*, 17, 103, 1981.
21. Bridge, T.P., Wise, C.D., Corash, L.M. et al., Lymphocytic monoamine oxidase: activity and thermoability in younger and older subjects, *Biol. Psychiatry*, 19, 599, 1984.
22. Brock, M.A., Temporal order vs. variability in activation of lymphocytes from aging mice, *Mech. Age. Dev.*, 37, 197, 1987.
23. Brocklehurst, J.C., Ed., *Textbook of Geriatric Medicine and Gerontology*, Churchill Livingstone, New York, 1985.
24. Brouwer, A. and Knook, D.L., The reticuloendothelial system and aging: a review, *Mech. Age. Dev.*, 21, 205, 1983.
25. Brunauer, L.S. and Clarke, S., Age dependent accumulation of protein residues which can be hydrolyzed to D-aspartic acid in human erythrocytes, *J. Biol. Chem.*, 201, 12538, 1986.
26. Burchinsky, S.G., Neurotransmitter receptors in the central nervous system and aging: pharmacological aspect (review), *Exp. Gerontol.*, 19, 227, 1984.
27. Buys, C.H., Osinga, J., and Anders, J.P.A., Age dependent variability of ribosomal activity in man as determined from frequencies of silver staining nucleolus organizing regions on metaphase chromosomes of lymphocytes and fibroblasts, *Mech. Age. Dev.*, 11, 55, 1979.
28. Calderini, G., Bonetti, A.C., Battistella, A. et al., Biochemical changes of rat brain membranes with aging, *Neurochem. Res.*, 8, 483, 1983.
29. Cao Danh, H., Strolin Beneditti, M., and Dostert, P., Age-related changes in glutamine synthetase activity of rat brain, liver and heart, *Gerontology*, 31, 95, 1985.
30. Cerami, A., Accumulation of advanced glycosylation end products on proteins and nucleic acids role in aging, in *Cellular and Molecular Aspects of Aging, The Red Cell as a Model*, Eaton, J.W., Konzen, D.K., and White, J.G., Eds., Alan R. Liss, New York, 1984, 79.
31. Chapuy, M.C., Durr, F., and Chapuy, P. Age-related changes in parathyroid hormone and 25 hydroxycalciferol levels, *J. Gerontol.*, 38, 19, 1983.
32. Chen, K.Y. and Chang, Z.F., Age dependence of the metabolic conversion of polyamines into amino acids in IMR-90 human embryonic lung diploid fibroblasts, *J. Cell Physiol.*, 128, 27, 1986.
33. Chodzko-Zajko, W.J. and Ringel, R.L., Physiological fitness measures and sensory and motor performance in aging, *Exp. Gerontol.*, 22, 317, 1987.
34. Cinader, B., Clandinin, B.T., Koh, S.W. et al., Dietary fat alters progression of some age-related changes of the immune system, *Immunol. Lett.*, 12, 175, 1986.
35. Cohen, B.J., Danon, D., and Roth, G.S., Wound repair in mice as influenced by age and anti-macrophage serum, *J. Gerontol.*, 47, 295, 1987.
36. Conover, C.A., Rosenfeld, R.G., and Hintz, R.L., Somatomedin C/insulin like growth factor I binding and action in

human fibroblasts aged in culture: impaired synergism with dexamethasone, *J. Gerontol.*, 42, 308, 1987.

37. Costanzo, R.M., Mann, D.M.A., Tucker, C.M., and Yates, P.O., Alzheimer's disease: an olfactory connection, *Mech. Age. Dev.*, 42, 1, 1988.
38. Couch, J.L., Konrao, M.W., and Glaser, D.A., Analysis of images of colonies of tissue culture cells and microorganisms, in *Pattern Recognition and Image Processing*, Institute of Electrical and Electronic Engineers, IEEE, New York, 1979, 473.
39. Cristofalo, V.J., Cellular biomarkers in aging, *J. Gerontol.*, 23, 297, 1988.
40. Cutler, R., Antioxidants and aging, *Am. J. Clin. Nutr.,* 53 (1 suppl.), 3735, 1991.
41. Dahl, K.D., Bicsak, T.A., and Hsueh, A.J.W., Naturally occurring anti-hormones: Secretion of FSH antagonists by women treated with a GnRH analog, *Science*, 239, 72, 1988.
42. Damle, N.K. and Gupta, S., Colony forming lymphocytes in man, *Gerontology.*, 29, 108, 1983.
43. Das, B.C., Rani, R., Mitra, A.B. et al., The number of silver staining NOR's (or DNA) in lymphocytes of newborns and its relationship to human development, *Mech. Age. Dev.*, 36, 117, 1986.
44. Dean, W., *Biological Aging Measurement — Clinical Applications,* The Center for Bio-Gerontology, Los Angeles, 1988.
45. deLeon, M.J., Ferris, S.H., George, A.E. et al., Position emission tomography and computed tomography evaluations in regional brain metabolism in senile dementia, *Age*, 4, 146, 1981.
46. DeMaertelaer, V., Calay, R., and Nerve, P., Thyroid, lipid and other biological variables in elderly patients with asymptomatic autoimmune thyroiditis: a statistical analysis, *Gerontology*, 33, 315, 1987.
47. deWeck, A.L., Kirstensen, F., Joncourt, F. et al., Lymphocyte proliferation, lymphokine production and lymphocyte receptors in aging and various clinical conditions, *Springer Semin. Immunol. Pathol.*, 7, 273, 1984.
48. Dick, J.E., and Wright, J.W., Human diploid fibroblasts with alterations in ribonucleotide reductase activity, deoxyribonucleotide pools and in vitro lifespan, *Mech. Age. Dev.*, 26, 37, 1984.
49. Dilman, V.M. and Bernstein, L.M., Hypothalamic mechanism of aging and specific age pathology. IV. Sensitivity threshold of the hypothalamo-pituitary complex to homeostatic inhibition by the thyroid, *Exp. Gerontol.*, 14, 225, 1979.
50. Doepel, L.K., From the NIH. Looking at the menopause's role in osteoporosis, *JAMA*, 254, 2379, 1985.
51. Doherty, P.C., Diminished T cell surveillance function in old mice infected with lymphocyte choriomeningitis virus, *Immunology*, 32, 751, 1977.
52. Dominice, J., Levasseur, C., Larno, S. et al., Age-related changes in rabbit articular chondrocytes, *Mech. Age. Dev.*, 37, 231, 1986.
53. Doria, G., Adorini, L., Sabbadini, E. et al., Immunoregulation in aging, *Ann. N.Y. Acad. Sci.*, 521, 182, 1987.
54. Dye, C.J., Age-related changes in taste and smell that affect nutritional adequacy, in *Nutritional Intervention in the Aging Process*, Armbrecht, H.J., Prendergast, J.M., and Coe, R.M., Eds., Springer-Verlag, New York, 1984, 13.
55. Dyundikova, V.A., Silvon, Z.K., and Dubina, T.I., Biological age and its estimation. I. Studies of some physiological parameters in albino rats and their validity as biological age tests, *Exp. Gerontol.*, 16, 13, 1981.
56. Edwards, C.K., III, Ghiasuddin, S.M., Schepper, J.M. et al., A newly defined property of somatotropin: priming of macrophages for production of superoxide anion, *Science*, 239, 769, 1988.
57. Ehrsam, R. E., Perruchoud, A., Oberholzer, M. et al., Influence of age on pulmonary haemodynamics at rest and during supine exercise, *Clin. Sci.*, 65, 653, 1983.
58. Eithe, M.E., Hermiller, J.B., Magorien, R.D. et al., The effect of age on central and regional hemodynamics, *Gerontology*, 30, 240, 1984.
59. Elcombe, C., personal communication, 1987.
60. Fabris, N.W., Pierpaoli, W., and Sorkin, E., Lymphocytes, hormones and aging, *Nature*, 240, 557, 1972.
61. Fabris, N., Amadio, L., Licastro, F. et al., Thymic hormone deficiency in normal aging and Down's syndrome: is there a primary failure of the thymus?, *Lancet*, 1, 983, 1984.

62. Fabris, N., Mocchegiani, E., Muzzioli, M. et al., Neuroendocrine-thymus interactions: perspectives for intervention in aging, *Ann. N.Y. Acad. Sci.*, 521, 72, 1987.
63. Finch, C. and Schneider, E., Eds., *Handbook of the Biology of Aging*, 2nd ed., Van Nostrand Reinhold, New York, 1985.
64. Finch, C.E. and Landfield, D.W., Neuroendocrine and autonomic functions in aging animals, in *Handbook of the Biology of Aging*, 2nd ed., Finch, C.E. and Schneider, E.L., Eds., Von Nostrand Reinhold, New York, 1985, 567.
65. Frolkis, V.V., Ed., *Physiology of Cell Aging*, S. Karger, New York, 1984.
66. Furukawa, T., Meydani, S.N., and Blumberg, J.B., Reversal of age associated decline in immune responsiveness by dietary glutathione supplementation in mice, *Mech. Age. Dev.*, 38, 107, 1987.
67. Gates, S.C., Provancal, S.J., Webb, J.W. et al., Metabolic profiles on rats of different ages, *Exp. Gerontol.*, 19, 279, 1984.
68. Gee, D.L. and Tappel, A.L., The effect of exhaustive exercise on expired pentane as a measure of in vivo lipid peroxidation in the rat, *Life Sci.*, 28, 2425, 1981.
69. Gensler, H.L. and Bernstein, H., DNA damage as the primary cause of aging, *Q. Rev. Biol.*, 56, 279, 1981.
70. Gensler, H.L., The effect of hamster age on UV-induced unscheduled DNA synthesis of freshly isolated lung and kidney cells, *Exp. Gerontol.*, 16, 59, 1981.
71. George, A.E., deLeon, M.J., Rosenbloom, S. et al., CT ventricular volume and its relationship to cognitive impairment in dementia, *AGE*, 4, 146, 1981.
72. Gershfeld, N.L., Selective phospholipid absorption and atherosclerosis, *Science*, 204, 506, 1979.
73. Gerstenblith, G., Cardiovascular aging, in *Biological Markers of Aging*, Reff, M.E. and Scheider, E.L., Eds., NIH Publ. #82-2221, National Institutes of Health, Bethesda, MD, 1982, 138.
74. Goldstein, S. and Shmookler-Reis, R.J., Amplification of extrachromosomal circular copies of an inter-ALU unstable DNA sequence during in vitro and in vivo aging, *Mol. Basis Aging*, pp. 1, 1984.
75. Goldstein, R.S., Tarloff, J.B., and Hook, J.B., Age-related nephropathy in laboratory rats, *FASEB J.*, 2, 2241, 1988.
76. Gonzalez, E. and Quapri, S.K., Effect of aging on the pituitary-thyroid axis in the dog, *Exp. Gerontol.*, 23, 151, 1988.
77. Goodwin, J.S. and Messner, R.P., Sensitivity of lymphocytes to prostaglandin E_2 increases in subjects over age 70, *J. Clin. Invest.*, 64, 434, 1979.
78. Gordon, M.N., Mobbs, C.V., Morgan, D.G. et al., Effects on age and estradiol on brain and pituitary glucose 6 phosphate dehydrogenase and 6 phosphogluconate activities, *Soc. Neurosci. Abstr.*, 10, 477, 1984.
79. Gordon, S.M., Szidon, J.P., and Krotoszynski, B.K., Volatile organic compounds in exhaled air from patients with lung cancer, *Clin. Chem.*, 31, 1278, 1985.
80. Gosnell, B.A., Levine, A.S., and Morley, J.E., The effect of aging on opioid modulation of feeding in rats, *Life Sci.*, 32, 2793, 1983.
81. Grahn, D., Norman, D.C., and Yoshikawa, T.T., Fever and aging: central nervous system prostaglandin E2 in response to endotoxin, *Exp. Gerontol.*, 22, 249, 1987.
82. Gullo, L., Priori, P., Daniele, C. et al., Exocrine pancreatic function in the elderly, *Gerontology*, 29, 407, 1983.
83. Hagihara, M., Hishkaki, I., Maseki, M. et al., Age-dependent changes in lipid peroxide levels in the lipoprotein fractions of human serum, *J. Gerontol.*, 39, 269, 1984.
84. Hards, R.G. and Patterson, D., Variation of glycinamide ribonucleotide synthetase levels during in vitro aging of human fibroblasts: implications for gene dosage studies, *Mech. Age. Dev.*, 36, 65, 1986.
85. Harper, R.A. and Grove, G., Human skin fibroblasts derived from papillary and reticular dermis. Differences in growth potential in vitro, *Science*, 204, 526, 1979.
86. Harris, C.C., Future directions for research on the use of carcinogen-DNA adducts as dosimeters to monitor human exposure to environmental mutagens and carcinogens (Genetic Toxicology Association Abstr.), *Cell Biol. Toxicol.*, 3, 84, 1987.
87. Harrison, D.E. and Archer, J.R., Biomarkers of aging: tissue markers, future research needs, strategies, directions and priorities, *Exp. Gerontol.*, 23, 309, 1988.
88. Hart, R.W., Benirschke, A.K., and Walford, R.W., Correlation between ultraviolet induced DNA repair in primate lymphocytes and fibroblasts and species maximum achievable life span, *Mech. Age. Dev.*, 24, 163, 1984.

89. Hartwig, M., and Korner, I.J., Age-related changes of DNA winding and repair in human peripheral lymphocytes, *Mech Age. Dev.*, 38, 73, 19??.
90. Hausman, P.B., and Weksler, M.E., Changes in the immune response with age, in *Handbook of the Biology of Aging*, Finch C.E., and Schneider, E.L., Eds., Von Nostrand Reinhold, New York, 1985, 414.
91. Heaney, R.P., Age-related bone loss, in *Biological Markers in Aging*, Reff, M.E. and Schneider, E.L., NIH Publ. #82-2221, National Institutes of Health, Bethesda, MD, 1982, 161.
92. Hershey, D. Whole body calorimeter, Basal-Tech, Inc., Cincinnati, 1988.
93. Hershey, D. and Lee III, W.E., Entropy as a biological marker in human aging, in *Practical Handbook of Human Biologic Age Determination*, Balin, A.K., Ed., CRC Press, Boca Raton, FL, 1994, 231.
94. Hijmans, W., Radl, J., Bottazzo, F.G. et al., Auto-antibodies in highly aged humans, *Mech. Age. Dev.*, 26, 83, 1984.
95. Hochschild, R., The H-Scan: an instrument for the automatic measurement of physiological markers of aging, in *Intervention in the Aging Process*, Regelson, W. and Sinex, F.M., Eds., Alan R. Liss, New York, 1983, 113.
95a. Hochschild, R., Validating biomarkers of aging — mathematical approaches and results of a 2462-person study, in *Practical Handbook of Human Biologic Age Determination*, Balin, A.K., Ed., CRC Press, Boca Raton, FL, 1994, 93.
96. Hoenders, H.J. and Bloemendal, H., Lens protein and aging, *J. Gerontol.*, 38, 278, 1983.
97. Hofecker, G., Skalicky, M., Kment, A. et al., Models of the biological age of the rat. I. A factor model of age parameters, *Mech. Age. Dev.*, 14, 345, 1980.
98. Hollander, D. and Dadufalza, D.V., Increased intestinal absorption of oleic acid with aging in the rat, *Exp. Gerontol.*, 18, 287, 1983.
99. Horan, M.A. and Fox, R.A., Aging and the immune response — a unifying hypothesis, *Mech. Age. Dev.*, 26, 165, 1984.
100. Hornquist, R., Henriksson, R., Balk, O. et al., Iontrophoretic study of adrenergic and cholinergic skin vessel reactivity in normal aging and Alzheimer's disease, *Gerontology*, 23, 374, 1987.
101. Houben, A., Raes, M., Houbion, A. et al., Alteration of enzymes in aging human fibroblasts in culture. I. Conditions for the appearance of an alteration in glucose-6-phosphate dehydrogenase, *Mech. Age. Dev.*, 25, 23, 1984.
102. Husokawa, M., Phillips, T.D., and Cristofalo, V.J., The effect of dexamethasone on epidermal growth factor binding and stimulation of proliferation in young and senescent W138 cells, *Exp. Cell Res.*, 164, 408, 1986.
103. Imre, S. and Jahasz, G., The effect of oxidative stress on inbred mice of different ages, *Mech. Age. Dev.*, 38, 259, 1987.
104. Inkeles, B., Innes, J.B., Kuntz, M.M. et al., Immunologic studies of aging. III. Cytokinetic basis for the impaired response of lymphocytes from aged humans to plant lectins, *J. Exp. Med.*, 145, 1176, 1977.
105. Ito, M. and McLimans, W.F., Ammonia inhibition of interferon synthesis, *Cell Biol. Int. Rep.*, 5, 661, 1981.
106. Jacques, C., Schlienger, J.L., Kissel, C. et al, TRH-induced TSH and prolactin responses in the elderly, *Age Aging*, 16(3), 181, 1987.
107. Jarvik, C.F., Greenblatt, D.J., and Harman, D., Eds., *Aging*, Vol. 16, *Clinical Pharmacology and the Aged Patient*, Raven Press, New York, 1981.
108. John, E.R., Prichep, L.S., Fridman, J. et al., Neurometrics: computer-assisted differential diagnosis of brain dysfunction, *Science*, 239, 162, 1988.
109. Johnson, J.E., Effects of hypophysectomy on age-related changes in rat kidney glomerulus: observations by scanning and transmission electron microscopy, *Mech. Age. Dev.*, 13, 63, 1980.
110. Jozwiak, Z. and Jasnowska, B., Changes in oxygen metabolizing enzymes and lipid peroxidation in human erythrocytes as a function of age of donor, *Mech. Age. Dev.*, 32, 77, 1985.
111. Kaiser, F.E., Variability of response to thyroid releasing hormone in normal elderly, *Age Aging*, 16, 345, 1987.
112. Kaiya, H., Tanaka, T., Takeuchi, K. et al., Decreased level of B-endorphin-like immunoreactivity in cerebrospinal fluid of patients with senile dementia of Alzheimer type, *Life Sci.*, 33, 1039, 1983.
113. Kalimi, M., Gupta, S., Hubbard, J. et al., Glucocorticoid receptors in adult and se-

nescent rat liver, *Endocrinology*, 112, 341, 1983.
114. Kannel, W. and Hubert, H., *Biological Markers of Aging*, Reff, M.E. and Schneider, E.L., Eds., NIH Publ. #82-2221, National Institutes of Health, Bethesda, MD, 1982, 145.
115. Kasjanova, D. and Balaz, U., Age-related changes in human platelet function in vitro, *Mech. Age. Dev.*, 37, 175, 1986.
116. Kavaliers, M., Hirst, M., and Teskey, G.C., Aging, opioid analgesia and the pineal gland, *Life Sci.*, 32, 2279, 1983.
117. Kay, M.M.B., Aging of cell membrane molecules leads to appearance of an aging antigen and removal of senescent cells, *Gerontology*, 31, 215, 1985.
118. Kelley, K.W., Immunological consequences of changing environmental stimuli, in *Animal Stress*, Koberg, G.P., Ed., American Physiological Society, Williams & Wilkins, Baltimore, MD, 1985, 193.
119. Kihara, F., Tsuji, Y., Miura, M. et al., Events blocked in prereplicative phase in senescent human diploid cells, TIG-1, following serum stimulation, *Mech. Age. Dev.*, 37, 103, 1986.
120. Kihara, F., Ninomiya-Tsuji, J., Ishibashi, S. et al., Failure in S6 protein phosphorylation by serum stimulation of senescent human diploid fibroblasts, *Mech. Age. Dev.*, 37, 27, 1986.
121. Kim, S.K., Calkins, D.W., Weinhold, P.A. et al., Changes in the synthesis of exportable and nonexportable proteins in parotid glands during aging, *Mech. Age. Dev.*, 18, 239, 1982.
122. Kishi, K., Homma, A., Kawa, A. et al., Age-related change in the frequency of ARA-C induced chromosome aberrations in human peripheral blood lymphocytes, *Mech. Age. Dev.*, 37, 211, 1987.
123. Koistinaho, A., Sorvaniem, M., Alho, H. et al., Microspectrofluorometric quantitation of autofluorescent lipopigment in human sympathetic ganglia, *Mech. Age. Dev.*, 37, 79, 1986.
124. Koizumi, A., Hasegawa, L., Walford, R.L. et al., H2, Ah and aging. The immune response and the inducibility of P-450 mediated monooxygenase activities, xanthine oxidase and lipid peroxidation in H-2 congenic mice on C57Bl/10, C3H and A strain background, *Mech. Age. Dev.*, 37, 199, 1986.
125. Kontermann, K. and Bayreuther, K., The cellular aging of rat fibroblasts in vitro is a differentiation process, *Gerontology*, 25, 261, 1979.
126. Krotoszynski, B.K., O'Neill, G.G., and Claudio, H.J., Characterization of human expired air: a promising investigative and diagnostic technique, *J. Chromatogr. Sci.*, 15, 239, 1977.
127. Kulhemeier, K.V., Age-related changes in sympathetic function, in *Experimental and Clinical Interventions in Aging*, Walker, R.F. and Cooper, R.L., Eds., Marcel Dekker, New York, 1983, 355.
128. Kusiak, J.W. and Pitha, J., Decreased response with age of cardiac catecholamine sensitive adenylate cyclase system, *Life Sci.*, 33, 1679, 1983.
129. Lakatta, E.G., Heart and circulation, in *Handbook of the Biology of Aging*, 2nd ed., Finch, C.E. and Schneider, E.L., Van Nostrand Reinhold, New York, 1985, 377.
130. Lakatta, E.G., Cardiovascular system aging, in *Human Aging Research: Concepts and Techniques*, Kent, B. and Butler, R.N., Eds., Raven Press, New York, 1988, 199.
131. Landfield, P.W., Adrenocortical hypothesis of the brain and somatic aging, in *Biological Mechanisms of Aging*, Schimke, E.R.T., Ed., NIH Publ. #81-2194, National Institutes of Health, Bethesda, MD, 1981, 658.
132. Landfield, P.W., Commentary on biomarkers of aging in the nervous system, *Exp. Gerontol.*, 23, 413, 1988.
133. Lee, S.-C., Bemiller, P.M., Bemiller, J.N. et al., Nuclear area changes in senescing human diploid fibroblasts, *Mech. Age. Dev.*, 7, 417, 1978.
134. Lim, M., Jacobson-Kram, D., Bowman, R.E., and Williams, J.R., Effects of chronic exposure of 2,3,7,8-tetrachlorodibenzo-P-dioxin on sister chromatid exchange and chromosomal aberration, *Cell Biol. Toxicol.*, 3, 87, 1987.
135. Litwin, S.D., Zehr, B.D., and Rogers, S.K., There is marked age-related decline in human sera IgD, *Aging Immunol. Infect. Dis.*, 1, 41, 1988.
136. Loo, D.T., Fuquay, J.I., Rawson, C.L. et al., Extended culture of mouse embryo cells without senescence: inhibition by serum, *Science*, 236, 200, 1987.
137. Loria, R., Inge, T., Cook, S.S. et al., Protection against acute lethal viral infections

with the native steroid dehydro-epiandrosterone (DHEA), *J. Med. Virol.*, 12, 301, 1988.

138. Lucivero, G., Surico, G., Mazzini, G. et al., Age-related changes in the proliferative kinetics of phytohemagglutinin stimulated lymphocytes. Analysis by uptake of tritiated precursors of DNA, RNA and proteins and by flow cytometry, *Mech. Age. Dev.*, 43, 259, 1988.

139. Ludwig, F.G. and Smoke, M.C., The measurement of biological age, *Exp. Age Res.*, 6, 497, 1980.

140. Lurie, M.B., Resistance to tuberculosis, in *Experimental Studies in Active and Acquired Defensive Mechanisms*, Harvard University Press, Cambridge, MA, 1984, 265.

141. Lymangrover, J.R., Valeco, N.K., and Shilling, R.D., Rat adrenal zona fasciculated cell electrophysiological responses to ACTH and MSH vary with age, *Mech. Age. Dev.*, 43, 269, 1988.

142. Maestroni, G.J.M., Conti, A., and Pierpaoli, W., Pineal melatonin, its fundamental immunoregulatory role in aging and cancer., *Ann. N.Y. Acad. Sci.*, 521, 140, 1987.

143. Mahley, R.W., Apolipoprotein E: cholesterol transport protein with expanding role in cell biology, *Science*, 240, 622, 1988.

144. Makinodan, T., James, T.J., Inamizu, T. et al., Immunologic basis for susceptibility to infection in the aged, *Gerontology.*, 30, 279, 1984.

145. Marcus, D.L., Ibrahim, N.G., and Freedman, M.L., Age-related decline in the biosynthesis of mitochondrial inner membrane proteins, *Exp. Gerontol.*, 17, 333, 1982.

146. Marcus, R., Understanding and preventing osteoporosis, *Hosp. Pract.*, 24, 189, 1989.

147. Massie, H.R., Aieuo, V., and Banziger, V., Iron accumulation and lipid peroxidation in aging C57 B1/6J mice, *Exp. Gerontol.*, 18, 277, 1983.

148. May-Hoopes, L.L., Cleland, G., and Bochantin, J., Function and fidelity of aging tRNA: in vivo acylation discrimination, synthetase binding and in vitro translation, *Mech. Age. Dev.*, 22, 135, 1983.

149. Mazzeo, R.S., Colburn, R.W., and Horvath, S.M., Effect of aging and endurance training on tissue catecholamine response to strenuous exercise in Fischer 344 rats, *Metabolism*, 35, 602, 1986.

150. McKay, M.J. and Hipkiss, A.R., The subcellular distribution and proteolysis of abnormal proteins in aging rabbit reticulocytes, in *Cellular and Molecular Aspects of Aging: The Red Cell as a Model*, Eaton, J.G., Konzen, D.K., and White, J.C., Eds., Alan R. Liss, New York, 1984, 29.

151. Meco, M., Bonifati, V., Collier, W.L. et al., Enzyme histochemistry of monoamine oxidase in the heart of aged rats, *Mech. Age. Dev.*, 38, 145, 1987.

152. Meites, J., Neuroendocrine biomarkers of aging in the rat, *Exp. Gerontol.*, 23, 349, 1988.

153. Meneilly, G.S., Minaker, K.L., Elahi, D. et al., Insulin action in aging mice: evidence for tissue specific differences at low physiologic insulin levels, *J. Gerontol.*, 42, 196, 1987.

154. Merril, C. and Sunderland, T., personal communication, 1988.

155. Mets, T., Bekaert, E., and Verponk, G., Similarity between in vitro and in vivo cellular aging, *Mech. Age. Dev.*, 22, 71, 1983.

156. Michalski, J.P., Razandi, M., McCombs, C.C. et al., Surface properties of lymphocyte subpopulations in autoimmune WZB/NZW F_1 hybrid mice: alterations correlated with the immunodeficiency of aging, *Clin. Immunol. Immunopathol.*, 29, 15, 1983.

157. Migeon, C.J., Keller, A.R., Lawrence, B. et al., Dehydroepiandrosterone and androsterone levels in human plasma. Effect of age and sex; day-to-day and diurnal variations, *J. Clin. Endocrinol. Metab.*, 17, 1051, 1957.

158. Miller, J.M., Moxham, J., and Green, M., The maximal sniff in the assessment of diaphragm function in man, *Clin. Sci.*, 69, 91, 1985.

159. Miller, M., Increased vasopressin secretion: an early manifestation of aging in the rat, *J. Gerontol.*, 43, 3, 1987.

160. Minkowitz, S., Minkowitz, F., and Conklin, D., Quantitative assay of enzyme activity in skin: a new approach to the correlation of cell biology and physiology, *Age*, 1, 74, 1978.

161. Mittman, C., Edelman, N.H., Norris, A.H. et al., Relationship between chest wall and pulmonary compliance and age, *J. Appl. Physiol.*, 20, 1211, 1965.

162. Monnier, V.M., and Cerami, A., Nonenzymatic browning in vivo: possible process for aging of long-lived proteins, *Science*, 211, 491, 1981.
163. Murasko, D.M., Weiner, P., and Kaye, D., Association of lack of mitogen induced lymphocyte proliferation with increased mortality in elderly, *Aging Immunol. Infect. Dis.*, 1, 1, 1988.
164. Murthy, V.K., Oredipe, O.A., Stiles, M.R. et al., Increased fatty acid uptake, a factor in increased hepatic triacylglycerol synthesis in aging rats, *Mech. Age. Dev.*, 37, 49, 1986.
165. Musilova, J., Michalova, K., and Pacovsky, V., Induction of sister chromatid exchanges by mitomycin C in lymphocytes of young and old human donors, *Gerontology*, 30, 365, 1984.
166. Oimomi, M., Kitamuna, Y., Nishiboto, S. et al., Age-related acceleration of generation of tissue proteins in rats, *J. Gerontol.*, 41, 695, 1986.
167. Orentreich, N., Markofsky, J., and Vogelman, J.H., The effect on aging on the rate of linear nail growth, *J. Invest. Dermatol.,* 73, 126, 1979.
168. Orentreich, N., Brind, J.L., Rizer, R.L. et al., Age changes and sex differences in serum dehydroepiandrosterone sulfate concentrations throughout adulthood, *J. Clin. Endocrinol. Metab.*, 59, 551, 1984.
169. Oyeyinka, G.O., Age and sex differences in immunocompetence, *Gerontology*, 30, 188, 1984.
170. Papavasiliou, P.S., Miller, S.T., Thal, L.J. et al., Age-related motor and catecholamine alterations in mice on levodopa supplemented diet, *Life Sci.*, 28, 2945, 1981.
171. Patel, P.J., Aging and antimicrobial immunity impaired production of mediator T cells as a basis for the decreased resistance of senescent mice to listeriosis, *J. Exp. Med.*, 154, 821, 1981.
172. Paterniti, J.R., Lin, C.-I., and Beattie, D.S., Delta amino levulinic synthetase regulation of activity in various tissues of the aging rat, *Arch. Biochem. Biophys.*, 191, 792, 1978.
173. Pathy, M.S.J., Ed., *Principles and Practices of Geriatric Medicine*, John Wiley & Sons, New York, 1982.
174. Pereira-Smith, O.M., Fisher, S.F., and Smith, J.R., Senescent and quiescent cell inhibitions of DNA synthesis, *Exp. Cell Res.*, 160, 297, 1985.
175. Pfeiffer, M.A., Halter, J.B., and Wilkie, F., Autonomic nervous system. Function and age-related increases of blood pressure and heart rate in man, *Clin. Res.*, 28, 335, 1980.
176. Pfeiffer, M.A., Weinberg, C.R., Cook, D. et al., Differential changes of autonomic nervous system function with age in man, *Am. J. Med.*, 75, 249, 1983.
177. Phillips, P.D., Kaji, K., and Cristofalo, V.J., Progressive loss of the proliferative response of senescing WI-38 cells to platelet-derived growth factor, epidermal growth factor, insulin, transferrin, and dexamethasone, *J. Gerontol.*, 39, 11, 1984.
178. Pierpaoli, W. and Sorkin, E., Relationship between thymus and hypophysis, *Nature*, 215, 834, 1967.
179. Pierpaoli, W., Kopp, H.G., and Bianchi, E., Interpendence of thymic and neuroendocrine functions in ontogeny, *Clin. Exp. Immunol.*, 24, 501, 1976.
180. Piko, L., Hougham, A.L., and Bulpitt, K.J., Studies of sequence heterogeneity of mitochondrial DNA from rat and mouse tissue, evidence for an increased frequency of deletions/additions with aging, *Mech. Age. Dev.*, 43, 279, 1988.
181. Platt, D., Ed., *Geriatrics*, Vol. 1 and 2, Springer-Verlag, New York, 1982.
182. Plesko, M.M. and Richardson, A., Age-related changes in unscheduled DNA synthesis by rat hepatocytes, *Biochem. Biophys. Res. Commun.*, 118, 730, 1984.
183. Proust, J., Rosenzweig, P., ReBouzy C. et al., Lymphopenia induced by acute bacterial infections in the elderly: a sign of age-related immune dysfunction of major prognostic significance, *Gerontology*, 31, 178, 1985.
184. Purdy, R.H. and Goldheizer, J.W., Toward a safer estrogen in aging, in *Intervention in the Aging Process*, Part A, Regelson, W. and Sinex, F.M., Eds., Alan R. Liss, New York, 1983, 247.
185. Regelson, W., Biomarkers in aging, in *Intervention in the Aging Process*, Part A, *Quantitation, Epidemiology and Clinical Research*, Regelson, W. and Sinex, F.M., Eds., Alan R. Liss, New York, 1983, 3.
186. Regelson, W., The evidence for pituitary and thyroid control of aging: is age reversal a myth or reality? The search for a "death hormone", in *Intervention in the Aging Process*, Regelson, W. and Sinex, F.M., Eds., Alan R. Liss, New York, 1983, 3.

187. Regelson, W. and Pierpaoli, W., Melatonin: a rediscovered antitumor hormone? Its relation to surface receptors; sex steroid metabolism, immunologic response and chronobiologic factors in tumor growth and therapy, *Cancer Invest.*, 5, 379, 1987.

188. Regelson, W., Loria, R., and Kalimi, M., Hormonal intervention: "buffer hormones" or "state dependency". The role of dehydroepiandrosterone (DHEA) thyroid hormone, estrogen and hypophysectomy in aging, *Ann. N.Y. Acad. Sci.*, 518, 260, 1987.

188a. Kalini, M. and Regelson, W., Eds., in *The Biologic Role of Dehydroepiandrosterone (DHEA)*, Walter de Gruyter, Berlin, 1990.

188b. Regelson, W., Loria, R., and Kalini, M., Dehydroepiandrosterone (DHEA) the "mother steroid," PT I, immunologic action, *Ann. N.Y. Acad. Sci.*, in press, 1994.

188c. Regelson, W., Kalini, M., Loria, R. et al., Dehydroepiandrosterone (DHEA): a pleiotropic steroid, *Ann. N.Y. Acad. Sci.*, in press, 1994.

189. Ries, W. and Pethig, D., Chronological and biological age, *Exp. Gerontol.*, 19, 211, 1984.

190. Rikans, L.E., Influence of aging on the susceptibility of rats to hepatoxic injury, *Toxicol. Appl. Pharmacol.*, 73, 243, 1984.

191. Riley, V. and Spackman, D., Pacific NW Research Foundation. Report to the Murdoch Foundation and Fund for Integrative Biomedical Research (FIBER), 1982.

192. Rivnay, B., Orbital-Harel, T., Shinitzky, M. et al., Enhancement of the response of aging mouse lymphocytes by in vitro treatment with lecithin, *Mech. Age. Dev.*, 23, 329, 1983.

193. Roberts, J.M. and D'Urso, G., An origin unwinding activity regulates initiation of DNA replication during mammalian cell cycle, *Science*, 241, 1486, 1988.

194. Robinson, A.B., Dirren, H., Sheets, A. et al., Quantitative aging pattern in mouse urine vapor as measured by gas-liquid chromatography, *Exp. Gerontol.*, 11, 11, 1976.

195. Robinson, A.B. and Robinson, L.R., Quantitative measurement of human physiologic age by profiling of body fluids and pattern recognition, *Mech. Ageing Dev.*, 59, 47, 1991.

196. Robinson, A.B., Molecular clocks, molecular profiles, and optimum diets: three approaches to the problem of aging, *Mech. Age. Dev.*, 9, 225, 1979.

197. Robinson, A.B. and Robinson, L.R., Quantitative measurement of human physiological age by profiling of body fluids and pattern recognition, in *Practical Handbook of Human Biologic Age Determination*, Balin, A.K., Ed., CRC Press, Boca Raton, FL, 1994, 263.

198. Robinson, S., Bill, D.B., Tzankoff, S.P. et al., Longitudinal studies of aging in 37 men, *J. Appl. Physiol.*, 39, 263, 1975.

199. Rolandi, E., Franceschini, R., Messina, V. et al., Somatostatin in the elderly: diurnal plasma profile and secretory response to meal stimulation, *Gerontology*, 33, 296, 1987.

200. Rosenthal, J., Aging and the cardiovascular system, *Gerontology*, 33, 3, 1987.

201. Rousen, G. and Solomon, R.D., Changes in phospholipid composition of human aorta with age, *Lipids*, 4, 232, 1969.

202. Rowe, J.W., Renal function in aging, in *Biological Markers of Aging*, Reff, M.E. and Schneider, E.L., Eds., NIH Publ. #82-2221, National Institutes of Health, Bethesda, MD, 1982, 228.

203. Ruwe, W.D., Naylor, A.M., and Dinarello, C.A., Characteristics of pyrogen fevers are altered in the aged rabbit, *Exp. Gerontol.*, 23, 103, 1988.

204. Sastry, B.V., Owens, L.K., and Janson, V.E., Enhancement of the responsiveness of the rat diaphragm DL-methionine and phospholipid methylation and their relationships to aging, *J. Pharmacol. Exp. Ther.*, 221, 629, 1982.

205. Saunders, D.R., Prolino, R.M., Bousquet, W.F. et al., Age-related responsiveness of the rat to drugs affecting the central nervous system, *Proc. Soc. Exp. Biol. Med.*, 147, 593, 1974.

206. Sawada, K., Hummel, B.C.W. and Walfish, P.G., Age-related changes in rat hepatic and renal thyroid sensitive enzymes — different responses to acute and chronic L-triodothyronie stimulation, *Mech. Age. Dev.*, 42, 229, 1988.

207. Scarpace, P.J. and Abrass, I.B., Decreased beta-adrenergic agonist affinity and adenylate cyclase activity in senescent rat lung, *J. Gerontol.*, 38, 143, 1983.

208. Schinitzky, M., Lyte, M., Heron, D.S. et al., Intervention in membrane aging: the development and application of active lipid, in *Intervention in the Aging Process*, Part B: *Basic Research and Preclinical Screening*, Regelson, W. and Sinex, F.M., Eds., Alan R. Liss, New York, 1983, 175.
209. Schmidt-Ullrich, R., Lin, P.S., Mikkelsen, R.B. et al., Proliferative rates of cloned malignant mammary epithelial cells as a measure of clonal heterogeneity in human breast carcinomas, *JNCI*, 77, 1001, 1986.
210. Sclabrino, G. and Ferioci, M.A., Polyamines in mammalian aging: an oncological problem, too? A review, *Mech. Age. Dev.*, 26, 149, 1984.
211. Scotto, A.W., Rinehart, R.W., and Beattie, D.S., Aging-related decreases in hepatic mitochondrial and cytosolic delta-aminolevulinic acid synthetase during experimental porphyria, *Arch. Biochem. Biophys.*, 222, 150, 1983.
212. Sharma, R. and Timaris, P.S., Regulatory changes in glucocorticoid receptors in the skeletal muscle of immature and mature male rats, *Mech. Age. Dev.*, 37, 249, 1987.
213. Shephard, R.J., Cardiovascular limitations in the aged, in *Exercise and Aging*, Smith, E.L. and Serfass, R.C., Eds., Enslow Publishing, Hillside, NJ, 1981, 19.
214. Shock, N.W., Longitudinal studies of aging in humans, in *Handbook of the Biology of Aging*, 2nd ed., Finch C.E. and Schneider, E.L., Eds., Von Nostrand Reinhold, New York, 1985, 721.
215. Short, R., Williams, D.D., and Bowden, D.M., Cross sectional evaluation of potential biological markers of aging in pigtailed macaques: effects of age, sex and diet, *J. Gerontol.*, 42, 644, 1987.
216. Silverberg, A.B., Carbohydrate metabolism in diabetes in the aged, in *Nutritional Intervention in the Aging Process*, Armbrecht, H.J., Pendergast, J.M., and Coe, R.M., Eds., Springer-Verlag, New York, 1984, 191.
217. Singh, V.K., Fudenberg, H.H., and Brown, F.R. III, Immunologic dysfunction: simultaneous study of Alzheimer's and older Down's patients, *Mech. Age. Dev.*, 37, 257, 1987.
218. Smith, E.L., Sempos, C.T., and Purvis, R.W., Bone mass and strength decline with age, in *Exercise and Aging*, Smith, E.L. and Serfass, R.C., Eds., Enslow Publishing, Hillside, NJ, 1981, 59.
219. Sonntag, W.E., Steger, R.W., Forman, S.J. et al., Decreased pulsatile release of growth hormone in old male rats, *Endocrinology*, 107, 1875, 1980.
220. Sourander, L.B. and Rowe, J.W., The genitourinary system — the aging kidney, in *Textbook of Geriatric Medicine and Gerontology*, Brocklehurst, J.C., Churchill Livingstone, New York, 1985, 608.
221. Sprott, R.L., Ed., Biomarkers in aging, *Exp. Gerontol.*, 23 (Issues 4, 5), 1988.
222. Stadtman, E.R., Biochemical markers of aging, *Exp. Gerontol.*, 23, 327, 1988.
223. Stadtman, E.R., Protein modification in aging, *J. Gerontol. Biol. Sci.*, 43, 112, 1988.
224. Stephens, R.E. and Lipetz, P.D., Higher order DNA repair in human peripheral leukocytes: a factor in aging and cancer, in *Intervention in the Aging Process*, Part B, Regelson, W. and Sinex, F.M., Eds., Alan R. Liss, New York, 1983, 155.
225. Sun, A.S. and Holland, J.F., Implications of 5' nucleotidase and its inhibitor for cellular aging and cancer, in *Molecular Biology of Aging*, Woodhead, A.D., Blackett, D., and Hollander, A., Eds., Plenum Press, New York, 1985, 163.
226. Tack, M., Actose, M.D., and Cherniak, N.S., Effects of aging on sensation of respiratory force and displacement, *J. Appl. Physiol. Resp. Environ. Exercise Physiol.*, 55, 1433, 1983.
227. Thakur, M.M., Age-related changes in the structure and function of chromatin: a review, *Mech. Age. Dev.*, 27, 263, 1984.
228. Tolmasoff, J.M., Ono, T., and Cutler, R.G., Superoxide dismutase: correlation with life span and specific metabolic rate in primate species, *Proc. Natl. Acad. Sci. U.S.A.*, 77, 2777, 1980.
229. Torrelio, B.M., Paz, M.A., and Gallop, P.M., Modulation of purine synthesis and phosphoribosyl pyrophosphate content in aging human fibroblasts, *Age*, 4, 134, 1981.
230. Van Bezooijen, C.F.A., Influence of age-related changes in rodent liver morphology and physiology or drug metabolism — a review, *Mech. Age. Dev.*, 25, 122, 1984.
231. Vargas, E., Rothwell, C., Weinkove, C. et al., The measurement of plasma noradrenaline before and after tilt in young and old healthy subjects, *Gerontology*, 30, 253, 1984.

232. Vistines, A.I., Henriksen, T., Nicolaissen, B. et al., Free radicals and aging: electron spin resonance studies on neuronal lipopigments and cells grown in vitro, *Mech. Age. Dev.*, 22, 335, 1983.
233. Von Zglinicki, T. and Bimmler, M., Intracellular water and ionic shifts during growth and aging of rats, *Mech. Age. Dev.*, 38, 179, 1987.
234. Wagner, J.A., Horvath, S.M., Kitagawa, K. et al., Comparisons of blood and urinary responses to cold exposures in young and older men and women, *J. Gerontol.*, 42, 173, 1987.
235. Walker, R.F. and Cooper, R.L., *Experimental and Clinical Interventions in Aging*, Marcel Dekker, New York, 1983.
236. Walsh, R.A., Cardiovascular Effects on the aging process, *Am. J. Med.*, 82(Suppl. 1B), 34, 1987.
237. Weksler, M.E., A search for immunological markers of aging in man, in *Biological Markers of Aging*, Reff, M.E. and Schneider, E.L., NIH Publ. #88-2221, National Institutes of Health, Bethesda, MD, 1982, 320.
238. Wiederanders, B., Ansorge, S., Bohley, P. et al., The age dependence of intracellular proteolysis: changes of substrate proteins, *Mech. Age. Dev.*, 8, 355, 1978.
239. Wilkinson, C.W. and Dorsa, D.M., The effect of aging on molecular forms of beta and gamma endorphins in rat hypothalamus, *Neuroendocrinology*, 43, 124, 1986.
240. Williams, J.R., Alterations in DNA chromatin structure during aging, in *Intervention in the Aging Process*, Part B, Regelson, W. and Sinex, M., Eds., Alan R. Liss, New York, 1983, 145.
241. Williamson, J.R. and Kilo, C., Comparative pathobiology of major age-related diseases: current status and research frontiers, in *Extracellular Matrix Changes in Diabetes Mellitus*, Migaki, G. and Scarpelli, D.G., Eds., Alan R. Liss, New York, 1984, 269.
242. Wilson, V.L. and Jones, P.A., DNA methylation decreases in aging but not in immortal cells, *Science*, 220, 1055, 1983.
243. Winkelmann, J.C., Mariash, C.N., Towle, C.N. et al., Thyroidectomy increases rat hepatic ferritin iron, *Science*, 213, 569, 1981.
244. Wollner, L. and Spalding, J.M.K., The autonomic nervous system, in *Textbook of Geriatric Medicine and Gerontology*, Brocklehurst, J.C., Ed., Churchill Livingstone, New York, 1985, 449.
245. Wongsurawat, N. and Armbrecht, H.J., Comparison of calcium effect on *in vitro* calcitonin and parathyroid hormone release by young and aged thyroparathyroid glands, *Exp. Gerontol.*, 22, 263, 1987.
246. Rosens, S.W. and Reichsteiner, M.C., Microinjection studies on selective protein degradation: relationship between stability, structure and location, *Biomed. Biochim. Acta*, 45, 1611, 1986.
247. Wright, H.T., Non-enzymatic deamidation of asparaginyl and glutaminyl residues in proteins, *Crit. Rev. Biochem. Mol. Biol.*, 26, 1, 1993.
247a. Wright, H.T., Nonenzymatic degradation of asparaginyl and glutamyl residues in proteins, *Crit. Rev. Biochem. Mol. Biol.*, 26, 1, 1991.
248. Yamamoto, I., Fuji, I., Yoshida, T. et al., Age dependency of base modification in rabbit liver DNA, *J. Gerontol.*, 43, B132, 1988.
249. Yin, F.C.P., Spurgeon, H.A., Rakusan, K. et al., Use of tibial length to quantify cardiac hypertrophy: application in the aging rat, *Am. J. Physiol.*, 243(Heart Circ. Physiol. 12), H941, 1982.
250. Zbuzek, V.K. and Wu, W.-H., Age-related changes of vasopressin in rat plasma and the hypothalamo-hypophyseal system, *Exp. Gerontol.*, 17, 133, 1987.
251. Zebrower, M., Kieras, F.J., and Brown, W.T., Urinary hyaluronic acid elevation in Hutchinson-Gilford progeric syndrome, *Mech. Age. Dev.*, 35, 39, 1986.
252. Zepelin, H. and McDonald, C.S., Age differences in autonomic variables during sleep, *J. Gerontol.*, 42, 142, 1987.
253. Drentreich, N.D., Zimmerman, J.A., and Matias, J.R., Dehydroepiandrosterone: marker or modifier of aging?, in *Practical Handbook of Human Biologic Age Determination*, Balin, A.K., Ed., CRC Press, Boca Raton, FL, 1994, 385.
254. Zubenko, G.S., Wusylko, M., Cohen, B.M. et al., Family study of platelet membrane fluidity in Alzheimer's disease, *Science*, 238, 539, 1987.
255. Papaconstantinou, J., A unifying model of the programmed (intrinsic) and stochastic (extrinsic) theories of aging: the stress response genes and aging, *Ann. N.Y. Acad. Sci.*, in press, 1994.

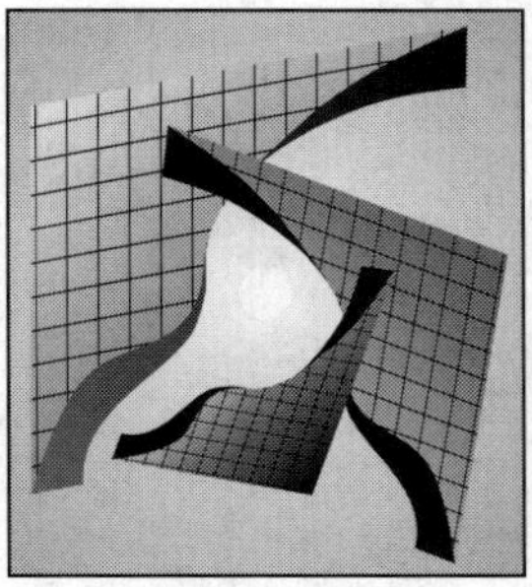

RISK APPRAISAL

CHAPTER 4
HISTORICAL COMMENTS

Lewis C. Robbins

You are decision makers looking for new ways to estimate risk.

Back in 1949, as we began to see the Framingham heart disease study unfold, I realized that we would someday face the job of reaching the ultimate decision maker — the patient himself. I began to understand that we needed to give information directly to the patient so that he can make an informed decision, because we cannot make decisions for him, but this idea was recognized long before 1949.

In about 1760, Lloyds of London decided that ships of commerce were in great need of insurance. In order to improve the life expectancy of these ships, an army of ship inspectors was employed. These inspectors followed every ship from the laying of her keel to annual inspections in order to determine how seaworthy the ship was. Their annual report "Registry of Ships" led them also to design the "load line" for ships. The "load line" is a line painted horizontally on the lower hull of the ship to mark where the maximum water line should be for safe loading. By reducing the ship's chance of early demise due to overloading, they were able to make her a "younger ship", and, of course, they also limited their liability.

F. Buckminster Fuller, the statistician–philosopher, was a great man who also understood the need for prevention. When he bought a new 17-ton sloop, he was carried away with man's progress over the years with sailing ships. The demands and hazards of sailing brought more scientific progress for man than anything we see today. His book *Intuition* has been very useful to me in interpreting the individual patient. Fuller advised us to be more adequately anticipatory regarding the probable re-occurrence of yesterday's experience with excess death. In this regard, I have found it useful to involve the individual patient in anticipating disease or injury instead of waiting for it to occur.

Before 1938, Raymond Pearle, of The Johns Hopkins University, admonished us to find the determinants of disease and to study them. From this understanding, he believed we would be able to extend the average life span. Therefore life span extension is a matter of anticipating future disease outcomes and intervening before they happen.

When I came out of Johns Hopkins in 1938, I began working as a local health officer primarily in the area of communicable disease. Things changed when I joined the Public Health Service. I had some "Uncle Dudleys" who had ideas of their own and they tried to involve me.

One of those "Uncles" was Dudley Jackson, a cancer surgeon who was frustrated by his field because he had so many failures. He felt that only the U.S. Government had the money to start a cancer research institute and do something about this problem. Subsequently, I became Chief of Cancer Control for the U.S. Public Health Service.

Another was Paul Dudley White, who believed that heart disease was a public health problem and raised the question of what was to be done about it. I entered his arena when I took over a heart demonstration project for the U.S. Public Health Service and helped to start the Framingham Study. Joe Mountin, one of my chiefs and the founder of what is now the Centers for Disease Control, had to justify the budget of the Public Health Service to Congress. They told him that "we have all this money for cancer because we have a cancer institute which Dudley Jackson started."

0-8493-0129-7/94/$0.00+$.50

They said, "Joe Mountin, we don't want you to come back here next year without a program for heart disease." So Joe developed a prospective study for heart disease and that led to my involvement in heart disease.

In 1965 I started a special study for the Public Health Service on health hazard appraisal. It seemed that the only real interest in health hazard appraisal was in primary care, so I worked in that area. I gradually developed some methods of demonstration, which is the only real method for bringing about change. I wasn't trying to estimate health age but I had to define the problem. I believed that the higher your health risk, the greater your health age in comparison to your chronological age.

Contributing to this effort was the work of Harvey Geller and his development of tables of average risks. He classified all deaths in the U.S. by age, sex, and race to determine the individual's risk of dying. Then he looked at deviations from average risks. From the Geller tables all that an individual can be told is the average risk for a person of his age, sex, and race. To help reduce the average risk we need to take it a step farther. This involves several things.

We must quantify and stratify individual precursors because the person who has smoked 2000 packs of cigarettes in a lifetime is different from one who smoked 12,000 packs of cigarettes. It has been said that after 10,000 packs of cigarettes the effects of smoking go up geometrically.

Then it is our responsibility to make a *prognosis* that lets us identify precursors and reduce them by *treating* them. Too often we wait until the individual shows signs of disease and injury. Our concern should be to target the individual and find ways to give him information to help reduce personal risks.

By estimating the probability of future disease or injury, the individual can know what his *priorities* are and thereby preclude what might otherwise be a *fait accompli* precipitated by external forces. By knowing the determinants of disease and injury, surveying them to know the degree to which the individual deviates, estimating individual total risk, individual health age, and health age of the comparable age group, we can then engage in risk reduction. By so doing we can hope to add years to life.

CHAPTER 5
LIFE INSURANCE AND BIOLOGIC AGING

W. John Elder

The life insurance industry is always seeking better ways to predict survival. Premiums are based on the predictability of mortality rates for populations; thus, the better the understanding of longevity, the more accurate the pricing of life insurance. Attention has been focused almost exclusively on chronological age as the knowledge of biological aging has been too imprecise to be used for insurance purposes. Even though the concept of biological aging intrigues actuaries and insurance physicians, not enough information has been reported to stimulate their own research as yet.

Life insurance is founded on empirical observations on survival rates in populations. This dates back to Roman, perhaps even to Babylonian times, through Halley's study of births and funerals in Breslau, on to the first official English life tables prepared by William Farr (1843) and the mathematical works of Gompertz in the mid-1800s. For well over a century it has been accepted that mortality increases geometrically after childhood.

Through the years there has been an attempt to separate healthy from unhealthy lives. From the life insurance point of view, the early objective was to insure healthy people at a standard premium and to decline the unhealthy. As mortality rates associated with disease became better understood, it became possible to offer insurance to less healthy people at a higher premium. One hypothesis is that if the effects of accident and disease can be removed, the residual curve may represent mortality caused by the natural aging process. In recent decades, the idea of risk factors predisposing people to disease has come into vogue. Risk factors include raised levels of serum lipids, elevated blood pressure, obesity, and smoking. By removing these from the populations studied, the resulting mortality curve may be nearer to natural aging. More recently, concepts of positive health and fitness, regular exercise, and periodic medical examinations have been used in a similar way to produce a rash of preferred life insurance products.

In the past few years there has been much actuarial attention to the mortality of older (over 65) age groups. Present evidence reveals a flattening of the mortality curve at ages over 85 with conflicting evidence of a possible crossing over of the male/female curves a few years above 100 years of age. Controversy, however, surrounds the actuarial methodologies used and the populations studied.

Actuaries have conducted studies on various population groups (including general, insured, and social security). In some, there is a definite bias toward the middle socioeconomic class. Although previous studies addressed chronological age, the increased understanding of the effects of disease, risk factors, and health may bring a time when the process of aging itself can be addressed. The aging patterns of many subgroups present some intriguing discoveries, such as the unusual findings among the very old, the difference between male and female longevity, the Amish (where men live longer than women), and the exceptional longevity of some, including English, clergymen.

Aging occasionally crops up as a topic at actuarial, underwriting, or insurance medical meetings. These discussions almost never get beyond chronological aging. In 1980 the Society of Actuaries organized a meeting called "The Future of Life Expectancy", which included a brief discussion of

0-8493-0129-7/94/$0.00+$.50

the theories of aging.[1] The notable exception on the insurance scene is the study by Richard Hochschild, "Biomarkers of Age", in insurance company employees[2] and his continuing attempt to persuade insurance companies to apply his results to an insurance product (see Chapter 8). This has been done in a very limited way by only two companies. Unfortunately, not enough policies have been placed to produce any worthwhile mortality studies, mostly because of pricing and marketing problems.

The explanation for the lack of insurance attention to the aging process itself is twofold. First, the effects on mortality of disease, risk factors, and lifestyles have only recently become more fully understood. Second, and probably more important, no definitions of biologic aging have enabled the industry to investigate the question.

Research into aging is of real intellectual and professional interest to actuaries and insurance medical directors, both at the individual and the organizational levels. How could the life insurance industry help in the investigation of biologic aging? Life insurance companies are devoting increasing attention to the older age market because of the increasing age of the population. Consequently, there is support for efforts aimed at improving the industry's understanding of all aspects of aging, including the aging process itself. Many examples of this support can be given. David R. Carpenter, CEO of Transamerica Life Companies, is national chairman of the Washington, DC-based Alliance for Aging Research. We have just completed a national survey on how the middle and older ages view their financial future and security.[3] We also give financial support to gerontology centers in Southern California.

On the negative side, it should be mentioned that life insurance companies find it difficult to be profitable these days. Many companies are very budget conscious and cost control is widely emphasized. Despite the size of some companies, resources are not limitless. A research project must have a reasonably sound chance of success in order to receive financial support. In addition, the following items should be considered when discussing possible insurance research programs:

1. It would be unwise to suggest a study that involves giving any substance or medication, however bland, to any individual.
2. The chances of success are poor if results depend on changing an individual's way of life, diet, etc.
3. It would be wise to think of "pure" research in the first instance and not something linked with a special product or a reduced premium.
4. There would be better prospects for support of a program aimed at older ages. Earlier results are one aspect, but more important is the present predisposition of the industry to support investigation aimed at understanding the older population.
5. The research must be simple, such as a question or two on a form, a single laboratory test, or an easily performed physical test.

One possible insurance research approach is a demographic study of existing or routinely obtained data. Any subgroup of the insured population could be investigated. Many of the obvious ones (chronological age, sex, geographic location, socioeconomic status, to name a few) are routinely evaluated now. Any of the items obtained at the time of insurance application could be analyzed. This information routinely includes a health history (usually with a family history), a medical examination (often limited to a paramedical), a urinalysis, and a blood test. Currently, an HIV test and a blood profile (glucose, urea nitrogen, creatinine, liver enzymes, lipids, etc.) are done on most applicants for insurance coverage of $100,000 or more.

This opens another possible avenue for gathering information. The addition of a question or two on the medical history, a simple physical test easily performed by a paramedical examiner, or even laboratory testing could be included. With the present sophistication of actuarial methodology in addressing mortality experience, it should be possible to begin to obtain useful information within 5 years of beginning a prospective study of this type, although the time will vary with the population group studied. For example, meaningful results can be obtained earlier if an older population group is under investigation because of the higher mortality rates.

Despite the prospect of having large population groups available for study, there are immense difficulties in setting up investigations of this type. These may include soliciting a company to participate and persuading it to cooperate, possible legislative and regulatory restrictions, consumer resistance, and funding. Separately, none of these problems are insurmountable, but to have a chance at success, a proposed investigation requires sound ideas, to be thought through in depth, and well presented.

Finally, a few words about the future, biologic aging, and insurance. If aging research discovers wide variation in the rates of aging among the general population, there will be problems for the insurance industry. If those who age more quickly and presumably have a shorter life span can modify this by attention to lifestyle, medication, or some other technique, the outcome will be good. The insurance approach will be thought of as little more than extending the present approach to known risk factors. However, if those who age more slowly (and presumably have a longer life span) can be identified and offered lower insurance premiums, there will be difficulties, as such differences in longevity would probably stem from differences in genetic coding. I pass on a slightly paraphrased quote made at a recent conference on genetics by Aubrey Milunsky, Director of the Center for Human Genetics at Boston University: "You know what the insurance industry will want to do with these genetic tests...give some of us a terrific break on our premiums, and screw the rest".[4] Horrifying as this sounds, I do not think society will allow insurance companies to get away with this approach. Legislation and regulation will force the industry to find another way.

REFERENCES

1. The Future of Life Expectancy, Symposium Proc., Society of Actuaries, Chicago, 1980.
2. Hochschild, R., Validating biomarkers of aging — mathematical approaches and results of a 2462-person study, in *Practical Handbook of Human Biologic Age Determination,* Balin, A.K., Ed., CRC Press, Boca Raton, FL, 1994, 93.
3. Pollock, J.C. and Heidt, P.E., Transamerica Life Companies Retirement Report, Transamerica Life Companies, Los Angeles, 1988.
4. Milunsky, A., Managing our Genetic Miracles, paper presented at conference, DePaul University College of Law, Chicago, 1988.

CHAPTER 6
AGING AND THE APPRAISAL OF HEALTH RISKS

Edwin B. Hutchins

TABLE OF CONTENTS

I. BACKGROUND

If the eventual goal of aging research is to develop interventions useful in delaying the rate of aging or improving the healthy functional life span of people, then the work on health risk appraisal is relevant to this goal.

The effort to make statements about the probability of dying from specific causes of death has a long history in a variety of disciplines. The effort to modify general estimates of mortality based on measurement of specific precursors is a relatively recent undertaking. Dr. Lewis C. Robbins, a proponent of prospective appraisal of health risks for over 4 decades, described some of this history. One landmark in this history was a health chart developed in 1966 by the outpatient department of the U.S. Public Health Service, which provided individual total present risks and presented a method of calculating survival advantage. Many of the health risks were assigned weights that derived from early work done in the Framingham and other prospective studies. This was followed in 1970 by the book *How To Practice Prospective Medicine*, authored by Robbins and Hall.[8] In 1979 the translation of the Robbins and Hall algorithms into computer code by Health and Welfare Canada facilitated the computational tasks involved in making individual estimates.[9] The subsequent adoption and updating of the method by the Centers for Disease Control began the widescale adoption of the health risk appraisal methodology in the U.S. *The Risk Factor Update Project* by Breslow et al.[2] dealt specifically with coronary heart disease and trauma. More recently, the Health Risk Appraisal Update Project, directed by Amler and Moriarty, a collaboration between the Centers for Disease Control and the Carter Center of Emory University, resulted in the 1988 release of an updated public domain health risk appraisal (HRA) instrument supported by a modularized C language computer program.[1]

0-8493-0129-7/94/$0.00+$.50

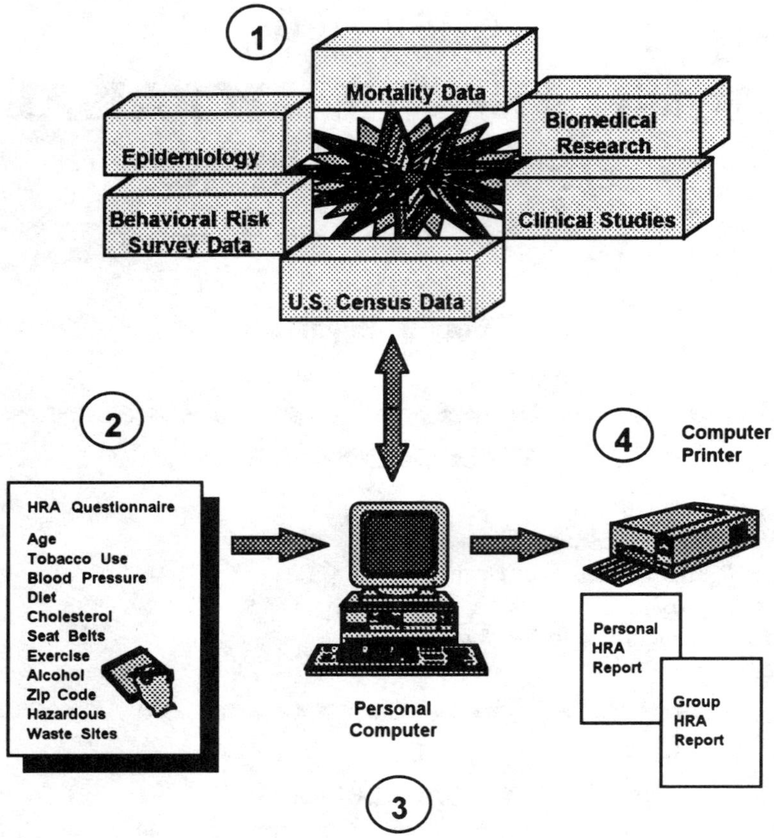

Figure 1 The four components defining a health risk appraisal (HRA).

II. THE HEALTH RISK APPRAISAL INSTRUMENT

A HRA is a multiphasic assessment that endeavors to estimate an individual's probability of dying, usually in the next 10 years. It is based upon factors known to be predictive of mortality outcomes for specific causes of death. A technical definition of a HRA includes four major components (Figure 1).

The first is a normative scientific database including mortality statistics by cause of death, epidemiological data, and biomedical, clinical, and behavioral studies focused on an understanding of the natural history of disease. The second component is an assessment of an individual's status on a number of precursors of mortality. This assessment can be accomplished in a variety of ways, but is most often done with a self-report questionnaire in tandem with some physiologic measures, most notably cholesterol and blood pressure. The third component is a set of quantitative algorithms that allow evaluation of the individual's status on the selected precursors according to the normative scientific database. The application of these algorithms results in the fourth component, the individual report, or personal HRA. A derivative of the data questionnaire obtained from the cohort being tested is a group or summary report which serves as a local behavioral risk factor surveillance report.

The form the individual report takes may vary depending on what information one intends to communicate to the client, but the basic information on which the report messages are based is generally in the form of estimates of the probability of dying from a specific cause of death sometime in the next 10 years. Typically these probabilities are rank ordered and customarily only the most

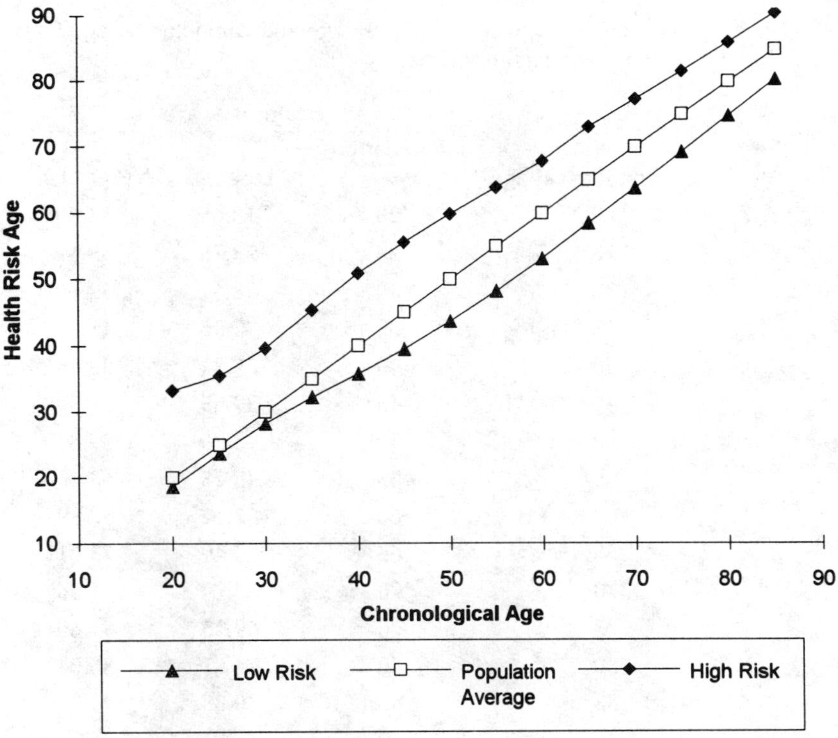

Figure 2 The relationship between health risk age and chronological age for low risk and high risk cohorts.

probable causes of death for that participant are presented. In addition, a total probability of dying from all causes of death is also computed. This metric is often transformed into a score called "health risk age", which presents the total 10-year risk of dying in terms comparable to chronological age. Thus, a 45-year-old American male who has a number of elevated risk factors may have his health risk age computed at 56 years. This means that his probability of dying in the next 10 years is essentially the same as that of an average 56-year-old American male. Conversely, if the individual has lower than average risk factors, his health risk age may be less than his chronological age.

Figure 2 illustrates the concept of health risk age and its relationship to chronological age. When the population average risk is converted to a health risk age, this is exactly equivalent to chronological age because population average risk derives from national mortality data presented by chronological age. When these probability estimates are adjusted according to elevated or reduced risk factors, health risk age will increase or decrease compared to chronological age. In Figure 2, for the average American male the relationship between these two measures is represented by the straight diagonal line. The higher curve represents a cohort of individuals who carry a variety of risk factors: overweight, elevated blood pressure, high cholesterol, smoker, and risky driving habits (no seatbelt use, over the speed limit, and driving under the influence). Risk ages for a cohort with no known risk factors are below chronological age and are represented by the lower curve. Data for Figure 2 are presented in Table 1. Data for the population average curve fall between the high and low risk age curves because of the known prevalence of risk factors among the general population, e.g., one out of four Americans are smokers. Table 2 presents the values of the risk factors used in the estimation of health risk age along with the attributable risk years lost at ages 20, 40, and 60 for the high-risk male group.

Table 1 Relationship between health risk age and chronological age for low risk and high risk cohorts

	Health risk age		
Chronological age	**Population av.**	**Low risk**	**High risk**
20	20	18.65	33.30
25	25	23.73	35.49
30	30	28.31	39.60
35	35	32.26	45.34
40	40	35.84	50.85
45	45	39.55	55.59
50	50	43.70	59.82
55	55	48.23	63.85
60	60	53.12	67.89
65	65	58.49	73.01
70	70	63.79	77.26
75	75	69.25	81.60
80	80	74.81	86.04
85	85	80.38	90.57

Table 2 Risk factor values and attributable risk years lost for high risk males at ages 20, 40, and 60[a]

		Risk years gained[b]		
Risk factor	**Value**	**Age 20**	**Age 40**	**Age 60**
Smoking	1 pack/d	0.21	2.86	4.13
Blood pressure	150/110	0.13	1.80	1.72
Total cholesterol	300	0.30	3.39	2.35
HDL[c]	35	0.07	0.98	0.84
Weight	235 lb (47% overweight)	0.03	0.37	0.32
Alcohol, drunk driving	12 Beers/week Drink and drive 4 times/week	5.52	1.21	0.33
Driving speed	11-15 MPH over speed limit	4.27	0.78	0.15
Seat belt usage	0% Usage	4.02	0.74	0.14
Total risk years gained		14.55	12.13	9.97
Total 10-year probability of dying		0.05	0.09	0.40

[a] *All computations were performed using algorithms presented in Reference 1.*
[b] *Number of risk years to be gained if risk factor is reduced to optimum level.*
[c] *HDL = high density lipoprotein.*

The appraisal of health risks begins with population mortality data and focuses on the amelioration of the causal factors associated with premature death. Variance attributable to an underlying rate of aging is included because age-specific death rates are employed, although this variance is not explicitly accounted for.

III. HEALTH RISKS AND CAUSES OF DEATH

Currently a number of HRA instruments are available through private companies. Because these are considered generally proprietary, the algorithms underlying the risk computations are often not documented. These instruments are periodically catalogued by the federal Office of Disease Prevention and Health Promotion[6] and by the Society of Prospective Medicine.[7]

The current public domain HRA identifies 42 cause of death groupings from the International Classification of Diseases (ICD) Ninth Revision plus a 43rd category that grouped all other causes of death.[5] The list of 42 causes of death is based on criteria of importance, including modifiability and incidence, e.g., each of the 42 causes of death accounted for at least 3000 deaths annually. The 42 groupings account for three fourths of all deaths in the U.S. as reported in the 1986 to 1988 mortality tables. Most heavily represented are circulatory diseases, cancer, and trauma. Of the 42 ICD groupings, quantifiable precursors can be identified for 19 causes of death. Table 3 illustrates the intersections among 42 cause of death outcomes and the 29 precursor questions covering 23 risk factors. A dot entered in a cell of the matrix indicates that there is a known quantifiable relationship between precursor and outcome. Sex and age are included in all cause of death groupings because the mortality tables are sex and age specific. Some of these precursors are implicated in more than one cause of death category. For example, smoking is entered in the algorithms for 13 of the 19 causes of death which could be appraised quantitatively.

The various precursors fall into three classes: modifiable, semimodifiable, and nonmodifiable. Modifiable or malleable precursors are of primary interest because they allow prospective interventions aimed at reducing those years of life lost unnecessarily. Nonmodifiable or fixed precursors are of interest because they interact synergistically with the modifiable precursors to alter the risk estimates, thereby raising or lowering the payoff function. Nonmodifiable precursors may take the form of personal history factors such as hysterectomy, as it weights the estimate for uterine cancer, or these fixed factors may be genetic in origin, whether directly measured or indirectly assessed through family history. Thus, mother-sister history of breast cancer may serve as a surrogate measure of genetic propensity for breast cancer. Recollection of first drinking experience may stand in as a genetic indicator of abnormal metabolism of alcohol. Genetic and other biomarkers along with dosimetry for measures of environmental exposure ultimately may be employed as part of the data set obtained to assess health risks. At present, these represent promising technologic additions to be employed in future developments of the HRA. In the meantime proxy measures serve the useful function of allowing incorporation of genetic information.

IV. ESTIMATING RISKS

Having chosen the cause of death groupings and identified the related precursors, the next requirement is specification of the algorithm for each cause of death to allow an individualized estimate of the 10-year risk of dying based on that person's profile on the relevant precursors. The nature of these algorithms varies according to the methodologic sophistication of the studies in the literature or the databases supporting the precursor outcome relationships.

Table 3 Precursors Healthier People Network uses to predict causes of death

Precursors	1 Sex	2 Age	3 Height	4 Weight	5 Frame size	6 Diabetes	8 Systolic blood pressure	9 BP high or normal	10 Serum total cholesterol	11 Serum HDL cholesterol	12 Cigars per day	13 Pipes per day	14 Smokeless tobacco use	15 Smoking habit	16 Current cigarettes per day	17a Years since quit cigs	17b Cigs a day before quit	18a Car miles travel per year	18b Motorcycle miles per year	19 Travel mode/car size	20 Safety belt use	21 MPH over speed limit	22 Drive/ride after drink	23 Drinks per week	24 Menarche	25 Age at first birth	26 Mammogram (if over 50)	27 Breast cancer family history	28 Hysterectomy	29 Pap smear
1 HIV/AIDS	•	•																												
2 Mouth cancer	•	•									•	•	•	•	•	•								•						
3 Throat cancer	•	•									•	•	•	•	•	•								•						
4 Esophageal cancer	•	•												•	•	•														
5 Stomach cancer	•	•																												
6 Colon cancer	•	•																												
7 Rectal cancer	•	•																												
8 Pancreatic cancer	•	•												•	•															
9 Laryngeal cancer	•	•												•	•	•								•						
10 Lung cancer	•	•												•	•	•	•													
11 Skin cancer/ melanoma	•	•																												
12 Breast cancer	•	•																							•	•	•	•		
13 Cervical cancer	•	•												•	•														•	•
14 Uterine cancer	•	•																											•	
15 Ovarian cancer	•	•																												
16 Prostatic cancer	•	•																												
17 Bladder cancer	•	•												•	•	•														
18 Brain cancer	•	•																												
19 Lymphoma	•	•																												
20 Leukemia	•	•																												
21 Diabetes mellitus	•	•				•																								
22 Alcohol toxicity	•	•																												
23 Rheumatic heart disease	•	•																												
24 Hypertensive heart disease	•	•																												
25 Heart attack	•	•	•	•	•	•	•	•	•	•				•	•															
26 Stroke	•	•				•	•	•						•	•															
27 Arterial vascular disease	•	•																												
28 Influenza/ pneumonia	•	•												•	•															
29 Emphysema/ chronic bronchitis	•	•												•	•															

Table 3 Precursors Healthier People Network uses to predict causes of death (continued)

	Precursors	1 Sex	2 Age	3 Height	4 Weight	5 Frame size	6 Diabetes	8 Systolic blood pressure	9 BP high or normal	10 Serum total cholesterol	11 Serum HDL cholesterol	12 Cigars per day	13 Pipes per day	14 Smokeless tobacco use	15 Smoking habit	16 Current cigarettes per day	17a Years since quit cigs	17b Cigs a day before quit	18a Car miles travel per year	18b Motorcycle miles per year	19 Travel mode/car size	20 Safety belt use	21 MPH over speed limit	22 Drive/ride after drink	23 Drinks per week	24 Menarche	25 Age at first birth	26 Mammogram (if over 50)	27 Breast cancer family history	28 Hysterectomy	29 Pap smear
30	Pneumoconioses	•	•																												
31	Peptic ulcer	•	•									•	•		•																
32	Liver cirrhosis	•	•																						•						
33	Kidney failure	•	•				•																								
34	Motor vehicle injury	•	•																•	•	•	•	•	•							
35	Pedestrian injury	•	•																												
36	Poisoning	•	•																												
37	Falling	•	•																												
38	Fire injury	•	•																												
39	Drowning	•	•																												
40	Suicide	•	•																												
41	Homicide/assault	•	•																												
42	All other unintentional injury	•	•																												

Five methods of risk estimation are employed by the current public domain HRA:[1]

1. Through collaboration with the Framingham Heart Study, logistic regression equations were developed for estimating the 10-year probabilities of dying from either a heart attack or stroke.[3] This method was also used to estimate the risk of an incident case in the initial step of computation for breast cancer.[4] Seven precursors were weighted in the equation for heart attack, five for stroke, and six for breast cancer. These three causes of dealth — heart attack, stroke, and breast cancer — account for two out of every five U.S. deaths.
2. Composite relative risk times baseline estimates is the second method of computation used to estimate an individual's risk of death from nine cancer sites and six other cause of death groupings. These 15 causes of death account for nearly one in five of all U.S. deaths annually.
3. The third method uses a composite risk multiplier multiplied by the age- and sex-specific population death rate to estimate risk of dying from a motor vehicle accident. Motor vehicle accidents account for 1 in 50 deaths but are the first cause of death for people under age 40.
4. These three principal methods are supplemented by branching logic chains for breast cancer, cervical cancer, and diabetes mellitus.
5. Finally age- and sex-specific population death rates are used to estimate risk of dying for the remaining 23 cause of death groupings. These 23 causes of death had no quantifiable and modifiable precursors identified.

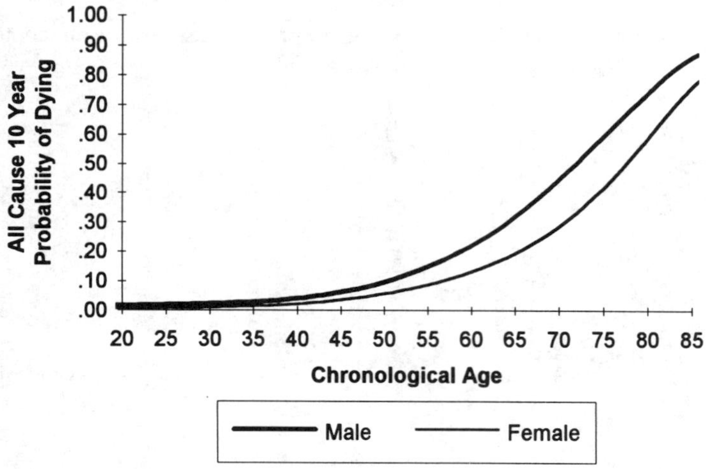

Figure 3 All cause 10-year probability of dying by gender.

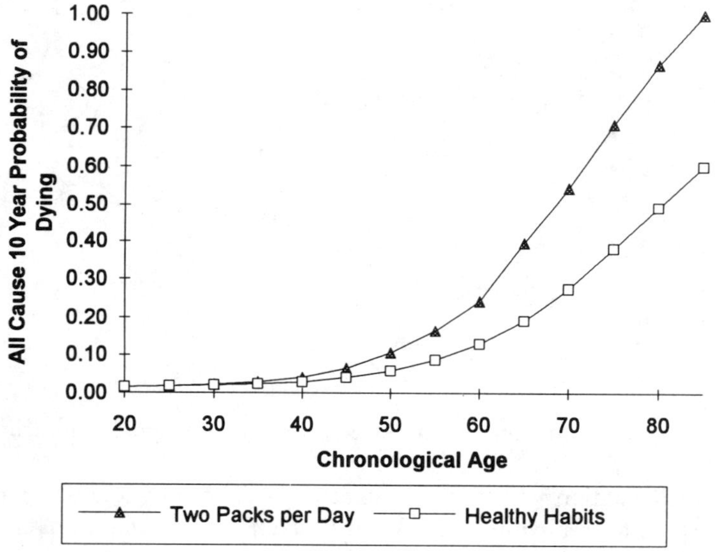

Figure 4 Ten-year probability of dying for male smokers vs. males with healthy habits.

Once the algorithms have been computed, the contribution to total 10-year risk of dying can be summarized by both cause of death, for which the various prediction algorithms were developed, and by specific precursor. Examples were computed for the contribution to elevated health risk age made by smoking two packs of cigarettes per day. Computations were made of the overall attributable risk derived from the 13 algorithms implicating smoking as a risk factor. In these examples all other risk factors were entered at ideal levels so that the comparisons presented reflect only the contribution of smoking. As a basis for comparison the all cause probability of dying is first presented for males and females in Figure 3. As is generally known, the female probabilitites are lower throughout the life span. Figure 4 compares the total 10-year probability of dying for males who smoke two packs a day but have no other health risks with males who have no known health risk at all. Similar data are presented in Figure 5 for females. The actual data supporting Figures 4 and 5 are presented in Table 4.

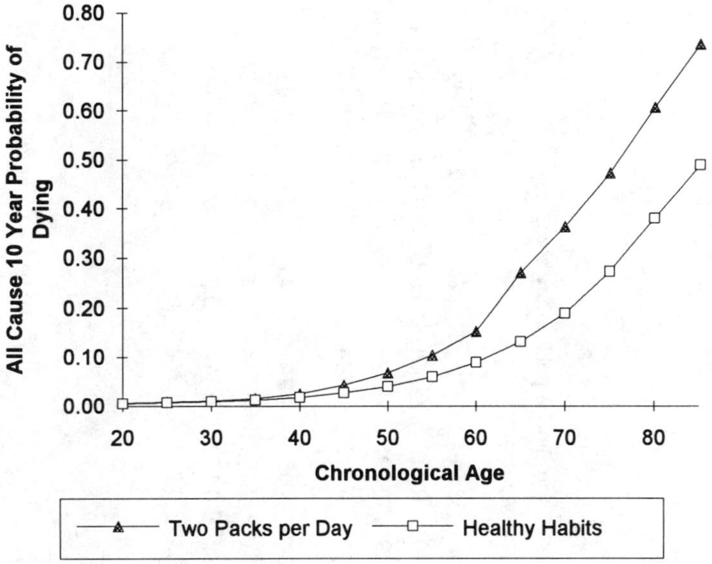

Figure 5 Ten-year probability of dying for female smokers vs. females with healthy habits.

Two other observations regarding methodology are worthy of note. Perusal of the scientific literature in search of quantifiable precursors of morbidity or mortality lays bare the unevenness of scientific rigor and methodological sophistication and the lack of comparability across studies. Because HRA has been a derived method dependent on the synthesis of other scientific endeavors, its ultimate validity is also dependent on the quality of the science supporting it. Where conservative science prevails, the burden falls on the cross-validation of findings across multiple studies. The first correlational study implicating cigarette smoking in lung cancer appeared in 1954. The number of scientific studies supporting the finding that smoking is a causal factor is now estimated to be in the tens of thousands. By contrast, the literature supporting a quantifiable relationship between dietary fiber and colorectal cancer is still rudimentary, as is the science relating normal nutrition to specific mortality outcomes. By comparison to the total product of the biomedical sciences, the literature relevant to an understanding of the natural history of disease and of the malleable precursors of premature death is sparse. Nevertheless, the work devoted to appraising health risks has progressed rapidly over the last 2 decades.

Using actuarial methods in 1970, the Robbins and Hall appraisal included a limited number of mortality outcomes with known modifiable precursors. By 1984, the Centers for Disease Control had expanded the matrix to include additional causes of death. The present public domain instrument addresses 19 causes of death with known modifiable precursors. These 19 outcomes account for 59% of all deaths. Thus progress has been made in filling in the precursor by cause of death matrix with valid predictive algorithms. Given the complexity of the human organism and the range of insults to which it is subjected, it is likely that for some time the largest component of the total variance in mortality outcomes will remain the residual or unexplained variance term. What proportion of this is attributable to heredity or to "biological aging" may ultimately be answered through the research on aging described in other papers presented in this volume. Resolution of this issue may remain elusive, with the upper limits of age constantly moving beyond attempts to define it as more is learned about the malleable precursors of mortality and how to reduce them. As these phenomena are better understood and health promotion interventions serve to stretch the life span beyond today's accepted norm, studies of the process of aging may assume other forms and directions of inquiry.

Table 4 All causes 10-year probability of dying by age and sex for population average, healthy habits cohort, and 2 pack a day smokers

	Age													
Group males	**20**	**25**	**30**	**35**	**40**	**45**	**50**	**55**	**60**	**65**	**70**	**75**	**80**	**85**
Population average	0.017	0.019	0.023	0.029	0.040	0.062	0.096	0.148	0.220	0.317	0.444	0.591	0.735	0.857
Healthy habits	0.016	0.018	0.021	0.024	0.029	0.041	0.059	0.088	0.129	0.192	0.275	0.380	0.493	0.600
2 Packs a day	0.016	0.018	0.023	0.029	0.041	0.066	0.106	0.165	0.244	0.395	0.544	0.710	0.868	0.999
Group females	**20**	**25**	**30**	**35**	**40**	**45**	**50**	**55**	**60**	**65**	**70**	**75**	**80**	**85**
Population average	0.006	0.007	0.010	0.012	0.022	0.036	0.056	0.087	0.131	0.194	0.284	0.416	0.585	0.758
Healthy habits	0.005	0.007	0.009	0.012	0.018	0.027	0.040	0.060	0.089	0.132	0.190	0.274	0.380	0.489
2 Packs a day	0.006	0.008	0.010	0.016	0.025	0.043	0.068	0.104	0.153	0.272	0.363	0.473	0.606	0.737

V. MORBIDITY OUTCOMES AND AGING

The escalation of morbidity with the advance of age is a phenomenon that has also received increased attention in the health sciences. The social implications that attend this increase include not only decline in functional autonomy and quality of life for the older person but increased demand on the supporting caregivers, on social support systems, and, as health care costs also escalate, a heightened economic burden on the total society. Per capita personal health expenditures for hospital care nearly double from age 65 to 85 while expenditures for nursing home care quadruple.

Much of the work on the midlife HRA has heretofore been mortality based. When we focus on the older age groups, it is clear that the conceptual model must be expanded to include not only mortality-based estimates, but also morbidity-based models, functional status assessments, and ultimately, quality of life issues. While 65-year-olds have an average of 16.4 years of life remaining, they have only 12 years of healthy life remaing, a factor reflecting on the definition of quality of life. Still another indicator of quality of life is an individual's ability to perform activities of daily living, such as bathing, dressing, and eating. Loss of ability to perform these tasks leads to the need for assistance and a subsequent decrement in independent living. Although people 85 and above constitute the substantial share of all those who are not independent in physical functioning, many of the health problems of this group are preventable. While the major causes of death for the over-65 age group are similar to those for the midlife group, (i.e., heart disease, cancer, stroke, chronic obstructive pulmonary disease, pneumonia, and influenza), chronic problems such as arthritis, osteoporosis, incontinence, visual and hearing impairments, and dementia are of concern because of their impact on day-to-day living. The challenge is to prevent the ill from becoming disabled, to help people with disabilities preserve or increase what functional capacity they have, and to prevent further disability. In the statement of national goals for the year 2000, Healthy People 2000 focuses on physical activity, preventive health services, and social networks for the older age groups.[10]

Of necessity, short-term and intermediate approaches to health care for the elderly will seek ways to serve the immediate needs of an elderly population growing numerically and proportionately larger with each succeeding decade. Yet the data are clear. Geometric growth functions in the utilization of resources cannot continue indefinitely. It is imperative that interventions be developed in the near term that can successfully forestall the onset of morbidity and the loss of functional autonomy.

To accomplish this requires that several things must happen. First, it is critical that the causal pathways to the onset of illness and diminished functional status be identified. As an ever-more sophisticated understanding of the pathophysiology of geriatric diseases develops, the second requirement involves the ability to predict, *a priori,* who is at risk for negative health outcomes and what that individual's modifiable factors are that can be reduced or eliminated. Finally, the interventions and supports necessary to assure reduction of these causal factors need to be made accessible to all who need them.

Recent efforts to develop a HRA for the elderly have identified 30 outcome measures having some supporting evidence that they would be amenable to the development of predictive models. These 30 outcomes are categorized into seven clusters (Table 5).

As prediction models are derived from existing literature or through reanalysis of existing databases, precursors are identified and collected in a questionnaire. The present research version of the questionnaire has 185 items. Reduction in the length of the questionnaire will be required to make it amenable for practical use in health care settings.

A library of report messages that can be stored in a computer program to be triggered by the risk algorithms was created through technical advisory committee participation, from the National Institute on Aging AGE PAGE materials and other health education materials. These messages emphasize malleable risk factors and the interventions that can be employed to reduce them.

Table 5 Selected outcome measures for development of a HRA for elderly populations

Clusters	Mortality/morbidity/ functional status outcomes	Clusters	Mortality/morbidity/ functional status outcomes
I	Cardiovascular diseases	IV	Injuries
II	Cancers		Falls
	Breast		Adverse drug events
	Lung		Motor vehicle injuries
	Bladder		Burns and fire-related injuries
	Cervical	V	Sensory impairments
	Esophageal		Hearing impairments
	Laryngeal		Vision impairments
	Mouth and throat		Senile cataracts
	Pancreatic		Senile macular degeneration
	Uterine		Primary open-angle glaucoma
	Colon		Diabetic retinopathy
	Rectal	VI	Functioning
	Skin/melanoma		Physical disability
	Prostatic		Urinary incontinence
	Other, without malleable risks		Nutrition
	Leukemia		Institutionalization
	Lymphoma	VII	Social and mental health
	Brain		Depression
	Liver		Cognitive impairments/advance directives
	Ovarian		Social networks
	Stomach		
III	Vaccine preventable diseases		
	Influenza and pneumonia		
	Tetanus		

As our understanding of the aging process progresses, a concern for life span extension should incorporate equal concern for the factors that preclude or facilitate enjoyment of these extended years. A compelling concern for underlying values requires that the added years are years of quality living as research on aging continues to contribute to increased life expectancy.

REFERENCES

1. Amler, R.W., Moriarty, D.G., and Hutchins, E.B., *Healthier People*, Carter Center of Emory University, Health Risk Appraisal Program, Decatur, GA, 1988.
2. Breslow, L., Fielding, J., and Affifi, A.A., *Risk Factor Update Project: Final Report*, U.S. Department of Health and Human Services, Centers for Disease Control, Center for Health Promotion and Education, Atlanta, 1985.
3. Hutchins, E.B., Amler, R.W., Evans, R.C., Jacobs, T.A., Sceigaj, M., and Sligh, D., *Healthier People Health Risk Appraisal Version 4.0*, Carter Center of Emory University, Health Risk Appraisal Program, Atlanta, 1991, 6:44.
4. Hutchins, E.B., Amler, R.W., Evans, R.C., Jacobs, T.A., Sceigaj, M., and Sligh, D., *Healthier People Health Risk Appraisal Version 4.0*, Carter Center of Emory University, Health Risk Appraisal Program, Atlanta, 1991, 6:77.
5. *International Classification of Diseases*, 9th rev., *Clinical Modification (ICD-9-CM)*, U.S. Department of Health and Human Services, Public Health Service, 1980.
6. Office of Disease Prevention and Health Promotion, *Healthfinder on Health Risk Appraisals*, Department of Health and Human Services, Washington, D.C., 1988.
7. Peterson, K.W. and Hilles, S.B., Eds., *The SPM Directory of Health Risk Appraisals*, The Society of Prospective Medicine, Indianapolis, IN, 1992.
8. Robbins, L.D. and Hall, J.H., *How to Practice Prospective Medicine*, Slaymaker Enterprises, Indianapolis, IN, 1970.
9. Task Force on the Periodic Health Examination, Periodic Health Examination Monograph, Canadian Government Publishing Centre, Montreal, 1980.
10. U.S. Department of Health and Human Services, Public Health Service, *Healthy People 2000*, Washington, D.C., 1990.

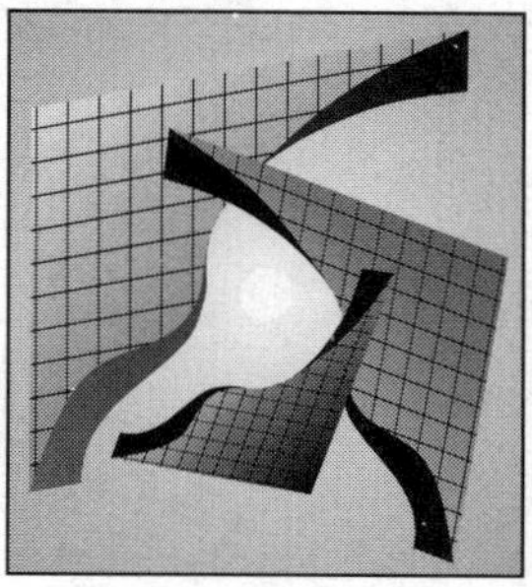

PHYSIOLOGIC ASSESSMENT

CHAPTER 7

VARIATIONS IN AGING PARAMETERS, THEIR SOURCES, AND POSSIBILITIES OF PREDICTING PHYSIOLOGICAL AGE

Eino Heikkinen, Harri Suominen, Pertti Era, and Anna-Liisa Lyyra

TABLE OF CONTENTS

I. INTRODUCTION

Over the past 20 years interest has been growing in research dealing with the assessment of physiological age. In the earlier studies the parameters selected for the assessments were chosen on the basis of their correlation with chronological age. It was assumed that an index of biological (or physiological) age can be constructed by combining the results of different tests into a single figure, which could be interpreted as a yardstick of biological age.[3,4,20-23] Studies applying basically similar designs were subsequently performed in a number of different populations.[5,13,14,16,34,50] These studies have produced information about the levels of various functions in different age groups, but due to the cross-sectional design of the studies it was not possible to elucidate the predictive role of the assessments with respect to life expectancy or nearness of death. Furthermore, it was observed that the suggested decrement model of functions was not true for all the parameters included in the studies, as relations to chronological age were not always linear and very little was known about the relative importance of various aging parameters in relation to their ability to predict life expectancy. Therefore, more information about the parameters of aging and about the sources of their variation is required.

II. JYVÄSKYLÄ STUDIES ON FUNCTIONAL AGING

In 1971 the authors initiated a series of studies with the aim of describing levels of functional capacity and certain biological properties in population samples drawn from different age groups.

0-8493-0129-7/94/$0.00+$.50

Developmental work on methods was also included in these research projects; new methods were developed and many tests were modified on the basis of the experience gained. The first study was done among population samples of 460 men aged 25 to 27, 35 to 37, 45 to 47, and 55 to 57 years living in southwest Finland and in North Carelia, Finland.[14] Of the 460 men, 86% participated in the laboratory examinations, which included tests on vital capacity, vibratory threshold, hearing, reaction time, cognitive capacity, and thickness of cortical bone.

Despite large differences in life expectancy between men in the two areas (higher mortality in North Carelia[28]) the single parameters or the indices of biological aging investigated did not show significant differences between the two areas. On the other hand, when analyses on biological aging were undertaken in different occupational groups, it was observed that men with lighter occupations had better test results as compared to the results for industrial and mine workers.[15]

In 1972 we commenced a number of longitudinal surveys on the health, functional abilities, and lifestyles of 66-year-old residents of Jyväskylä. Participating in the interviews were 392 people (137 men and 255 women), 92% of this 1-year birth cohort. Of this number, 73 men and 64 women took part in 1973 in laboratory investigations in which health status and various indices of physiological aging (the above-mentioned parameters plus an indirect assessment of $VO_{2\ max}$) were examined.[2] In 1977 44 men and 48 women participated in the follow-up study on health and physiological aging. The results of these studies showed that physically active men had better index values of physiological aging than sedentary men.[42]

The next populations studied were men aged 40 to 50 years working in two industrial enterprises. All together 390 men (87% of all the male workers) participated in the study. Of these, 156 worked in a mechanical wood processing factory in Jyväskylä, and 234 in a shipbuilding yard in Turku (southwest Finland). The main observation was that physically active men showed better values in several indicators of physiological aging as compared to their more sedentary counterparts. Better results were also observed for managerial employees as compared to the results of the other occupational groups.[26]

In a later study dealing with the functional capacity of male and female employees in the metal industry, a total of 341 subjects were studied.[27] Here again, managerial workers showed better performance than the manual workers, particularly in the tests of psychomotor and cognitive functions. This was observed among both men and women.

Because the level of physical exercise appeared to be among the factors causing variation in the parameters of physiological aging, the next study was performed among middle-aged endurance athletes with a history of "lifelong" endurance training, and their results were compared with sedentary men of the same age.[41] The endurance athletes showed better values in several tests of physiological aging, and also in the indices which comprised the results of six tests (systolic blood pressure, digit symbol test, vibratory threshold, hearing threshold at 4000 Hz, vital capacity, and $VO_{2\ max}$. A major part of the difference in the indices, however, could be explained on the basis of functional tests which are directly influenced by physical exercise (particularly $VO_{2\ max}$).

III. FUNCTIONAL CAPACITY AMONG MEN OF DIFFERENT AGES

On the basis of the above-mentioned studies a major population study among men at different ages was implemented in 1981 and 1982. The results and experiences of our previous studies had clearly shown a need for a more comprehensive assessment of aging and better knowledge of variation in the parameters of aging and on the possible sources of this variation.

A structural model of functional capacity was adopted for the conceptual framework; i.e., physical, psychic, and social functions were categorized on a scale from simple to complex (Figure 1). In the theoretical working models it was assumed (Figure 2) that functional capacity is affected by the processes of aging, which in turn vary with differences in health status, lifestyle, and socioeconomic conditions.

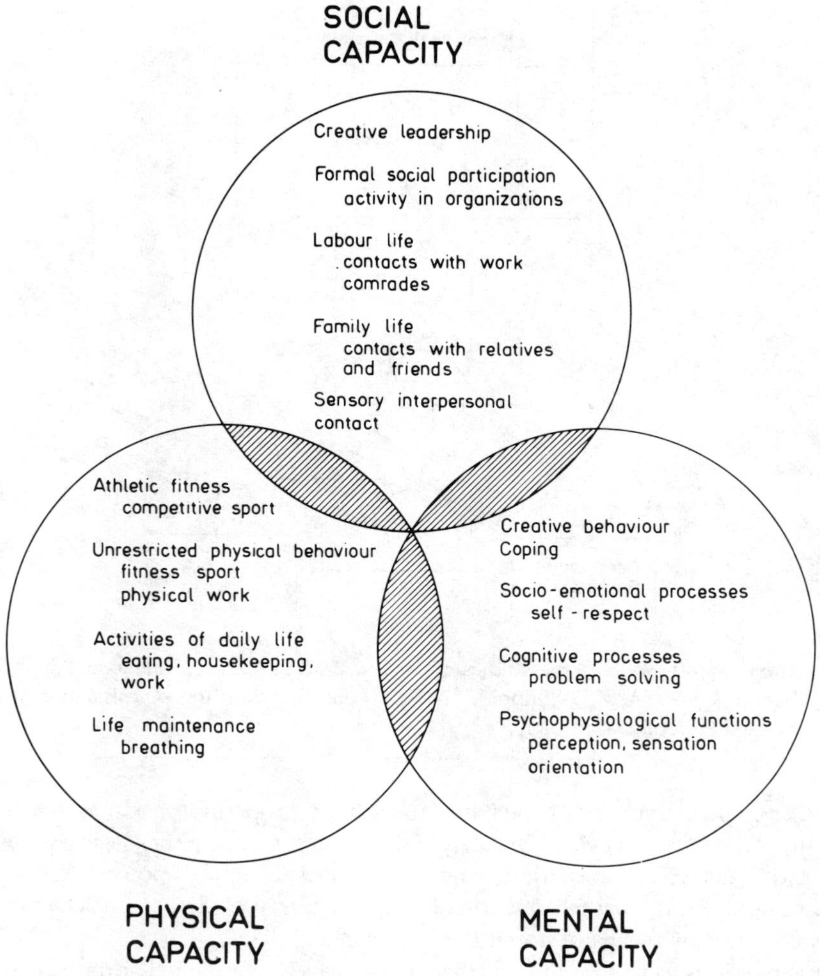

Figure 1 Schematic diagram of the sublevels of an individual's physical, mental, and social capacity and their interactions.[17]

The study material consisted of samples of men aged 31 to 35, 51 to 55, and 71 to 75 years. The samples were drawn from the local population register. All together 388 men, 71%, participated in the laboratory examinations. No major differences were observed between the participants and non-participants in certain basic sociodemographic parameters (age, civilian status, level of education, status of health), although in the oldest age group the nonrespondents tended to have somewhat poorer health status compared to that of those who took part in the study.

Functional capacity was assessed under normal laboratory conditions. A detailed description of the study process, the methods used, and reports on several aging parameters have been published elsewhere.[6-9,17,39,51] Therefore, only the main methodological features of the study are given here.

The men were invited to the laboratory examinations by a letter in which instructions were given on living habits concerning the 24-h period preceding the examinations. The length of the laboratory examinations was about 4 h. The sequence of the tests was as follows: cognitive performance (vocabulary, arithmetic, digit span, block design), sensory performance (pure tone thresholds, speech understanding, dark adaptation, lens accommodation and adaptation, vibratory threshold, postural control), psychomotor and motor capacity (reaction and movement time, tapping rate, leg extension velocity), anthropometric properties (body height, total body weight,

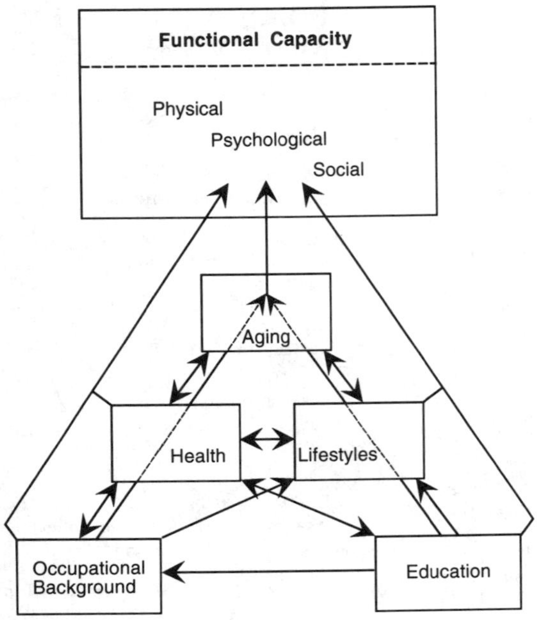

Figure 2 The working model of the studies of the Jyväskylä Studies on Functional Aging. (From Era, P., Scand. J. Soc. Med., 39(Suppl.), 1, 1987. Published with the permission of the Almqvist & Wiksell Periodical Company.)

skeletal widths, skinfold thickness at four sites, mechanical properties of skin *in vivo*, bone mineral density), status of the musculoskeletal system (physiotherapist's assessment), health status (physician's assessment, blood analyses), isometric strength of muscles, anaerobic power, aerobic power, and anaerobic threshold. Additional information on health status, lifestyles, social activities, and mental balance was collected by means of postal questionnaire.

The same methods were applied in further studies which were aimed at describing the levels of physiological aging among two groups of male athletes, 46 to 60 years of age[42] and 70 to 81 years of age,[12,39,45] in relation to the functional capacity of population samples of men of corresponding ages.

Analysis of variance and Student *t*-tests were used for the comparisons of the means in various subject subgroups. In addition to conventional cross-tabulations, the frequency data were also analyzed using log-linear and logit models. In addition to traditional multivariate methods (discriminant analysis, regression analysis), various methods combining the different areas of the study were constructed within the framework of linear structural relationships (LISREL)-models.[25]

In this chapter we first present data on intra- and interindividual variation in certain physical fitness parameters and in sensory, psychomotor, and motor functions before dealing with possible sources of the observed variation.

A. VARIATION IN THE PARAMETERS OF AGING

The existence of a large variation in functional capacity both within a single individual and between individuals belonging to the same age group has been widely documented in the gerontological literature.[38,47,48,52] In our study a few persons in the age group 31 to 35 years achieved results which were typical of men aged 71 to 75 years and vice versa. The frequency distributions of selected parameters will serve to concretize the variations between and within the age groups (Figures 3 to 12).[19]

The overlapping of the test results between the age groups is indeed marked, but differences also occurred between the parameters in this respect. This can be seen in Figure 13, in which the

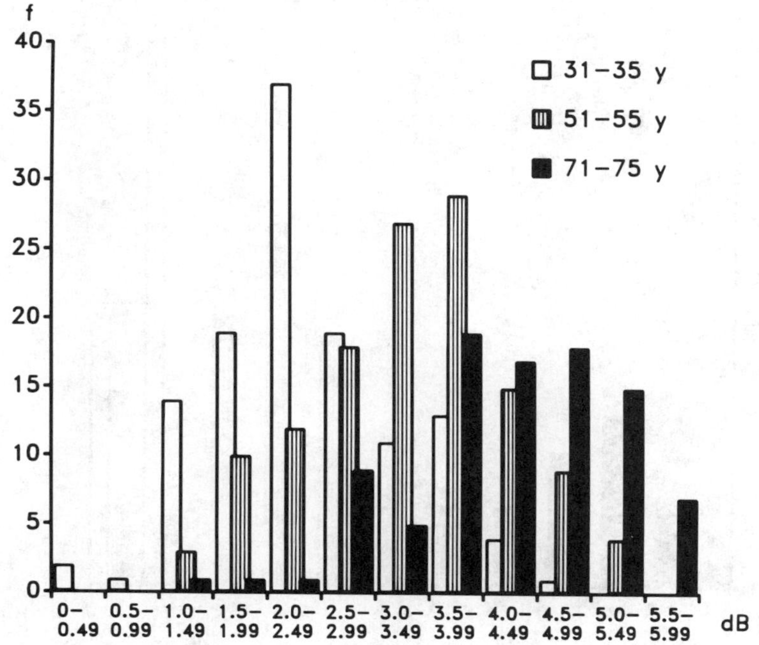

Figure 3 Frequency distributions of the results of vibrotactile threshold at 100 Hz in different age groups. (From Heikkinen, E. et al., in *Aging, Health and Competence,* Schroots, H.J.F., Ed., Elsevier, Amsterdam, 1993, 65. Published with the permission of Elsevier Science Publishers.)

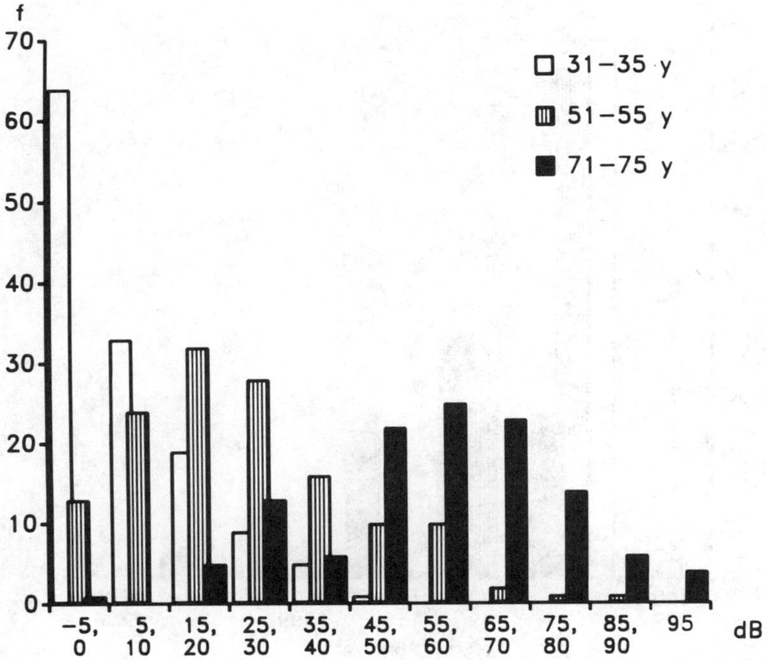

Figure 4 Frequency distributions of the results on air-conducted pure tone thresholds at 4000 Hz in different age groups.

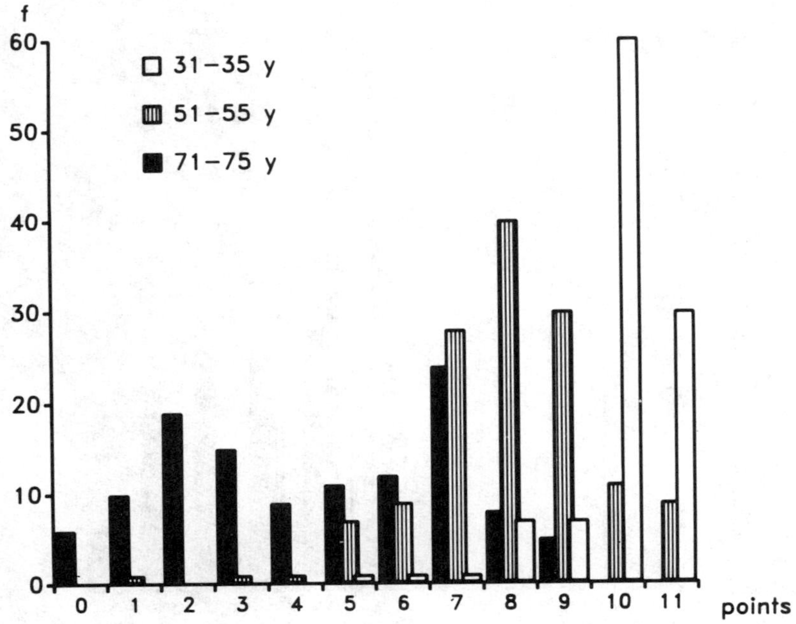

Figure 5 Frequency distributions of the results on the speech understanding test in different age groups.

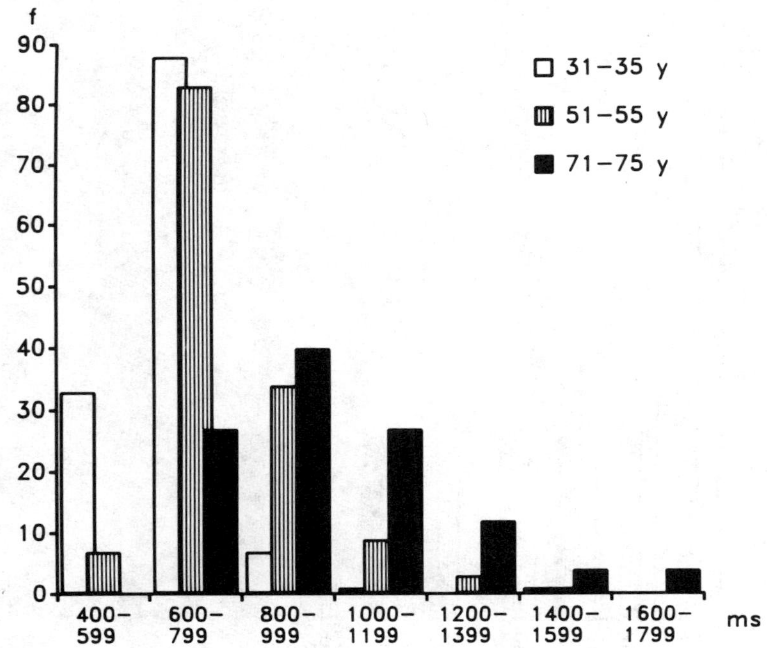

Figure 6 Frequency distributions of the results on choice reaction and movement times (visual stimuli) in different age groups.

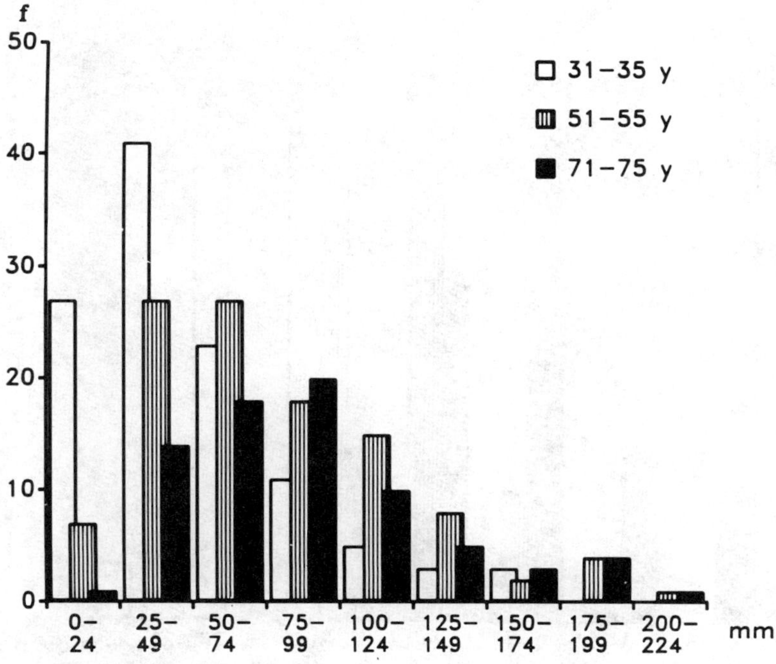

Figure 7 Frequency distributions of the extent of postural sway over 8 s while normal standing and eyes open in different age groups. (From Heikkinen, E. et al., in *Aging, Health and Competence,* Schroots, H.J.F., Ed., Elsevier, Amsterdam, 1993, 65. Published with the permission of Elsevier Science Publishers.)

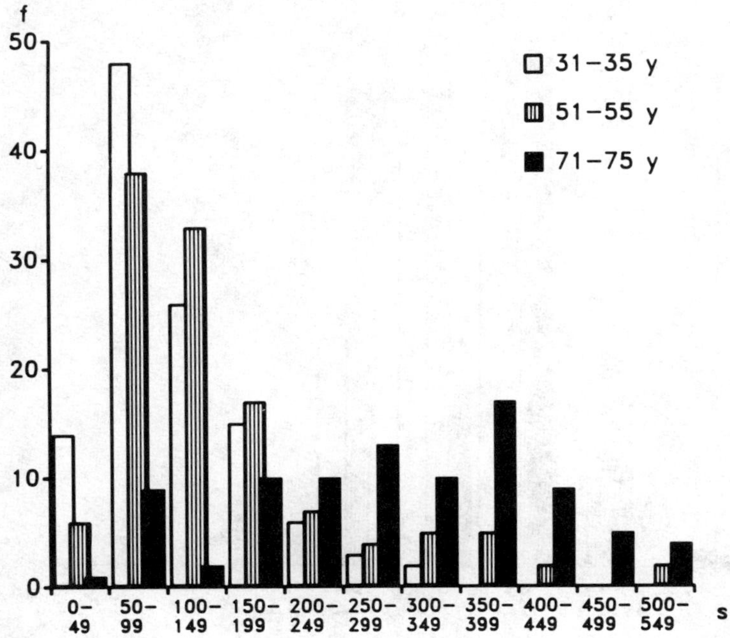

Figure 8 Frequency distributions of the results on dark adaptation in different age groups.

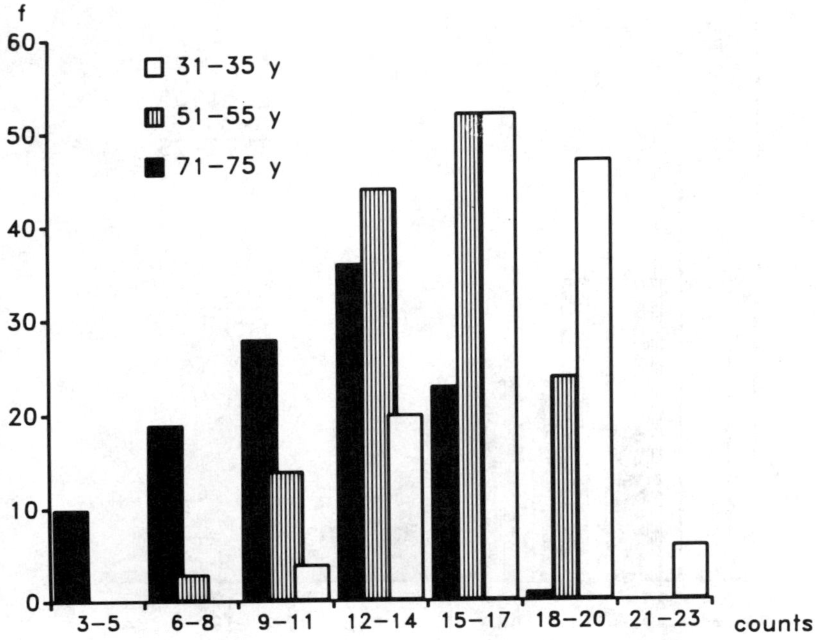

Figure 9 Frequency distributions of the results on the tapping rate of the fingers of the dominant hand over 2.5 s in different age groups.

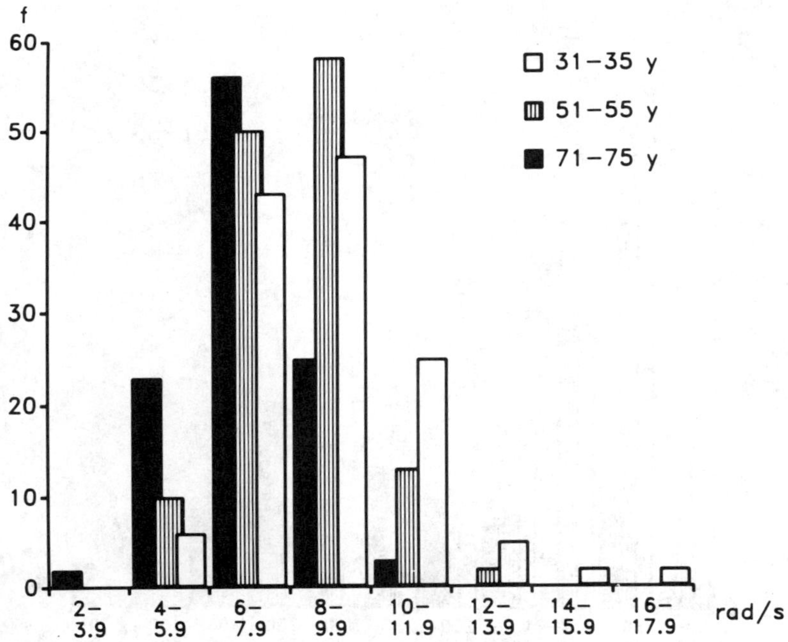

Figure 10 Frequency distributions of the results on maximal knee extension velocity in different age groups.

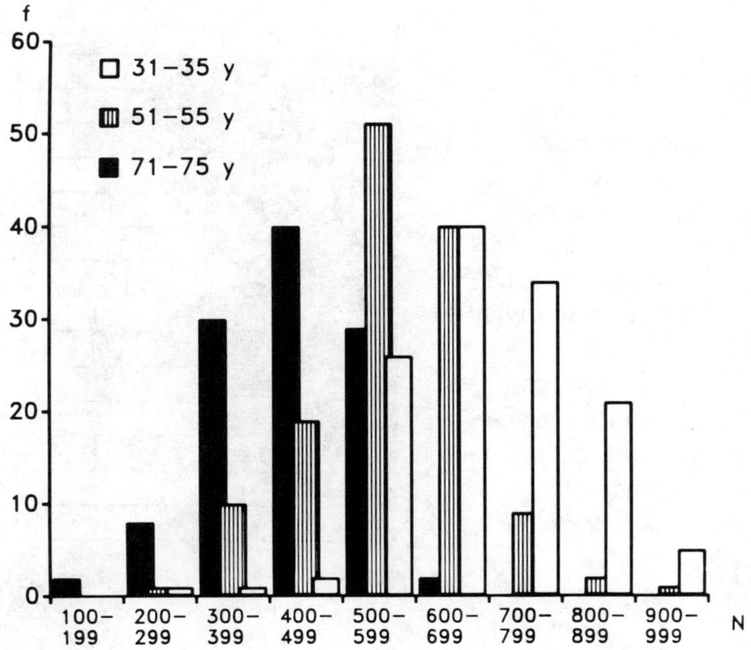

Figure 11 Frequency distributions of the results on hand grip strength in different age groups. (From Heikkinen, E. et al., in *Aging, Health and Competence*, Schroots, H.J.F., Ed., Elsevier, Amsterdam, 1993, 65. Published with the permission of Elsevier Science Publishers.)

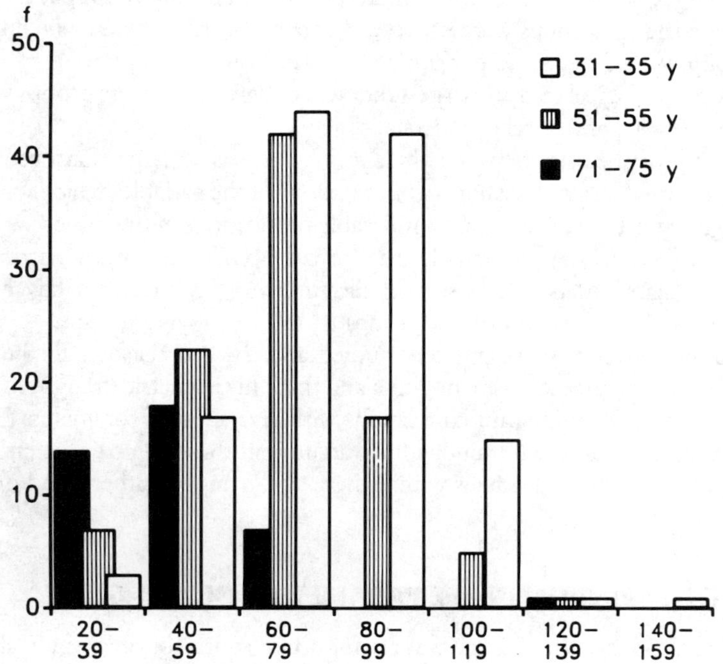

Figure 12 Frequency distributions of the indices of physical fitness (calculated on the basis of work and heart rates during recovery in bicycle ergometer test) in different age groups.

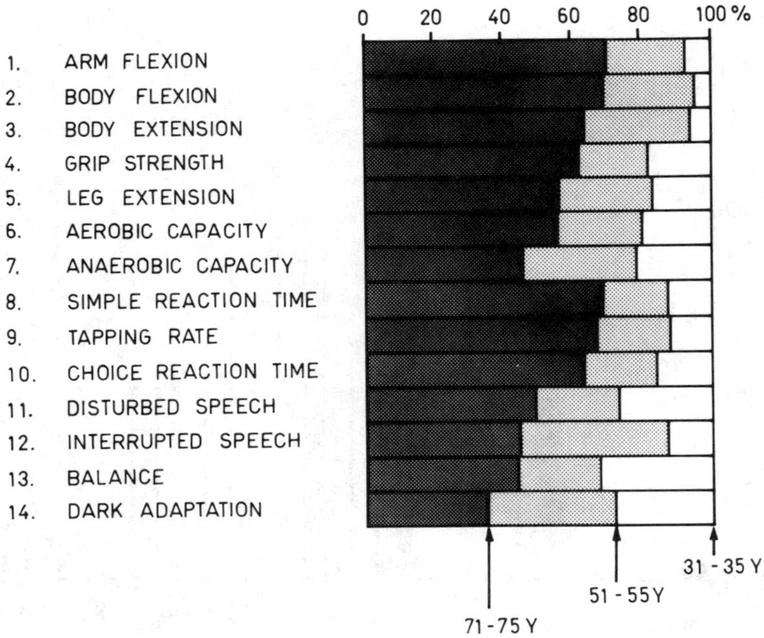

Figure 13 Profiles of certain test results of physical performance and psychophysiological performance in different age groups.

test results of the youngest group is defined as 100%, and the results of the other two groups are counted as percentages of the results of the youngest group. In the area of physical fitness the largest differences between the age groups were observed in anaerobic capacity, in which the performance of the oldest group was <50% of the performance of the youngest group.

In the psychophysiological tests the largest differences between the age groups were seen in dark adaptation, postural sway, and speech understanding.

The overlapping of the data between the age groups was so large that even in discriminant analyses, which were used to produce linear combinations of the variables which would differentiate the age groups in the most effective ways, considerable proportions of the subjects were not assigned to the right categories. This was particularly true for the isometric strength discriminant function, but even the discriminant function for a sensory discriminator assigned respectively 20 and 25% of the subjects in the middle-aged and oldest groups to the wrong age groups.

The correlations between the parameters studied also showed that within the age groups the associations between the parameters were not high and that only isometric strength measurements and reaction time had statistically significant correlations with several other parameters (Tables 1 to 3).[19]

The findings suggest that the intraindividual variation in the aging parameters is high and that the performance of not many individuals within these age groups is either good or poor in several parameters of aging.

B. SOURCES OF VARIATION IN THE PARAMETERS OF AGING

As shown in the previous paragraphs, age was an important source of variation in all the parameters investigated. In addition to age, our working model, based on the findings of the previous studies, suggests that there are many other sources of variation. These include differences in lifestyles, in levels of education and occupational status, and in the levels of different indicators of functional capacity.

Table 1 Pearson's product moment correlation coefficients among variables studied in 31- to 35-year-old men (only statistically significant correlations shown)

Variable	1	2	3	4	5	6	7	8	9	10
Body extension	1.00									
Hand grip	0.37[a]	1.00								
Postural sway			1.00							
Reaction time	–0.32[a]	–0.22[b]		1.00						
Knee extension velocity	0.22[b]			0.26[c]	1.00					
Tapping	0.28[c]	0.19[b]		0.26[c]	0.17[b]	1.00				
Hearing thresholds (4000 Hz)							1.00			
Speech understanding	0.22[b]			–0.23[c]		0.19[b]	–0.32[a]	1.00		
Dark adaptation									1.00	
Vibrotactile thresholds										1.00

[a] $p < 0.001$.
[b] $p < 0.05$.
[c] $p < 0.01$.

From Heikkinen, E. et al., in Aging, Health and Competence, *Schroots, H.J.F., Ed., Elsevier, Amsterdam, 1993, 65. Published with the permission of Elsevier Science Publishers.*

Table 2 Pearson's product moment correlation coefficients among variables studied in 51- to 55-year-old men (only statistically significant correlations are shown)

Variable	1	2	3	4	5	6	7	8	9	10
Body extension	1.00									
Hand grip	0.29[a]	1.00								
Postural sway			1.00							
Reaction time	–0.21[b]	–0.31[a]		1.00						
Knee extension velocity	0.23[b]				1.00					
Tapping	0.21[b]	0.35[a]		–0.44[a]	0.34[a]	1.00				
Hearing thresholds (4000 Hz)							1.00			
Speech understanding				–0.24[c]		0.24[c]	–0.33[a]	1.00		
Dark adaptation			0.20[b]				0.22[b]		1.00	
Vibrotactile thresholds		0.26[c]		–0.27[c]						1.00

[a] $p < 0.001$.
[b] $p < 0.05$.
[c] $p < 0.01$.

From Heikkinen, E. et al., in Aging, Health and Competence, *Schroots, H.J.F., Ed., Elsevier, Amsterdam, 1993, 65. Published with the permission of Elsevier Science Publishers.*

The sensory functions, cognitive capacity, and psychomotor speed within the age groups appeared to be associated within the age groups, whereas the sensory functions themselves appeared to be mostly independent of each other.[10]

The effects of different parameters on functional capacity within the age groups were analyzed by constructing multivariate linear structural equation models for each age group. In constructing

Table 3 Pearson's product moment correlation coefficients among variables studied in 71- to 75-year-old men (only statistically significant correlations shown)

Variable	1	2	3	4	5	6	7	8	9	10
Body extension	1.00									
Hand grip	0.48[a]	1.00								
Postural sway		–0.34[b]	1.00							
Reaction time	–0.41[a]	–0.33[a]		1.00						
Knee extension velocity	0.28[b]	0.31[a]		–0.31[b]	1.00					
Tapping	0.37[a]	0.30[b]		–0.39[a]	0.29[b]	1.00				
Hearing thresholds (4000 Hz)							1.00			
Speech understanding				–0.29[b]		0.23[c]	–0.57[a]	1.00		
Dark adaptation				0.28[b]					1.00	
Vibrotactile thresholds				0.25[c]						1.00

[a] $p < 0.001$.
[b] $p < 0.05$.
[c] $p < 0.01$.

From Heikkinen, E. et al., in Aging, Health and Competence, *Schroots, H.J.F., Ed., Elsevier, Amsterdam, 1993, 65. Published with the permission of Elsevier Science Publishers.*

the models it was assumed that socioeconomic status in combination with cognitive capacity forms the basis of the living conditions that affect people's health and lifestyles and which, in turn, affect the investigated parameters of physical and mental capacity. The models were estimated and tested by a LISREL program.[25]

It appeared that in all age groups that data fit the models well (Figures 14 to 16). Also, the determination coefficient, which is a characteristic of the proportion of the total variation of the data explained by the model, was satisfactory for each age group.

In general, the estimated models corresponded well to the assumptions differing from each other in details according to the typical features of the respective age groups. In the youngest age group the overall level of functional capacity was good and varied only slightly, the differences in health status showing the strongest effect on functional capacity. The estimated model for the middle-aged men corresponded most distinctly to the hypothetical model. The effect of the level of cognitive performance appeared to be an important predictor of functional capacity in the oldest age group.

The effects of physical exercise on functional capacity were not marked in the samples of men investigated. The impact of physical exercise was much more pronounced when comparisons were made between 70- to 81-year-old athletes and a population sample of the same age (Figure 17). The subjects of the study were 97 athletes aged 70 to 81 years still actively engaged in physical exercises and most of them taking part in competitive sports. The control group consisted of a population sample of men ($n = 67$) of the same age. Taking part in the laboratory assessments was 64% of the sample.[45] The test results of the control sample were defined as 100%, and the results of the two groups of athletes were counted as percentages of the results of the control sample. The endurance athletes received significantly better values in all the parameters of aging as compared to the controls. The same finding was true for most of the parameters among the power athletes as well. Physical exercise also affects body composition.

When the bone mineral content in the calcaneus of the middle-aged athletes was compared to that of the population sample of the same age, higher values up to 40% were observed among the athletes (Table 4).

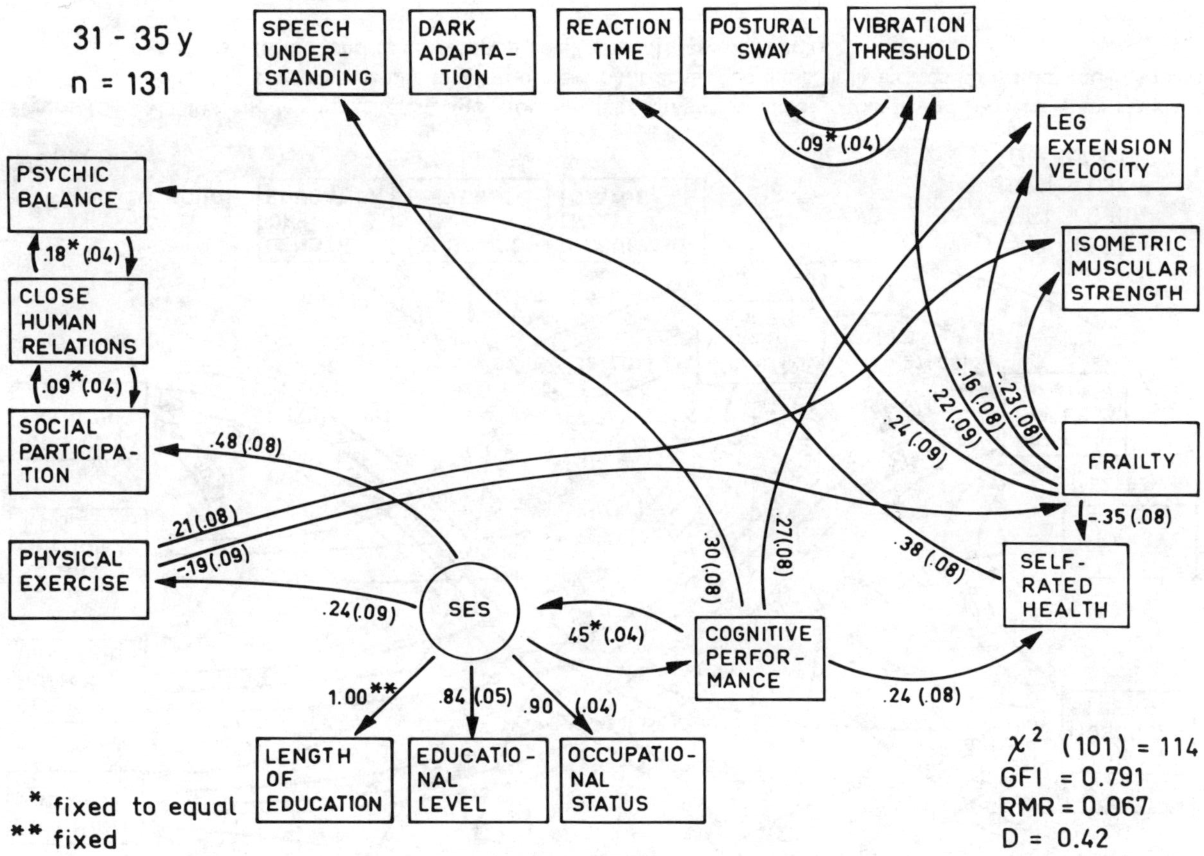

Figure 14 LISREL models for different age groups. ML, estimates of factor loadings and β-coefficients (standard errors in brackets); results of χ^2 goodness of fit tests, goodness of fit indices (GFI), root mean square residuals (RMR), and determination coefficients (D) are presented.

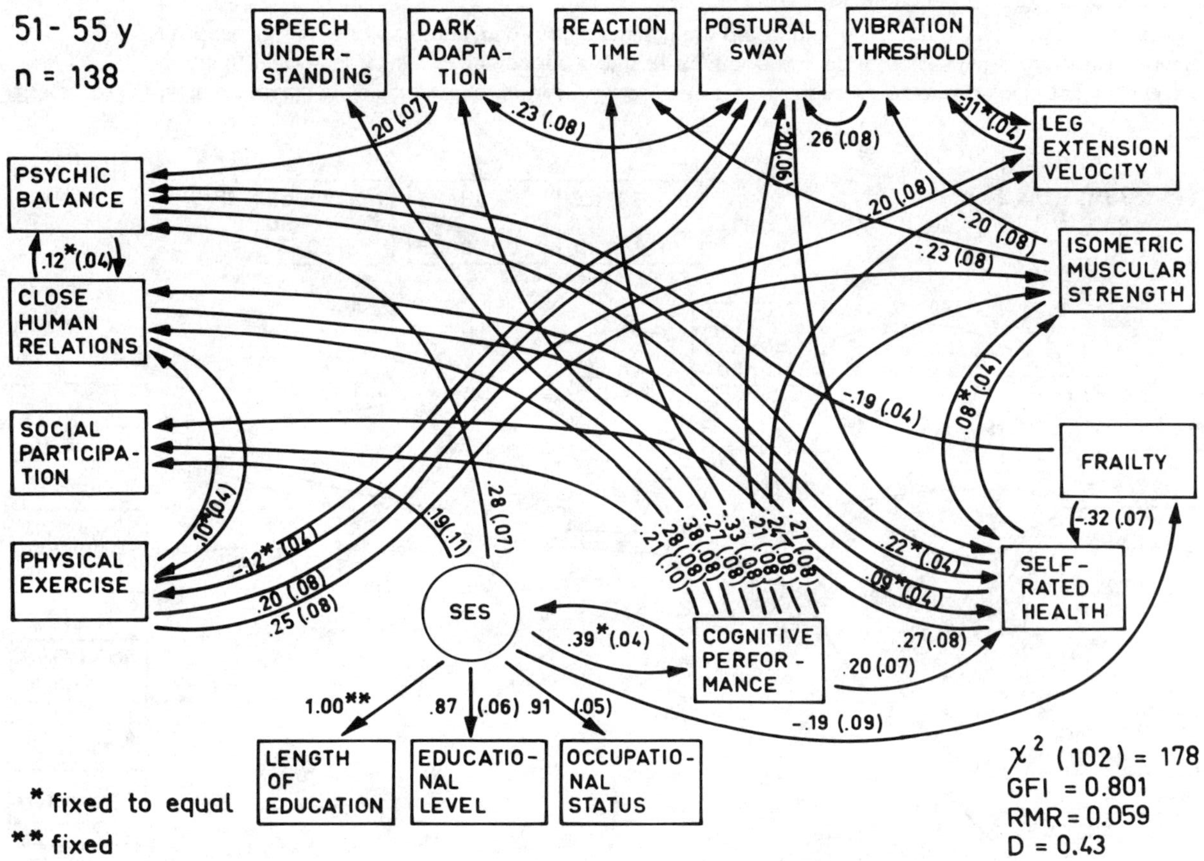

Figure 15 LISREL models for different age groups. ML, estimates of factor loadings and β-coefficients (standard errors in brackets); results of χ^2 goodness of fit tests, goodness of fit indices (GFI), root mean square residuals (RMR), and determination coefficients (D) are presented.

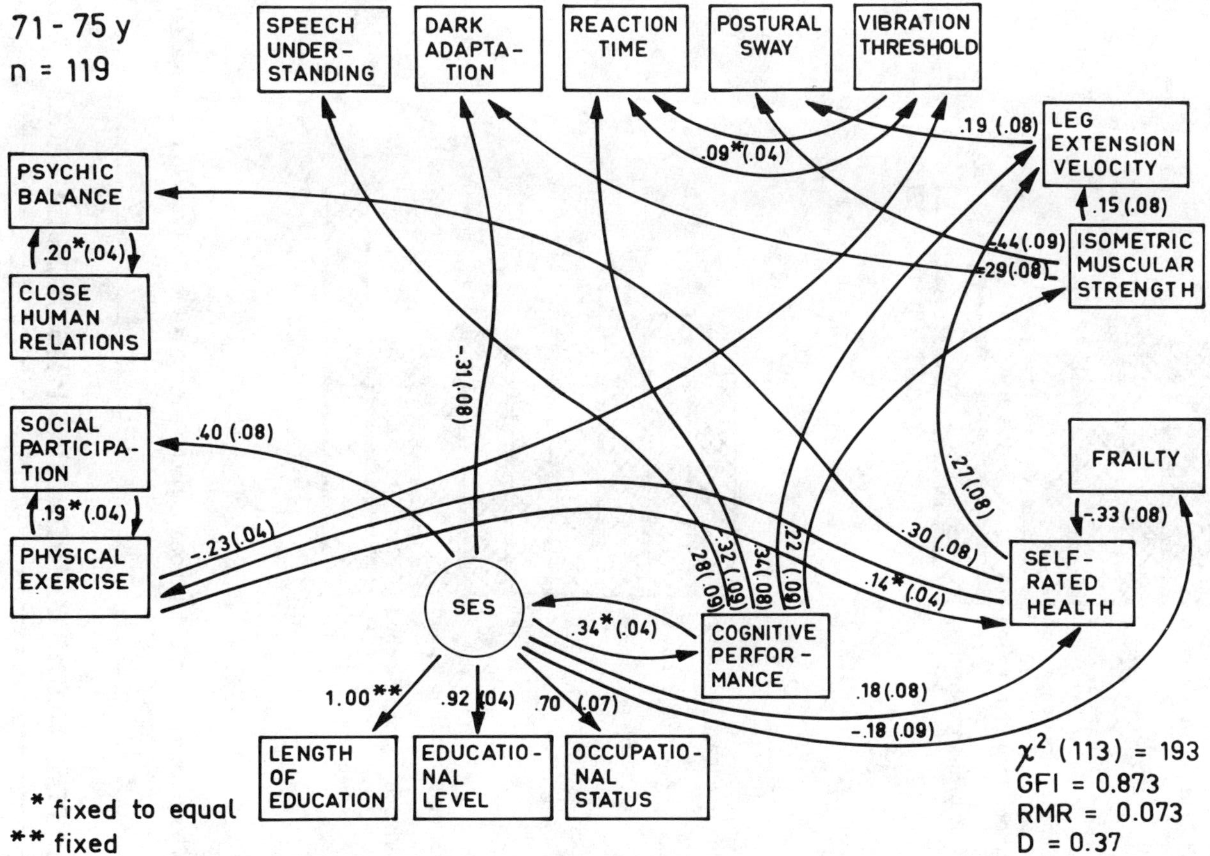

Figure 16 LISREL models for different age groups. ML, estimates of factor loadings and β-coefficients (standard errors in brackets); results of χ^2 goodness of fit tests, goodness of fit indices (GFI), root mean square residuals (RMR), and determination coefficients (D) are presented.

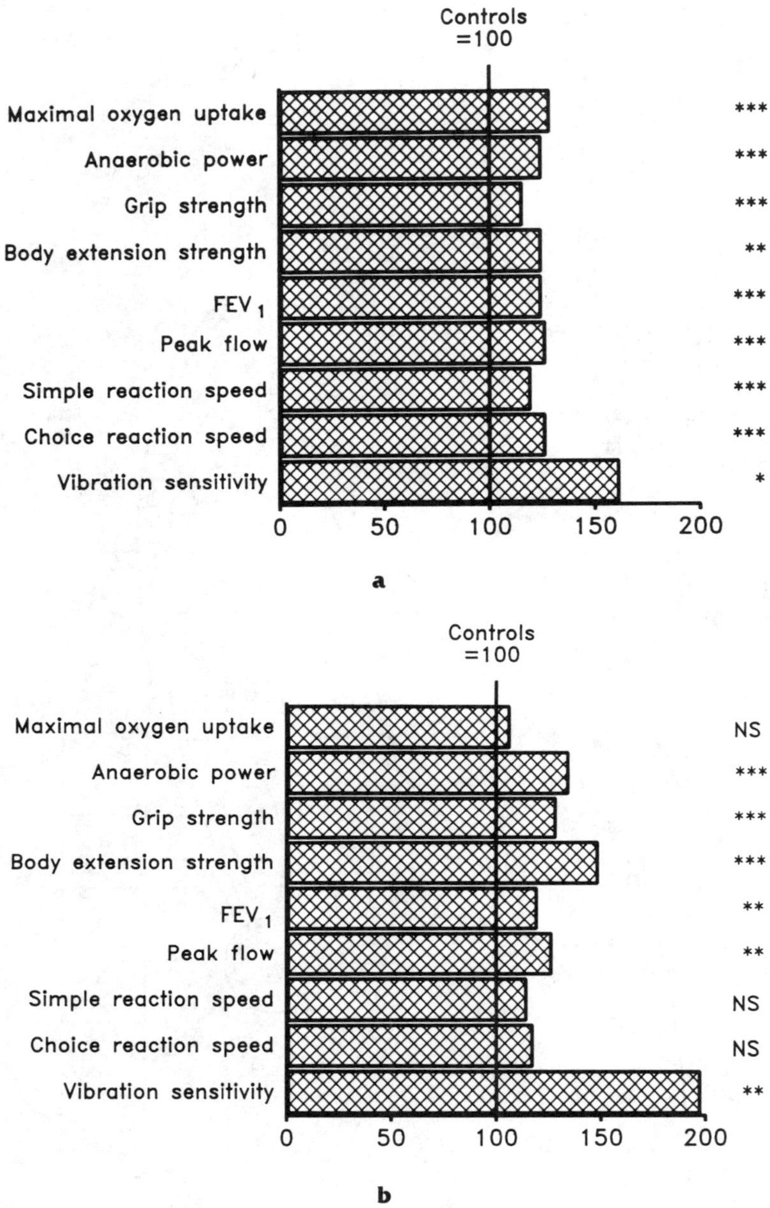

Figure 17 Profiles of certain tests of functional capacity among 70- to 81-year-old endurance (a) and power (b) athletes.

IV. POSSIBILITIES OF PREDICTING PHYSIOLOGICAL AGE

With respect to the results of our studies, certain general conclusions and hypotheses can be put forward. The means of all the parameters investigated showed significant differences between the age groups which covered 40 years of chronological age. In several tests, the decline from the middle-aged group (51 to 55 years) to the elderly (71 to 75 years) was larger than the corresponding decline from the youngest (31 to 35 years) to the middle-aged group. This phenomenon, i.e., different rates of change in different aging parameters when proceeding from younger to older age groups, is well documented in the gerontological literature, and information from the few longi-

Table 4 Bone mineral density (BMD) of calcaneus in middle-aged endurance and power athletes and population sample in different age groups (mean ± S.D.)[43,45]

Subjects	*n*	Age group	BMD (g/cm^{-3})
Endurance athletes	10	46–60	0.210 ± 0.024[a]
Power athletes	8	48–57	0.199 ± 0.022[a]
Population sample	59	31–35	0.162 ± 0.024
	52	51–55	0.147 ± 0.029
	31	71–75	0.133 ± 0.029

[a] *Significantly different* ($p < 0.001$) *from the values for the three population samples.*

tudinal studies confirms these observations.[31,32,46] Differences both within and between the age groups presumably would be even larger if the assessments could be made on all individuals. The largest decline with aging can be observed in tests that measure tolerance to stress. These tests in particular might be good choices for predicting biological aging, but only a few individuals in old age are fit enough to take part in the assessments. For example, it was only possible to do a direct assessment of $VO_{2\,max}$ in an epidemiological study among a small proportion (about 20%) of people over 70 years of age, and an even smaller proportion are able to perform a test for anaerobic capacity.[16]

In principle, some of the parameters described above might appear to be useful in predicting biological or physiological age. We do not, however, have sufficient knowledge about the relationships between life expectancy and a certain level or certain rate of change in any of the parameters used to predict biological age. Such information may not be easy to achieve because most people die from diseases, not as a result of aging. If the parameters of aging showed worse results in individuals suffering from certain chronic diseases (e.g., diabetes, hypertension), this may suggest "accelerated aging" in the affected people as suggested by Ries et al.[34] and Ries and Pöthig.[35] Reliable research findings to support this suggestion have not, however, been published.

The situation is further complicated by the fact that there are significant intraindividual variations in the parameters of aging. The relative independence of the results for several functions suggests that no single factor can be regarded as a general indicator of biological or physiological age. This also makes it difficult to combine their information by statistical calculations, whether by summative or regression methods. A high value for one variable may be compensated by a poor value for another and vice versa. In addition, giving different weights to different variables, which may be necessary, is difficult to soundly perform. Thus, we can say a person who is old in one respect may yet be young in other respects.

Different types of factors cause variation in the parameters of aging within an individual and also in population groups. Some of these associations are self-explanatory. Certain diseases, for example, decrease the functional capacity of the affected organs or physiological systems. Logically, a good level of functioning can be maintained by continuous training of the respective system. The effects of physical exercise clearly show that even in old age functions that are directly influenced by physical exercise in particular show significantly higher levels compared to the results of sedentary people of the same age. In addition, our data suggest that the impact of physical exercise also can be seen in functions in which the training effect is not logically expected (e.g., vibratory threshold, sensitivity of visual field.[11] The interpretation of these findings is, however, rendered difficult by observations that indicate that physically active and sedentary people often differ from each other in other respects such as smoking, obesity, and nutritional habits.[37]

It can be assumed, however, that in functions such as aerobic and anaerobic capacity and muscle strength a significant part of the differences between physically active and sedentary people can be attributed to differences in the level of physical exercise. Whether these effects also would add years to life is still controversial. The findings of longitudinal studies suggest that lifestyle factors are important predictors of longevity.[31] Our own findings on the basis of the 10-year follow-up of the 60- to 89-year-old residents of Tampere, Finland also suggest that a high level of habitual physical exercise contributes to an increased life expectancy. In addition, the available evidence from intervention studies has shown that various functions often included in the assessment of physiological aging can be improved by physical exercise even in old age,[1,40] leading to a better quality of life.

Reduction of bone mineral density is apparently one aging phenomenon that may lead to osteoporotic changes in the skeleton and contribute to an increased incidence of bone fractures with advancing age. Smoking, excessive drinking, lack of physical exercise, and deficiencies in nutrition are among the lifestyle factors that seem to accelerate the loss of bone in aging.[30,36,43,45] There is no conclusive evidence, however, that an accelerated loss of bone is an indicator of a more generalized acceleration of biological aging or that it would predict a below-average life expectancy.

The effects of level of education and of cognitive capacity on several parameters of aging also need further clarification. It can be assumed that a high cognitive capacity is an important factor in selecting individuals for different life courses and different occupations which may further develop their skills and functional abilities. Also, educated people have more test experience and are perhaps also better motivated to perform different tests compared to their less educated age peers. Furthermore, there are marked differences in life expectancies between different social groups. For example, in Finland the mortality rate for teachers and clergymen is about 50 vs. the standard mortality rate of 100 for men aged 15 to 64 years. This kind of social inequality in the face of death must be taken into account when predicting findings on health and the functional capacity of aging populations.[49]

V. CONCLUDING REMARKS

Our results support the findings of certain other studies[28,33] which suggest that no single factor, but rather a combination of biological, psychological, and social factors featuring what could be called elite status, contribute to healthy aging. Therefore, any assessment of single or even multiple parameters of aging with the purpose of assessing an individual's biological age is premature and the concept of biological age will have to be regarded as an empty abstraction until we know more about the ecological validity of various assessments and their predictive value with respect to the development of health, unrestricted functioning, and life expectancy.

However, as Mark Twain said of Wagner's music, "It is not as bad as it sounds." Concepts of functional or biological age as statistical entities may be useful in making comparisons of different populations or between larger groups of individuals as shown by our studies on different age and occupational groups. In addition, assessments of physiological age might be useful if some parameters of aging were associated with abilities to cope with the activities of daily life. Even for these purposes a need exists for methodological development and more information is required, particularly from interdisciplinary longitudinal studies among representative population samples, on different aspects of physiological aging and on the sources of variation within.

What is said above does not, however, necessarily mean that we should wait for the results of more conclusive studies before any intervention programs can be initiated or any actions recommended to decision makers. The present evidence on the sources of variation in biological aging is not strong and there are quite definite doubts which, if proved true, would lead to the restructuring of a number of established theoretical frameworks. On the other hand, as suggested above, there is evidence of factors affecting biological aging that can be regarded as highly plausible. This kind of evidence could be used as a point of departure for intervention and program evaluation studies and for decision making aimed at promoting the physical and mental capacity of aging populations and reducing inequalities in health.[18]

ACKNOWLEDGMENTS

Grants from the National Medical Research Council in the Academy of Finland and Research Council for Sport and Physical Culture of the Ministry of Education are gratefully acknowledged.

REFERENCES

1. Aniansson, A. and Gustafsson, E., Physical training in elderly men with special reference to quadriceps muscle strength and morphology, *Clin. Physiol.*, 1, 87, 1981.
2. Aunola, S., Käyhty-Seppänen, B., Heikkinen, E., Parvi, V., and Vuori, I., Functional capacity of 68-year old people in the town of Jyväskylä, *Z. Alternsforsch.*, 31, 439, 1976.
3. Comfort, A., Test-battery to measure ageing-rate in man, *Lancet*, 2, 1411, 1969.
4. Dirken, J., Ed., *Functional Age of Industrial Workers*, Wolters-Noordhoff, Gröningen, 1972.
5. Dubina, T.L., Mints, A.Ya., and Zhuk, E.V., Biological age and its estimation. III. Introduction of a correction to the multiple regression model of biological age and assessment of biological age in cross-sectional and longitudinal studies, *Exp. Gerontol.*, 19, 133, 1984.
6. Era, P. and Heikkinen, E., Postural sway during standing and unexpected disturbance of balance in random samples of men of different ages, *J. Gerontol.*, 40, 287, 1985.
7. Era, P., Jokela, J., Suominen, H., and Heikkinen, E., Correlates of vibrotactile thresholds in men of different ages, *Acta Neurol. Scand.*, 74, 210, 1986.
8. Era, P., Jokela, J., and Heikkinen, E., Reaction and movement times in men of different ages, a population study, *Percept. Motor Skills*, 63, 111, 1986.
9. Era, P., Jokela, J., Qvarnberg, Y., and Heikkinen, E., Pure-tone thresholds, speech-understanding, and their correlates in samples of men of different ages, *Audiology*, 25, 338, 1986.
10. Era, P., Sensory, psychomotor, and motor functions in men of different ages, *Scand. J. Soc. Med.*, 39(Suppl.), 1, 1987.
11. Era, P., Pärssinen, O., Pykälä, P., Jokela, J., and Suominen, H., Sensitivity of the central visual field in 70 to 81-year-old male athletes and in a population sample, *Aging Clin. Exp.*, in press, 1994.
12. Era, P., Pärssinen, O., and Suominen, H., Neurophysiological aspects of exercise among the elderly, in *Sport for All*, Oja, P. and Telema, R., Eds., Elsevier, Amsterdam, 1991, 343.
13. Furukawa, T., Inoue, M., Kajiya, F., Inada, H., Takasugi, S., Fukui, S., Takeda, H., and Abe, H., Assessment of biological age by multiple regression analysis, *J. Gerontol.*, 30, 422, 1975.
14. Heikkinen, E., Kiiskinen, A., Käyhty, B., Rimpelä, M., and Vuori, I., Assessment of biological age, *Gerontologia*, 20, 33, 1974.
15. Heikkinen, E., Seppänen, B., and Rimpelä, M., Biological age, health, and health-risk in indicators among 25-57-year old men in two parts of Finland, *Scand. J. Soc. Med.*, 3, 105, 1975.
16. Heikkinen, E., Assessment of functional ageing, in *Lectures on Gerontology*, Vol. 1, *On Biology of Ageing*, Part B, Viidik, A., Ed., Academic Press, London, 1982, 481.
17. Heikkinen, E., Arajärvi, R.-L., Era, P., Jylhä, M., Kinnunen, V., Leskinen, A.-L., Leskinen, E., Mässeli, E., Pohjolainen, P., Rahkila, P., Suominen, H., Turpeinen, P., Väisänen, M., and Österback, L., Functional capacity of men born in 1906-1910, 1926-30 and 1946-50. A basic report, *Scand. J. Soc. Med.*, 33(Suppl.), 1, 1984.
18. Heikkinen, E., Health implications of population aging in Europe, *World Health Stat. Q.*, 40, 22, 1987.
19. Heikkinen, E., Era, P., Jokela, J., Jylhä, M., Lyyra, A.-L., and Pohjolainen, P., Socioeconomic and lifestyle factors as modulators of health and functional capacity with age, in *Aging, Health and Competence*, Schroots, H.J.F., Ed., Elsevier, Amsterdam, 1993, 65.
20. Heron, A. and Chown, S., *Age and Function*, J. & A. Churchill, London, 1967.
21. Hirayama, H., Some physical functions of aging people in an agricultural village, *Acta Med.*, 13, 187, 1969.

22. Hollingsworth, J.W., Hashizume, A., and Jablon, S., Correlations between tests of aging in Hiroshima subjects — an attempt to define "physiologic age", *Yale J. Biol. Med.*, 38, 11, 1965.
23. Jalavisto, E. and Makkonen, T., On the assessment of biological age, *Ann. Acad. Sci. Fenn. A,* 100, 1, 1963.
24. Jylhä, M., Jokela, J., Tolvanen, E., Heikkinen, E., Heikkinen, R.-L., Koskinen, S., Leskinen, E., Lyyra, A.-L., and Pohjolainen, P., The Tampere Longitudinal Study on Aging, *Scand. J. Soc. Med.*, 47(Suppl.), 1, 1992.
25. Joreskog, K.G. and Sorbom, D., Analysis of Linear Structural Relationships by Maximum Likelihood and Least Squares Methods, Res. Rep. 81-8, University of Uppsala, Uppsala, Sweden, 1981.
26. Kiiskinen, A., Heikkinen, E., Parkatti, T., Pohjolainen, P., and Vuori, I., Functional aging of 40-50-year old men in two industrial enterprises, *Scand. J. Soc. Med.*, 14, 12, 1980.
27. Kiiskinen, A., Era, P., and Parkatti, T., Functional age of relatively young and old female and male employees in the machine industry, *IRCS Med. Sci.*, 9, 6, 1981.
28. Lehr, U., Aging as fate and challenge: the influence of social, biological and psychological factors, in *Mental Health in the Elderly*, Häfner, H., Moschel, G., and Sartorius, N., Eds., Springer-Verlag, Berlin, 1986, 57.
29. Leppo, K., Lindgren, J., and Ritamies, M., *Mortality Trends in Finland in the 1960's*, Yearbook of Population Research in Finland, The Population Policy Research Institute, Vammala, 1972.
30. Lindsay, R., Prevention of osteoporosis, in *Prevention of Disease in the Elderly*, Gray, J.A.M., Ed., Churchill Livingstone, Edinburgh, 1985, 95.
31. Palmore, E., Predictors of the longevity difference: a 25-year follow-up, *Gerontologist*, 6, 513, 1982.
32. Palmore, E.B., Nowlin, J.B., and Wang, H.S., Predictors of function among the old-old: a 10-year follow-up, *J. Gerontol.*, 40, 244, 1985.
33. Pfeiffer, E., Survival in old age: physical, psychological and social correlates of longevity, *J. Am. Gerontol. Soc.*, 18, 273, 1970.
34. Ries, W., Pöthig, D., Hunecke, I., and Sauer, I., Untersuchungen über das biologische Alter von Menschen, *Z. Alternsforsch.*, 36, 255, 1981.
35. Ries, W., and Pöthig, D., Chronological and biological age, *Exp. Gerontol.*, 19, 211, 1984.
36. Riggs, B.L. and Melton, III, L.J., Involutional osteoporosis, *N. Engl. J. Med.*, 314, 1676, 1986.
37. Rose, C.L. and Cohen, M.L., Relative importance of physical activity for longevity, in *Physiological, Medical, Epidemiological, and Psychological Studies*, *Ann. N.Y. Acad. Sci.*, 301(Spec. Iss.), 671, 1977.
38. Shock, N.W., Indices of functional age, in *Aging: Challenge to Science and Society*, Vol. 1, *Biology*, Danon, D., Shock N.W., and Marois, M., Eds., Oxford University Press, Oxford, 1981, 270.
39. Sipilä, S., Viitasalo, J., Era, P., and Suominen, H. (1991). Muscle strength in male athletes aged 70-81 years and a population sample, *Eur. J. Appl. Physiol.,* 63, 399, 1991.
40. Suominen, H., Heikkinen, E., and Parkatti, T., Effect of eight weeks physical training on muscle and connective tissue of the m. vastus lateralis in 69-year-old men and women, *J. Gerontol.*, 32, 33, 1977.
41. Suominen, H., *Effects of Physical Training in Middle-Aged and Elderly People with Special Regard to Skeletal Muscle Connective Tissue and Functional Aging*, Studies in Sport, Physical Education and Health 11, University of Jyväskylä, Jyväskylä, Finland, 1978.
42. Suominen, H., Heikkinen, E., Pohjolainen, P., Parkatti, T., and Forsberg, S., Funktionell ålder hos 72-åriga män och kvinnor, in *Nordisk Gerontologi*, Beverfelt, E., Julsrud, A-Ch., Kjϕrstad, H., and Nygård, A.M., Norsk Selskap for Aldersforskning, Oslo, 1980, 53.
43. Suominen, H., Heikkinen, E., Vainio, P., and Lahtinen, T., Mineral density of calcaneus in men at different ages: a population study with special reference to lifestyle factors. *Age Ageing*, 13, 273, 1984.
44. Suominen, H., Rahkila, P., Era, P., Jaakkola, L., and Heikkinen, E., Functional capacity in middle-aged male endurance and power athletes, in *Physical Activity, Aging and Sports,* Vol. 1, *Scientific and Medical Research,* Harris, R., and Harris, S., Eds., Center for the Study of Aging, Albany, NY, 1989, 213.
45. Suominen, H. and Rahkila, P., Bone mineral density of the calcaneus in 70 to 81-year-old male athletes and a population sample, *Med. Sci. Sports Exercise,* 23, 1227, 1991.

46. Svanborg, A., Berg, S., Mellström, D., Nilsson, L., and Persson, G., Possibilities of preserving physical and mental fitness and autonomy in old age, in *Mental Health in the Elderly*, Häfner, H., Mosckel, G., and Sartorius, N., Springer-Verlag, Berlin, 1986, 195.
47. Thomae, H., Ed., *Patterns of Aging, Findings from the Bonn Longitudinal Study of Aging*, S. Karger, Basel, 1976.
48. Tobin, J.D., Physiological indices of aging, in *Aging: A Challenge to Science and Society*, Vol. 1, *Biology*, Danon, D., Shock N.W., and Marois, M., Eds., Oxford University Press, Oxford, 1981, 286.
49. Valkonen, T., Martelin, T., Rimpelä, A., Notkola, V., and Savela, S., Eds., *Socio-Economic Mortality Differences in Finland 1981–90,* Statistics Finland, Population 1, Helsinki, 1993.
50. Webster, I.W. and Logie, A.R., A relationship between functional age and health status in female subjects, *J. Gerontol.*, 31, 546, 1976.
51. Viitasalo, J.T., Era, P., Leskinen, A.-L., and Heikkinen, E., Muscular strength profiles and anthropometry in random samples of men aged 31-35, 51-55 and 71-75 years, *Ergonomics*, 28, 1563, 1985.
52. Weg, R.B., Changing physiology of aging: normal and pathological, in *Aging*, Woodruff, D.S. and Birren, J.E., Eds., Van Nostrand Co., New York, 1975, 229.

CHAPTER 8

VALIDATING BIOMARKERS OF AGING — MATHEMATICAL APPROACHES AND RESULTS OF A 2462-PERSON STUDY

RICHARD HOCHSCHILD

TABLE OF CONTENTS

ABSTRACT

Biomarkers of aging are needed to evaluate proposed treatments to retard aging rates. At present, the only validated biomarker of aging is maximum life span, which remains impractical for human use. Identification of other biomarkers awaits development of a method of biomarker validation. This chapter outlines an approach for this purpose intended for selecting biomarkers usable in humans. Prospective biomarkers are validated and weighted according to their correlation with interventions that, in healthy individuals, influence life span, namely mortality risk factors. A general mathematical method is presented for combining biomarker scores into an index of aging rate. This method addresses problems encountered with the traditional (multiple regression) method of calculating biological age and develops an index termed standardized biological age (SBA). In applying the method to 2462 office workers, SBA, based on 12 physiological tests under investigation as biomarkers of aging, was found to depend on most of the 17 surveyed dietary, exercise, lifestyle, and geographical risk factors for mortality or health, suggesting that many risk factors predict rates of common functional declines with age. The 12 candidate biomarkers of aging in this study differed widely in validity according to the criterion employed. The approach holds promise for assembling an experimentally useful battery of biomarkers of aging.

I. INTRODUCTION

By various measures, individuals of the same species age at different rates. This observation underlies the growing interest in biomarkers of aging and their possible use to explore why aging rate differences exist and what influences them. Valid biomarkers of aging are needed to investigate mechanisms of aging and to evaluate treatments for retarding the aging process.[4,10,15,30,31,80]

Only one biomarker of aging has been validated, namely maximum life span, which remains impractical for human use.[53] Nevertheless, it appears possible that many functional, biochemical, or morphological parameters will be found to be effective biomarkers of aging. Hollingsworth et al.,[36] Comfort,[15] and others have suggested that aging rate assessments can be based on measurements of a sufficiently large and diverse test battery of such parameters.

A. VALIDATING BIOMARKERS OF AGING

The fundamental problem in developing an arsenal of biomarkers of aging has been the lack of a method of biomarker validation. Validation criteria have varied from author to author.[4,26,31,37-40] Selection of criteria of biomarker validity remains a controversial area. Lack of any independent method of measuring the rate of aging to use as a standard of comparison leaves only a number of indirect approaches, none of which is quite satisfactory.

Proposed biomarker validation criteria include correlation of biomarker scores with (1) mortality rate, (2) interventions that influence mortality rate, and (3) the quality of later life. Few attempts have been made to apply biomarker validation criteria (other than correlation with chronological age, which is an insufficient criterion). In mice, correlation with life span was used to assess the validity of candidate biomarkers of aging by Harrison and Archer[28] and by Ingram and Reynolds.[40] Correlation with caloric restriction was used for this purpose by Harrison et al.[31] and Ingram.[38] In human studies, Furukawa et al.[22] investigated correlation with hypertension, and Webster and Logie[90] checked correlation with health status as independent variables against which to evaluate a biological age index. Correlation with mortality rate, which has been frequently proposed as a biomarker validation criterion, presents problems in longer-lived species because of its time requirement.

This study tested the criterion that to qualify as valid, a biomarker of aging should be responsive to interventions that influence the natural life span.[10,31,38,80] Examples of such interventions are caloric restriction in rodents, body temperature modulation in poikilotherms, and, in humans, a variety of dietary and lifestyle practices that are recognized as mortality risk factors. This criterion was tested by applying it, in a study of 2462 office workers, to 12 physiological tests under investigation as potential biomarkers of aging. Associations were studied between each of the 12 tests individually and composite validation variable (CVV), a composite index of risk based on 8 of 17 surveyed mortality and health risk factors. The 12 physiological tests are listed in Table 1; the 8 risk factors are listed in Table 2. All 17 surveyed risk factors are listed in the captions of Figures 13 to 31. In addition, associations were studied between the 17 risk factors individually and standardized biological age (SBA), a composite index of aging based on the 12 tests.

The first study of the sensitivity of putative biomarkers of aging to life span interventions, albeit not for the purpose of validating the biomarkers, was reported by Hollingsworth et al.,[36] who studied survivors of Hiroshima some 15 years after radiation exposure. Other investigators have used various physiological tests to study aging effects of life span interventions in mice, such as hypophysectomy[30] and caloric restriction.[31] Harrison and Archer[29] demonstrated the value of this approach by observing that dietary restriction produced different aging effects in different strains of mice.

B. RATIONALE FOR USING CORRELATION WITH RISK FACTORS FOR VALIDATING BIOMARKERS

In humans, many proposed risk factors are unreliably correlated with mortality. Even for risk factors that are significantly related to mortality rate, correlations tend to be low, due in part to the large number of risk factors at work and in part to the high variability of age at death, death tending to be triggered by a chance event. A composite index of several risk factors can be expected to have a somewhat higher, but still not particularly high, correlation with mortality. That being the situation, is correlation with risk factors a useful criterion for purposes of validating biomarkers of aging?

Table 1 Physiological tests administered by H-SCAN

j	Test	Unit
1	Vibrotactile sensitivity, fingertip	×1.5 dB
2	Memory, sequence of lamps	# of jumps
3	FVC	10 ml
4	FEV-1	10 ml
5	Alternate button tapping time, 30×	0.1 s
6	Highest audible pitch	100 Hz
7	Visual accommodation	0.1 diopter
8	Auditory reaction time	ms
9	Visual reaction time without decision	ms
10	Movement time without decision	ms
11	Visual reaction time with decision	ms
12	Movement time with decision	ms

Note: j *is test number.*

It is difficult to make a case for the use of risk factor data solely as a substitute for mortality data. However, an additional rationale exists for using correlation with risk factors, and with mortality interventions in general, as a validating criterion: many interventions that in healthy individuals biologically alter the natural life span may do so by their primary action on the rate of aging, thereby altering disease probability. Interventions that operate this way will be more closely related to the rate of aging than to the rate of death.

To illustrate this point, suppose that the task is to evaluate respiratory quotient (RQ) as a potential biomarker of aging in rats. RQ, or specifically its 48-h range, is highly correlated with a mortality intervention, caloric restriction (CR).[21] Changes in RQ signal changes in main metabolic pathway (carbohydrate vs. fatty acid metabolism). The 48-h range of RQ can be used reliably to separate restricted from *ad libitum*-fed animals,[20] except for a small proportion of borderline animals such as those that are self-restricting in the *ad libitum* group (as indicated by low fat to lean body mass ratio) or overfeeders in the CR group. Much evidence indicates that CR retards the rate of decline of age-associated physiological parameters and delays the onset of degenerative diseases (reviewed by Weindruch and Walford[91]). If the effects of CR on mortality rate are secondary to its effects on aging rate, CR would be a more appropriate variable against which to validate a biomarker of aging than is mortality rate. Correlation with CR offers an additional advantage. According to

Table 2 Mortality risk factors included in composite validation variable, CVV

	Risk factor	Weight
1	Cigarettes smoked per day	4
2	High fat foods, servings per day	2
3	Emphasis on red meat in diet	3
4	Exercise intensity level	2
5	Combined exercise score based on hours/week + years + intensity	2
6	State life expectancy at birth	1
7	State life expectancy at age 45	1
8	Years of school completed	4

the data from the above example, the correlation between RQ and CR is higher than the correlation between RQ and mortality, partly because of the high variability of the latter. In this example, correlation with a mortality intervention is probably the more appropriate, and evidently the more sensitive, validation criterion.

The point is not quite so clear cut when applied to human studies, with risk factors in the role of interventions. No risk factor in humans — with some possible exceptions such as the composite of risk factors at work in being a practicing Seventh Day Adventist — has nearly the dramatic relationship with life expectancy that caloric restriction has in rodents. However, that does not invalidate the proposition that correlation with an intervention that biologically alters the natural life span can be a more appropriate and sensitive validation criterion for a biomarker of aging than is correlation with mortality, and that the former does more than serve as an estimate of the latter.

C. CORRELATION WITH MORTALITY RATE AS A VALIDATION CRITERION

Mortality rate differences between groups are generally considered to be closely related to aging rate differences, at least in the laboratory, where the variable influences of predatorial activity, accidents, natural disasters, and (with exceptions) infectious diseases are not likely to be important factors. Accordingly, mortality rate, when available and accurate, remains a viable validating variable for biomarkers of aging. In the above example, if RQ were found to be associated with mortality rate among the *ad libitum*-fed animals (or among the CR animals), this would further support the validity of RQ as a biomarker of aging.

Because collecting mortality data tends to be a 20-year or longer undertaking in the case of humans, little data exist that can be used to evaluate human prospective biomarkers of aging for correlation with mortality rate. Exceptions to this are the lung function parameters, forced vital capacity (FVC), and forced expiratory volume-1 s (FEV-1). Much evidence has accumulated from various studies that lower than normal values of FVC and FEV-1 during times of health are associated with increased deaths from most major causes, not just lung disease.[2,3,5,6,9,32,45,46,54,69,71] Lower than normal FVC was found to be associated with earlier mortality in the elderly as well as the young, in both sexes, and in nonsmokers as well as smokers. In some studies lung function was more predictive of mortality than were smoking status, history of ischemic heart disease, blood pressure, or gender, and was second only to chronological age as a predictor of survival.

D. CORRELATION WITH QUALITY OF LATER LIFE AS A VALIDATION CRITERION

A third proposed biomarker validation criterion is correlation of candidate biomarker scores with the quality of later life in healthy persons.[27] Humans perceive aging as the decline of characteristics that contribute to quality of life. That perception may be sufficient to validate, as human biomarkers of aging, those physiological functions and appearance features that decline with age in healthy individuals and are commonly (though not necessarily) linked to quality of life, such as acuity of hearing, memory, lung function, the speed of reactions and movement, and, to the extent that they undermine self-image, skin laxity, hair graying, and muscle sagging. Such functions and features probably integrate the effects of multiple aging mechanisms.

The 12 physiological functions in Table 1 were selected in part because of their evident role in determining the quality of later life. Age decrements in these functions are associated with some of the more noticeable and troublesome intellectual and physical deficits that commonly accompany human aging. The 12 functions are involved in physically demanding activities such as sports, travel, some occupations, and self-care in old age, and mentally demanding activities such as work, social interactions, and intellectual pursuits.

E. IS BIOLOGICAL AGE A VALID CONCEPT?

A more powerful approach for estimating aging rates than examining data from individual biomarkers is to combine scores from a battery of biomarkers into a single index of aging. When in units of time, such an index is conventionally (but not necessarily appropriately) called biological, physiological, or functional age. The problem with any of these designations is that they promise more than they can deliver.

As will be seen for biomarkers in current use, such as those examined in this study, the amount of variance of biomarker scores explained by the aging process tends to be low. Part of the reason for this is that people are born with relatively faster or slower nervous systems, smaller or larger lung capacities, and with a range of other physiological and psychological characteristics that influence biomarker scores, yet do not necessarily reflect the participant's age. Other contributors to variance are such temporary factors as diurnal and day to day fluctuations in mood, alertness, fatigue, etc.

An individual's rate of aging can be estimated more gainfully from the rate of change of his or her biomarker scores, or of a composite index of such scores, over a number of years. In such long-term studies, further reliability can be gained by repeating testing sessions twice or three times over a span of a few days and averaging results to suppress diurnal and other short-term influences.

Such sources of variance cause fewer problems in group studies, where they partially tend to wash out or lend themselves to statistical control (see below). As will be seen, scores for biomarkers of aging can be combined into a useful composite index of aging for comparisons among groups of individuals that demonstrates relationships to dietary and lifestyle factors and can be used to evaluate proposed interventions in aging.

F. CRITICAL EVALUATION OF PRIOR MATHEMATICAL METHODS OF CALCULATING BIOLOGICAL AGE

Attempts to estimate human biological age from physiological tests include those of Dirken,[18] Dubina et al.,[19] Furukawa et al.,[22] Hollingsworth et al.,[36] Nakamura et al.,[62] Voitenko and Tokar,[89] and Webster and Logie.[90]

In all of these studies, (1) an insufficient criterion, namely association with chronological age, was used to validate tests as biomarkers of aging; (2) a method inappropriate for the purpose, namely multiple regression, was used to calculate biological age from test scores; and (3) no attempt was made to reduce unwanted variance in calculating biological age. These three criticisms are now examined in some detail.

1. Association with Chronological Age Is Insufficient as a Validation Criterion

That association with chronological age (CA) is not a sufficient criterion for validating biomarkers of aging has been pointed out by Costa and McCrea[16] and Ingram.[37,39] This follows from the consideration that a hypothetical biomarker that approaches perfect correlation with CA (and would therefore receive the highest validation) could be replaced by a calendar and would be insensitive to differences in aging rates between individuals. Many physiological parameters that are correlated with CA may be irrelevant to aging. For example, degree of baldness increases with age, especially in men, but men who grow bald early do not necessarily show signs of accelerated aging nor is baldness a risk factor for early death.

This does not mean that CA can be ignored in calculating an index of aging from physiological tests that depend on age (as do practically all functional tests that have been proposed as possible biomarkers of aging at present). For age-dependent tests, the relevant information is not the subject's absolute score but the deviation of that score from the norm for the subject's age and sex (based on some chosen norm group). These norms can be determined by regressing test scores on CA (as in this chapter). If CA were not used in combining scores from age-dependent tests, as was tried by Chodzko-Zajko and Ringel,[14] who substituted principal component analysis and weighted scores according to the resulting eigenvalues, it would constitute an unwelcome source of additional variance.

2. Multiple Regression Leads to Errors in Calculating Biological Age

Multiple regression, used in all of the cited studies of human biological age (BA) and in many animal studies as well, leads to errors in calculating BA from physiological test scores because of three, and under some conditions, four problems:[34]

a. Multiple Regression Calls for an Inappropriate Step, Equating BA to Predicted-CA, Causing Regression to Sample Mean Age

In all of the cited prior biological age studies, BA was calculated analogously to the following procedure. Let j be an integer identifying one of n physiological tests whose scores, Y_j, for a subject of chronological age are to be combined into biological age. The multiple linear regression equation is

$$\text{CA} = a + \Sigma b_j Y_j \qquad (1)$$

the summation being over test number $j = 1$ to n. Running the regression using norm group data produces coefficients a and the set of b_j from which Predicted-CA can be calculated for an individual's set of scores as:

$$\text{Predicted-CA} = a + \Sigma b_j Y_j \qquad (2)$$

The final step, and the one questioned here, is to define BA as follows:

$$\text{BA} = \text{Predicted - CA} \qquad (3)$$

At least since 1972, a troublesome side effect of the above traditional approach has been recognized, namely regression to sample mean age.[16,18,19,37,62,90] This effect causes BA values calculated for persons younger than the sample mean age to tend to be too old, and those for persons older than the sample mean age, too young. The effect will be considered further under "Methods" and "Results", and is illustrated in Figure 4, which shows that the sample's Predicted-CA values cover less of an age range than does sample CA.

Corrections were proposed by Dirken[18] and Dubina et al.,[19] in which an artificial change in slope and intercept were calculated separately for each physiological test in order to rotate the too nearly horizontal regression lines to 45° to the horizontal. This made the problem disappear cosmetically without, however, addressing its cause.

In the above procedure, CA is considered to be the dependent variable and scores the independent variables on the notion that CA is to be predicted from scores. However, CA does not depend on test scores but on the calendar. Therefore, it is meaningless to make CA the dependent variable and to use a regression equation designed to predict it. If predicted CA has no meaning, it is equally meaningless to equate BA to it. This applies to both simple and multiple regression.

Reversing the direction of the regression should solve the problem and is the approach used in this study. Regressing scores on CA precludes the use of multiple regression, requiring the substitution of individual regressions, one per measured variable. Later in this chapter, results obtained using the two methods are compared and the issue of whether reversing the regression eliminates the problem of regression to the mean is discussed.

b. Multiple Regression Automatically and Inappropriately Weights the Contributions of the Included Tests According to Their Correlation with CA

If correlation with CA is not a sufficient validation criterion, then it is inappropriate to weight biomarker scores according to this criterion in combining them into a single index, as occurs with multiple regression. Reversing the regression avoids this by avoiding multiple regression and furthermore permits the optional use of alternative weighting criteria. In this study, weights are based on each test's validation rating.

c. *Multiple Regression Produces "Wrong" Signs for Some Coefficients*

Frequently, when multiple regression is used to calculate biological age, one or more of the resulting regression coefficients in Equation 1 carries a sign that is opposite to the sign of the coefficient for the same physiological test obtained from a simple regression of CA on scores for that test alone. For tests that contribute to the multiple regression with the "wrong" sign, scores characteristic of older individuals in simple regressions inappropriately correspond to younger biological ages in multiple regressions, and vice versa, a consequence of applying the method of least squares fit. It does not make sense to use computational methods that equate poorer (adult) scores on any test to a younger biological age. The problem is removed by substituting individual regressions of scores on CA.

d. *Multicollinearity Can Confound Results of Multiple Regression*

Multicollinearity occurs when two or more of the independent variables in a multiple regression are strongly (but not perfectly) related to one another. This condition can lead to unstable and misleading estimates of the multiple regression coefficients. Examples are given by FVC and FEV-1. These tests are used in this study and have not infrequently been included in BA assessments. Not only are FVC and FEV-1 strongly correlated with each other, but each is correlated with a third variable, height, which must also be included on the right side of Equation 1. (Thus, multicollinearity would be a problem even if scores from only one lung function test plus height were included in a multiple regression.) Regressing scores on CA individually by test avoids this problem because scores and height can be placed on opposite sides of the equation.

3. *No Attempt was Made to Reduce Unwanted Variance in Calculating Biological Age*

The physiological tests used in this and prior studies of BA tend to differ markedly in variance. Table 5 illustrates this for the tests of this study. Standard deviations (S.D.) of the (transformed) test scores cover a 4 to 1 range. A problem arises when scores from tests that differ appreciably in variance are combined into a single index. An unknown part of each test's variance is "useful" in the sense that it represents genuine aging differences between individuals, while another part is "useless", originating from such sources as measurement error, baseline (e.g., inborn) differences between individuals, and short-term variations in test subject responses (e.g., differences in alertness, fatigue, etc.).[35] The problem is that combining scores from tests differing in variance can lead to information loss.

If (transformed) scores from the various tests were simply averaged in calculating a composite index of aging, the tests would contribute to the variance of their mean in proportion to their individual variances, quite the opposite of what is desired if most of the variability is useless rather than useful. This leads to the undesired condition that the useless variance contributed to the mean by high-variance tests will swamp the useful variance contributed by all tests. The result is information loss and a reduction of the ratio of useful to useless variance of the mean. This matter seems to have received little prior attention.

Standardization and weighting are variance control techniques. In the approach used in this study, transformed test scores are standardized (i.e., transformed to z-scores) before combining them. Because standardized transforms are in units of standard deviations, they contribute equal (i.e., unity) variance to their mean. Second, the approach optionally provides for weighting the contribution that each test makes to the mean according to any selected variable. In analyzing the study data, the weights used are the score each test earns on the biomarker validation criterion. The weighted mean, after being restandardized to put it into units of standard deviations, is designated "standardized biological age", SBA, the index of aging developed in this study. A method is added for calculating BA from SBA.

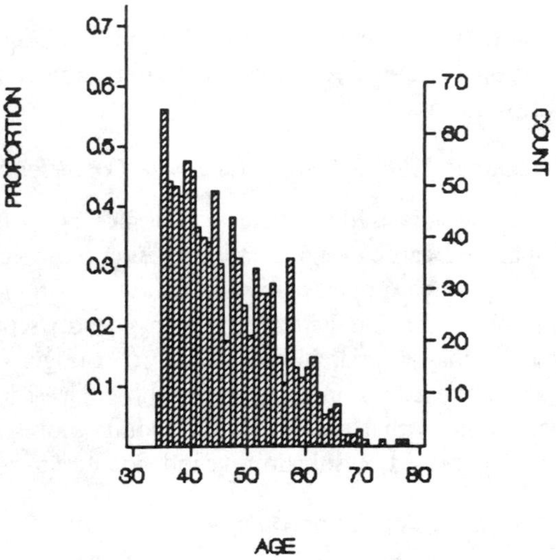

Figure 1 Age distribution of 977 male participants.

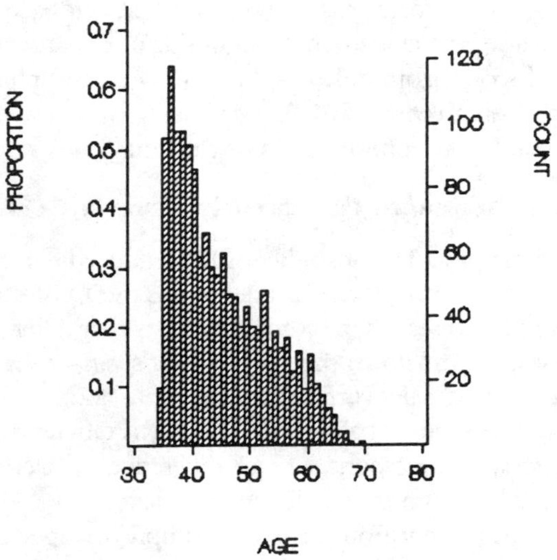

Figure 2 Age distribution of 1485 female participants.

II. METHOD

A. SAMPLE

Seventeen life insurance companies in various parts of the U.S. contributed a total of 2462 headquarters office employees as study subjects. Of the 1485 females, 1344 were white, 86 black, 23 asian, and 29 other, or declined to say. Of the 977 males, 931 were white, 22 black, 15 asian, and 9 other, or declined to say. Figures 1 and 2 show the age distributions of males and females, respectively. Test locations were selected to cover a range of different state life expectancies to allow investigation of the relationship between geographical factors and aging rate.

Table 3 Companies that made employees available for testing, number of participants of each sex, and state life expectancies at birth and age 45 by sex

	No. of subjects			State life expectancy[63]			
				At birth		At age 45	
Company	**Males**	**Females**	**State**	**Males**	**Females**	**Males**	**Females**
Allstate	53	110	Illinois	69.6	77.1	28.8	34.8
American General	58	139	Tennessee	69.2	77.5	28.4	35.1
American States	72	115	Indiana	70.2	77.5	29.0	34.8
American United	69	103	Indiana	70.2	77.5	29.0	34.8
Business Men's Assur.	67	86	Missouri	69.9	77.7	29.0	35.3
Chubb LifeAmerica	75	141	New Hampshire	71.4	78.4	29.7	35.5
Cuna Mutual	77	107	Wisconsin	71.9	78.9	30.2	36.0
E.F. Hutton Life	34	62	California	71.1	78.0	30.1	35.5
Gulf Life	84	112	Florida	70.1	78.0	29.9	36.0
Maccabees Mutual	35	40	Michigan	70.1	77.3	29.0	34.9
National Fidelity	20	43	Kansas	71.6	79.0	30.4	36.4
National Life of Vt.	50	68	Vermont	71.1	78.5	29.5	35.6
Pacific Mutual	82	128	California	71.1	78.0	30.1	35.5
Prudential	45	59	New Jersey	70.5	77.4	29.2	34.7
Southern Farm Bureau	96	106	Mississippi	67.6	76.4	27.9	34.6
United Insurance	39	38	Illinois	69.6	77.1	28.8	34.8
Unity Life	22	28	New York	70.0	77.2	29.1	34.7
Totals	977	1485					

Participating companies are listed in Table 3 together with number of subjects by sex, the state in which testing took place, and male and female life expectancies at birth and at age 45 in each test state. Each company was asked to select randomly up to 200 subjects from headquarters office employees aged 35 and above and to avoid volunteers (who might constitute a self-selected, healthier than average group). Participation was not mandatory, but most companies reported that only a small proportion of those asked to participate declined to do so. Use of life insurance company headquarters employees had the advantage of providing a study sample that was widely distributed geographically while being rather well matched educationally, occupationally, and socioeconomically.

B. PHYSIOLOGICAL TESTS AND INSTRUMENTATION

Table 1 lists the 12 physiological tests that were evaluated in this study as prospective biomarkers of aging. All had been included in one or more of the cited prior human studies of BA. They were selected for this study because they met the criteria for age-sensitive tests according to the earlier studies, were judged to meet the "quality of life" criterion, and could be made to fit the format of the automatic instrument the author developed to measure them. In addition, two of the selected functions, FVC and FEV-1, were judged to meet the "correlation with mortality rate" criterion.

The instrumentation used to administer the 12 physiological tests and the risk factor questionnaire was the H-SCAN (Hoch Company, Corona del Mar, CA), developed by the author. This instrument operates automatically, requiring no operators to be in attendance. Thus, data variance associated with differences in the quality of instructions and the degree of motivation provided by operators (important in performance-oriented tests) is eliminated. The instrument fits on a table top, is designed for field use, and can be set up quickly by untrained persons.

The H-SCAN includes headphones, a pulmonary flow transducer, a vibrotactile transducer, a viewer containing a computer-controlled lens system, a module with six push buttons and six lamps, and the electronic circuits that drive these transducers and components, collect and process data, and link the system to a desktop computer which provides the graphical user interface.

Subjects follow simple instructions that appear in large letters on the screen. Instructions are designed particularly to motivate subjects to perform maximally. Messages tend to be friendly, sometimes humorous, and have been revised many times as it was learned, over several thousand testing sessions conducted prior to this study, what mistakes participants were making. The program is designed to catch procedural errors or attempts to cheat and responds appropriately, prompting the participant to correct the error.

About 40 min are required to complete the 12 physiological tests, 10 min more for the risk factor questionnaire. Results are automatically printed out immediately after testing, and all data are stored on floppy disks from which the information was transferred to statistics software for analysis. To keep data from being lost during a power failure or other interruption in testing, data are stored after each test. The program remembers where it left off and, after the interruption is ended, resumes automatically from that point. For each of the 12 physiological tests, correlations with CA and their significance, variance, and other characteristics have been described by Hochschild.[35]

To gather the data for this study, H-SCANs were sent to the participating insurance companies for several weeks without accompanying personnel. Each company appointed an employee to the part-time task of overseeing the equipment and scheduling participants.

In the author's experience, the investment made in automating the tests produced the following returns:

1. Test operators were eliminated as a source of data variance
2. Repeatability of the procedure was improved over nonautomated tests, permitting data collected at different times and locations to be reliably compared and combined
3. The test format facilitated testing large numbers of subjects efficiently
4. There were almost no staff costs
5. There was no need to train operators or send personnel to test sites
6. Participants found the format attractive, resulting in high rates of participation among randomly selected subjects

C. DESCRIPTION OF TESTS

1. Vibrotactile Sensitivity at Fingertip

A finger is placed on a small metal bar vibrating at a frequency of 120 Hz. The vibration goes on and off unpredictably, and the task is to depress a button only while the vibration is felt. As long as the vibration is correctly identified, it continues to drop in amplitude. Button depression when the vibration is off causes an error message, restarts the test with a somewhat stronger vibration, and upon the fourth such error, cancels the test, resulting in a deleted score for this test. The program makes several passes through the limit of perception in order to define the boundary.

2. Memory

This spacial memory test is independent of verbal, color, or tone clues that tend to favor individuals with verbal, visual, or musical abilities. Six lamps light momentarily in random succession over six push buttons set in a row at a 1.5-in. spacing. The participant is asked to repeat the sequence a moment later by pushing the corresponding buttons in the same order. The first sequence is two buttons long. With each correct repetition, the prior sequence repeats and one position is added for a maximum sequence length of 16, which if reached terminates the test. After any miss, there is a chance to review the last sequence and to try again. If an error is made on two successive attempts, the test is ended. A different random sequence is generated for each test participant.

3. Vital Capacity and FEV-1

The participant is instructed to take the deepest breath possible, then blow it out forcefully and exhaustively through a small hand-held tube. The rotation of a very light impeller blade (moment of inertia 0.00148 g) on sapphire bearings is measured to $^1/_{16}$ rotation from pulses generated by four photoemitter-detector pairs encircling the tube, whose beams are broken by the blade. Volume accuracy is 2% of reading, repeatability 0.5%. The tube is fitted with disposable cardboard mouthpieces and is submersible for washing.

Forced vital capacity is the total volume of air exhaled during the effort while FEV-1 is the volume exhaled during the first second. Just prior to each of three efforts, a target time-volume curve appears on the screen. This is the average curve predicted for the participant's sex, age, and height. A real-time curve for the actual effort is traced instantaneously during exhalation next to the target curve, permitting comparison and providing motivation to try to beat the target curve. Faulty procedure produces helpful messages and prompts a repeat of the effort. If the participant is aware of a lung impairment, the test can be skipped by pushing a button.

4. Highest Audible Pitch

The H-SCANs headphones are capable of reproducing 30,000 Hz (well above the human auditory frequency range) and are provided with earcups to seal out external noise. A binaural tone in the headphones goes on and off at arbitrary times while it rises in pitch. The participant responds by depressing a button as long as the tone is heard. Button depression when the tone is off produces an error message and requires the test to be repeated up to four times, after which the test is abandoned, resulting in a deleted score. The program determines the boundary frequency at which the tone becomes inaudible, making several passes through that boundary. Persons who believe that they have a hearing impairment can push a button to skip the test.

5. Visual Accommodation

This test of the focal range of the eye is partly a measure of lens and lens-capsule elasticity and is largely independent of refractive errors. The program first establishes the kind of glasses (if any) the participant has brought. Contact lenses may be worn during the test, as may glasses correcting distance vision. Not permitted are multifocal or reading glasses. Persons who cannot read the instructions without them can push a button to skip the test, as can anyone who has difficulty with the first few steps.

The objective is to identify a small symbol visible in a 13-in.-long viewer containing an actuator-driven lens system under program control. The symbol, either a 0 or an 8, flashes on for 0.2 s, then off, at 1.3-s intervals. Usually a 0 comes up, but at random times there is an 8. The 0s are to be ignored and a button is to pressed whenever an 8 is seen.

Starting at the point of clearest vision (set by the participant before start of the test by a push button focusing procedure), the program advances the image in small steps toward infinity, reversing the motion slightly and narrowing the steps at each error until several errors have been made. The far point limit of focus, where the ability to distinguish the symbols is lost, is determined by several passes through that boundary. The near point limit of focus is determined in similar fashion. The score is the difference in diopters between the near and far points.

6. Psychomotor Indices

In the test of auditory reaction time, a button is pressed as quickly as possible in responses to a tone on the headphones. After a short practice session, the best five responses (measured to an accuracy of 0.001 s) in ten trials are averaged for the score.

Visual reaction time (VRT) and visual movement time (VMT), both without decision, are measured in a single procedure. A button is depressed until the illuminated lamp above it goes out, whereupon the finger is jumped as quickly as possible to a second, predetermined button. VRT is the time to release the first button, VMT the travel time to the second button. Each is measured to 0.001 s. In each case, the score is the average of the five best of ten tries. A short practice session precedes the scored run.

Reaction and movement time with decision are measured similarly except that six lamps light one at a time in an unpredictable sequence of the six buttons. The participant follows the jumping light by jumping a finger as quickly as possible from button to button. The light waits for the participant to jump, then proceeds after a short, unpredictable delay. Release time and travel time to the new button are the two measured parameters. Again for each parameter, the best five scores obtained in ten jumps are averaged for the final scores.

Alternate button tapping time is the time required to jump with one finger back and forth 30 times between two buttons spaced 7.5 in. apart. In all six of the psychomotor tests, program detection of faulty procedure or attempts to cheat prompts appropriate messages and sets up a repeat of the mismanaged step.

D. MISSING DATA

Scores for the physiological tests were listed as missing if a test was skipped at the election of the participant (usually for certain impairments), abandoned by the H-SCAN program due to excessive errors by the participant, or if the score was deleted for being sufficiently beyond expected limits to suggest a physical handicap, an improperly conducted test, or a testing malfunction. Conditions for score deletions were as follows, with the total number of male/female scores missing given in parentheses: vibrotactile sensitivity score if under 6 dB (38/45), memory if less than three jumps (34/126), both lung function scores if vital capacity was under 1 l or height was outside the working range of 140 to 220 cm (2/8), button tapping time if under 10 s (24/61), highest audible pitch if under 5 kHz (91/60), and accommodation if under 1.3 diopter (224/475). The large number of missing accommodation scores was due to malfunctioning viewers at 3 of the 17 test sites. No reaction or movement time scores were missing. All 12 test scores were available for 645 males and 881 females. No other outliers were deleted, nor were deletions made for any reason not stated. To avoid bias, all deletions were made before data analysis began.

E. RISK FACTOR QUESTIONNAIRE

Programmed into the H-SCAN to continuously follow the physiological tests, 33 multiple choice questions appear one at a time on the H-SCAN screen, answerable by the push of one of six buttons. No questionnaire answers were missing because the computer does not go on until it gets an answer. Information on two additional factors, namely life expectancy at birth and at age 45 in the states of residence (Table 3), was obtained from the National Center for Health Statistics.[63]

F. SELECTION OF MORTALITY RISK FACTORS IN TABLE 2

Table 2 lists the eight surveyed risk factors that were combined into composite validation variable, CVV. Their selection and the listed assigned weights were based on evidence of the association of these factors in healthy individuals with subsequent mortality. Weights represent subjective judgment of the strength of such evidence, based largely on literature cited under "Results" in separate "Background" subsections for each risk factor. When aspects of the same risk factor were represented twice in the list, the assigned weights (4 for exercise and 2 for state life expectancy) were split 50-50 between the two similar factors. To avoid bias, weights were assigned before data analysis began.

Evidence of relationships to mortality in healthy individuals exists for four other of the surveyed factors which were, however, excluded from CVV for the following reasons. Parental longevity was surveyed by asking whether a subject's natural mother or father or both had died before age 75. For most subjects, one or both parents remained alive and under 75. To have included these two factors would have reduced sample size by about 60% and would have introduced a bias favoring older subjects. A relatively weak predictor of mortality, parental longevity was further weakened in our survey by being limited to a simple determination of whether parents had reached age 75. Race (black/white) is a strong predictor of mortality, but the representation of blacks in our sample (4.5%) was too low for the effective use of that factor. Nevertheless, data for all races were retained for all analyses. The relationship between alcohol consumption and mortality remains ambiguous and apparently disease specific, being positively associated with cancer, negatively (in moderate quantities) with coronary heart disease, according to the cited evidence.

G. COMPOSITE VALIDATION VARIABLE (CVV)

In the description of the mathematical method to follow, virtually all variables are sex dependent. For this reason, all steps of the analysis are carried out separately by sex, whether explicitly stated.

To evaluate the 12 physiological tests of Table 1 as biomarkers of aging, the criterion in this study was correlation with CVV based on the eight mortality risk factors of Table 2. The following mathematical method, however, can be generally applied to any selected set of validation variables. Let m be an integer identifying one of N validation variables F_m (such as risk factor scores) which are to be combined into a single variable, CVV. Standardization (transformation to z-scores) is a useful method for putting differently scaled variables all on the same scale.

Designating the standardized transform of F_m as SF_m,

$$SF_m = \frac{F_m - \overline{F}_m}{\sigma_m} \tag{4}$$

where $\overline{F}_m$ is the mean and σ_m is the standard deviation of F_m for the norm group (in this study, the sample as a whole). Because a distribution of standardized scores always has a mean of 0 and an S.D. of 1, SF_m indicates how far F_m deviates from the norm group mean in units of standard deviations.

Weighting the SF_m in calculating their mean is appropriate when the included factors differ in quality as validators or when two closely related variables each deserve half-weight. Designated as mean validation variable (MVV), the weighted mean is

$$\text{MVV} = \frac{\Sigma W_m SF_m}{\Sigma W_m} \tag{5}$$

The weighting coefficients, W_m, used in this study are listed in Table 2. Summations are over the N values of m.

$$\text{CVV} = \frac{\text{MVV} - \overline{\text{MVV}}}{\sigma_{\text{MVV}}} \tag{6}$$

Having CVV in standardized form makes it possible (for example) to use normal curve scales to express results in percentiles of the norm group when results are nearly normally distributed. This is useful if CVV has additional applications such as estimating relative risk in a health risk appraisal (HRA).

Plotting SBA (calculated below) against CVV results in a scatterplot. One way to make such a plot more intelligible is to graph mean SBA by CVV decile (as in Figures 13 and 14).

$$\text{CVV - decile} = INT\left(10\frac{R}{S}+1\right) \tag{7}$$

Here, $INT(x)$ is the largest integer that is less than or equal to x, R is the rank of each CVV score, and S is the total number of sample cases. Higher rank and higher deciles correspond to higher risk. The number of cases per decile may not be exactly $S/10$ because cases having identical CVV scores will carry the same rank and all cases of equal rank are sorted into one decile.

H. AGE/SEX NORMS OF PHYSIOLOGICAL TEST SCORES IN TERMS OF CHRONOLOGICAL AGE

Standardized biological age is the composite index of aging to be developed. It is calculated from a subject's n physiological test scores, Y_j, where j is test number. For the 12 tests and over the age range 35 to 65+ of this study, eyeball examination indicates that the scatterplots of the Y_j vs. CA do not depart perceptibly from linear. Hence, n linear regression equations of scores on CA replace the multiple regression of CA on scores of Equation (1):

$$Y_j = d_j + e_j\text{CA} \quad \left(+f_jH\right) \tag{8}$$

where j = 1 to n, H is height, and the term in parentheses is added only when j designates a height-dependent test (FVC and FEV-1 in this study). No multicollinearity results because H is not on the same side of the equation as Y_j.

I. TEST AGE (TA_j)

Running the regressions of Equation 8 with the norm group data produces regression coefficients d_j, e_j, and as needed, f_j that can be used to calculate Predicted-Y_j for age CA on test j:

$$\text{Predicted-}Y_j = d_j + e_j\text{CA} \quad \left(+f_jH\right) \tag{9}$$

Equation (9) can be used in reverse to estimate the age equivalent of a participant's score on test j. This estimate will be termed "test age", TA_j, defined as follows:

$$\text{TA}_j = \text{CA for which the norm group's Predicted-}Y_j \text{ equals obtained score } Y_j \tag{10}$$

In effect, TA_j is the norm group age that is typical of score Y_j. Substituting TA_j for CA and Y_j for Predicted-Y_j in Equation 9 yields

$$\text{TA}_j = -\frac{d_j}{e_j} + \frac{1}{e_j}Y_j \quad \left(-\frac{f_j}{e_j}H\right) \tag{11}$$

with the term in parentheses again applying only when j is a height-dependent parameter. Equation 11 can be rewritten

$$\text{TA}_j = a_j + b_jY_j \quad \left(+c_jH\right) \tag{12}$$

using the definitions

$$a_j = -d_j / e_j \tag{13}$$

$$b_j = 1 / e_j \tag{14}$$

$$c_j = -f_j / e_j \quad \text{(lung function only)} \tag{15}$$

where the coefficients d_j, e_j and, as needed, f_j, are generated by the n regressions of Equation 8. Equation 12 represents n equations defining a participant's set of test ages, TA_j. For the 12 tests of Table 1 and the study group, the coefficients a_j, b_j, and c_j are listed by sex in Table 4 and can be used to plot score vs. age by test. These coefficients are based on the units of measurement listed in Table 1.

J. RELATIVE TEST AGE (RTA_j)

Differences in variance by test can be examined by dividing TA_j by CA to remove CA as a variable. Calling the result RTA_j for "relative test age",

$$RTA_j = \frac{TA_j}{CA} \tag{16}$$

RTA_j expresses the deviation of a subject's TA_j from its age/sex norm, which is 1. For example, $RTA_j = 0.9$ indicates a score on test j that corresponds, in the norm group, to a test age that is 10% younger than the participant's CA.

K. VALUE OF STANDARDIZATION AND WEIGHTING IN CALCULATING A COMPOSITE INDEX

An age-independent composite index of aging could be produced by averaging a subject's set of RTA_j. However, this will lead to information loss when the RTA_j differ widely in variance, as they do in this and most other studies of biological age (see Introduction and Table 5). The RTA_j will contribute to the variance of their mean in proportion to their individual variances with the result that the useful variance (variance related to aging rate differences between subjects) contributed by each test will be swamped by the useless variance contributed by high-variance tests.

This potential for information loss can be limited by standardization and weighting. The standardized transforms, STA_j, of the RTA_j will each contribute equal (unity) variance to their unweighted mean

$$STA_j = \frac{RTA_j - \overline{RTA}_j}{\sigma_j} \tag{17}$$

As usual, $\overline{RTA}_j$ and σ_j are the norm group mean and standard deviation of RTA_j for test j.

Even though the STA_j all have the same variance, they still differ in ratio of useful to useless variance. Variance in the composite index can be further reduced by weighting the STA_j according to a selected biomarker validation criterion, allowing relatively more valid biomarkers to contribute more heavily. Designating the weighted mean as MSTA,

$$MSTA = \frac{\Sigma w_j STA_j}{\Sigma w_j} \tag{18}$$

The summations are over the n values of j and the weights w_j are "biomarker validation scores" earned by the individual tests. In this study, these weights were the Pearson correlations, r, between STA_j and CVV as listed in Table 6. (It might have been as appropriate to use r^2, the F-ratios, or some other parameter describing the relationship.)

L. STANDARDIZED BIOLOGICAL AGE (SBA)

Standardizing MSTA produces the composite index of aging employed in this study, termed standardized biological age, SBA. Thus

Table 4 Norm coefficients, by sex, for calculating test age (TA_j) using Equation 12

j	1	2	3	4	5	6	7	8	9	10	11	12
						Males						
a_j	176.6	141.9	−66.54	−34.71	−144.1	113.8	109.8	−209.0	−327.1	−64.44	−273.7	−79.31
b_j	−6.894	−9.437	−0.223	−0.275	0.927	−0.530	−1.475	1.947	1.833	0.713	1.298	1.034
c_j			1.239	1.058								
						Females						
a_j	170.0	149.4	−55.44	−38.99	−140.6	127.7	111.0	−139.8	−358.3	−75.21	−227.5	−58.65
b_j	−6.31	−11.74	−0.280	−0.329	0.834	−0.619	−1.656	1.286	1.925	0.651	1.129	0.688
c_j			1.201	1.075								

Note: *Applicable units are given in Table 1. Height is in centimeters.*

$$\text{SBA} = \frac{\text{MSTA} - \overline{\text{MSTA}}}{\sigma_{\text{MSTA}}} \tag{19}$$

Although it is not in units of years, SBA is a particularly useful way to express an individual's BA or comparative aging rate. SBA expresses, in units of standard deviations, how far a subject's composite test score deviates from the norm for the subject's age and sex. At any age, SBA has a norm group mean of 0 and S.D. of 1. Positive values of SBA indicate subjects who are aging more rapidly than average by the included tests, negative values corresponding to slower than average aging. Contrary to the traditional concept of BA in units of time, SBA is age independent. Thus, it facilitates comparisons between experimental groups comprising individuals of mixed ages.

Our data indicate that SBA distributions are nearly normal over the age range of the study sample, essentially 35 to 65. Therefore, to good approximation, the usual normal curve percentile scales apply,[41] whereby 68.26% of individuals selected randomly from the norm population will have SBA scores between –1 and +1 S.D., and 95.44% of individuals will score between SBA = –2 and +2 S.D. SBA < –1.28 S.D. identifies individuals testing in the youngest (conventionally designated as the highest) decile for their age. The other decile boundaries occur at SBA = –0.84, –0.53, –0.25, 0, 0.25, 0.53, 0.84 and 1.28 S.D.

Mean standardized biological age, $\overline{\text{SBA}}$, can be calculated for mixed-age groups characterized by different levels of a factor of interest. For example, in Figures 13 through 31, $\overline{\text{SBA}}$ is the variable used to illustrate the relationship between 12-function aging rate and 17 surveyed health risk factors.

M. BIOLOGICAL AGE (BA)

Clarity is gained in describing $\overline{\text{SBA}}$ differences by additionally expressing these differences as differences in BA in units of years at some given age. Therefore, a method of calculating BA is needed. In deriving BA from SBA and CA, we are free to select any desired norm group mean, $\overline{\text{BA}}$, and standard deviation, σ_{BA}, for the following reason. Let z be the standardized transform of X:

$$z = \frac{X - \overline{X}}{\sigma} \tag{20}$$

This transformation also can be run in reverse. Any standardized variable, z, can be transformed into a new variable, X, having any selected mean $\overline{X}$, and standard deviation, σ,

$$X = \sigma z + \overline{X} \tag{21}$$

or, in terms of SBA and BA,

$$\text{BA} = \sigma_{\text{BA}}\text{SBA} + \overline{\text{BA}} \tag{22}$$

Here, $\overline{\text{BA}}$ and σ_{BA} can be given any appropriate values. The situation is similar to that encountered in defining the Stanford-Binet IQ scale, which also required the selection of an arbitrary mean and standard deviation. In that case, raw test scores, X, obtained on an IQ test by a norm population were first standardized to z-scores by Equation 20. IQ was defined in terms of these z-scores to have a mean of 100 and S.D. of 16,[41]

$$\text{IQ} = 16z + 100 \tag{23}$$

The choice of $\overline{\text{BA}}$ is not an issue. The concept of biological age implies that the average-scoring individual in the norm group should test his or her CA, i.e.,

$$\overline{\text{BA}} = \text{CA} \tag{24}$$

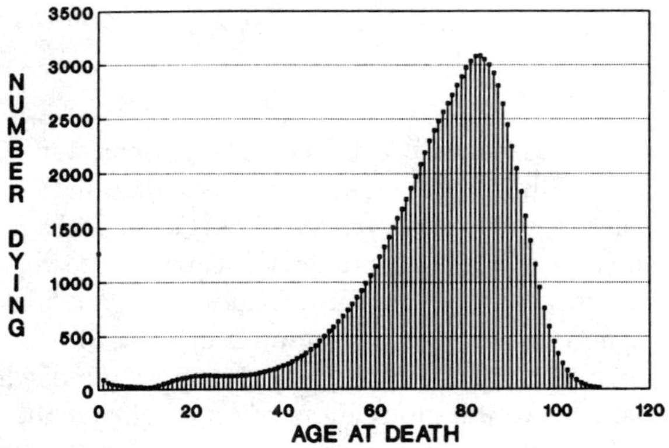

Figure 3 Distribution of U.S. total deaths per 100,000 live births, by age, males and females combined, 1979 to 1981.[88] Mean age at death is 73.4 years. The distribution has an S.D. of 18.1 years and a marked negative skewness.

No such obvious choice exists in selecting σ_{BA}. The preceding standardization and weighting steps wiped out any guidelines the data may have provided for determining σ_{BA}. As a first condition on σ_{BA}, it seems reasonable that it should be a function of CA because no postulated mechanism of aging can account for groups of young and old individuals having the same σ_{BA}. The simplest expression of this condition is to make σ_{BA} a linear function of CA with a zero intercept at CA = 0, i.e.,

$$\sigma_{BA} = c\text{CA} \tag{25}$$

As a second condition, the constant c remains to be selected. There is nothing critical about the choice of c any more than there was about the standard deviation of IQ scores. It seems reasonable, however, that the distribution of BAs around the mean age at death of the population under study should be similar to the distribution of deaths around the mean age at death. The latter is reproduced in Figure 3, which shows deaths at each age per 100,000 live births from U.S. Life Tables for 1979 to 1981 for males and females combined.[88]

The curve deviates appreciably from normal, having a marked negative skewness, and offers no more than a starting point for selecting c. Mean age at death is 73.4 years and the distribution has a S.D. of 18.1 years. Substituting these values, respectively, for CA and σ_{BA} in Equation 25 gives $c = 0.25$. To compensate for the skewness, the contribution of deaths below age 35 and the greater homogeneity of typical study populations, the author revised this value downward, setting $c = 0.16$ for human populations similar to the one of this study. Using Equations 22, 24, and 25, the definition of BA for human studies becomes

$$\text{BA} = \text{CA}(0.16\,\text{SBA} + 1) \tag{26}$$

How this choice of c works out in practice is illustrated in Figure 4. Here, the frequency distribution of BA values obtained by all females in the study aged 45 ±1 year, and for whom all 12 scores were available, is shown superimposed on the distribution of U.S. deaths. (For this illustration, all w_j in Equation 18 were set = 1.)

By selecting other values of c, custom tailoring of BA distributions is possible. Because the BA values are nearly normally distributed, normal curve percentile scales apply, and c can be selected so that a specified percentage of norm population members whose age is CA will obtain BA values that are within a specified number of years of CA. For example, in the distribution of 45-year-olds in Figure 4, 68.3% (±1 S.D.) of the norm population will obtain BA values that are within 7.2 years (0.16 x 45) of age 45. If c were assigned a value of 0.08 instead, then 68.3% of these 45-year-olds would have tested within 3.6 years of their age.

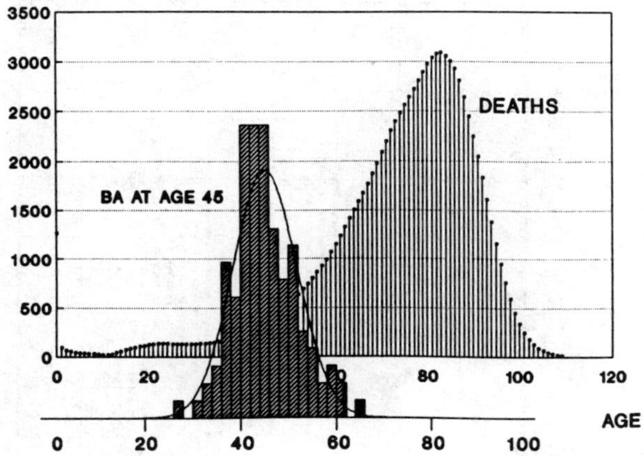

Figure 4 Frequency distribution of BA scored by all females in the study aged 45 ±1 years for whom all 12 test scores were available, superimposed on the distribution of U.S. total deaths by age.

III. RESULTS

A. ILLUSTRATION OF REGRESSION TO SAMPLE MEAN AGE

Using as an example only female data for test $j = 6$, highest audible pitch, Figures 5 to 8 illustrate results by the traditional method and by the method of this chapter, i.e., before and after reversing the regression. Figure 5 is a scatterplot of highest audible pitch scores, Y_6, (in units of kilohertz) vertically vs. CA horizontally. Of the two lines in Figure 5, the steeper represents the traditional direction of the regression (CA on scores) as in Equation 1 with $j = 6$ and the summation omitted because only one test is involved. The less steep line represents the reversed regression (scores on CA) of Equation 8.

Using the steeper line to convert an obtained score to predicted CA indicates that younger subjects tend to test too old and older subjects too young, a characteristic of the problem of regression to sample mean age. This effect is illustrated when predicted CA is plotted vertically against actual CA horizontally, as in Figure 6. For each data point in Figure 6, predicted CA is the X-axis coordinate of the point on the steeper line in Figure 5, whose Y-axis coordinate is the subject's highest audible pitch score. The distribution of points in Figure 6 is wider than it is high. The line shown in Figure 6 is the regression line of predicted CA on CA (not the reverse because CA is considered as the independent variable). This line fails to pass through coordinates 30,30 and 70,70 as it would if regression to sample mean age were absent.

B. RESULTS WHEN REGRESSION IS REVERSED

In contrast, the method of this chapter is based on the regression of test scores on CA, Equation 8, which defines the less steep line in Figure 5. The scatterplot in Figure 7 of test age, TA_6, vertically vs. CA horizontally, is generated using Equation 12 and the coefficients listed for $j = 6$ for females in Table 4. For each data point in Figure 7, test age is the X-axis coordinate of the point on the less steep line in Figure 5, whose Y-axis coordinate is the subject's highest audible pitch score.

In comparison to Figure 6, Figure 7 illustrates that regression to sample mean age is absent when test ages are predicted by the less steep line. (Note the contraction of the vertical scale in Figure 7. Some points lying beyond the upper and lower limits were cut off.) The line shown in Figure 7 is the regression line of TA_6 on CA. It satisfies the condition that it should coincide with the line between coordinates 30,30 and 70,70. (The reverse regression line, CA on TA_6, would regress away

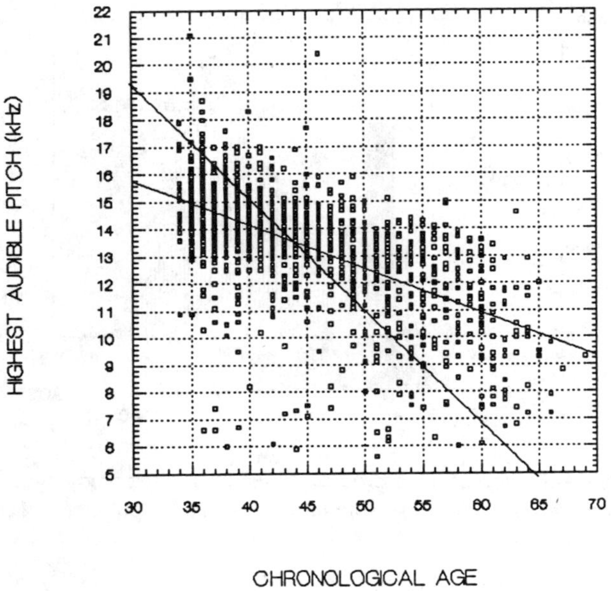

Figure 5 Highest audible pitch scores (in KHz) vs. CA for females. Steeper line is the regression line of CA on scores (Equation 1). Less step line is the regression line of scores on CA (Equation 8).

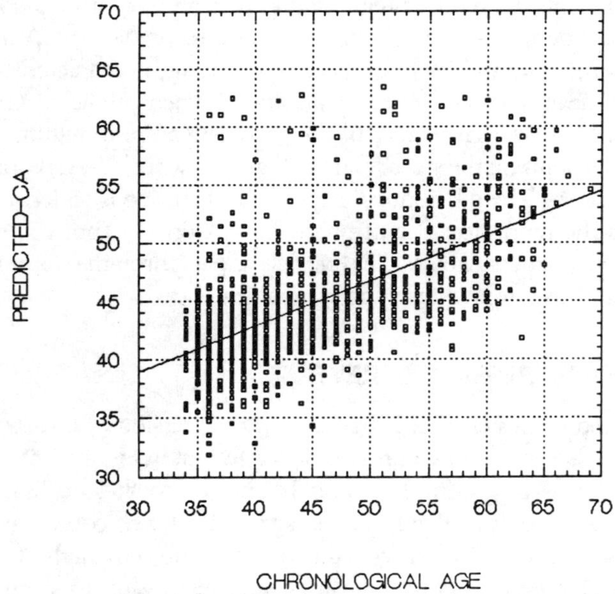

Figure 6 Predicted-CA, based on the steeper line in Figure 5, vs. CA for each data point in Figure 5. By failing to pass through coordinates 30,30 and 70,70, the regression line of Predicted-CA on CA illustrates regression to sample mean age.

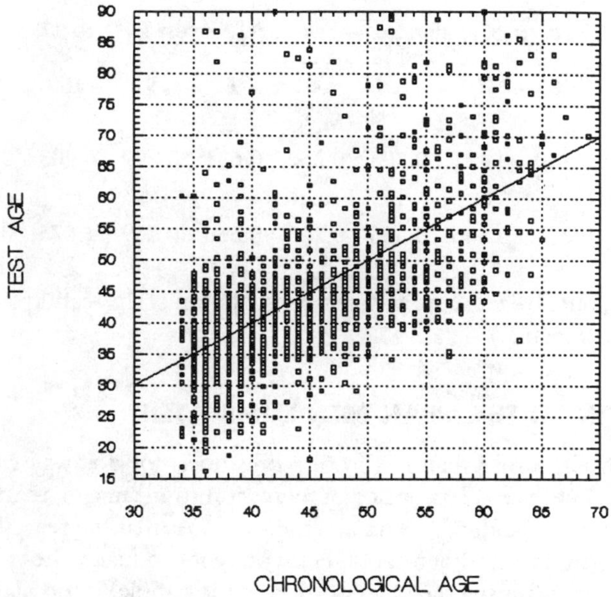

Figure 7 Test age, TA_j, based on the less steep line in Figure 5, vs. CA for each data point in Figure 5. By passing through coordinates 30,30 and 70,70, the regression line of TA_j on CA indicates absence of regression to sample mean age.

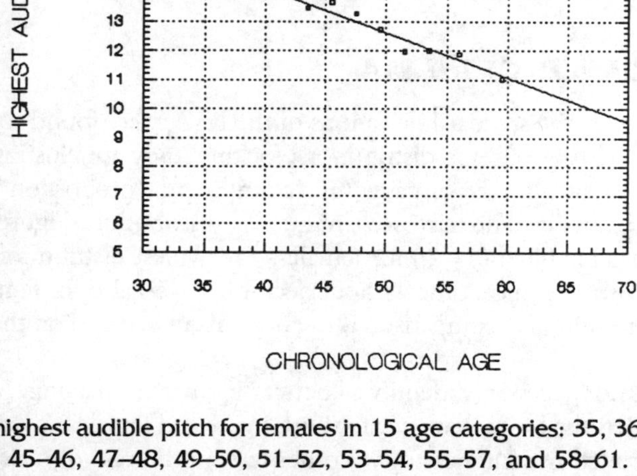

Figure 8 Mean highest audible pitch for females in 15 age categories: 35, 36, 37, 38, 39, 40, 41–42, 43–44, 45–46, 47–48, 49–50, 51–52, 53–54, 55–57, and 58–61. Regression line of mean pitch on median category age almost coincides with less step line in Figure 5.

Table 5 Standard deviations of relative test ages (RTA_j) for test j = 1 to 12

j	1	2	3	4	5	6	7	8	9	10	11	12
						Males						
S.D.	0.683	0.749	0.410	0.421	0.708	0.262	0.631	0.799	0.905	0.689	0.869	0.775
						Females						
S.D.	0.636	0.890	0.374	0.366	0.660	0.226	0.660	0.809	1.075	0.706	0.788	0.609

from sample mean age, but is not an appropriate representation of the scatterplot in Figure 4 because CA is the independent variable.)

C. HAS REGRESSION TO THE MEAN BEEN ELIMINATED?

Predicting scores from CA rather than CA from scores does not do away with regression to the mean, which occurs whenever $r < 1$. In place of regression to mean age, regression to mean score occurs instead. Lower-scoring individuals on average have CAs that the regression line of scores on age predicts to be associated with somewhat higher scoring individuals. The average predicted score of lower-scoring individuals (mostly the older portion of the sample) is too high (typical of younger individuals), and vice versa. Does this mean that results calculated for older persons still tend to make them score younger on average, and vice versa, as before?

Figure 7 illustrates that this does not happen, the explanation being that $r = 1$ (the condition for no regression to sample mean age) applies to the regression of estimated mean scores at each CA on CA. Estimated mean score at each CA is given by Equation 9, which is the equation of the less steep line in Figure 5. Predicted-Y_6 is an estimate of sample-mean Y_6 at each CA. This is demonstrated in Figure 8, which shows a regression line fit through 15 plotted points that are the actual sample means of Y_6 in 15 CA categories (category age range being adjusted to contain at least 80 points), namely 35, 36, 37, 38, 39, 40, 41–42, 43–44, 45–46, 47–48, 49–50, 51–52, 53–54, 55–57, and 58–61. The regression line of Figure 8 nearly coincides with the less step line in Figure 5.

In Figure 8, the correlation between the plotted means and CA is close to $r = 1$. For the less steep line of Figure 5, it reaches $r = 1$ (because the means are predicted) and regression to sample mean age is absent. It has been replaced by regression to sample mean score. (If the objective were instead to predict scores from age, it would be appropriate to trade regression to mean score for regression to mean age and use the steeper line in Figure 5. This can be accomplished by applying Equations 8 through 11 analogously, replacing age by score and score by age everywhere.)

D. RANGE OF VARIANCES OF THE RTA_j

For the 12 tests in Table 1, the standard deviations of the RTA_j were found to differ by more than 4 to 1 (see Table 5). The two extreme distributions for this study are illustrated in Figures 9 and 10. Both are histograms of number of cases (as "count" and "proportion" per standard unit) vertically vs. RTA_j horizontally. The narrowest frequency distribution, Figure 9, with $\sigma = 0.226$, occurred for highest audible pitch ($j = 6$) for females. The widest distribution, Figure 10, with $\sigma = 1.075$, occurred for visual reaction time without decision ($j = 9$) also for females. (Superimposed on each frequency distribution for comparison is the normal curve based on the sample's mean and standard deviation.)

Low variance does not necessarily identify a "better" biomarker of aging. An example is highest audible pitch. While it has the lowest variance for both males and females among the 12 tests of this study, highest audible pitch was inferior to two other tests in the case of males and to three other tests in the case of females in correlation with CVV (see Table 6).

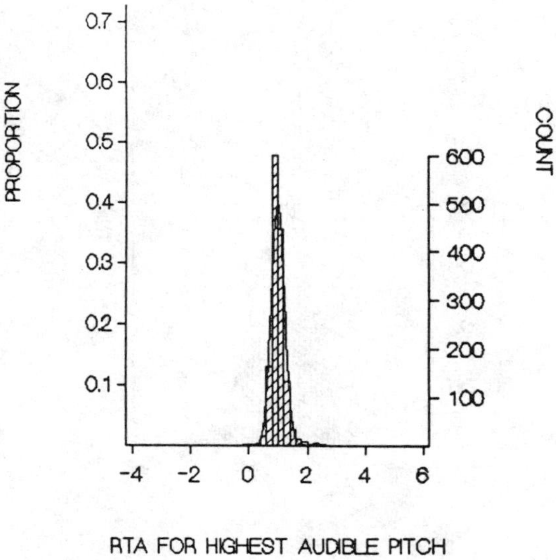

Figure 9 Frequency distribution of RTA_6, the relative test age for highest audible pitch, in females, before standardization. Mean = 1. S.D. = 0.226 (narrowest distribution in study). Normal curve with same mean and S.D. is superimposed.

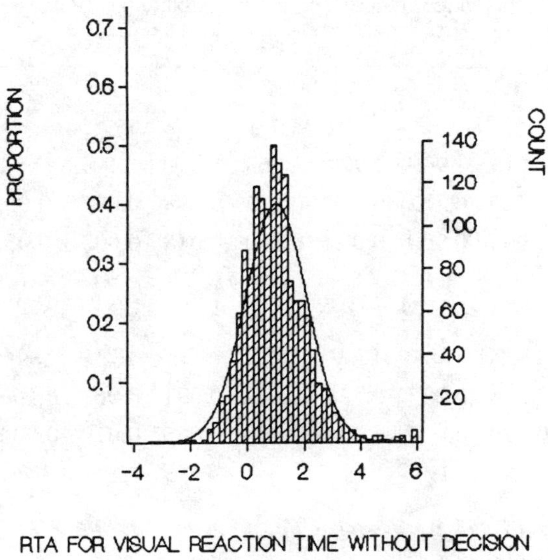

Figure 10 Frequency distribution of RTA_9, the relative test age for visual reaction time without decision, in females, before standardization. Mean = 1. S.D. = 1.075 (widest distribution in study). Normal curve with same mean and S.D. is superimposed.

E. EFFECT OF STANDARDIZATION

Two methods are used in this study to control the variance contributed by the individual tests to SBA, namely standardization and weighting. How standardization contributes to variance control is illustrated in Figures 11 and 12. Corresponding to Figures 9 and 10, respectively, these figures show the frequency distributions of the STA_j, the standardized transforms of the RTA_j, given by

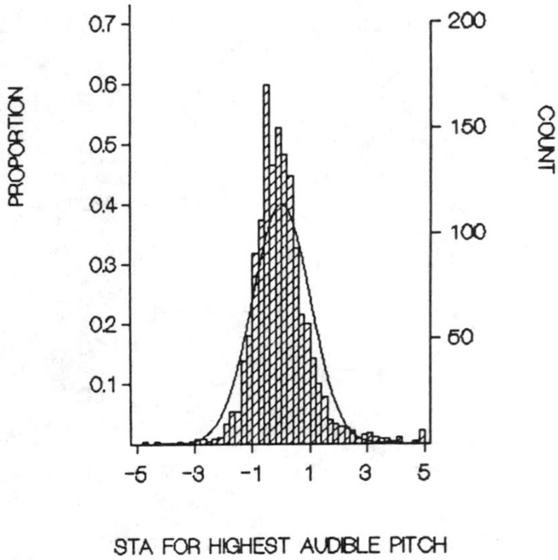

Figure 11 The frequency distribution of Figure 9 after standardization. STA_6, the standardized transform of RTA_6, has mean = 0, S.D. = 1.0.

Table 6 Number of subjects (*N*), correlation (*r*), and probability (*p*) for linear regression of CVV on STA_j for each test, *j*

j	1	2	3	4	5	6	7	8	9	10	11	12
						Males						
N	912	917	945	945	924	863	731	947	947	947	947	947
r	0.028	0.027	0.220	0.272	0.094	0.136	0.018	0.097	0.068	0.081	0.037	0.061
p	0.405	0.413	0.000	0.000	0.004	0.000	0.618	0.003	0.037	0.013	0.260	0.059
W%	2	2	19	24	8	12	2	9	6	7	3	5
						Females						
N	1355	1279	1387	1387	1337	1338	956	1394	1394	1394	1394	1394
r	0.016	0.103	0.216	0.227	0.128	0.102	0.091	0.063	0.166	0.096	0.093	0.059
p	0.550	0.000	0.000	0.000	0.000	0.000	0.005	0.019	0.000	0.000	0.001	0.028
W%	1	8	16	17	9	8	7	5	12	7	7	4

Note: The tabulated values of r *are used as weighting coefficients to calculate SBA.* W% *is the percentage of total weight contributed by each test to SBA.*

Equation 17, for the same two sets of data, $j = 6$ and $j = 9$, respectively, for females. Number of cases is plotted vertically vs. STA_j horizontally, in units of S.D. Both distributions have S.D. = 1 and a mean of 0. The STA_j contribute equal variance to their unweighted mean.

F. WEIGHTS BASED ON CORRELATION BETWEEN STA_j AND CVV

As a second method of variance control, Equation 18 provides for the weighted mean of the STA_j, where the weights w_j can be based on some measure of the validity of each test as a biomarker of aging. The selected validation and weighting criterion is the Pearson correlation between STA_j and CVV. For each test, this correlation is listed as *r* in Table 6, along with number of subjects, *N*, and

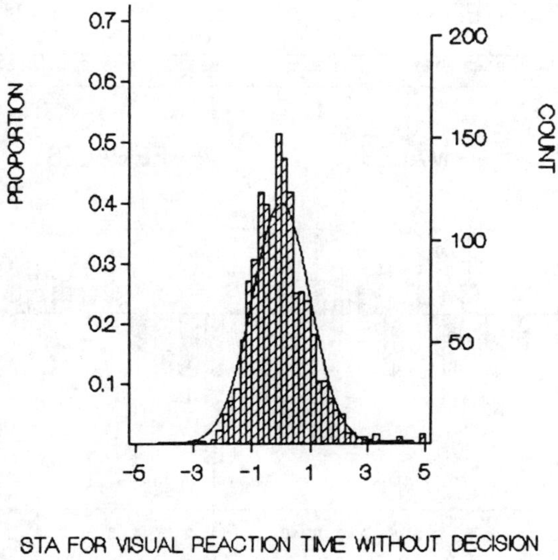

Figure 12 The frequency distribution of Figure 10 after standardization. STA_9, the standardized transform of RTA_9, has mean = 0, S.D. = 1.0.

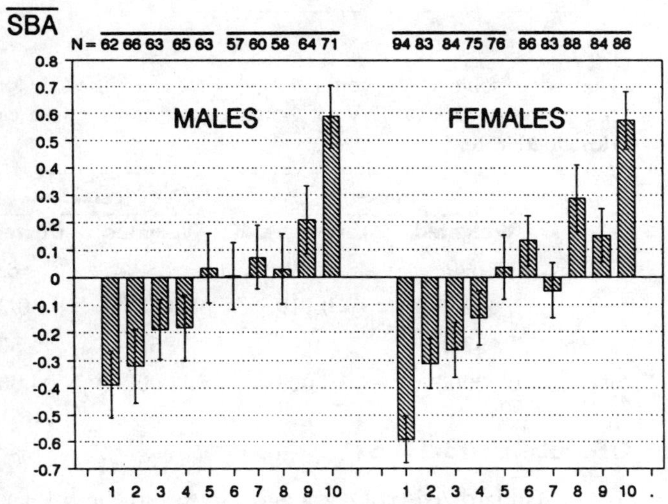

	r	F-ratio	P	r	F-ratio	P
REGR'N	.260	45.5	.0000000	.309	88.4	.0000000
ANOVA		25.7	.0000005		54.7	.0000000

Figure 13 Mortality risk decile.

probability, p, for each relationship. The high values of N account for the large number of significant p values despite low r values. Whether or not the r values, and the variation of CVV explained by each test, are trivial is considered in the Discussion. The W% line was added to show more clearly the percentage weight that each test contributes to SBA.

How the weighting step affects results is illustrated below in comparisons between Figure 13 (weighted case) and Figure 14 (unweighted case) and between columns marked "weighted" and "unweighted" in Table 7.

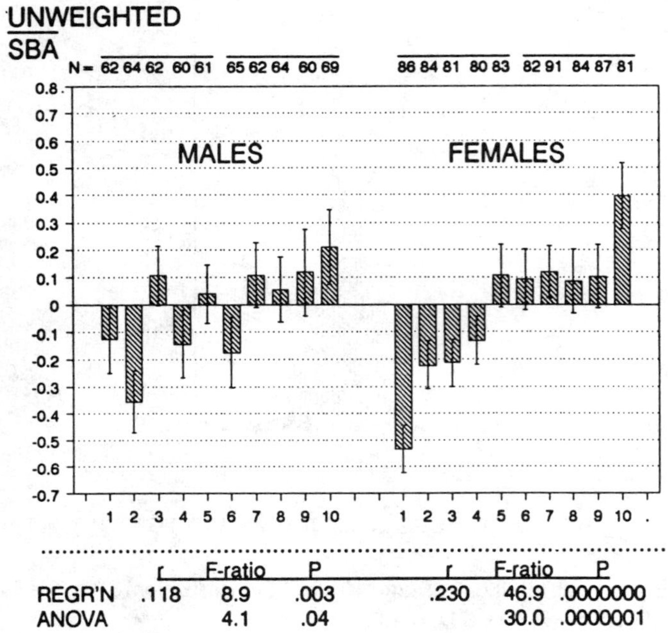

Figure 14 Unweighted mortality risk decile.

Table 7 Number of subjects (*N*), correlation (*r*), *F*-ratio, and *p* value for linear regression of SBA on CVV for weighted and unweighted cases as described in text

	Males		Females	
	Weighted	**Unweighted**	**Weighted**	**Unweighted**
N	629	629	839	839
r	0.277	0.119	0.321	0.238
F-ratio	52.2	9.0	96.1	50.1
p	0.0000000	0.003	0.0000000	0.0000000

G. EXPLANATION OF FIGURES 13 TO 31

Relationships between mean standardized biological age, $\overline{SBA}$, and the risk factors are presented as bar graphs in Figures 13 through 31. In all of these figures, $\overline{SBA}$ is the vertical axis coordinate, while the figure captions label the horizontal axis and identify the plotted factor levels. Because the risk factor questionnaire offered from two to six possible answers per question, horizontal axes have from two to six levels per sex, except for Figures 19 and 30, which are based on combinations of factors. Codes, when used to identify factor levels, are explained in the figure captions. Data for males are grouped in the left half of each chart, data for females are at right. Error bars designate standard error of the mean of SBA. The number of subjects, *N*, represented by each bar, is shown centered above the corresponding bar across the top of each chart (line beginning "N=").

No questionnaire answers were missing for any participant. However, in Figures 17, 23, 27, and 28, bars for "other" replies were omitted for clarity. Accordingly, the numbers listed across the top of these figures add up to fewer than the 645 males and 881 females for whom a complete set of all 12 physiological test scores was available (see "Missing data").

H. A WALK THROUGH FIGURE 15

Figures 13 to 32 attempt to condense more than the usual amount of information into a small space and, for this reason, an examination of one representative figure may help to clarify what is being shown in all figures.

The data for males in Figure 15 are used as the example. Of the 645 males for whom all 12 test scores were available, 518 were current nonsmokers. The first entry on the line labeled "N =" above the chart is 518. It is the entry above the bar labeled "0", designating no packs smoked, on the horizontal axis. This first bar extends downward, indicating a negative (younger than average) $\overline{\text{SBA}}$ and a lower than average aging rate. The other bars for males extend upward, indicating that a positive or older than average $\overline{\text{SBA}}$ and a higher than average aging rate was scored by men who smoke 0.5, 1, 1.5, and 2 packs per day on average as labeled on the horizontal axis.

The first bar extends downward to $\overline{\text{SBA}} = -0.08$ S.D. Using normal curve percentiles, this puts nonsmoking males at the 47 percentile level in terms of aging rate (which is as close to 50% as it is because 518/645 or 80% of sample males were nonsmokers). Using Equation 26 to convert to units of years and designating mean BA, for example, at CA = 45 as $\overline{\text{BA}}_{45}$, 45-year-old nonsmoking men scored $\overline{\text{BA}}_{45} = 44.4$ years. In contrast, the 40 men who said they smoke 1 pack per day on average (third bar) scored $\overline{\text{SBA}} = +0.33$ S.D., which gives $\overline{\text{BA}}_{45} = 47.4$ years, corresponding to a difference of 0.41 S.D. (3.0 years at age 45) between male nonsmokers and 1 pack per day smokers. For 70-year-old men, this difference in mean BA, $\overline{\text{BA}}_{70}$, corresponds to 4.6 years. Results for women are generally similar, as shown in the right half of Figure 15.

I. EXPLANATION OF TABLE BELOW EACH FIGURE

A small table below each figure shows the relationship, by sex, between SBA (not $\overline{\text{SBA}}$) and the horizontal axis factor levels, looking at the factor levels in two ways: as a continuum and categorically. Data in the left half of each table refer to males, data in the right half, to females.

The line labeled "REGR'N" lists the Pearson correlation, *r*, for the linear regression of SBA on the horizontal axis factor (designated in the figure caption). Also shown is the *F*-ratio which tests the significance, listed as *p*, of the relationship between SBA and the horizontal axis variable. All numerical data in these tables (as well as the bar graphs) are based on the w_j in Equation 18 being set equal to the *r* values in Table 6, except for data applying to the unweighted case in Figure 14 and Table 7. As a point of interest, one or two asterisks, representing $p < 0.05$ and $p < 0.01$, respectively, have been added to the *p* values to indicate relationships that are significant without this added weighting step, i.e., for all $w_j = 1$ in Equation 18.

Regression analysis is appropriate for those questions for which the factor levels are more or less continuous (e.g., 0, 0.5, 1, 1.5, and 2 packs of cigarettes smoked per day). Regression is less appropriate, although it can be used, for risk factor questions that produce categorical factor levels (e.g., dietary preference for chicken and fish over red meat), in which case analysis of variance is the more suitable test. The table below each figure gives results for both regression and one-way ANOVA, with contrasts, for all factors regardless of their continuous or categorical nature. In most cases, both are applicable, regression being the more sensitive test.

The data on the ANOVA line were based on estimation of contrasts,[66] in order to determine the probability that the SBA means were equal for two selected factor levels or, more commonly, for two selected groups of factor levels. In each figure, for each sex, the factor levels (bars) that are grouped together for the ANOVA contrast are designated by solid lines overscoring the number of subjects per bar across the top of each figure (the "N=" line).

For example, in Figure 15 the first level (nonsmokers) is contrasted with the remaining four levels (smokers) for each sex. The data on the ANOVA line are the corresponding *F*-ratio and probability, *p*, testing the significance of the selected contrast. As before, one or two asterisks on the p value indicate that the equivalent contrast in the unweighted case was significant at $p < 0.05$ or $p < 0.01$, respectively. For factors having only two levels, results for regression and ANOVA are identical and are combined into one line.

J. EXCLUSION OF RISK FACTORS FROM WEIGHTING STEPS

Absence of an asterisk on any p value in the tables under Figures 15 through 31 indicates a result that is not significant for the unweighted version of SBA. This occurred for three of the eight risk factors listed in Table 2 that make up CVV, namely the first three (Figures 15, 16, and 17). For these risk factors, it is necessary to determine whether an observed significance in the weighted case is dependent on inclusion of that risk factor in CVV. This was done by recalculating SBA substituting new weights in Equation 18, the new weights being set equal to the correlation between STA_j and a new value of CVV calculated by excluding, in Equation 5, the risk factor in question. These results are reported in the text describing Figures 15 through 22, which apply to the eight risk factors in CVV.

K. STANDARDIZED BIOLOGICAL AGE VS. MORTALITY RISK DECILE

Because it comprises eight mortality risk factor scores, CVV can be interpreted as an index of composite mortality risk. In Figures 13 and 14, CVV scores have been ranked into ten approximately equally populated "mortality risk deciles" using Equation 7. Decile 1 represents the 10% of the sample at lowest risk. The height of the bars shows $\overline{SBA}$ per decile, negative values representing younger than average results and positive values, older. A significant relationship was found between $\overline{SBA}$ and mortality risk decile whether or not SBA was calculated by the routine weighted method (Figure 13) or all weights in both Equations 5 and 18 were set = 1 (Figure 14). For men, the difference in BA between the lowest and highest mortality risk decile for the weighted case is about 1.0 S.D. (equivalent to 7 years at age 45). For women, it is 1.2 S.D. (9 years at age 45).

Comparing these figures illustrates the degree by which weighting sharpened the relationships. Referring to the tables below the figures, weighting increased the correlation between SBA and mortality risk decile for males from 0.118 to 0.260. For females, the increase was from 0.230 to 0.309. While not listed in the tables, weighting increased the correlation between $\overline{SBA}$ (the value designated by the bars) and mortality risk decile from 0.694 to 0.931 for males, and from 0.914 to 0.934 for females.

L. SBA VS. CVV (TABLE 7)

Some information is lost in exchange for the graphical clarity gained in ranking CVV into deciles. Table 7 gives the results of the regression of SBA (not $\overline{SBA}$) on CVV, listing number of subjects (N), correlation (r), F-ratio, and p value, by sex, for the weighted and unweighted cases. Weighting increased the correlation between SBA and CVV from 0.119 to 0.277 for males and from 0.238 to 0.321 for females.

M. CIGARETTE SMOKING (FIGURE 15)

In this and the following sections, 17 individual risk factors are examined briefly for how they relate to disease and death (see "Background") and how they relate to calculated BA (see "Results").

1. Background

According to the Surgeon General's annual report on smoking,[87] smoking is responsible for one out of every six deaths in the U.S. Many studies have identified cigarette smoking as strongly associated with subsequent all-cause mortality. These include the 6928-person Alameda County, CA, study,[11,95] the 5209-person Framingham Heart Study,[44,74] and the 5041-person Honolulu Heart Program.[7]

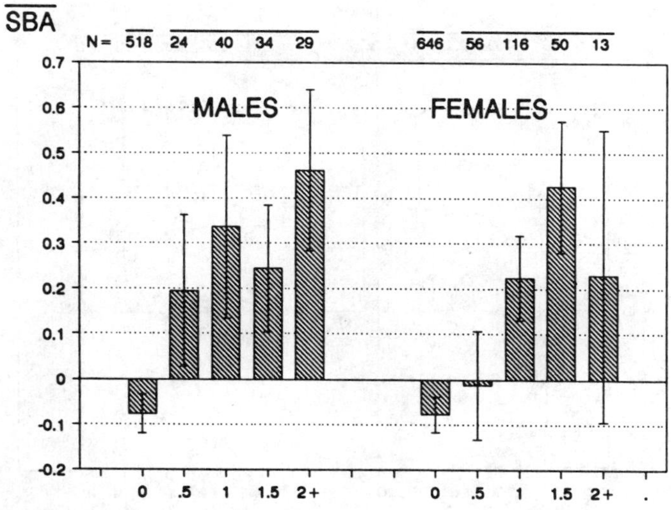

	r	F-ratio	P	r	F-ratio	P
REGR'N	.154	15.6	.00009	.143	18.2	.00002
ANOVA		15.0	.0001		9.5	.002

Figure 15 Cigarettes smoked per day (packs).

In the Alameda County Study, current smokers had a 51 (females) to 69% (males) greater age-adjusted mortality rate than never-smokers.

Virtually all life insurance companies have used separate premium tables for smokers and nonsmokers since shortly after 1979, when State Mutual Life announced the results of its 15 years of smoker vs. nonsmoker mortality experience, showing that the average 32-year-old male who smokes takes 7.3 years off his life compared to nonsmoking males.[17]

2. Results

Cigarette smoking was found to be a predictor of BA in both males and females (see Figure 15). The mean BA of both men and women who did not smoke at the time of the study was younger by about 0.4 S.D. (3 years at age 45) than that of current smokers as a group. In both sexes, the smokers' BA disadvantage tended to increase with number of cigarettes smoked per day. Asterisks missing in the table of Figure 15 indicate that results were not significant for the unweighted version of SBA. Standardized biological age, recalculated as described, eliminating cigarette smoking from the weighting step, remained significantly correlated with smoking level (for males, $r = 0.135$, $p = 0.0006$; for females, $r = 0.111$, $p = 0.0009$).

N. HIGH FAT FOODS (FIGURE 16)

1. Background

All-cause mortality among 12,763 men under age 60 was found to be directly related to percent calories from saturated fatty acids.[47] Kahn et al.[42] report increases in all-cause mortality with increased consumption of specific (but not all) high fat foods surveyed among 27,530 Seventh-Day Adventists. Enhancement of tumorigenesis by fat is discussed by Carroll,[13] who also graphs per capita breast cancer mortality in different countries vs. dietary fat intake. In a recent study of 250 Italian women with breast cancer and 499 controls, relative risks of breast cancer between the highest and lowest quartiles of consumption were a significant 2.1 for total dietary fat and 3.0 for saturated fat.[86]

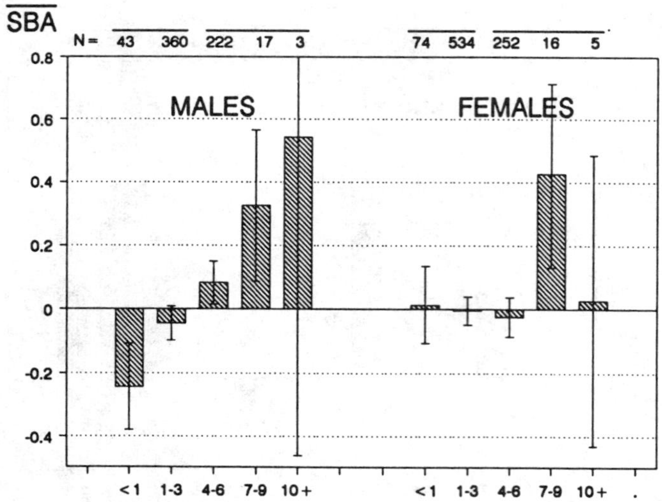

	r	F-ratio	P	r	F-ratio	P
REGR'N	.105	7.2	.007	.013	0.1	N.S.
ANOVA		4.2	.04		0.6	N.S.*

Figure 16 High-fat foods per day (average number of servings).

The suggested causal association of fat intake with breast cancer is supported by Phillips,[72] Miller et al.,[60] and Lubin et al.,[51] but not by a cohort study of nearly 90,000 U.S. nurses.[93] Butrum et al.[12] offer an up to date review of some of the abundant evidence linking fat consumption to cancer incidence, including some studies that demonstrated no association. Willcox and Lei[92] review the link between dietary fat and coronary heart disease.

2. Results

Figure 16 reports results of answers to the following question: "Consider the foods you eat that are high in fats, such as meat, cheese, fried foods, salad dressings, french fries, creamy soups, ice cream, etc. How many servings of high-fat foods do you eat per day on average?" Number of servings of high fat foods per day was found to be a significant predictor of BA in men but not in women (although the ANOVA relationship reached significance for women for the unweighted version of SBA).

On average, men who generally consumed ten or more servings of high fat foods per day tested older by 0.8 S.D. (6 years at age 45) than did men who consumed less than one serving per day. The rather smooth dependence in Figure 16 of $\overline{\text{SBA}}$ on number of servings between these two extremes may be something of a statistical quirk considering the standard errors. Similar results were not significant for the unweighted version of SBA. However, when servings of high fat foods were eliminated from influence on the calculation of the weighted version of SBA, the relationship between SBA and servings of high fat foods for males remained virtually unchanged ($r = 0.106$, $p = 0.007$).

O. PREFERENCE FOR RED MEAT VS. CHICKEN AND FISH (FIGURE 17)

1. Background

In a paper reviewing several studies of 27,529 California Seventh-Day Adventists, meat consumption was positively associated with all-cause mortality in males ($p < 0.001$) but not in females, with

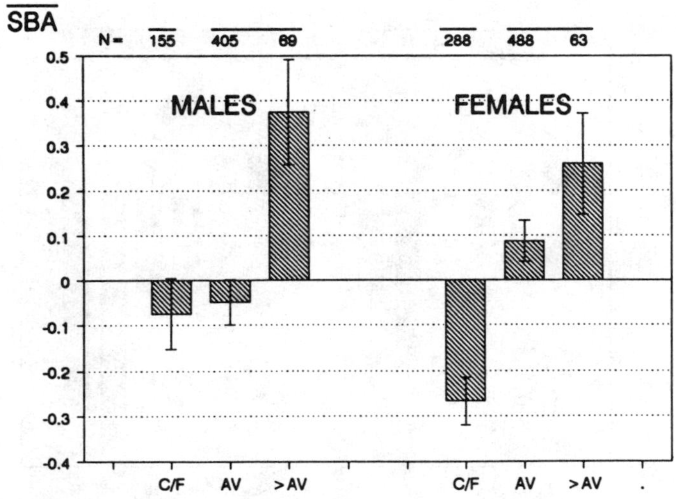

	r	F-ratio	P	r	F-ratio	P
REGR'N	.100	6.4	.01	.183	29.1	.0000001**
ANOVA		5.4	.02		26.3	.0000004**

Figure 17 Which best describes your diet? C/F: chicken and fish, but little red meat; AV: average amount of red meat; >AV: greater than average amount of red meat; "other" reply omitted.

coronary heart disease in males and females, and with diabetes in males.[81] Males consuming meat 6 d/week had a relative risk of death from all causes that was 1.7 times that of males consuming no meat. There is similar evidence that meat consumption is associated with fatal ischemic heart disease in men and women.[73,82]

In the study by Toniolo et al.[86] of 499 healthy women and 250 women with breast cancer, relative risks of breast cancer between the highest and lowest quartiles of consumption were a significant 2.9 for animal protein (which included dairy products) and nonsignificant risks of 1.4 for meat, 0.9 for poultry, and 1.0 for fish.

2. Results

As shown in Figure 17, the relationship between mean BA and dietary emphasis on red meat is significant for both men and women. Participants who characterized their diet as consisting of "above average amounts of red meat" tested biologically older on average by 0.46 S.D. (3 years at age 45) for men and 0.53 S.D. (4 years at age 45) for women than persons of like sex who described their diet as "fish and chicken but little red meat". Males and females who said they consumed "average amounts of red meat" scored an intermediate mean BA. Diets that did not fall into these three categories were omitted from the analysis. Using the unweighted version of SBA, this relationship was significant for women but not for men. When emphasis on red meat was excluded from the calculation of the weighted version of SBA, the relationships remained significant and little changed (for males, $r = 0.091$, $p = 0.02$; for females, $r = 0.178$, $p = 0.0000002$).

P. PHYSICAL ACTIVITY (FIGURES 18 AND 19)

1. Background

Paffenbarger et al.[67] studied 16,936 Harvard alumni aged 35 to 74, of whom 1413 died during a 16-year follow-up period. Death rates of the alumni declined steadily and significantly as energy regularly expended in physical activity increased from under 500 to 3500 kcal/week, beyond which

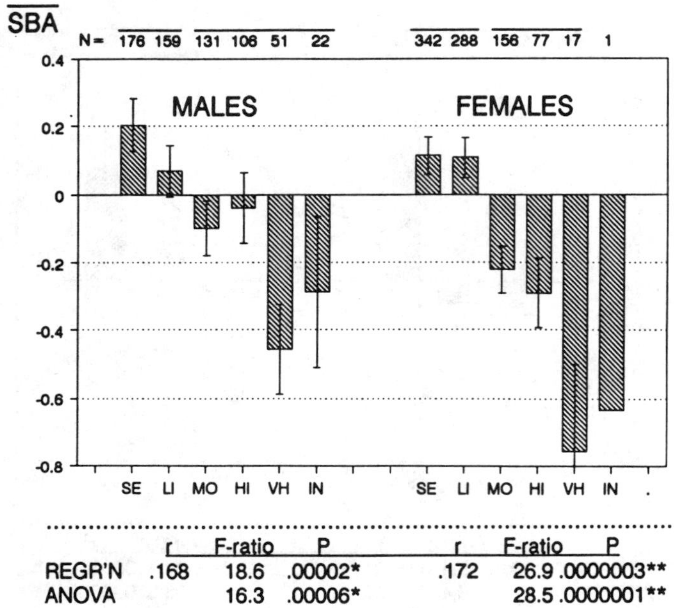

Figure 18 Average intensity of exercise. SE: sedentary; LI: light; MO: moderate; HI: high; VH: very high; IN: intense.

death rates increased slightly. Rates were ≈30% lower among alumni expending 2000 kcal or more per week than among less active men, with or without consideration of hypertension, cigarette smoking, extremes or gains in body weight or early parental death.

In the 6928-person Alameda County Study,[11,95] regular physical activity was associated with lower mortality from all causes. Among 16,882 British male civil servants, the incidence of coronary heart disease in those who engaged in vigorous exercise was about one third that in comparable men who did not.[61]

2. Results

Separate questions dealt with three measures of physical activity. Hours of physical activity per week were given as one of six levels: none, 1, 2, 3 to 4, 5 to 6, and >6. Aerobic intensity was selected from five levels: "light (like walking, golf), moderate (tennis, bicycling), high (jogging 10-min miles), very high (running 8 min/mi), and intense (more than above)." Five levels applied to the number of years the participant had been exercising: 0 to 1, 1 to 3, 3 to 6, 6 to 10, and >10.

Figure 18 shows results for the second of these three questions, namely average aerobic intensity. Significant inverse associations were found in both men and women, with and without weighting, between mean BA and aerobic intensity. These associations could not be confirmed at the highest intensity level, where $\overline{\text{SBA}}$ decreased nonsignificantly for men and was meaningless for women because only one woman classified herself in the "intense" category. The mean BA difference between persons who classified themselves as "sedentary" and "very high" was 0.66 S.D. for men and 0.87 S.D. for women (5 and 6 years at age 45).

In Figure 19, results are examined in terms of a composite exercise score, defined as the sum of the three exercise scores (hours/week + intensity + years, each on arbitrary scales from 1 to 5 or 1 to 6 corresponding to the levels listed above) divided by 2. There is a significant inverse dependence of mean BA on increasing composite exercise score for both sexes, regardless of weighting. On average, men whose composite score was <3 tested biologically older by 0.70 S.D. (5 years at age 45) than men who scored 8, the highest level. For women, the mean BA difference between the same two categories was 0.52 S.D. (4 years at age 45).

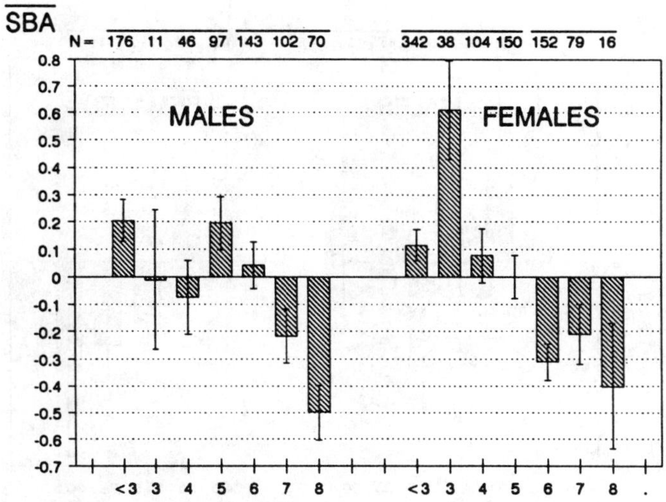

	r	F-ratio	P	r	F-ratio	P
REGR'N	.182	22.1	.000003*	.164	24.3	.000001**
ANOVA		8.3	.004		22.6	.000002**

Figure 19 Exercise, total of 3 scores ÷2 (hours/week + intensity + years, on arbitrary scales).

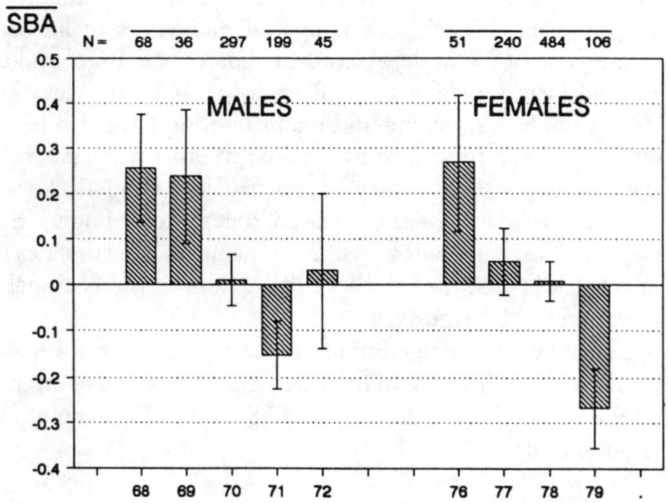

	r	F-ratio	P	r	F-ratio	P
REGR'N	.108	7.6	.006	.103	9.4	.002**
ANOVA		5.5	.02		9.5	.002**

Figure 20 Life expectancy at birth in state of residence (years).

Q. LIFE EXPECTANCY IN STATE OF RESIDENCE (FIGURES 20 AND 21)

1. Background

Sizable geographical variations exist in all-cause death rates in the U.S. These have been examined by county[77,78] and by state.[58,63] For men, U.S. state life expectancies at birth range from 67.6 years

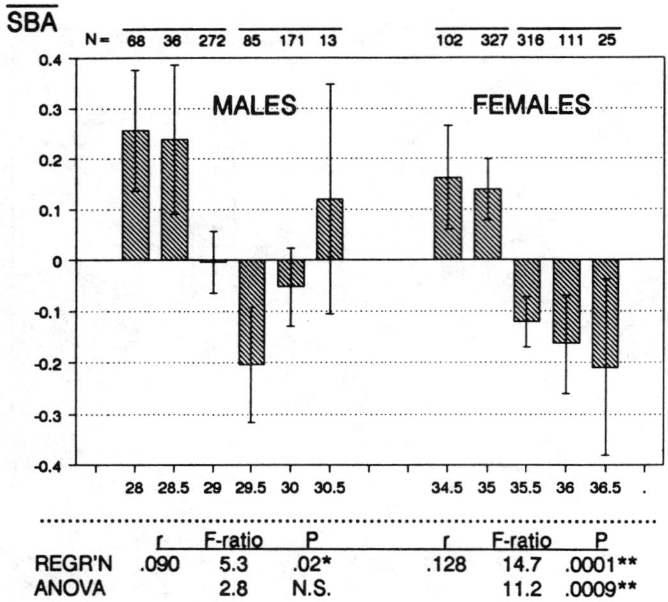

Figure 21 Life expectancy at age 45 in state of residence (years).

(Louisiana, Mississippi, South Carolina) to 74.1 years (Hawaii). For women, they range from 75.9 years (Louisiana) to 80.3 years (Hawaii). Geographical differences in life expectancy reflect a combination of variables, some of the more obvious candidates being race and ethnic origin, years of education, and regional dietary preferences. Effects associated with elevation above sea level, drinking water hardness, rural living, mining and manufacturing have also been observed.[78]

In organizing this study, it was of interest to examine whether persons residing in longer-lived states age less rapidly in the sense that they experience less rapid declines of the measured physiological functions than residents of shorter-lived states. Accordingly, in inviting insurance companies to participate, an effort was made to select companies located in states representing a wide distribution of life expectancies based on 1979 to 1981 data from the National Center for Health Statistics.[63] This goal was met only partially.

As Table 3 shows, our test states ranged in life expectancy at birth for males from 67.6 years (Mississippi) to 71.9 years (Wisconsin), 66% of the U.S. range. For females, our range was from 76.4 years (Mississippi) to 79.0 years (Kansas), 59% of the U.S. range. These ranges were, nevertheless, sufficient to show significant effects.

2. Results

Figure 20 shows the relationship between mean BA and state life expectancy at birth rounded to the nearest 0.5 year. Both men and women residing in longer-lived states tested significantly younger on average than men and women living in shorter-lived states. The mean BA of men living in states with a male life expectancy of 71 ± 0.5 years was younger by 0.40 S.D. (3 years at age 45) than that of men living in states with a male life expectancy of 68 ± 0.5 years. Women living in states with a female life expectancy of 79 ± 0.5 years were found to have a mean BA that was 0.54 S.D. (4 years at age 45) younger than women living in states with a female life expectancy of 76 ± 0.5 years.

Similar results were found in analyzing data for state life expectancy at age 45, (Figure 21). In this case, life expectancies were rounded to the nearest 0.25 year. BA relationship became more significant for women but less so for men. For both sexes, significance was reached regardless of weighting.

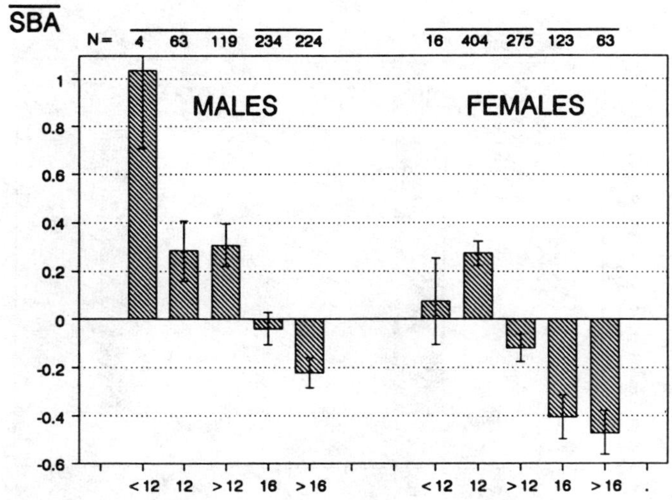

	r	F-ratio	P	r	F-ratio	P
REGR'N	.211	29.9	.0000001**	.264	65.8	.0000000**
ANOVA		14.5	.0002**		20.9	.000006**

Figure 22 Years of school completed. <12: less than grade 12; 12: high school graduate.; >12: less than 4 years of college; 16: college graduate; >16: more.

R. EDUCATIONAL LEVEL (FIGURE 22)

1. Background

Among 312 Catholic nuns in Minnesota assessed from 1936 to 1987, nuns with at least a bachelor's degree lived to a median age of 89.2 years, compared to 81.4 years for nuns with less than a bachelor's degree.[83] This study of the association of educational level with mortality rate is of particular interest because many of the usual correlates of low education in the general population, such as limited access to medical care, low income, poor housing, and smoking were not present in this population. Occupation was a factor, however. All of the more highly educated nuns were teachers, half of the less educated nuns did domestic work. The authors conclude that education is a robust marker for surviving, the causes remaining obscure.

Of 23 factors studied among 1474 Framingham Heart Study participants, education was one of five significant predictors of "survival with good function" in men, while in women, education was the only significant predictor besides age.[74] A Metropolitan Life study[56] of nearly 40,000 men demonstrated that college graduates lived an average 5 years longer than the population as a whole, while men graduating with honors lived an average 7 years longer, an observation that has been confirmed by more recent studies.[57]

Among 270,000 men employed by the Bell System, coronary heart disease (incidence and death) was 30% lower among college men than noncollege men regardless of age or occupation, the difference in risk seeming to be traceable to biological differences between college and noncollege men existing at the time they were hired.[33]

2. Results

Educational level was found to be a significant predictor of BA in both sexes regardless of weighting (see Figure 22). On average, male college graduates tested 0.33 S.D. (2 years at age 45) younger than males who stopped their formal schooling after graduating from high school. Female college graduates, on average, tested 0.67 S.D. (5 years at age 45) younger than females who stopped after

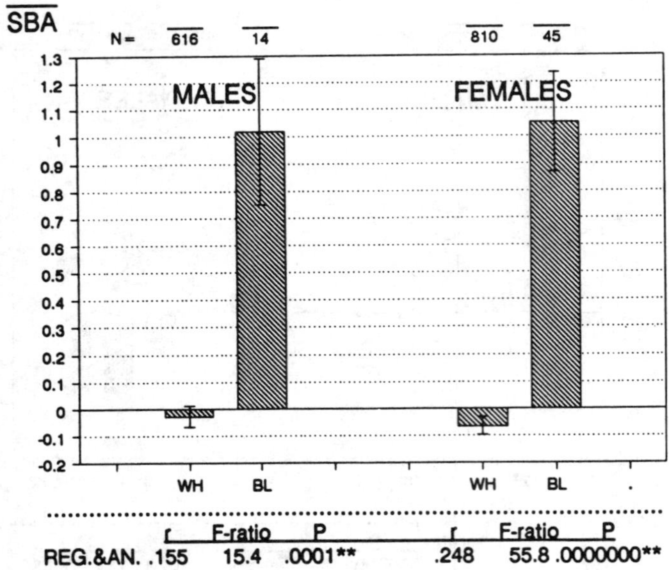

Figure 23 Race, black/white. "Other races" and "no reply" omitted.

earning a high school diploma. Additional education beyond college boosted these differences further but nonsignificantly.

S. RACE (FIGURE 23)

1. Background

Racial differences in mortality in the U.S. are substantial.[63] The issue is complicated by the large number of risk factors which tend to weigh more heavily on blacks than on whites, including nutrition, preventive care, high blood pressure, smoking, and injury control.[64]

2. Results

Figure 23 shows a mean BA difference of 1.04 S.D. (8 years at age 45) between black and white males, white males testing younger. Results were significant regardless of weighting. The standard error of this result is quite large due to the fact that the analysis included only 14 black males. White females, on average, tested 1.12 S.D. (8 years at age 45) younger than black females, based on 45 black females.

T. COFFEE CONSUMPTION (FIGURE 24)

1. Background

Investigations of the relationship between coffee intake and the risk of coronary heart disease have given inconsistent results. Positive associations were reported in three publications and no association in seven publications cited by Yano et al.,[96] who reported that a positive association among 7705 Japanese men living in Hawaii became insignificant when cigarette smoking was taken into account. A review by Leonard and Watson[50] cites two studies that showed positive associations of intakes of five, six, or more cups of coffee per day with risk of myocardial infarction, one study relating coffee consumption to all-cause death, and five studies showing no such associations.

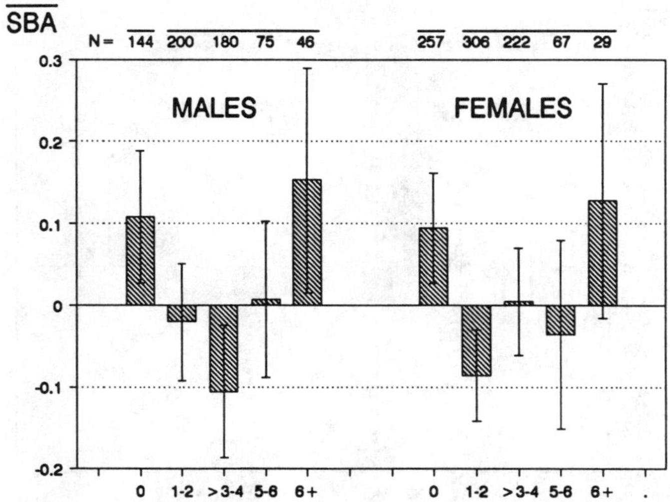

	r	F-ratio	P	r	F-ratio	P
REGR'N	.017	0.2	N.S.	.018	0.3	N.S.
ANOVA		1.0	N.S.		1.1	N.S.

Figure 24 Coffee consumption (average number of cups per day).

2. Results

Figure 24 indicates that BA was not significantly associated with average number of cups of coffee consumed per day. The possibility of a U-shaped relationship is suggested because, for both sexes, mean BA was older at the two extremes of consuming no coffee and consuming the highest amounts (more than six cups per day). However, standard errors were large at all levels of consumption, ruling out significance regardless of hypotheses as to shape.

U. CONTENTMENT SCALE (FIGURE 25)

1. Background

Of 22 variables that were found to be significant predictors of longevity among 252 participants aged 60 to 94 at the start of a 25-year longitudinal study at Duke University, work satisfaction was one of the three strongest predictors in men, and health satisfaction was one of the three strongest predictors in women (Palmore, 1982). In the same study, a weaker but nevertheless significant predictor of longevity was happiness based on a choice of one of 6 statements such as "these are the best years of my life" and "this is the saddest time of my life".

2. Results

Subjects were asked: "Where would you place yourself on the following contentment scale? 1 – Quite a bit happier than average. 2 – Happier than average. 3 – Average. 4 – More often depressed than average. 5 – Depressed most of the time." Regardless of weighting, BA was found to be significantly associated with contentment self-rating in women but not in men (see Figure 25). Compared to women who answered "more often depressed than average", women who answered "quite a bit happier than average" had a mean BA that was younger by 0.55 S.D. (4 years at age 45).

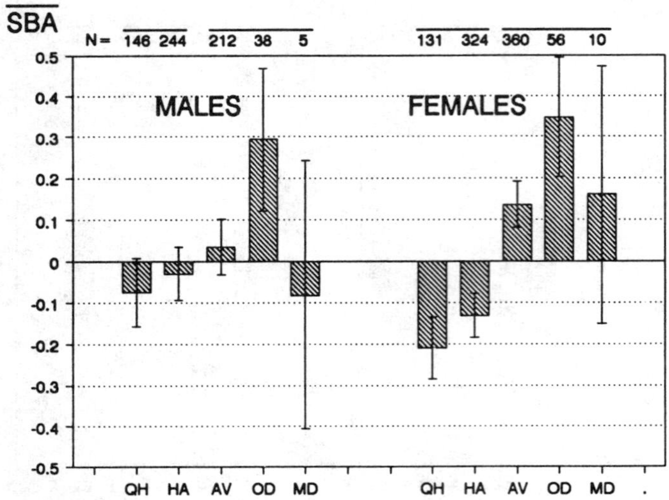

	r	F-ratio	P	r	F-ratio	P
REGR'N	.069	3.0	N.S.	.159	22.8	.000002**
ANOVA		0.6	N.S.		9.5	.002*

Figure 25 Contentment scale. QH: quite a bit happier than average; HA: happier than average; AV: average; OD: often depressed; MD: mostly depressed.

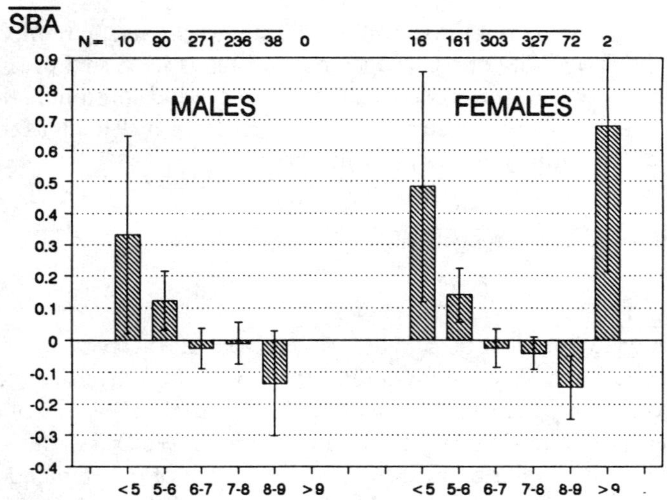

	r	F-ratio	P	r	F-ratio	P
REGR'N	.056	2.0	N.S.	.084	6.2	.01**
ANOVA		2.6	N.S.		7.6	.006*

Figure 26 Hours of sleep (average per night).

V. HOURS OF SLEEP (FIGURE 26)

1. Background

In a prospective study of 1,064,004 American men and women, sleeping <5 h/night was associated with a large decrease in life expectancy, <6 h/night with a small decrease.[25] In the Alameda County

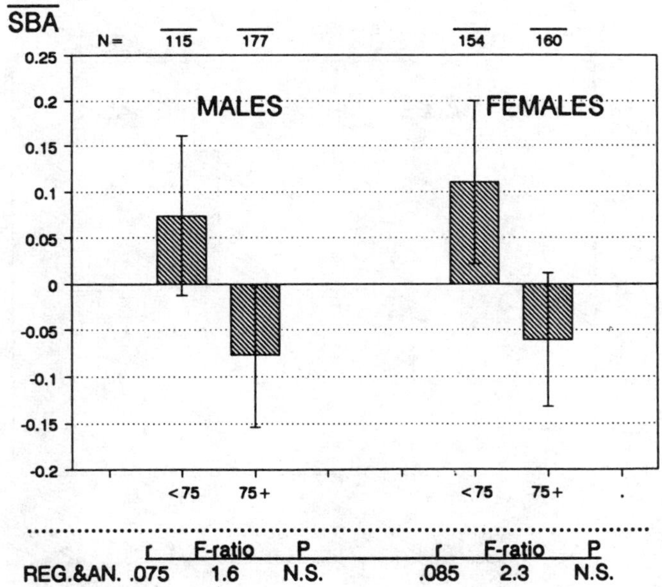

Figure 27 Natural mother's age at death. "Not yet 75" and "not sure" replies omitted.

Study, the 6928 participants were classified into two categories based on usual number of hours of sleep per night, namely "7 or 8 h" and "≤6 or ≥9". Both males and females sleeping 7 to 8 h/night had a significant ≈25% lower age-adjusted mortality rate then those sleeping ≤6 or ≥9 h.[11,95] In the Honolulu Heart Program study of 5041 men of Japanese ancestry, hours of sleep were not associated with health during a 12-year follow-up period.[7]

2. *Results*

In both sexes, BA was inversely associated with average hours of sleep per night, but the association was significant only in females (regardless of weighting). As illustrated in Figure 26, women who slept 5 to 6 h/night on average had a mean BA that was older by 0.29 S.D. (2 years at age 45) than that of women who got 8 to 9 hours of sleep per night on average. Women who slept <5 h/night tended to score older still. (The reversal for >9 h of sleep is not significant because only two females slept that long on average.)

W. PARENTAL LONGEVITY (FIGURES 27 AND 28)

1. *Background*

Long life runs in families, and a number of studies have explored genetic factors as contributors to longevity.[1,70,84,85] While mother's age at death was not a significant predictor, father's age at death was one of the weaker of 22 predictors of longevity for men (not women) identified by Palmore[68] in the Duke 25-year follow-up study of 252 ambulatory, noninstitutionalized residents of North Carolina aged 60 to 94 at the start of the study. Each additional year the father lived predicted about one third year more longevity for the men in the study.

2. *Results*

Participants were asked separately about the longevity of their natural mother and father. Those who answered "died under age 75" were categorized as "<75" in Figure 27 (mother) and Figure 28 (father). Subjects who answered "living and 75 or older" or "died at age 75 or older" were

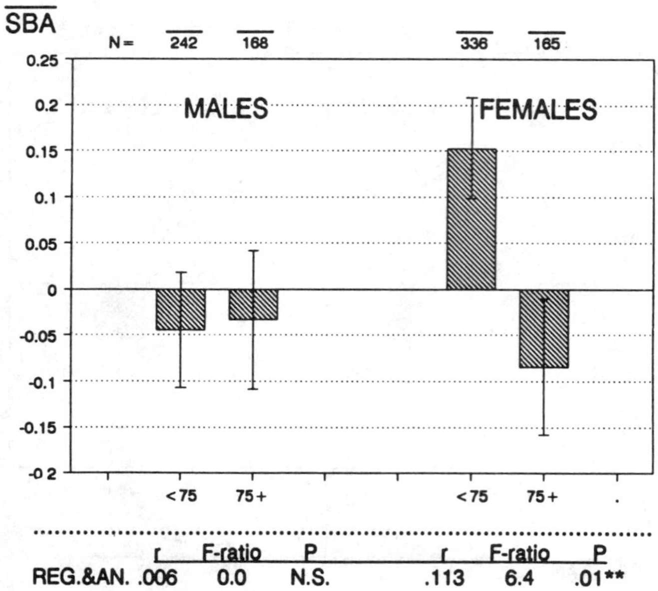

Figure 28 Natural father's age at death. "Not yet 75" and "not sure" replies omitted.

categorized as "75+". In both figures, subjects who answered "living; not yet age 75" or "not sure" were excluded. In consequence, 55% of the male subjects and 64% of the female subjects were excluded from the data in Figure 27. Likewise 36% of the male subjects and 43% of the female subjects were excluded from Figure 28.

Of the four relationships shown in these two figures, only one reached significance. On average, women whose father lived to age 75 or older scored younger biologically by 0.23 S.D. (2 years at age 45) than women whose father died at a younger age (significant regardless of weighting). No such trend was detectable in males. Mother's age at death produced trends in both males and females, but these were not significant.

X. VITAMIN SUPPLEMENTS (FIGURES 29 AND 30)

1. Background

A number of studies have shown that a decrease in risk of some types of cancer is associated with dietary intake of vitamin A,[24,49,59] β-carotene,[48,55,75,97] and vitamin E.[8] Results for vitamin C are inconsistent, protective effects against cancer being found in some studies,[43] but not in others.[65,76] A review of the literature and the current position of the National Cancer Institute on the subject of vitamins and β-carotene is given by Butrum et al.[12]

2. Results

Compared to persons of like sex who answered "no", mean BA was found to be significantly younger for women but not men who answered "yes" to the question "do you take any vitamin or mineral supplements (tablets, capsules, etc.)?". As illustrated in Figure 29, the difference for women came to 0.16 S.D. (1 year at age 45), which was significant regardless of weighting.

There was also a significant dose-dependent relationship (regardless of weighting) between mean BA and intake of vitamin C in women but not men. Figure 30 shows that women who listed their vitamin C intake as "high" (but below "megadose" levels) had a mean BA that was 0.57 S.D. (4 years at age 45) younger than women who said they took no vitamins.

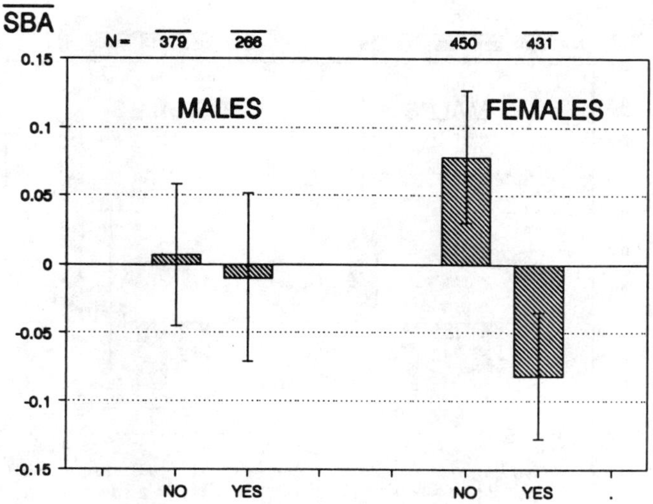

	r	F-ratio	P	r	F-ratio	P
REG.&AN.	.008	0.0	N.S.	.080	5.7	.02*

Figure 29 Are you taking vitamin or mineral supplements?

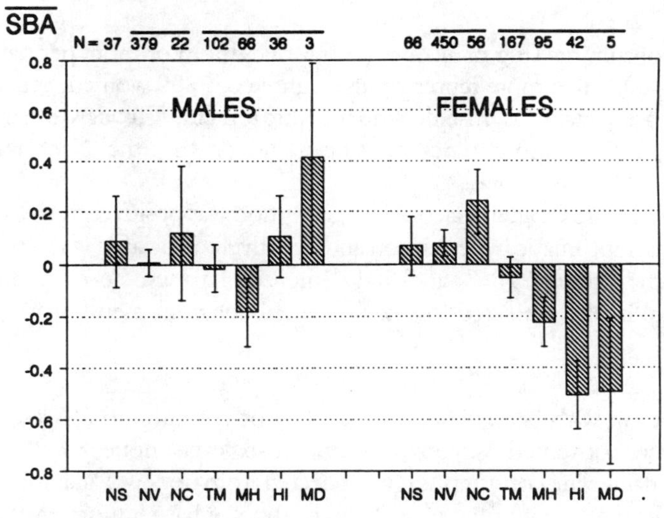

	r	F-ratio	P	r	F-ratio	P
REGR'N	.020	0.3	N.S.	.137	16.9	.00004**
ANOVA		0.0	N.S.		11.6	.0007**

Figure 30 Vitamin C supplements, daily intake. NS: not sure; NV: no vitamins of any kind; NC: no C, but other vitamins; TM: amount in typical multivitamin; MH: moderately higher; HI: high; MD: megadose.

Y. ALCOHOL CONSUMPTION (FIGURE 31)

1. Background

Of 17 cohort and case-control studies, almost all found a positive association between alcohol consumption and risk of breast cancer.[23] In a recent large cohort study of 89,538 nurses, Willett

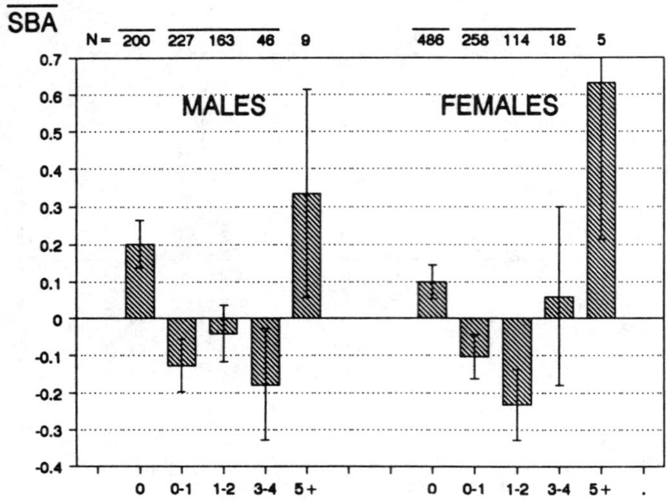

	r	F-ratio	P	r	F-ratio	P
REGR'N	.086†	4.8	.03*	.087†	6.7	.01
ANOVA		1.8	N.S.		2.6	N.S.

†Correlations are positive.

Figure 31 Total alcohol consumption (average number of drinks per day).

et al.[94] found that consuming 15 g of alcohol (about one drink) or more per day increased the risk of breast cancer by ≈60%. In a more representative sample of 7200 women, Schatzkin et al.[79] found a similar ≈60% increase which was dose dependent. Butrum et al.[12] review the association between alcohol consumption and various types of cancer and present the National Cancer Institute guidelines.

In the Honolulu Heart Program, alcohol consumption was positively associated with the risk of cancer, stroke, and asymptomatic hypertension and negatively associated with coronary heart disease (incidence and death) among 7705[96] and 5041[7] men of Japanese ancestry. In the Framingham Heart Study, alcohol intake predicted loss of functional ability in men but not in women.[74]

2. Results

Separate questions dealt with beer, wine, and hard liquor consumption. Average daily number of bottles or cans of beer consumed were given as one of six levels: none, <1, 1, 2, or 3, 4 or 5, and 6 or more. Average daily wine consumption was selected from none, <1 glass, 1 glass, 2 to 3 glasses, half bottle, full bottle. Average number of cocktails or shots of hard liquor per day was selected from none, <1, 1, 2, 3, 4, or more. Estimates[94] put the alcohol content of a bottle or can of beer at 13.2 g, a glass of wine at 10.8 g, and a shot of liquor at 15.1 g. Because all three are within 15% of 13 g and poured drink sizes tend to vary by more, 13 g was taken here as the unit "drink" size for each beverage, which allowed cans of beer, glasses of wine, and shots of liquor to be added to obtain average number of drinks per day. This is the horizontal axis coordinate of Figure 31.

A positive linear regression relationship was found between BA and alcohol consumption which was barely significant in men and only slightly more significant in women. Results are difficult to interpret because both relationships appear U-shaped. On average, persons consuming five or more drinks per day scored oldest biologically, while persons who drank no alcohol scored next oldest. Moderate drinkers tended to score younger biologically than the sample average. Relatively few persons said they consumed three to four or five and above drinks per day, which suggests that if all categories had been more nearly equally populated, the significance of the linear regression for both men and women would have disappeared.

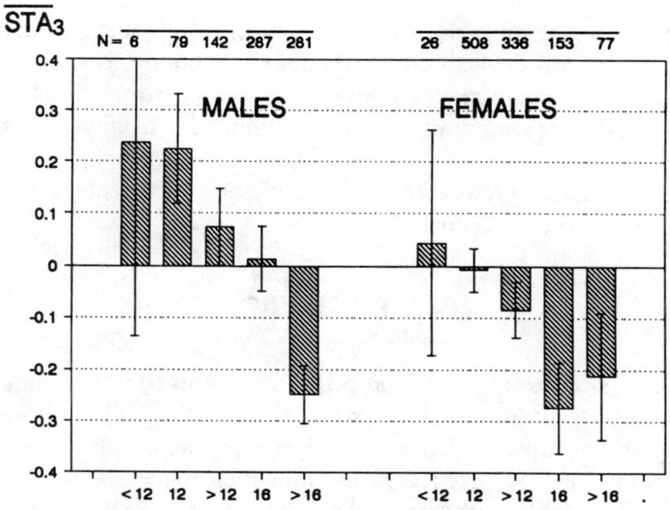

	r	F-ratio	P	r	F-ratio	P
REGR'N	.157	20.1	.000008	.089	8.8	.003
ANOVA		4.2	.04		5.5	.02

Figure 32 $\overline{STA}$ for vital capacity vs. years of school completed — nonsmokers. See Figure 22 for explanation of horizontal scale.

Z. RELATIONSHIP BETWEEN EDUCATION AND LUNG FUNCTION (FIGURE 32)

Additional insights can be gained by examining interventions in terms of their relationships to the individual physiological tests under study. In this study, 12 tests × 17 risk factors = 204 additional relationships that might be examined. A 204-item correlation matrix is not very meaningful unless supported by other analyses. In its place, just one of these 204 relationships will be examined in this article to demonstrate the potential value of this approach.

The selected relationship is not one of the most highly correlated relationships but it is one of the more interesting, namely FVC vs. years of school completed among nonsmokers. There is no obvious reason why level of education and lung function should be linked for nonsmokers except that both predict mortality rate (see Section III.R and Section I.C).

1. Background

Possible causes of the relationship between education and mortality rate are poorly understood. The cited study of 312 Catholic nuns[83] removed as variables some of the common correlates of education (socioeconomic status, housing, smoking, access to health care), but left a number of other correlates of education (occupation, intelligence, degree of life control, stress and stress hormones, diet).

2. Results

Figure 32 illustrates the relationship between vital capacity and level of education. Cigarette smokers have been excluded. This figure differs from the other figures in that the vertical axis coordinate is $\overline{STA}_3$, the mean value of standardized test age for vital capacity ($j = 3$) at each listed educational level. $STA_3 = 0$ designates subjects whose vital capacity is average for their age and sex. Positive values of STA_3 represent poorer vital capacities (an "older lung age") in units of standard deviations, and vice versa. The horizontal axis coordinate of Figure 32 is the same as that of Figure 22.

The data graphed and tabulated in Figure 32 indicate that when cigarette smoking is excluded, level of education predicts lung age. Among nonsmokers, more highly educated men and women had significantly better average lung function for their age, height, and sex than did less educated persons. On average, men with a college education but no additional formal schooling had a "lung age" that was 0.22 S.D. (2 years at age 45) younger than men who quit school after receiving a high school degree. For women, the same comparison corresponded to a difference of 0.27 S.D. (2 years at age 45).

The observed association suggests a link between physical and mental development. Nutrition may be a factor, as may genetic influences.

IV. DISCUSSION

Biomarkers of aging are needed to evaluate proposed treatments to retard aging rates. While there are many age-sensitive physiological tests, age sensitivity is not a sufficient condition to validate a biomarker of aging. A fundamental problem in assembling an experimentally useful battery of biomarkers has been the lack of a practical method for their validation.

This study sought to investigate the criterion that a valid biomarker of aging should be responsive to interventions that influence the natural life span. Twelve physiological tests (Table 1) were investigated as potential biomarkers of aging, being administered to 2462 study subjects who were also surveyed for 17 health and mortality risk factor "interventions". A mathematical approach was introduced for calculating a composite index of aging, standardized biological age, SBA. The approach addressed a variety of problems which, for reasons given in the Introduction, appear to invalidate traditional methods of calculating BA that used multiple regression. Relationships between the 12 prospective biomarkers, 17 risk factors, SBA, and a composite validation variable, CVV were examined in various aspects.

A. TOTAL VARIANCE OF CVV EXPLAINED BY THE 12 TESTED FUNCTIONS

The correlation between STA_j (Equation 17), and CVV (Equation 6), was used as the relative measure of the validity of test j as a biomarker of aging and to weight the STA_j in combining them into SBA (Equations 18 and 19). These correlations are given in the "r" lines of Table 6 by test number and sex.

For each sex, only 2 of 12 such correlations were found to exceed $r = 0.2$. The rest ranged from 0.027 to 0.136 for males and 0.016 to 0.166 for females. Squaring and summing these r show that the total variation of CVV explained by the 12 tested functions is 18% for males and 20% for females. Of these amounts, the amount attributable to the two best-correlated functions, FVC and FEV-1 ($j = 3$ and 4), taken together is 12% for males and 10% for females. The remaining ten functions explain 6% for males and 10% for females of the variability of CVV. These values err on the high side because the tested functions are interrelated. When the correlations for the weighted case given in Table 7 are squared, SBA is found to account for 8% of CVV variance for males, 10% for females.

Are some of the physiological tests included in this study experimentally useful biomarkers of aging, and if so, at what r^2 are we to draw the line? To answer this question, it is useful to estimate the highest r^2 that might be expected in terms of correlations of biomarker scores, transformed to STA_j, with CVV.

In this connection, an important issue is how well CVV predicts mortality. CVV comprises eight of a much larger number of possible mortality risk factors that were not surveyed. The eight factors are, to some extent, interrelated. Moreover, they represent crude estimates of risk because questions had a limit of six possible answers and, in most cases, provided only a rough assessment of the factor in question. There is also the unknown element of how accurately the questions were answered.

In summary, CVV is an imperfect measure of the risk factors which it incorporates and CVV is largely insensitive to many other influences on mortality risk, including known and unknown risk factors, genetic influences, chance events (illnesses, exposure to damaging agents), etc. Therefore, CVV, as constituted in this study, realistically cannot be expected to explain more than perhaps one fourth or one third of the variance of mortality rate, nor can a hypothetical battery of ideal biomarkers of aging be expected to explain more than that proportion of the variance of CVV. While this helps to put in perspective the finding that the variance shared between SBA and CVV in this study was only about 10%, it suggests considerable room for improvement in the selection of the battery of biomarkers composing SBA and the selection and scoring of risk factors (or other interventions) composing CVV.

B. TRIAL ACCEPTANCE CRITERION FOR A VALID BIOMARKER OF AGING

The results provide some guidelines for establishing a tentative quantitative acceptance criterion for a useful biomarker of aging based on CVV as composed in this study. If a value of $r^2 = 0.20$ were set as the lowest acceptance limit for SBA as an index of aging, then 12 unrelated tests constituting SBA would make an average individual contribution of $r^2 = 0.017$ which corresponds to $r = 0.129$. This number is low as an individual biomarker acceptance limit because actual biomarkers are likely to be interrelated, but it is high considering that it represents the average and that it may be useful to accept tests that are as much as 50% below average, particularly if they meet other criteria such as the quality of life criterion (See Introduction). In round numbers, $r = 0.1$ may be a reasonable trial acceptance limit for a biomarker of aging. Of the 12 physiological tests included in this study, only three qualify as biomarkers of aging under this criterion for males, while six qualify for females.

Certainly the 12 selected tests do not make up an ideal test battery for determining SBA. A few tests seem to be next to useless for the purpose. Likewise, the risk factor composition of CVV might be considerably improved. Despite these limitations, the study demonstrated the application of a quantitative approach for validating biomarkers of aging. This general approach might be used to evaluate other candidate biomarkers of aging in the future, leading to improved biomarker batteries.

C. RISK FACTOR BEHAVIORS PREDICT RATES OF FUNCTIONAL DECLINES IN HEALTHY PERSONS

Secondary to its main objective, the study asked whether risk factors that predict mortality also predict rates of functional decline with age. In looking at the results from this perspective, biomarker validation is not an issue. Rather than as putative biomarkers of aging, the 12 tests are viewed as what they are: tests of function. Likewise, SBA is seen not as a composite index of aging but as a composite index of function.

SBA was found to be responsive to a number of health risk behaviors of healthy persons. On average, individuals who scored more favorably with respect to various risk factors were found to have better function at any age than individuals who scored less favorably. Results suggest that on average, individuals who modify their diet and lifestyle in the direction of lower risk of major diseases are also delaying or retarding the onset of important functional declines in healthy persons.

Figures 15 to 31 show that many risk factors are significantly associated with SBA for both sexes, providing a split-sample validation of results. These risk factors were cigarette smoking, consumption of red meat, alcohol intake, intensity of exercise, a composite exercise score, life expectancy at birth and age 45 in the state of residence, years of school completed, and race. In males only, SBA was significantly associated with consumption of high fat foods, while in females only, significant associations were found with contentment score, hours of sleep, father living to age 75, intake of vitamin/mineral supplements, and intake of vitamin C supplements. SBA was not significantly related in either sex to mother living to age 75 or coffee drinking.

D. CAUSATION

Clearly, none of the reported relationships can be considered as causative. For example, persons emphasizing fish and chicken instead of red meat might be taking better care of themselves in other ways. Some of these ways could have influenced test scores. Some persons who engage in little physical activity might be disinclined to exercise for reasons of health or heredity, the reasons rather than the lack of exercise accounting for poorer functional scores. (Do runners have better lung function because they run or do they become runners because they have better lung function?) Nor is it clear that alcohol consumption in any quantity has beneficial effects on the aging process. Distinctions represented by alcohol may be cultural, socioeconomic, educational, genetic, or based on personality, all of which have been linked to life expectancy.

E. CAN A HANDFUL OF PHYSIOLOGICAL TESTS BE USEFUL IN EVALUATING TREATMENTS TO RETARD AGING?

Assuming that it becomes possible, as seems consistent with the results of this study, to identify a dozen or more biomarkers of aging that are valid by the proposed criterion or by a stricter one, and to base SBA on these, can such an index be expected to be experimentally useful in evaluating treatments to retard aging rates? It is reasonable to argue that the aging process is too complex and too limitless in its diversity of expression to be defined by a battery of biomarker tests, whatever its size. Ludwig[52] responds to this argument with the suggestion that "in science, not only pure reason governs, but also common sense (Max Planck), and common sense tells us that if the rate of progress of a variety of unrelated markers that correlate with chronological age is demonstrably decelerated by a given experimental variable (e.g., caloric restriction), the role of aging of the entire organism... has been modified too."

Ludwig[52] suggests that a relatively small number of biomarkers can be representative of many and that it is unnecessary to look at the full spectrum of age changes to know what is going on. The results of this study support that view. While the selection of the 12 physiological tests investigated in this study was far from ideal, results show that even an inferior index of aging is responsive to interventions that predict life expectancy in healthy persons. This suggests that the same index may also be responsive to other than the tested interventions. As additional tests are qualified as biomarkers of aging, it should be possible to develop increasingly sensitive tools for evaluating treatments to retard aging rates.

It is interesting that physiological correlates of risk factor behaviors can be detected by a handful of tests that were selected as generalized indicators of aging. The sensitivity of SBA to the risk factors suggests that SBA is measuring an aspect of aging beyond the obvious decline in the measured functions.

ACKNOWLEDGMENTS

I wish to thank Dr. David E. Harrison, Jackson Laboratories, Bar Harbor, ME; Dr. Donald K. Ingram, National Institute on Aging, Baltimore, MD; Dr. Frederic C. Ludwig, University of California, Irvine; and Dr. Matthew Witten, University of Texas, Austin, for stimulating and helpful discussions; and Drs. Harrison and Witten for their thoughtful review of this chapter and the valuable ideas they offered, many of which were incorporated in the manuscript. Thanks also go to the 17 life insurance companies listed in Table 3 who made employees available for testing and provided facilities and supervisory staff. Without their willingness to cooperate, this study could not have been done.

This chapter, with minor modifications, was previously published under the title "Can an index of aging be constructed for evaluating treatments to retard aging rates? A 2,462-person study," in the *Journal of Gerontology: Biological Sciences,* 45(6), B187-214, 1990. Reprinted with permission of The Gerontological Society of America.

REFERENCES

1. Abbott, M.H., Murphy, E.A., Bolling, D.R. et al., The familial component in longevity: a study of offspring of nonagenarians II. Preliminary analysis of the complete study, *Johns Hopkins Med. J.*, 134, 1, 1974.
2. Anderson, H.R., Respiratory abnormalities, smoking habits and ventilatory capacity in a highland community in Papua New Guinea: prevalence and effect on mortality, *Int. J. Epidemiol.*, 8, 127, 1979.
3. Ashley, F., Kannel, W.B., Sorlie, P.D., and Masson, R., Pulmonary function: relation to aging, cigarette habit, and mortality, *Ann. Intern. Med.*, 82, 739, 1975.
4. Baker, G.T. and Sprott, R.L., Biomarkers of aging, *Exp. Gerontol.*, 23, 223, 1988.
5. Beaty, T.H., Cohen, B.H., Newill, C.A. et al., Impaired pulmonary function as a risk for mortality, *Am. J. Epidemiol.*, 116, 102, 1982.
6. Beaty, T.H., Newill, C.A., Cohen, B.H. et al., Effects of pulmonary function on mortality, *J. Chronic Dis.*, 38, 703, 1985.
7. Benfante, R., Reed, D., and Brody, J., Biological and social predictors of health in an aging cohort, *J. Chronic Dis.*, 38, 385, 1985.
8. Bjelke, E., Dietary factors and the epidemiology of cancer of the stomach and large bowel, *Aktuel. Ernaehrungsmed. Klin. Prax.*, 2(Suppl.), 10, 1978.
9. Borkan, G.A. and Norris, A.H., Assessment of biological age using a profile of physical parameters, *J. Gerontol.*, 35, 177, 1980.
10. Bowden, D.M., Short, R., and Williams, D.D., Constructing an instrument to measure the rate of aging in female pigtailed macaques (*Macaca nemestrina*), *J. Gerontol. Biol. Sci.*, 45, 859, 1990.
11. Breslow, L. and Enstrom, J.E., Persistence of health habits and their relationship to mortality, *Prev. Med.*, 9, 469, 1980.
12. Butrum, R.R., Clifford, C.K., and Lanza, E., NCI dietary guidelines: rationale, *Am. J. Clin. Nutr.*, 48, 888, 1988.
13. Carroll, K.K., Experimental evidence of dietary factors and hormone-dependent cancers, *Cancer Res.*, 35, 3374, 1975.
14. Chodzko-Zajko, W.J. and Ringel, R.L., Physiological fitness measures and sensory and motor performance in aging, *Exp. Gerontol.*, 22, 317, 1987.
15. Comfort, A., Test-battery to measure ageing-rate in man, *Lancet*, 2, 1411, 1969.
16. Costa, P.T. and McCrae, R.R., Functional age: a conceptual and empirical critique, in *Epidemiology of Aging*, NIH Publ. No. 80-969, Haynes, S. G. and Feinleib, M., Eds., U.S. Government Printing Office, Washington, D.C., 1980, 23.
17. Cowell, M.J. and Hirst, B.L., Mortality Differences between Smokers and Non-Smokers, Report, October 22, 1979, State Mutual Life Assurance Company of America, Worcester, MA, 1979.
18. Dirken, J.M., Ed., *Functional Age of Industrial Workers,* Wolters-Noordhoff, Gröningen, 1972, 173 and 201.
19. Dubina, T.L., Mints, A.Ya., and Zhuk, E.V., Biological age and its estimation. III. Introduction of a correction to the multiple regression model of BA in cross-sectional and longitudinal studies, *Exp. Gerontol.*, 19, 133, 1984.
20. Duffy, P.H., personal communication, 1990.
21. Duffy, P.H., Feuers, R.J., Leakey, J.A., Nakamura, K.D., Turturro, A., and Hart, R.W., Effect of chronic caloric restriction on physiological variables related to energy metabolism in the male Fischer 344 rat, *Mech, Ageing Dev.*, 48, 117, 1989.
22. Furukawa, T., Inuoe, M., Kajija, F. et al., Assessment of BA by multiple regression analysis, *J. Gerontol.*, 30, 422, 1975.
23. Graham, S., Alcohol and breast cancer (editorial), *N. Engl. J. Med.*, 316, 1211, 1987.
24. Gregor, A., Lee, P.M., Roe, F.C., Wislon, M.J., and Melton, A., Comparison of dietary histories in lung cancer cases and controls with special reference to vitamin A, *Nutr. Cancer*, 2, 93, 1980.
25. Hammond, E.C., Some preliminary findings on physical complaints from a prospective study of 1,064,004 men and women, *Am. J. Public Health*, 54, 11, 1964.
26. Harrison, D.E., Experience with developing assays of physiological age, in *Biological Markers of Aging*, NIH Publ. No. 82-2221, Reff, M.E. and Schneider, E.L., Eds., National Institutes of Health, Bethesda, MD, 1982, 237.
27. Harrison, D.E., personal communication, 1988.

28. Harrison, D.E. and Archer, J.R., Physiological assays for biological age in mice: relationship of collagen, renal function, and longevity, *Exp. Aging Res.*, 9, 245, 1983.
29. Harrison, D.E. and Archer, J.R., Genetic differences in effects of food restriction on aging in mice, *J. Nutr.*, 117, 376, 1987.
30. Harrison, D.E., Archer, J.R., and Astle, C.M., The effect of hypophysectomy on thymic aging in mice, *J. Immunol.*, 129, 2673, 1982.
31. Harrison, D.E., Archer, J.R., Astle, C.M., Effects of food restriction on aging: separation of food intake and adiposity, *Proc. Natl. Acad. Sci. U.S.A.*, 81, 1835, 1984.
32. Higgins, M.W. and Keller, J.B., Predictors of mortality in the adult population of Tecumseh, *Arch. Environ. Health*, 21, 418, 1970.
33. Hinkle, L.E., Whitney, L.H., Lehman, E.W. et al., Occupation, education and coronary heart disease, *Science*, 161, 238, 1968.
34. Hochschild, R., Improving the precision of biological age determinations. I. A new approach to calculating biological age, *Exp. Gerontol.*, 24, 289, 1989.
35. Hochschild, R., Improving the precision of biological age determinations. II. Automatic human tests, age norms and variability, *Exp. Gerontol.*, 24, 301, 1989.
36. Hollingsworth, J.W., Hashizume, A., and Jablon, S., Correlations between tests of aging in Hiroshima subjects: an attempt to define "physiologic age," *Yale J. Biol. Med.*, 38, 11, 1965.
37. Ingram, D.K., Toward the behavioral assessment of biological aging in the laboratory mouse: concepts, terminology, and objectives, *Exp. Aging Res.*, 9, 225, 1983.
38. Ingram, D.K., Biological age: a strategy for assessment, in *Geriatrics and Gerontology Yearbook (U.S.S.R.)*, Chebortarev, F., Tokar, A. V., and Voitenko, V. P., Eds., Institute for Gerontology, Kiev, 1984, 30.
39. Ingram, D.K. Key questions in developing biomarkers of aging, *Exp. Gerontol.*, 23, 429, 1988.
40. Ingram, D.K. and Reynolds, M.A., Assessing the predictive validity of psychomotor tests as measures of biological age in mice, *Exp. Aging Res.*, 12, 155, 1986.
41. Jensen, A.R., *Bias in Mental Testing*, The Free Press, New York, 1980, 85.
42. Kahn, H.A., Phillips, R.L., Snowdon, D.A., and Choi, W., Association between reported diet and all-cause mortality. 21 year follow-up on 27,530 adult Seventh-Day Adventists, *Am. J. Epidemiol.*, 119, 775, 1984.
43. Kallistratos, G., and Fasske, E., Inhibition of benzo[a]pyrene carcinogenesis in rats with vitamin C, *J. Cancer Res. Clin. Oncol.*, 97, 91, 1980.
44. Kannel, W.B., Habits and heart disease, in *Prediction of Life Span*, Palmore, E. and Jeffers, F.C., Eds., Health, Lexington, MA, 1971.
45. Kannel, W.B. and Hubert, H., Vital capacity as a biomarker of aging, in *Biological Markers of Aging*, NIH Publ. No. 82-2221, Reff, M.E. and Schneider, E.L., Eds., National Institutes of Health, Bethesda, MD, 1982.
46. Kannel, W.B., Lew, E.A., Hubert, H.B., and Castelli, W.P., The value of measuring vital capacity for prognostic purposes, *Trans. Assoc. Life Insur. Med. Dir. Am.*, 64, 66, 1980.
47. Keys, A., Aravanis, C., van Buchem, F.S.P. et al., The diet and all-causes death rate in the Seven Counties Study, *Lancet*, 2, 58, 1981.
48. Kvale, G., Bjelke, E., and Gart, J.J., Dietary habits and lung cancer risk, *Int. J. Cancer*, 62, 1435, 1979.
49. Kvale, G., Bjelke, E., and Gart, J.J., Dietary habits and lung cancer risk, *Int. J. Cancer*, 31, 397, 1983.
50. Leonard, T.K. and Watson, R.R., The cardiovascular effects of caffeine, in *Nutrition and Heart Disease*, Vol. 2, Watson, R.R., Ed., CRC Press, Boca Raton, FL, 1987, 101.
51. Lubin, J.H., Burns, P.E., Blot, W.J. et al., Dietary factors and breast cancer risk, *Int. J. Cancer*, 28, 685, 1981.
52. Ludwig, F.C., Personal communication, 1989.
53. Masoro, E.J., A physiological approach to the study of aging, *Med. Times*, 117(5), 63, 1989.
54. Menkes, H.A., Cohen, B.H., Beaty, T.H., Newill, C.A., and Khoury, M.J., Risk factors, pulmonary function, and mortality, *Prog. Clin. Biol. Res.*, 147, 501, 1984.
55. Menkes, M.S., Comstock, G.W., Vuilleumier, J.P., Helsing, K.J., Rider, A.A., and Brookmeyer, R. Serum beta-carotene, vitamins A, and E, selenium, and the risk of lung cancer, *N. Engl. J. Med.*, 315, 1250, 1986.

56. College Honor Men Longer-Lived, Metropolitan Life Stat. Bull. No. 13, Metropolitan Life, New York, 1932, 5.
57. Socioeconomic Mortality Differentials, Metropolitan Life Stat. Bull. No. 56, Metropolitan Life, New York, 1975, 3.
58. Longevity Gains by State, Metropolitan Life Stat. Bull. No. 67(4), Metropolitan Life, New York, 1986, 12.
59. Middleton, B., Byers, T., Marshall, J., and Graham, S., Dietary vitamin A and cancer — a multisite case-control study, *Nutr. Cancer,* 8, 107, 1986.
60. Miller, A.B., Kelly, A., Choi, N.W. et al., A study of diet and breast cancer, *Am. J. Epidemiol.,* 107, 499, 1978.
61. Morris, J.N., Chave, S.P., Adam, C., Sirey, C., Epstein, L., and Sheehan, D.J., Vigorous exercise in leisure-time and the incidence of coronary heart-disease, *Lancet,* 1, 333, 1973.
62. Nakamura, E., Kimura, M., Nagata, H., Miyao, K., and Ozeki, T., Evaluation of the progress of aging based on specific biological age as estimated by various physiological functions, *Nippon Eiseigaku Zasshi,* 36, 853, 1982.
63. National Center for Health Statistics, U.S. Decennial Life Tables 1979-81, Vol. 1, No. 1 and Vol. 2, No. 1 to 51, U.S. Department of Health and Human Services Publ. No. (PHS) 85-1150-1 and (PHS) 86-1151-1-51, DHHS, Hyattsville, MD, 1985.
64. National Center for Health Statistics, Health Promotion and Disease Prevention, United States, 1985, Data from the National Health Survey, Vital and Health Statistics Ser. 10, No. 163, U.S. Department of Health and Human Services Publ. No. (PHS) 88-1591, DHHS, Hyattsville, MD, 1988.
65. National Research Council, Assembly of Life Sciences, Committee on Diet, Nutrition and Cancer, *Diet, Nutrition and Cancer,* National Academy Press, Washington, D.C., 1982.
66. Neter, J., Wassermann, W., and Kutner, M.H., *Applied Linear Statistical Models,* 2nd ed., Richard D. Irwin, Homewood, IL, 1985, Sects. 16.2–16.9 and 17.1.
67. Paffenbarger, R.S., Hyde, R.T., Wing, A.L., Hsieh, C., Physical activity, all-cause mortality, and longevity of college alumni, *N. Engl. J. Med.,* 314, 605, 1986.
68. Palmore, E.B., Predictors of the longevity difference: a 25-year follow up, *Gerontologist,* 22, 513, 1982.
69. Pardee, N.E., Winterbauer, R.H., Morgan, E.H., and Allen, J.D., Determination of mortality risk in obstructive pulmonary syndromes: physical examination compared with measurement of forced expired volume in one second, *Thorax,* 36, 928, 1981.
70. Pearl, R. and Pearl, R. de W., *The Ancestry of the Long-Lived,* H. Milford, London, 1934.
71. Petty, T.I., Pierson, D.J., Dick, N.P., Hudson, L.D., and Walker, S.H., Follow-up evaluation of a prevalence study for chronic bronchitis and chronic airway obstruction, *Am. Rev. Resp. Dis.,* 114, 881, 1976.
72. Phillips, R. L., Role of life-style and dietary habits in risk of cancer among Seventh-Day Adventists, *Cancer Res.,* 35, 3513, 1975.
73. Phillips, R.L., Lemon, F.R., Beeson, L., and Kuzma, J.W., Coronary heart disease mortality among Seventh-Day Adventists with differing dietary habits: a preliminary report, *Am. J. Clin. Nutr.,* 31, S191, 1978.
74. Pinsky, J.L., Leaverton, P.E., and Stokes, J., Predictors of good function: the Framingham Study, *J. Chronic Dis.,* 40(Suppl. 1), 159S, 1987.
75. Pisani, P., Berrino, F., Macaluso, M. et al., Carrots, green vegetables and lung cancer: a case-control study, *Int. J. Epidemiol.,* 15, 463, 1986.
76. Reddy, B.S., Hirota, N., and Katayama, S., Effect of dietary sodium ascorbate on 1,2-dimethylhydrazine- or methylnitrosourea-induced colon carcinogenesis in rats, *Carcinogenesis,* 3, 1097, 1982.
77. Sauer, H., Geographic Patterns in the Risk of Dying and Associated Factors, Ages 35-74 Years, U.S. Department of Health and Human Services Publ. No. 80-1402, DHHS, Hyattsville, MD, 1980.
78. Sauer, H. and Parke, D.W., Counties with extreme death rates and associated factors, *Am. J. Epidemiol.,* 99, 258, 1974.
79. Schatzkin, A., Jones, D.Y., Hoover, R.N. et al., Alcohol consumption and breast cancer in the epidemiologic follow-up study of the first National Health and Nutrition Examination survey, *N. Engl. J. Med.,* 316, 1169, 1987.
80. Schneider, E.L., Finch, C.E., and Weksler, M., Potential application of biological markers for assessing interventions of physiological aging, in *Biological Markers of Aging,* NIH Publ. No. 82-2221, Reff, M.E. and Schneider, E.L., Eds., National Institutes of Health, Washington, D.C., 1982, 237.

81. Snowdon, D.A., Animal product consumption and mortality because of all causes combined, coronary heart disease, stroke, diabetes, and cancer in Seventh-Day Adventists, *Am. J. Clin. Nutr.,* 48, 739, 1988.
82. Snowdon, D.A., Phillips, R.L., and Fraser, G.E., Meat consumption and fatal ischemic heart disease, *Prev. Med.,* 13, 490, 1984.
83. Snowdon, D.A., Ostwald, S.K., and Kane, R.L., Education, survival and independence in elderly Catholic sisters, 1936-1987, *Am. J. Epidemiol.,* 130, 999, 1989.
84. Suzuki, M., Mori, H., Asato, T. et al., Medical researches upon centenarians on Okinawa. I. Case controlled study of family history as hereditary influence on longevity, *Jpn. J. Geriatr.,* 22, 457, 1985.
85. Takata, H., Suzuki, M., Ishii, T., Sekiguchi, S., and Iri, H., Influence of major histocompatibility complex region genes on human longevity among Okinawan-Japanese centenarians and nonagenarians, *Lancet,* 2, 824, 1987 (see also editorial, *ibid.,* 835).
86. Toniolo, P., Riboli, E., Protta, F. et al., Calorie-providing nutrients and risk of breast cancer, *J. Natl. Cancer Inst.,* 81, 278, 1989.
87. Reducing the Health Consequences of Smoking: 25 Years of Progress. A Report of the Surgeon General, Publ. No. (CDC) 89-8411, U.S. Department of Health and Human Services, Rockville, MD, 1989.
88. *Vital Statistics of the United States,* Vol. 2, Part A, Section 1, National Center for Health Statistics, Washington, D.C.. 1980.
89. Voitenko, V.P. and Tokar, A.V., The assessment of biological age and sex differences of human aging, *Exp. Aging Res.,* 9, 239, 1983.
90. Webster, I.A. and Logie, A.R., A relationship between functional age and health status in female subjects, *J. Gerontol.,* 31, 546, 1976.
91. Weindruch, R. and Walford, R.L., *The Retardation of Aging and Disease by Dietary Restriction,* Charles C Thomas, Springfield, IL, 1988.
92. Willcox, K.K. and Lei, K.Y., Dietary fats and the aging adult, in *Nutrition and Heart Disease,* Vol. 1, Watson, R.R., Ed., CRC Press, Boca Raton, FL, 1987, 23.
93. Willett, W.C., Stampfer, M.J., Colditz, G.A. et al., Dietary fat and the risk of breast cancer, *N. Engl. J. Med.,* 316, 22, 1987.
94. Willett, W.C., Stampfer, M.J., Colditz, G.A. et al., Moderate alcohol consumption and the risk of breast cancer, *N. Engl. J. Med.,* 316, 1174, 1987.
95. Wingard, D.L., Berkman, L.F., and Brand, R.J., A multivariate analysis of health-related practices. A nine-year mortality follow-up of the Alameda County Study, *Am. J. Epidemiol.,* 116, 765, 1982.
96. Yano, K., Rhoads, G.G., and Kagan, A., Coffee, alcohol and risk of coronary heart disease among Japanese men living in Hawaii, *N. Engl. J. Med.,* 297, 405, 1977.
97. Ziegler, R.G., Mason, T.J., Stemhagen, A. et al., Carotenoid intake, vegetables and the risk of lung cancer among white men in New Jersey, *Am. J. Epidemiol.,* 123, 1080, 1986.

CHAPTER 9

THE PHYSIOLOGICAL AGING OF HUMAN POPULATIONS: ESTIMATION METHODS FOR COMPARATIVE ANALYSIS

A. Ruiz-Torres

TABLE OF CONTENTS

I. INTRODUCTION

The main reason for studying population aging is health planning because the results of comparative analyses can provide a useful basis for such plans. Analyses of this sort give us the chance to conserve individuals' biological and social well-being during aging. When the individuals reach old age, there is the possibility of reducing the propensity to afflictions inherent to the aging process. Ultimately, these studies should help bring down some of the high costs associated with aging.[35]

II. MAXIMUM LIFE SPAN: BIOLOGICAL TIME AND PHYSICAL TIME

The human life span can probably be reckoned at a maximum of 120 calendar years,[176] which is the time that it takes for the phenomena intrinsic to growth and to aging to develop if the environment is suitable. If it is not, the chronological duration of life is proportionally reduced, even when the biological space is the same for all individuals. Biological space is understood as the totality of complete cycles of cellular or organic activities that an individual goes through from birth to physiological death. Thus, the reference unit is biological time. When this runs out, death occurs. For example, the human life span in biological time can correspond to 120 or 50 years of physical time.

0-8493-0129-7/94/$0.00+$.50

According to Hayflick,[18] longevity is expressed in two periods: the developmental period of roughly 30 years, and the postdevelopmental period of a maximum of 80 years. This latter period is when aging sets in and thus is of greatest interest in comparative population analyses. Nonetheless, developmental longevity can be very important for postdevelopmental longevity because if the developmental stage should end later in a population, this will not only influence the dynamics of the second period, but can also determine the extension of total longevity. The developmental period terminates when the organism completes and optimizes its functions; its objectivization will obviously depend on the parameters we use.

III. OBJECTIVIZATION OF AGING ACCORDING TO DEMOGRAPHY AND EPIDEMIOLOGY

Aging in human populations is a term that is currently almost exclusively used by demographists. In principle, it is based on the ratio between the population at both ends of the life span. Thus, the result does not only depend on the survival rate, but also on the birth and emigration rates; i.e., aging is not objectivized as a biological process of the members of a specific population. However, using the mortality rate for age groups in the initial population and applying the Gompertz equation, one obtains a curve whose slope can be identified as an indication of aging.

With the same method as above, we can use the incidence rate for age-related diseases, such as type II diabetes, broncho-pneumopathies, osteoporosis, etc., to obtain an upward curve that expresses the progressive vulnerability of the population as a function of aging. However, we should emphasize that aging is not a pathological process. Further, the higher the chronological age, the more mortality influences the results, and thus, natural selection biases the gerontological reality. On the other hand, the correlation of the age-related disease incidence reaches the highest significant coefficient in different life stages for different diseases, as is the case with strokes and cancer.[7]

Despite the limitations of the demographic and the epidemiological procedures, it is possible to obtain aging curves in very stable groups that are suitable for comparative studies and can be related to biological results.

IV. SOCIAL AND BEHAVIORAL AGING

The interaction between aging and society is well known. Thus, the social manifestations of aging are not just the outcome of the progressive diminishing of psychological and motor activities of individual members of a specific society, but also due to the effect this society exerts over its members. The result is seen in manifestations that are described in the encompassing term " sociological aging" and quantified by the degree of participation in the activities of the population in question with respect to the conservation of its culture. Recording data by decades gives us a curve whose upward slope can show the process of aging in a specific population. The disadvantage that this procedure may have is the heterogeneity of the cultural heritage of different peoples and populations, which will influence the number, type, and specificity of the indicators, making it hard to conduct comparative studies (Figure 1).

Some sociological indicators are more directly related to the intrinsic process, such as the individual's role in the world of work at different ages,[21] and others related more to the above-mentioned interaction, such as the degree of integration[10] or the social welfare situation.[9] Finally, there are those indicators that are more society specific, such as the degree of competitiveness, which also reflect the environment and its influence.

Within the scope of sociology, changes in individual behavior also can be seen as manifestations of aging. Here, too, interaction occurs between the environment and the individual, even if the

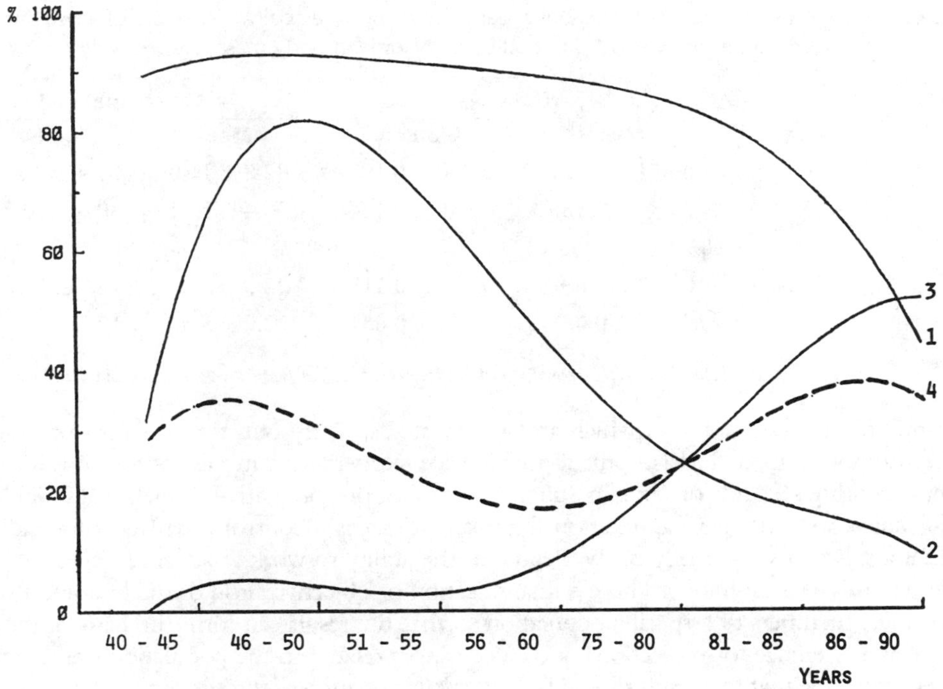

Figure 1 Sociological aging dynamics among a Spanish population,[28] according to indicators of political involvement. The graph represents the alternatives of each of the most meaningful variables from the gerontological point of view. (1) Participation last elections; (2) its assessment as very important; (3) political interest: none; (4) ideology: none.

result seems to be primarily conditioned by the intrinsic biological consequences of aging. This is so in the case of eating habits[27] and also in sexual behavior.[13] The results, collected individually by age groups in graphic form in a coordinates system, show changes in individual behavior as the age of a specific population advances. Using the multiple correlation procedure, it is possible to express the dynamics of a population's behavior from the gerontological point of view. The problem here is related to the difficulty of obtaining reliable, quantifiable data.

We have studied the sociological aging of a traditional agrarian population with a tendency to longevity, adding to the sociological indicators selected other behavioral indicators such as sexuality, physical exercise, and leisure activities. In this way, one can detect the moment when the values begin to diminish in a population. In the population studied, this is at 64 years of age.[28]

V. AGING ACCORDING TO FUNCTIONAL CAPACITY

Objectivization of aging is here based on carrying out functional tests on individual members of a group. As is well known, the functional expression of an organ (the heart or the brain, for example) is influenced by the aging process of the organ being studied. That aging in the organism as a whole does not evolve at the same rate in all its organs or everywhere at once, the functional results recorded for a specific organ will not represent the degree of aging throughout the entire organism. Moreover, especially in the case of the brain, there are different functions to consider when examining any one organ in order for the final result to express its functional capacity at a specific age. From all of this we can deduce that the functional method entails subjecting the individual to

Table 1 Late decrease of metabolic parameters by age: daily excretion of urea and creatinine per weight unit body weight or lean body mass, respectively[a]

	Urea		Creatinine	
Age	**Men**	**Women**	**Men**	**Women**
40–50	0.371 ± 0.121	0.360 ± 0.102	32.3 ± 11.0	31.4 ± 8.5
51–60	0.386 ± 0.135	0.350 ± 0.124	36.4 ± 10.1	30.8 ± 10.7
	$p < 0.02$	$p < 0.005$	$p < 0.005$	$p < 0.005$
75–85	0.282 ± 0.08	0.290 ± 0.115	22.3 ± 5.3	23.7 ± 5.4
>85	0.272 ± 0.03	0.242 ± 0.081	22.9 ± 5.5	17.7 ± 5.7

[a] *Calculated indirectly according to Reference 16. Data from a Spanish population.*[28]

a large number of tests, some of which are complicated to carry out, take up a lot of time, and therefore cannot be applied to a population-wide scale. Nonetheless, in this context, it is important to mention Pöthig's[22] study of aging in 365 individuals, carried out with 44 functional variables and 3 social indicators. The main application for this study is as a control population for individual biological assessments, especially of the degree of the ability to work at advanced ages.

Despite this, it is desirable to have a quantification or objectivization of the biological state of the individual members of a specific population so that the result can form the basis of the study and serve as a reference for projections of data or factors related to the population's environment. It is understandable that this result should be expressed in relation to the age of the individuals, such that one tries to get a curve that slopes downward from roughly 30 years of age, as would be expected due to the effect of aging. The methodological problem has two aspects: (1) in a transversal study, correcting the effect of selection by mortality, and (2) deciding the number of parameters open to study in numerous individuals. These values must reflect the overall biological state of the human organism.

VI. AGING ACCORDING TO LABORATORY RESEARCH

In the gerontological literature, the term "aging biomarkers" or "biological markers" is given to those parameters that, within the range of normality, vary with age. Despite the debate as to their usefulness for quantification of biological age (see, for example, Reference 12 vs. 14), there can be no doubt that human metabolic states vary with chronological age, influencing the result of the usual blood or urine tests. This is the case for albuminemia, uricemia, and glycemia, which is not simply observed in transversal studies but also in longitudinal ones.[8,25,32] However, eating immediately prior to the test or other exogenous factors can influence the result, thus making it difficult to use in determining the biological age of individuals. With the same limitations in interpretation as mentioned, but useful in population studies apart from those already referred to, we should mention among the metabolic expression parameters the daily elimination of urea or creatinine, with respect to body weight or muscular mass (Table 1 and Figure 2).

It is understandable that for population studies, the number of tests should be kept as low as possible. That is why we consider blood concentrations of effectors such as thyroid hormone (T_3), testosterone (Te), and low density lipoprotein-cholesterol (LDL), and of cyclic adenosine monophosphate (cAMP) to be useful in estimating biological aging. The results do not only regularly show age-related behavior,[36] but their overall expression is intimately linked to the intrinsic mechanisms of aging. Moreover, apart from the group of substances already mentioned, we should also add the terminal peptide of type III procollagen (PIIIP), whose blood concentration is directly proportional to the synthesis of type III collagen and is also age-related.[38] These measurements, although they need to be performed using a methodology suitable for detecting slight deviations

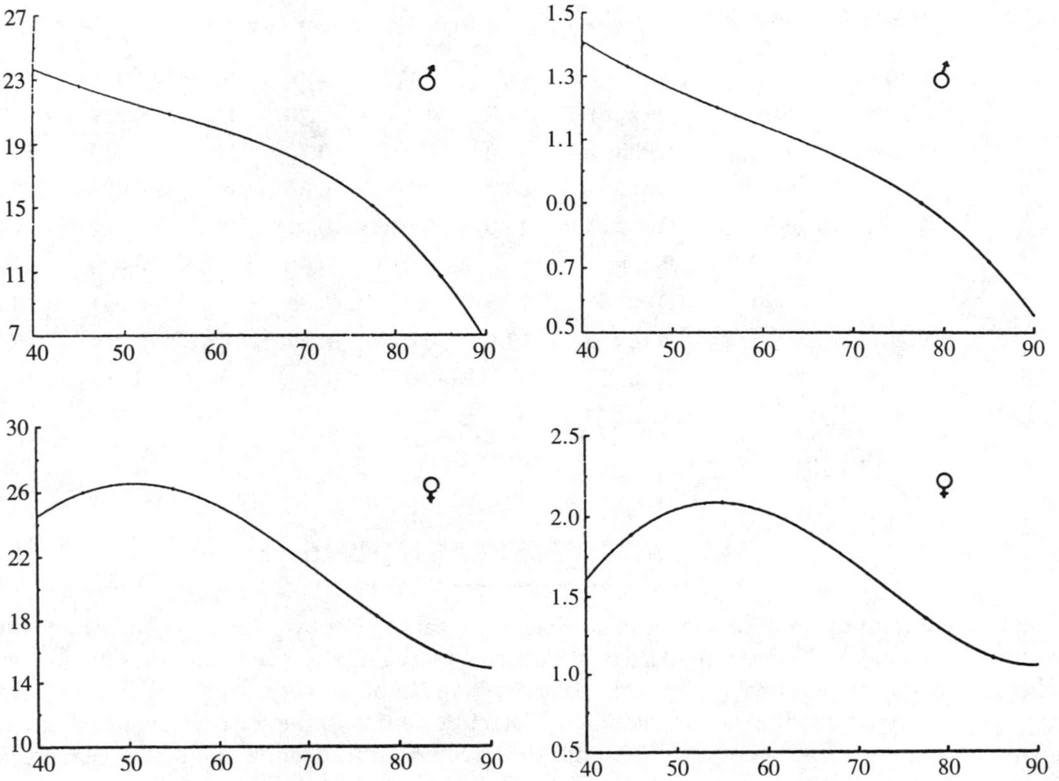

Figure 2 Graphic representation of the age-dependent absolute amounts of urea (left) and creatinine (right) urine excretion from which we can infer a similar behavior in terms of sex (above: males, below: females) (g/d vs. years of age).[27]

and controlled for reliability, are not complicated and can be performed using a few cubic centimeters of blood, duly conserved.

VII. BODY CHANGES AS AGING PARAMETERS

Anthropometric measurements, as Durnin and Womersley[16] have noted, give rise to results depending on chronological age, and therefore lead to deductions on the biological aging process of individual members of a specific population. The body mass index (BMI) rises during the first 30 years (approximately) of adulthood. Later, it decreases as age increases, but is closely related to the daily energy intake which, as is well known, also decreases with age. This behavior is linked to the involution of the muscle mass.

The decreased lean body mass (LBM) is usually accompanied by rising fat body mass (FBM) so that when their BMI is similar the body composition can be very different due to age. Consequently, BMI values are only valid for comparison in nutritional studies when the ages of the individuals are very similar. The reverse aging dependent behavior between LBM and FBM may be due to the corresponding degrees of growth hormone secretion.[24] The biological laboratory indicator of this could be the basal serum levels of IGF-1 which clearly show a decline as age advances.

Likewise, the body surface decreases with age. However, if one applies this measurement as a biological aging parameter, it needs to be corrected because the result is influenced by size, and this depends on secular growth.

Table 2 Age of maximum vitality (t_m) and the aging factor (B) by number of variables

Mathematical model		t_m	B	(r^2)	t_m	B	(r^2)
Multiple correlation	Own, 6[a]	34.8	−0.012	(0.90)	37.3	−0.009	(0.90)
Biological index	Pöthig, 47	33.2	−0.013	(0.73)	33.2	−0.013	(0.72)
	Own, 6	38.1	−0.009	(0.80)	39.6	−0.008	(0.82)
ADIMENS quotients	Own, 2[b]	26.0	−0.026	(0.81)	26.9	−0.024	(0.74)
	Pöthig, 5	—	−0.030	(0.90)	—	−0.020	(0.56)
	Own, 5[c]	16.6	−0.061	(0.83)	18.4	−0.051	(0.85)
Vector distances	Pöthig, 17	19.4	−0.047	(0.99)	16.0	−0.064	(0.97)
	Own, 6	33.7	−0.013	(0.47)	33.8	−0.013	(0.93)

[a] *T_3, T_E, LDL-chol., cAMP, PIIIP, CA.*
[b] *cAMP, PIIIP.*
[c] *T_3, T_E, LDL-chol., cAMP, PIIIP.*

VIII. MATHEMATICAL MODELS

The quantification of aging or its rate of acceleration is carried out by calculation procedures and mathematical models. All these are based on the concept that aging is an irreversible dynamic process whose increase is proportional to the physical survival time. In other words, they take chronological age as the reference axis for the variables used. Therefore, although the reasoning is based on the thermodynamic concept of entropy, the result that is intended to quantify the degree of aging is obtained by relation to chronological age (Table 2).

The procedure of multiple correlation has proved its validity in experimental work,[15,20,33,34] where multiple parameters have been considered (biochemical, structural, or behavioral) in direct relation to the chronological age of the animal. Using the same procedure, it is possible to obtain results on population aging which can be used for comparative studies.

Mathematical models drawn up to analyze aging of an individual can be applied to a population study. A good number of these are based on the concept of vitality, i.e., assuming that aging is a process of gradual loss of vitality as from the moment when the maximum value is reached, which in human beings is at an age of roughly 30 years.[1,2] It is deduced that vitality ($v(t)$) is the product of the stabilizing function ($\varepsilon(t)$) and destabilizing function ($P(t)$), the latter being the function expressing the deterioration of the organism's efficiency:

$$v(t) = \varepsilon(t) \cdot P(t)$$

From this one can deduce the importance of growth as a stabilizing factor, determinant of the first component of the curve represented by the function $\varepsilon(t)$, which according to Beier et al.[1] is a Gompertz function. However, the second component of the curve is a simple exponential function from the moment of maximum vitality.

The mathematical aging concept, according to the mathematical expression of vitality mentioned above, can be used in the direct application of the results or their prior elaboration of greater or lesser complexity. The most simple procedure is that of adapting the simple exponential function (which reflects aging through decreasing vitality) to the points obtained through multiple correlation, the variable of the order becoming a decreasing function. The biological index used by Ries[23] gives rise here to a standardization of the variables in order to finally be able to adjust the exponential curve[3] as in the previous case.

The adimensional quotients, a calculation procedure also introduced by Beier[4] in clinical gerontological studies, can be adapted as above to the concept of vitality. Finally, with vectorial

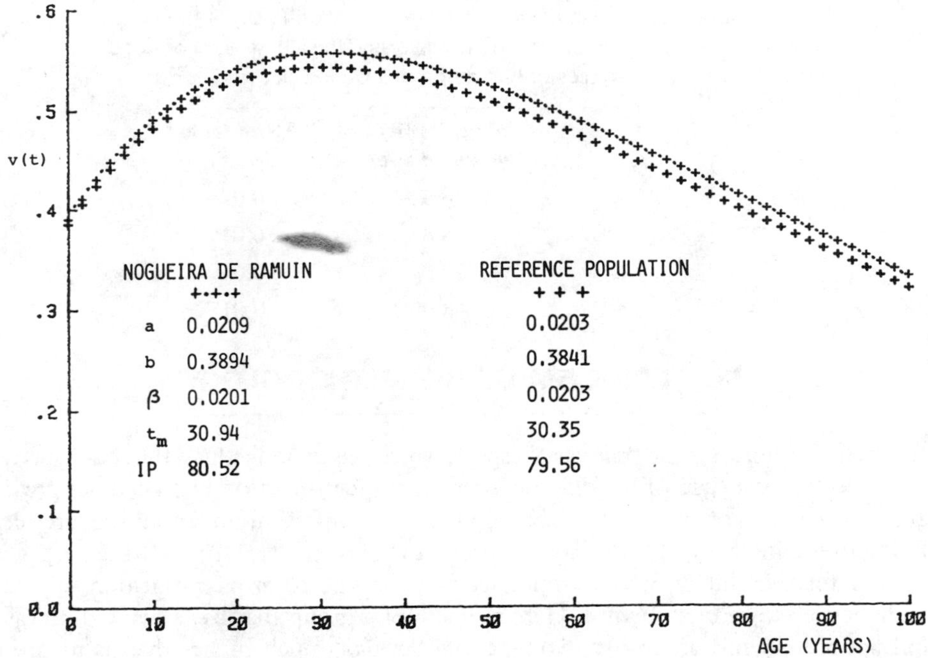

Figure 3 Vitality curve according to the mathematical bicompartmental model of a whole Spanish population[28] (both sexes) as compared to the reference population (see text). IP = inflection point or point changing declining velocity; Reference 29 explains more about mathematics.

calculation one has a mathematical model of greater coherence with the universal concept of aging. The principal method is in the determination of the distances between the vectors of individuals by age groups and the control vector which represents the mean of a young population, chronologically close to the age of maximum vitality.[5]

The author[27] has adapted the bicompartmental concept of the dynamic of aging to that of vitality (mentioned above) for the study of the biological aging of populations (Figure 3). Applying kinetic criteria, one can identify the variables with the corresponding compartments,[26] postulating that

$$v(t) = \text{REP} \cdot \text{PROD}$$

where REP (repairing or regulator compartment) $\hat{=}\ \varepsilon(t)$ and PROD (producer compartment) $\hat{=}\ P(t)$. The bicompartmental concept of the dynamics of aging is based on the assumption that all the involutional processes entail continuous regulation or repair in order to postpone the functional cataclysm, thereby guaranteeing survival. The involutional processes would be detrimental to the activities in the producer compartment, accompanied by an increase in those of the regulator compartment. Thus, the extension of one or other compartments would be in the function of the biological age of the organism in question. Adjusting a mathematical function to the behavior of the age-dependent variables (blood levels of PIIIP and LDL-cholesterol) in the REP compartment, one gets a linear equation instead of the Gompertz equation postulated by Beier for $\varepsilon(t)$. In the case of the values of the PROD variables (Te, T3, cAMP, and body surface), one obtains, as in $P(t)$, a simple exponential function, such that the original vitality equation varies as shown below:

$$v(t) = (at + b) \cdot e^{-\beta t}$$

Table 3 Mean (X) and standard deviation (S.D.) of the age of maximum vitality and the aging factor of studies of human groups carried out to date[30]

	Max. vitality (years of age)	Aging factor ($year^{-1}$)
X	28.4	0.026
S.D.	8.8	0.019
X	28.0	0.019
S.D.	8.0	0.017

IX. CRITICISM OF THE METHODOLOGY

The fundamental problem is the transversal aspect, which selects individuals that have survived and therefore are in the best state of biological conservation. This selection bias becomes greater with age. Thus, in a study of aging in a sub-population, Corpas[11] found that the prevalence of hyperalphalipoproteinemia [high density lipoprotein-cholesterol (HDL) >70 mg/dl], is significantly greater for the elderly, which would seem to be due to an accumulation of individuals biologically best endowed for survival. Here is a case of a group that has a marked prevalence of hyperalphalipoproteinemia among the younger age groups, much higher than is usual in other populations studied. Consequently, it is understandable that this observation should be the determining factor of the transversal behavior of the population's aging results. However, we have studied other populations where this circumstance is absent, but where one habitually sees a drop in the LDL-cholesterol concentrations after the age of 60.[19] Here it is also a transversally obtained result, which is therefore modified by natural selection.

The influence of natural selection on the methods for the calculation of aging rates is especially remarkable when the procedure is based on the regulation theory of aging. This is understandable because the two compartmental mathematical models deduced herefrom apply parameters that represent risk factors; i.e., the rise of LDL-cholesterol and the aminoterminal peptide of procollagen type III is combined with the appearance of arteriosclerosis, and thereafter the age-dependent slope of the corresponding function is linked with those values which may be related to precocious deaths. Consequently, when using a wide age range in cross-sectional population studies, i.e., including individuals living 90 years or more, the decay of the curve can be false. Put another way, the inflection point of the curve becomes shorter the longer the life of the selected population. Because of this the most logical results are obtained when the reference adult population is no older than 55 years, because in this population natural selection by aging does not play an important role.

On the other hand, in an earlier life period, the LDL-cholesterol levels increase as a function of age,[37] sometimes prematurely reaching atherogenous risk blood concentrations. Nonetheless, we have recently studied a population in which the lipoproteinic behavior seems to be independent of that of the reasons for the survival of its individuals.[28]

The main problem in the objectivization of biological aging of populations is the need to reduce the number and simplify the spectrum of tests. The individual study should include a sufficiently large number of persons equitably distributed in terms of age groups and sex for the sample to be representative of the population group. It is then necessary to make a selection of parameters to be used, with the risk that the final result may not give enough information to assess the biological state of the individual member of the sample. To avoid this, we have carried out this selection based on the bi-compartmental concept of the dynamics of aging, excluding direct interdependence of the parameters selected.[38]

Table 4 Results on the aging of a population[28] according to the estimation procedure and parameters used

Start (age in years)	Acceleration (year $^{-1}$)	Total life expectancy (years)	Method
64[a]	–	–	Sociological and behavioral indicators
33.5[b]	0.043[c]	80.4[d]	Mathematical vitality and compartment models with 5 effectors and body surface
44.8[b]	0.005[c]	–	Mathematical vitality models with daily urea/kg b.w.; daily creatinine/kg LBM and body surface corrected with the secular growth trend
–	–	78	Mean age of death in the locality in 1980
–	–	81	Idem, in 1990

[a] *From the age when the decline sets in regarding social participation, etc.*
[b] *Or from the age of maximum vitality.*
[c] *Speed of decrease in vitality (or aging factor).*
[d] *Period until the inflection point of exponential decrease of vitality in the corresponding curve obtained with the biocompartmental model.*

The question if a very long-lived population can be useful for biological studies related to the calculation of the maximal life span remains crucial, mainly after the above-mentioned results. In this relationship it seems to be logical to consider the fundamental role of functions which lead to the stabilization of the organism as the basic mechanism for reaching very advanced ages. Therefore, the mathematical model based on the concept that vitality ($v(t)$) depends not only on the accumulation of errors ($F(t)$) but also on the stabilization capacity ($\varepsilon(t)$) of the organism, seems to be helpful as the following function shows:

$$1/v(t) = \varepsilon(t) - F(t)$$

When assuming $\varepsilon(t)$ represents the capacity for repair (REP) for maintaining the organism and $F(t)$ should apply to those parameters that represent the organism output (PROD),

$$1/v(t) = k(\text{REP} - \text{PROD}); k = v(t_o)$$

the function obtained results in a curve with a declining part up to the age of 20 (approximately) and an increasing component with a maximum between 110 and 120 years.[31]

Another problem in objectivizing biological aging is to exclude ill persons from the sample, as it is based on the objectivization of the physiological process. At advanced ages, it can be very difficult to distinguish between physiological and pathological states. To such ends, we used very rigid sieving criteria, but with normal limits established according to a clinical approach based on experimental gerontology. The disadvantage that the selection can be extremely positive, especially when dealing with advanced ages, can be offset by having an epidemiological study of the same population and also by analyzing data from official records giving retrospective longitudinal information on the population over the last 9 to 10 decades. All this, as well as the results of a sociological study of the population, contributes not just to supporting the results with respect to its biological aging, but also makes interpretation easier when analyzing the differences between different populations.

X. CONCLUDING REMARKS

Apart from the diseases that shorten human life, there are definitely exogenous factors that contribute to the individuality of aging. The study of aging in populations that are standardizable according to habits, living conditions, and environment can clear up the enigma of why human beings especially do not show a homogeneous aging dynamic per time unit. However, this generally accepted assumption has yet to be demonstrated. To such ends we need methods that can be transversally applied to compensate for the problems of longitudinal studies.

Estimating when an organism has aged, one can determine its biological age, but irrespective of the importance of the parameters used as indicators of the biological state, the real problems are the controls for the results obtained. There is no one control population. Rather, we know that populations show different aging behavior. Thus, we think that instead of individualizing the problem, we should study the aging of carefully characterized populations in order to be able to establish comparisons. In order to obtain comparable results on the physiological aging of a specific population, we must study all the individuals in the sample. Therefore, we need a modest number of parameters to be determined. The disadvantages that reducing the number of measured parameters could entail can be relatively offset by a reasoned, meticulous selection of variables and their elaboration for the application of mathematical models coherent with the fundamental principles of gerontology. In all cases, any endeavor in this research should be undertaken using an interdisciplinary approach. Thus, the results, however modest and open to dispute they may be, could lead to some deductions that will not be important only for those interested in human aging, but also to state health and planning agencies.

ACKNOWLEDGMENTS

This work was initially supported by the Stiftung Volkswagenwerk, Hanover, Germany, and subsequently by the Ministry of Science and Education (Comisión Interministerial de Ciencia y Tecnologia, Plan Nacional I+D, Grant 89-1076-02-01), Spain.

REFERENCES

1. Beier, W., Brehme, K.-H., and Wregel, D., Vitalität, Altern und biologischer Wirkungsgrad eines multizellulären Systems, *Mech. Age. Dev.*, 1, 313, 1972.
2. Beier, W., Brehme, K.-H., and Wiegel, D., Biophysikalische Aspekte des Alterns multizellulärer Systeme, in *Fortschritte der Experimentellen und Theoretischen Biophysik*, Vol. 16, Beier, W., Ed., Georg Thieme Verlag, Leipzig, 1973.
3. Beier, W., Vitalitätskonzept und biologischer Index nach Ries, *Z. Gerontol.*, 18, 353, 1985.
4. Beier, W., Dimensionslose Kennzahlen des menschlichen Organismus und ihre Bedeutung für die Objektivierung der Vitalitat, *Z. Gerontol.*, 18, 358, 1985.
5. Beier, W., Vektoranalytische Auswertung klinisch-gerontologischer Daten, *Z. Gerontol.*, 20, 136, 1987.
6. Beier, W., Theoretische Lebensdauer und biologische Eigenzeit, *Z. Gerontol.*, 21, 110, 1988.
7. Benfante, R., Reed, D., and Brody, J., Biological and social predictors of health in an aging cohort, *J. Chronic Dis.*, 38, 385, 1955.
8. Borkan, G.A. and Norris, A.H., Assessment of biological age using a profile of physical parameters, *J. Gerontol.*, 35, 177, 1980.
9. Clausen, L., Anticipating death — old age as social process, in *Biological Age and Aging Risk Factors*, Ruiz-Torres, A., Ed., Tecnipublicaciones, Madrid, 1987, 191.

10. Cobb, S., Social support as a moderator of life stress, *Psychosom. Med.*, 38, 301, 1976.
11. Corpas, E., Estudio Transversal de una Poblacion Estable de Guadalajara. Aportación a la Investigación del Envejecimiento de Poblaciones, Ph.D. thesis, Universidad Autónoma de Madrid, Madrid, 1987.
12. Costa, P.T., Jr. and McCrae, R.R., Measures and markers of biological aging: "a great clamoring... of fleeting significance", *Arch Gerontol Geriatr.*, 7, 211, 1988.
13. Davidson, J.M., Chen, J.J., Crapo, L., Gray, G.D., Greenleaf, W.J., and Catania, J.A., Hormonal changes and sexual function in aging men, *J. Clin.. Endocrinol. Metab.*, 57, 71, 1983.
14. Dean, W., and Morgan, R.F., In defense of the concept of biological aging measurement — current status, *Arch. Gerontol. Geriatr.*, 7, 191, 1988.
15. Dubina, T.L., Biological age and its estimation. Introduction of a correction to the multiple regression model of biological age in cross-sectional and longitudinal studies, *Exp. Gerontol.*, 19, 133, 1984.
16. Durnin, J.V.G.A. and Womersley, J., Body fat assessed from total body density and its estimation from skinfold thickness: measurements on 481 men and women aged from 16 to 72 years, *Br. J. Nutr.*, 32, 77, 1974.
17. Franke, H., Theorien der Langlebigkeit, *Akta Gerontol*, 9, 167, 1979.
18. Hayflick, L., Origins of longevity, in *Modern Biological Theories of Aging*, Warner, H.R., Butler, R.N., Sprott, R.L., Schneider, E.L., Eds., Raven Press, New York, 1987, 21.
19. Heckers, H., Burkard, W., and Fuhrmann, W., Longevity syndrome hyper-alphalipoproteinemia?, in *Lipoproteins and Age*, Schneider, I. and Kaffarnik, H., Eds., Thieme Verlag, Stuttgart, 1982, 52.
20. Hofecker, G., Skalicky, M., Kment, A., and Niedermuller, H., Models of biological age of the rat. I. A factor model of age parameters, *Mech. Age Dev.*, 14, 345, 1980.
21. Palmore, E.B., Social risk factors, in *Risk Factors for Senility*, Rothschild H., Ed., Oxford University Press, New York, 1984, 3.
22. Pöthig, D., Experimentelle Entwicklung eines klinischen Diagnostikmodelles zur Objektivierung des biologischen Alters des Menschen, Dissertation Promotion B, Karl-Marx-University, Leipzig, 1982.
23. Ries, W., Problems associated with biological age, *Exp Gerontol.*, 9, 145, 1973.
24. Rudman, D., Feller, A.G., Cohn, L., Shetty, K.R., Rudman, I.W., Draper, M.W., Effects of human growth hormone on body composition in elderly men, *Horm. Res.*, 36(Suppl. 1), 73, 1991.
25. Ruiz-Torres, A. and Tapia, A., Altern als Umkehrung des Wachstums: Verhalten der Harnsaure, *Akt. Gerontol.*, 11, 129, 1981.
26. Ruiz-Torres A., Altern: Das Resultat einer Interaktion zwischen Aktivitätsminderung und Regulation?, in *Prozesses des Alterns*, 2nd ed., Beier, W., Laue, R., Leutert, G., Rotzsch, W., and Schmidt. U., Eds., Akademie Verlag, Berlin, 1987, 47.
27. Ruiz-Torres A., Ed., *Biological Age and Aging Risk Factors*, Tecnipublicaciones, Madrid, 1987.
28. Ruiz-Torres, A., *Multi-Disciplinary Study on Aging and Health Condition of the Population of Nogueira de Ramuin*, Tecnipublicaciones, Madrid, 1989.
29. Ruiz-Torres, A., Agudo, A., Vincent, D., and Beier, W., Two compartment mathematical model applying the vitality concept to measure the human aging, *Arch. Gerontol. Geriatr.*, 10, 69, 1990.
30. Ruiz-Torres, A., Agudo, A., Holzenberger, M., and Beier, W., Zur Objektivierung des biologischen Alters des Menschen: Ergebnisse, *Z. Gerontol.*, 22, 64, 1989.
31. Ruiz-Torres, A., Rajczy, K., Baún, C.P., and Beregi, E., On the age range for aging studies of populations with special reference to biological results obtained from centenarians, in *Modification of the Rate of Aging*, Vienna Aging Ser. Vol. 3, Ruiz-Torres, A. and Hofecker, G., Eds., Facultas Verlag, 1992
32. Shock, N.W., Normal Human Aging: The Baltimore Longitudinal Study of Aging. U.S. Department of Health and Human Services, Washington, D.C., 1984.
33. Skalicky, M., Hofecker, G., Kment, A., and Niedermüller, H., Models of the biological age of the rat. II. Multiple regression models in the study on influencing aging, *Mech. Age Dev.*, 14, 361, 19??.
34. Skalicky, M., Hofecker, G., Kment, A., and Niedermüller, H., Diskriminanzanalyse von Altersparametern der Ratte, *Akt. Gerontol.*, 11, 4, 1981.

35. Sommers, A.R., The high cost of health care for the elderly; diagnosis, prognosis and some suggestions for therapy, *J. Health Polit. Policy Law.*, 3, 163, 1978.
36. Sowers, J.R. and Felicetta, J.V., Eds., *The Endocrinology of Aging (Comprehensive Endocrinology)*, Raven Press, New York, 1988.
37. Takeuchi, N., Matsumoto, A., Katayama, Y., Arao, M., Koga, M., Nakao, H., and Uchida, K., Changes with aging in serum lipoproteins and apolipoprotein C subclasses, *Arch. Gerontol. Geriatr.*, 2, 41, 1983.
38. Vincent, D., Sérrano, S., and Ruiz-Torres, A., cAMP y procolágeno-III-péptido en el envejecimiento: ¿interdependencia fisiológica?, *Rev. Esp. Geriatr. Gerontol.*, 21, 303, 1986.

CHAPTER 10

A MULTIVARIATE APPROACH TO THE QUANTIFICATION OF PHYSIOLOGICAL STATUS IN OLD AGE

WOJTEK J. CHODZKO-ZAJKO

TABLE OF CONTENTS

I. INTRODUCTION

Although functional decline appears to be an inevitable and inescapable consequence of aging, there are often considerable differences between individuals with respect to the rate and extent of this decline.[27] In order to increase our understanding of the considerable variability between individuals with respect to the functional consequences of aging, gerontologists have attempted to take into account physiological parameters when studying senescent changes in behavior.

One of the most frequently adopted approaches for the assessment of physiological function in old age involves the computation of biological or functional age. While a variety of statistical

0-8493-0129-7/94/$0.00+$.50

models have been adopted in the generation of indices of biological age, the most common approach has utilized multiple regression analysis. In essence, the multiple regression approach generates the linear combination of physiological variables which maximizes the prediction of chronological age. This linear combination is subsequently used to predict the biological age of an individual (for a comprehensive review see Dean[22]).

A number of objections have been raised with respect to this approach, the most critical of which is the requirement that chronological age be selected as the criterion against which the biological variables be regressed. Because the decision to compute biological age implies a rejection of the adequacy of chronological age, it seems logically circular to subsequently adopt the rejected measure as the criterion in accordance with which biological age is to be defined.[18,34] This objection to the multiple regression approach is particularly difficult to overcome because there is no immediately apparent alternative external criterion to substitute for chronological age.

Several authors have adopted factor analytic approaches in an attempt to define biological age in the absence of an external criterion.[4,23,32,33,37] The major focus of these studies has been the identification of a general factor of biological aging in which a number of physiological variables load together with chronological age on a single independent factor. Although some authors have claimed that a unitary factor of biological aging can be identified,[32,37] the general consensus is that aging is a multidimensional process and that efforts to reduce physiological variables to a single factor are unlikely to meet with success..[9,18,34] It is worth noting that the decision to concentrate solely on the interpretation of physiological factors which have high loadings on chronological age de facto establishes chronological age as the criterion for the identification of biological aging factors. Such an approach does nothing to avoid the circular logic associated with the multiple regression model.

Regardless of whether multiple regression or factor analytic procedures are adopted, indices of biological age are seldom very efficient predictors of age-related declines in behavior.[34] Indeed, most studies suggest that the single most powerful predictor of functional decline in senescence remains chronological age. Consequently, it is probably of limited value for research to concentrate on the development of indices of biological age that are intended to be substitutes for chronological age and more useful to develop methods for evaluating physiological function in elderly populations which are intended to be complementary to chronological age.

Despite the large number of studies which have attempted to generate indices of biological age, there has been relatively little discussion of the purpose behind the derivation of such indices. Although many authors assume that the replacement of chronological age by some combination of physiological variables is intrinsically worthwhile, there appear to be strong grounds to challenge the utility of such a procedure. If, as seems likely, senescent changes in behavior are influenced by a combination of physiological and chronological factors, the *a priori* rejection of either domain is questionable. The tendency of biologically oriented gerontologists to deliberately ignore variance due to chronological age appears to be an error of similar proportion to that committed by others who unquestioningly attribute senescent changes in behavior to the passage of time.

The acknowledgment of the importance of both chronological age and physiological health status is imperative if we are to increase our understanding of the complex factors associated with senescence. Much of the author's more recent work has concentrated on the development of an index of physiological status (IPS) which has sufficient discriminatory power to be useful for the evaluation of physiological changes in geriatric populations. Our goal throughout these studies has been to increase our understanding of the vast intersubject variability that characterizes advancing age. In the author's experiments, the IPS is not intended to measure biological age; rather, we have attempted to use the instrument as a measure of overall physiological status which can be used in conjunction with chronological age. This chapter presents the results of several experiments which have examined the influence of physiological factors on age-related changes in sensory, motor, and cognitive performance. Throughout, we concentrate on the illustration of how both the IPS and chronological age can contribute to our understanding of these changes.

II. EXPERIMENT ONE

A. DEVELOPMENT OF THE INDEX OF PHYSIOLOGICAL STATUS (IPS)

In recent years a number of studies have presented evidence in support of the hypothesis that physiologically fit elderly individuals may experience less pronounced declines in selected sensory, motor, and cognitive behaviors than less healthy contemporaries. Specifically, high-fit individuals have been shown to experience less behavioral slowing,[10,26,25,58,60] improved auditory performance,[35] greater tactile sensitivity,[16] and less speech deterioration[51] than less fit individuals of the same chronological age. Unfortunately, the literature in this area is characterized by considerable inconsistencies with regard to the procedures adopted for the evaluation of physiological fitness. Accordingly, it is extremely difficult to compare the results of studies which have used quite different methodologies for the evaluation of fitness.

In most studies of physical fitness and aging, researchers have selected cardiovascular responses to exercise stress tests for the evaluation of physiological status.[11,54] This approach follows from the view that the integrity of biological systems is most effectively evaluated by gauging their ability to respond rapidly and appropriately to an external perturbation. Although cardiovascular measures such as maximal oxygen uptake ($VO_{2\ max}$) are generally acknowledged to be the most appropriate measures of overall physiological health, there are a number of objections to exclusive reliance on such measures for the evaluation of fitness in elderly populations.[56] The most serious objection is that large numbers of elderly subjects are unable to meet the relatively stringent medical criteria required for participation in even submaximal exercise stress tests.[2] As such, most studies of physical fitness in the elderly have been restricted to a relatively healthy subset of the elderly population capable of meeting the above criteria. Thus, the dependence upon exercise-based testing for the evaluation of fitness has effectively excluded less healthy subjects from participation in research, and (we suggest) has limited the extent to which findings can be generalized to the total aged population.

The goal of experiment one was to develop a simple, noninvasive instrument for the evaluation of physiological status which could be applied to virtually all elderly subjects. Although it is doubtful whether any single resting parameter can, by itself, adequately describe the complexity of physical fitness, we suggest that the information obtained from a diverse battery of resting physiological variables may be combined into a composite IPS which can be adopted as a measure of overall physiological health.

Because the procedure for the derivation of the IPS necessitates the reduction of a large number of physiological variables to a single score, there are obvious conceptual similarities between the IPS and the measures of biological age discussed earlier. However, there are several important differences between the IPS and most conventional measures of biological age: (1) the IPS is primarily a measure of fitness rather than a measure of biological age, (2) the IPS does not utilize chronological age as an external criterion, and (3) the IPS is intended to be complementary to, rather than in lieu of, chronological age.

B. METHOD

Seventy male volunteers (age 62 ± 12 years) participated in the study. Participants were recruited from a variety of residential institutions and senior citizen organizations. Because the tests chosen for the evaluation of physiological status were only minimally stressful, it was not necessary for subjects to meet overly stringent medical criteria in order to participate in the study. Less than 5% of the elderly subjects initially contacted were unable to complete the tests required for participation in the study. In all cases medical clearance was obtained from the individual's physician and informed consent was secured.

Table 1 Descriptive data: physiological variables

Variable	Mean	S.D.	*n*
Age (years)	62.9	11.8	70
SBP (mmHg; systolic blood pressure)	134.6	14.0	70
DBP (mmHg; diastolic blood pressure)	80.5	8.6	70
LWT (kg; lean body weight)	67.6	7.9	70
FVC (1; forced vital capacity)	3.9	0.9	70
FEV-1 (1/s; forced expiratory volume)	3.1	0.8	70
TRIG (mg/dl; triglycerides)	122.2	59.0	70
RISK (Chol/HDL; cardiac risk index)	5.0	1.3	70

In selecting physiological variables for inclusion in the IPS, we were guided by the thinking of Ludwig and Smoke,[44] who have suggested that variables selected for the evaluation of physiological status should be readily observable in virtually all individuals in the populations under study. Furthermore, they suggest that the chosen variables should be sufficiently diverse as to be unrelated to a single physiological process. In accordance with these criteria, we selected the following seven variables because they were known to be good indicators of general physiological health, and at the same time they could be obtained with virtually no risk in almost all elderly individuals:

Lean body weight (LWT)
Systolic blood pressure (SBP)
Diastolic blood pressure (DBP)
Forced vital capacity (FVC)
Forced expiratory volume-1s (FEV-1)
Serum triglycerides (TRIG)
Serum total cholesterol/high density lipoprotein (RISK)

Height, weight, and skin folds were recorded, and LWT was computed from these data in accordance with previously published procedures.[36] Following collection of anthropometric data, subjects were requested to recline on a bed for 10 min, after which resting heart rate, systolic, and diastolic blood pressure were recorded. Finally, pulmonary performance was determined by computerized spirometric analysis (MCG Microloop) using sterile disposable mouthpieces and standard experimental procedures. A more detailed description of the above protocols has been published elsewhere.[16]

The collection of blood for the biochemical analyses was performed on a separate day from the physiological testing. Blood, 100 ml, was collected between 07:00 and 08:00 while the subjects were in a 12-h fasting state. Serum analyses of cholesterol and triglycerides were determined using a commercial serum metabolite autoanalyzer (Technicon SMA II). Serum high density lipoprotein (HDL) analyses were performed using standard reagents (A-Gent, Abbott Laboratories).

C. RESULTS

1. Descriptive Data

Descriptive statistics for the physiological and biochemical variables are presented in Table 1. Examination of these data reveals that the mean scores reported for the subjects in this study are generally comparable to those reported elsewhere using similar elderly populations.[54]

Table 2 Factor analysis of the initial physiological variables

Variable	F1	F2	F3	h^2
LWT	0.16	–0.43	–0.14	0.22
SBP	–0.21	–0.05	–0.72	0.55
DBP	0.02	0.01	–0.80	0.64
FVC	0.96	0.04	0.11	0.92
FEV-1	0.97	0.08	0.10	0.96
TRIG	–0.14	–0.84	0.10	0.73
RISK	–0.16	–0.73	0.02	0.56
Eigenvalue	2.18	1.36	1.07	4.61
Percent variance	33.3	25.0	20.9	79.2

2. *Derivation of the IPS*

In order to reduce the seven physiological and biochemical variables to a single score, the correlation matrix for the physiological variables was factor analyzed. The principal axis form of solution was employed and the factors for each solution were rotated according to the varimax procedure.[39] A minimum eigenvalue of 1 was adopted as the criterion for factor extraction.

Three factors met the minimum eigenvalue criterion and these factors accounted for 79% of the initial variance (see Table 2). Factor one had high loadings on FVC and FEV-1 and was called "pulmonary function". Factor two was characterized by primary loadings on TRIG and RISK and secondary loadings on LWT. This factor was called "blood lipids and body weight". The third factor loaded almost exclusively on SBP and DBP and was called "blood pressure".

Factor scores were computed for each subject on each of the three factors. To account for the relative contribution of each of the three factors to the total solution, the pulmonary, blood lipid, and blood pressure factors were weighted in accordance with their respective eigenvalues. The weighted combination of factor scores was summed to generate the IPS according to the following equation:

$$\text{IPS} = E1F1 + E2F2 + E3F3$$

where, Ei is the eigenvalue associated with the *i*th factor.

IPS scores were computed for each participant in the study and normalized to T scores. Finally, in order to permit the simple generation of IPS scores in future experiments, a multiple linear regression analysis was performed with the factor analytically derived IPS scores as the dependent variable and the seven constituent measures as the independent variables. As expected, the seven physiological variables accounted for 100% of the variance associated with the IPS scores. The multiple regression equation is:

$$\text{IPS} = 6.95\ \text{FEV1} + 4.91\ \text{FVC} - 1.56\ \text{RISK} - .052\ \text{TRIG} - .100\ \text{LWT} - .197\ \text{SBP} + .063\ \text{DBP} + 46.06$$

D. DISCUSSION

Having developed our multivariate IPS it was necessary to evaluate the validity of the instrument as a measure of overall health status. Conceptually, we felt that it was appropriate that measures of physiological fitness designed for use with elderly subjects be evaluated in accordance with their sensitivity to a series of tasks that are important for health and effective functioning and that can be shown to be reflective of advancing age and physiological health. Accordingly, a series of experiments were performed to evaluate the sensitivity of the IPS with respect to the performances of elderly individuals on a broad variety of sensory, motor, and cognitive performance tasks.

III. EXPERIMENT TWO

This study sought to determine the strength of association between the IPS and a number of auditory, visual, somatosensory, speech, and reaction time measures. Previous research had established that performances of the above tasks could be shown to deteriorate appreciably with advancing age[7,26,51,55] and worsening health.[1,21,38,40] It seemed logical to expect that any measure of fitness designed for use with elderly subjects should also be sensitive to changes in performance of such tests. In this experiment we attempted to determine the extent to which knowledge of an individual's physiological status, as measured by the IPS, could contribute to our understanding of age-related changes in behavior.

A. METHOD

The 70 elderly adults described in experiment one were also tested on a variety of sensory, motor, and cognitive tasks selected for their sensitivity to both age and fitness effects. The protocols for this experiment have been reported in detail elsewhere,[16] however, a brief description of the variables is as follows:

1. Audiometric analyses: Pure tone air conduction sensitivity was determined using a standard clinical audiometer. Air conduction thresholds were obtained at 1000, 2000, and 4000 Hz for the left (L1, L2, L4) and right (R1, R2, R4) ears.
2. Visual analyses: Lens accommodation (LA) was determined in accordance with the "push-up method",[46] in which the subject was instructed to focus on a white target card which was moved towards him until blurring was reported.
3. Somatosensory analyses: Two-point touch discrimination (TP) procedures were used to determine tactile sensitivity in the pad of the middle finger of the dominant hand.
4. Acoustic analyses: Subjects were instructed to phonate the vowel "a" for as long as possible at a comfortable pitch and intensity level. Acoustic analyses of voice samples were performed using a computerized acoustic analysis program.[59] Data were obtained for the following acoustic parameters:

   Fundamental frequency (Fo)
   Frequency perturbation (jitter)
   Amplitude perturbation (shimmer)
   Harmonics-to-noise ratio (H/N)
5. Reaction time analyses: An 80-trial choice reaction time task was conducted in which subjects were asked to discriminate between colored stimuli presented on a computer screen. Half of the trials constituted a relatively easy discrimination task (RTeasy), whereas the other half of the trials consisted of a more difficult discrimination task (RTdiff).

B. RESULTS

1. Descriptive Data

Descriptive data for the sensory, motor and cognitive measures are presented in Table 3. Examination of these data reveals that the mean scores reported for subjects in this study are in broad agreement with those reported in previous studies using similar elderly populations.[26,51,52,55]

2. Correlations Between Chronological Age and Performance Items

In order to test the hypothesis that performances of the selected tasks did indeed deteriorate with advancing age, Pearson correlations were computed between these items and chronological age.

Table 3 Descriptive data: sensory and motor variables

Variable		Mean	S.D.	*n*
L1 (dB) Auditory threshold	Left 1000 Hz	22.6	8.3	68
L2	2000 Hz	26.8	11.8	68
L4	4000 Hz	42.6	18.9	68
R1	Right 1000 Hz	24.0	11.6	68
R2	2000 Hz	27.4	14.0	68
R4	4000 Hz	41.3	18.4	68
LA (cm; lens accommodation)		77.8	51.9	70
TP (mm; two-point touch)		3.0	0.9	70
Fo (Hz; fundamental frequency)		118.2	39.5	49
Jitter (%; frequency perturbation)		2.6	1.5	49
Shimmer (dB; amplitude perturbation)		3.3	1.9	49
H/N (harmonics-to-noise ratio)		18.2	4.3	49
RTeasy (s; reaction time, red/yellow)		0.70	0.14	64
RTdiff (s; reaction time, blue/green)		0.79	0.17	64

Table 4 Correlations between sensory and motor performance and chronological age

Variable	*r*	*n*	*p*
L1	0.19	68	0.05
L2	0.26	68	0.01
L4	0.45	68	0.001
R1	0.13	68	0.13
R2	0.25	68	0.02
R4	0.34	68	0.001
TP	0.35	70	0.001
LA	–0.42	70	0.001
Fo	0.14	49	0.16
Jitter	0.22	49	0.06
Shimmer	0.25	49	0.04
H/N	–0.26	49	0.03
RTeasy	0.53	64	0.001
RTdiff	0.61	64	0.001

Note: *The number of subjects in the individual correlations varies because a few subjects did not participate in all of the sensory and motor tests. In particular, due to the cost of the acoustic analyses, voice data are restricted to 49 subjects.*

Examination of Table 4 reveals that virtually all of the auditory, visual, somatosensory, speech, and reaction time tasks exhibited significant age-related performance declines. The choice reaction time measures were most strongly correlated with age, RTdiff exhibiting the higher correlation. Examination of the audiometric data revealed that the relationship between decreased auditory sensitivity and age was greatest for high frequency tones. Both TP and LA also deteriorated with age. Finally,

Table 5 Correlations between sensory and motor performance and the PS

Variable	*r*	*n*	*p*
L1	–0.17	68	0.07
L2	–0.20	68	0.04
L4	–0.37	68	0.001
R1	0.00	68	0.49
R2	–0.26	68	0.01
R4	–0.36	68	0.001
TP	–0.07	70	0.26
LA	0.30	70	0.01
Fo	–0.13	49	0.17
Jitter	–0.21	49	0.06
Shimmer	–0.25	49	0.03
H/N	–0.30	49	0.01
RTeasy	–0.36	64	0.001
RTdiff	–0.40	64	0.001

although vocal fundamental frequency was not significantly correlated with age, the more sensitive measures of voice perturbation (shimmer, H/N) were found to be related to chronological age.

Subject scores on the IPS were found to be inversely correlated with age ($r = -0.53$, $p < 0.001$), suggesting that overall physiological status declines with age. In addition, examination of Table 5 reveals significant correlations between the IPS and many of the sensory and motor performance tests. Higher levels of physiological fitness were associated with faster reaction times, increased LA, and decreased high frequency hearing loss. Although mean voice fundamental frequency was not related to fitness, both shimmer and H/N ratios were significantly correlated with IPS scores. In general, high scores on the IPS were associated with improved performances on the sensory and motor test battery.

3. *Discriminant Function Analysis*

It is tempting to suggest that the above data indicate that high levels of physiological health diminish the detrimental effects of age on sensory, motor, and cognitive performance. Unfortunately, the correlational data alone cannot be accepted as evidence for the influence of physiological fitness because performance differences between subjects are confounded by chronological age.

In order to control for differences in age between subjects, a multiple discriminant function procedure was adopted to determine whether a linear combination of the performance items could discriminate between two groups of high and low IPS subjects matched for chronological age. Subjects in group one (n = 10, mean age 65.4 years) scored at least one half a standard deviation above the mean on the IPS, whereas subjects in group two (n = 10, mean age 65.2 years) scored at least one half a standard deviation below the mean.

The results of the discriminant function analyses are presented in Table 6. These data reveal that a linear combination of visual, auditory, somatosensory, reaction time, and speech measures significantly discriminated between subjects in the good and poor condition groups. Furthermore, when the discriminant function canonical was used for classification purposes, subjects could be classified into the appropriate health group with 100% classification accuracy.

Table 6 Discriminant function analysis between high and low IPS groups matched for age

Variable		Standardized canonical discriminant function coefficients
TP		0.7397
LA		1.0105
Jitter		–0.5252
H/N		0.4684
RTeasy		–2.0987
RTdiff		1.6244
R4		0.0796
Chi squared	= 18.30	
Canonical correlation	= 0.87	
Wilk's lambda	= 0.23	
Probability	= 0.01	
Percent correct classification	= 100%	

C. DISCUSSION

As expected, performances on virtually all of the sensory, motor, and cognitive tasks deteriorated appreciably with advancing age. The strongest correlations were between age and reaction time measures, underscoring the importance of behavioral slowing which has frequently been referred to as one of the strongest and most ubiquitous characteristics of old age.[53] Similarly, LA and tactile sensitivity exhibited patterns of deterioration with age which were consistent with those reported by other investigators.[28,46,48] Examination of the auditory data revealed that age-related hearing impairment was greatest for the high frequency tones, a finding which has also been frequently reported elsewhere.[19,30] Finally, jitter, shimmer, and H/N ratios were found to be significantly correlated with age. These findings are similar to those reported by Ramig and Ringel,[51] who have suggested that fundamental frequency may be an insufficiently sensitive measure for the detection of age-related changes in the voice and that it is frequently necessary to sample finer aspects of vocal behavior in order to detect age changes in vocal performance.[50,51] In summary, for virtually all of the tests reported in this study, the observed relationships between age and sensory, motor, and cognitive performance were consistent with those previously reported in the literature.

With respect to the influence of physiological status on these age-related declines, examination of the correlations between IPS and the functional performance items revealed persistent associations between physiological health and functional performance. High scores on the IPS were associated with faster reaction times, improved hearing at high frequencies, greater phonatory control, and improved LA. Furthermore, when subjects were divided into discrete fitness groups which were matched for chronological age, discriminant analyses revealed reliable sensory, motor, and cognitive differences between the two groups. These results are supportive of Fries and Crapo's[27] notion of plasticity of response in human aging and suggest that individuals who are able to maintain high levels of physical fitness can apparently diminish the detrimental effects of aging and at least temporarily deviate from expected patterns of linear senescence.

IV. EXPERIMENT THREE

The goal of this experiment was to investigate the nature of interactions between chronological age, health status, and depressive tendencies in a group of elderly adults with no known history of psychiatric morbidity. The experimental examination of these relationships is of interest because considerable ambiguity exists within the literature with respect to the prevalence of depression in old age.[42] Some studies report depressive symptoms in as many as 30 to 65 percent of the elderly population.[12,24] whereas others have suggested that the prevalence of depression in old age may be considerably less.[20,41]

In addition to the confusion within the literature concerning the prevalence of depression in old age, some evidence suggests that any association that does exist may be confounded by differences among elderly individuals with respect to physical activity levels.[49] Unfortunately, relatively few studies have attempted to take into consideration physiological differences between subjects when examining the relationship between advancing age and depression.

This study was designed to shed light upon two specific experimental questions. First, is there a reliable relationship between advancing age and depressed mood in a nonclinical population? Second, is there an association between overall health status and mood state which might confound any relationship between depression and advancing age?

A. METHOD

Sixty adults (29 males, 31 females) ranging in age from 60 to 85 years volunteered to participate in the study. Participants represented a broad cross-section of the elderly population, not only with regard to education and social class but also with regard to overall health status. General health status was determined by the computation of the PS in accordance with the procedures described in experiment one.

Two psychometric instruments were selected for the evaluation of depression. The Beck Depression Inventory,[3] a well-established self-report index of clinical depression, was administered to screen subjects for significant levels of psychiatric depression. The group mean score on the Beck inventory was 4.2 (S.E. = 0.6) which fell within the normal ranges. No subject scored sufficiently high to be classified clinically depressed according to the criteria of Beck. In the present study, the Beck inventory was intended to be used solely as a pre-experimental screening procedure. Due to its low discriminatory power in the nonclinical population selected for this study, the Beck data were not included in subsequent analyses.

Depressive tendencies were evaluated by the depression scale of the Profile of Mood States Questionnaire (POMS).[45] POMS is a self-report inventory which has been shown to be a sensitive measure of feeling, effect, and mood state in normal subjects and other nonclinical populations.[47] The depression subscale is designed to assess feelings of personal worthlessness, emotional isolation, sadness, and guilt. In the present study, the psychometric tests were administered on a separate day from the physiological and biochemical testing.

B. RESULTS

No significant age or mood state differences were found between sexes. Accordingly, the data were pooled for subsequent analyses. Descriptive statistics for the physiological and psychometric data are presented in Table 7. Examination of these data reveal that participants scored within expected ranges for both physiological and psychological variables.

Pearson product moment correlations were computed in order to determine the nature and magnitude of relationships between chronological age, physiological health, and mood state. As expected, a small but statistically significant association was observed between chronological age and depression ($r = 0.25$, $p < 0.05$). At first glance, these data appear to be supportive of the widely accepted belief that depressive tendencies increase with advancing age. It is particularly interesting to note the presence of such an association in normal subjects with no evidence of psychiatric morbidity.

Table 7 Descriptive data (Experiment Three)

Variable	Mean	S.E.
Age (years)	67.9	1.05
IPS	50	1.30
SBP (mmHg)	129	1.57
DBP (mmHg)	76	1.16
FVC (1)	3.19	0.14
FEV1 (1/s)	2.35	0.13
TRIG (mg/dl)	130	7.70
RISK (TCHOL/HDL)	4.8	0.16
LWT (kg)	51.5	1.32
Depression (POMS)	42.9	0.88

Previous research has shown that changes in health status are frequently associated with related psychological manifestations.[13-15] Pearson product moment correlations were also computed to assess the strength of relationship between depression and general health status. High scores on the depression scale were found to be associated with low scores on the IPS ($r = -0.30$, $p < 0.01$).

Although small but significant relationships were observed between depression and both chronological age and the IPS, these data are difficult to interpret unambiguously because health status and chronological age are frequently confounded in the elderly population. In order to examine the strength of association between mood state and chronological age independent of differences in health status, partial correlation coefficients were computed for the relationship between the depression scale and chronological age while controlling for IPS differences. The association between chronological age and depression was no longer found to be significant when such an approach was adopted to control for health differences between subjects ($r = 0.15$, $p > 0.10$).

However, when similar approaches were adopted to test for the persistence of associations between the IPS and depression while controlling for chronological age, the association between the IPS and depression remained significant ($r = -0.23$, $p < 0.05$). These data suggest that for the nonclinical population studied, caution should be exerted when interpreting the relationship between chronological age and depressive tendencies since this association may be more a function of decreasing health status than a reflection of the passage of time.

C. DISCUSSION

The data presented in this study are in broad agreement with the findings of Berkman et al.[5] and Parent and Whall,[49] to the extent that the association between advancing age and depression appears to have been confounded by physiological health differences between subjects. It is important to note that in the current investigation, had physiological data not been collected, we would have concurred with the widely held belief that advancing age is associated with increased depression, at least with respect to the depression subscale of the POMS questionnaire. Such a conclusion would have been largely misleading because much of the above association could be due to health differences between subjects.

These data should not be attributed as evidence for a causal relationship between physiological health and depression in old age because the cross-sectional design of the study did not permit the experimental manipulation of physiological health. Nonetheless, a number of studies have suggested that regular physiological training may be effective in the reduction of depression, at least in clinical populations.[29,43] Ongoing research in the author's laboratory investigates the possibility of beneficial effects of exercise on affective state in nonclinical elderly individuals.

In summary, the data presented reveal the presence of a small but significant association between depression and advancing age in a group of asymptomatic elderly adults without a history of psychiatric illness. However, the passage of time per se should not be interpreted as the causative factor behind such a relationship. Rather, it is likely that chronological age effects are frequently confounded by coincident changes in physiological health, physical activity levels, and many other factors.

V. GENERAL DISCUSSION

The data presented in this chapter serve to underscore the tremendous variability with which selected sensory, motor, and cognitive functions decline with advancing age. While one person may exhibit profound deterioration in response to old age, another individual of the same chronological age may experience little or no loss of function.

It is the presence of precisely such variability that has led gerontologists to the realization that an understanding of physiological differences between subjects is imperative if we are to increase our understanding of the aging process. In an attempt to acknowledge the importance of physiological factors in the aging process, many researchers have developed indices for the computation of biological age. We have argued that in addition to the technical difficulties associated with the computation of such indices, there are also conceptual problems. In most instances, indices of biological age have been developed for use as physiological substitutes for chronological age. However, it is unclear why measures of biological age should be used as alternatives to chronological age, as it is apparent that both physiological and chronological factors contribute to intersubject variability.

Ingram[34] has pointed out that chronological age need not be considered simply a measure of the passage of time. Rather, it may be more appropriate to view chronological age as an exquisitely sensitive index which reflects a complex combination of biological processes that are usually, but not always, coincident with the passage of time. The persistent observation that chronological age is the single best predictor of functional deterioration in old age is testament to the power of the variable as an index of biological age. Research on aging benefits from an evaluation of both chronological and physiological factors and that the *a priori* exclusion of either is inadvisable.

The author's research has concentrated on the evaluation of the influence of physiological fitness on the degree of functional decline observed with advancing age. The procedures we have adopted for the evaluation of physiological health status mark a significant departure from more traditional approaches. Most measures of physiological fitness require an individual to participate in relatively strenuous exercise-stress protocols. As such, these measures are ill-suited for the evaluation of fitness in elderly populations because large numbers of the elderly cannot safely participate and must be excluded from the experimental group.

Our approach has involved the reduction of a battery of noninvasive physiological and biochemical measures to a single score, the IPS. A series of experiments have suggested that the IPS may have some utility as a measure of overall health status in old age. Specifically, subject scores on the IPS have been shown to be sensitive to performance changes in a wide variety of sensory, motor, cognitive, and affective attributes known to be sensitive to age-related deterioration. It is our belief that knowledge of IPS scores has contributed significantly to our understanding of intersubject variability in functional performance.

A persistent problem in our research, however, has been the statistical dissociation of age and fitness effects. As we have pointed out, because chronological age and physiological status are invariably highly correlated, it is difficult to isolate the influence of either variable. We have adopted several approaches in an attempt to account for this confound. In experiment three we reported partial correlations between age and depression while controlling for the IPS, and also partial correlations between the IPS and depression while controlling for age. While this procedure is probably statistically sound, we have persistent misgivings as to whether it is scientifically meaningful to consider either the influence of fitness in the absence of age or the influence of age in the absence of fitness. Indeed, such misgivings would appear to be prudent for any statistical design which attempts to partition variance between two manifestly nonindependent variables.

In experiment two we adopted an alternative procedure in that we attempted to differentiate between two discrete fitness groups on the basis of a battery of sensory, motor, and cognitive tests. Because we artificially manipulated the fitness groups to ensure that they did not differ on chronological age, we were able to conclude that IPS differences between subjects can be shown to be a factor in functional decline. Unfortunately, the weaknesses associated with this procedure are also apparent. Construction of the age-matched fitness groups required considerable manipulation after the fact. While these data show that it is *possible* for fitness to influence sensory, motor, and cognitive performance, the generalizability of these findings to the total elderly population is severely compromised due to the restricted sample on which they are based.

We have come to suspect that the experimental isolation of age and fitness effects, although theoretically possible, may be scientifically fruitless. In a recent experiment, we attempted to combine chronological age and physiological health measures in a multivariate design to evaluate the influence of senescence on cognitive performance.[17] In this experiment the overall physiological health status of 43 elderly individuals (age range 50 to 88 years) was determined using the IPS. In addition, cognitive performances were evaluated for these individuals for a battery of tasks distributed along an automatic to effortful processing continuum.[31] When these data were analyzed multivariately, a significant canonical correlation was found between a set of variables representing chronological and physiological aspects of senescence (age and IPS) and a set of measures representing cognitive performance. The time-dependent and effortful cognitive tasks were found to be most strongly associated with cognitive decline in senescence, whereas the more automatic tasks appeared to be less sensitive to senescent decline.

It seems likely that multivariate models similar to the above will become increasingly important in experimental gerontology. While these procedures may not have the interpretive simplicity associated with more traditional univariate designs, they have the distinct advantage of combining both physiological and chronological information in a single vector of senescence. Thus, these approaches are able to avoid many of the statistical pitfalls associated with the experimental isolation of confounded measures using univariate statistics which require assumptions of independence among variables.

In conclusion, we have presented an alternative approach to the evaluation of the influence of physiological health factors on functional decline in old age. Because the IPS has been established for a relatively small number of subjects it represents a preliminary solution and should not be regarded as a comprehensive blueprint for the measurement of physiological status. Nonetheless, it is our belief that the procedures reported here may provide the researcher with a useful alternative to more traditional measures for the evaluation of the influence of physiological factors in senescence.

REFERENCES

1. Albert, M.L., *Clinical Neurology of Aging*, Oxford University Press, New York, 1984.
2. American College of Sports Medicine, *Guidelines for Graded Exercise Testing and Exercise Prescription*, Lea & Febiger, New York, 1986.
3. Beck, A.T., Ward, C.H., Mendelson, M., and Mock, J., An inventory for measuring depression, *Arch Gen. Psych.*, 4, 561, 1961.
4. Bell, B., Significance of functional age for interdisciplinary and longitudinal research in aging, *Int. J. Aging Hum. Dev.*, 3, 145, 1972.
5. Berkman, L.F., Berkman, C.S., Kasl, S., Freeman, D.H., Leo, L., Ostfeld, A.M., Coroni-Huntley, J., and Brody, J., Depressive symptoms in relation to physical health and functioning in the elderly, *Am. J. Epidemiol.*, 124, 372, 1986.

6. Birren, J.E., Age changes in speed of behavior: its central nature and physiological correlates, in *Behavior, Aging and the Nervous System*, Weford, A.T. and Birren J.E., Eds., Charles C Thomas, Springfield, IL, 1965.
7. Birren, J.E., Woods, A.M., and Williams, M.V., Behavioral slowing with age: causes, organization and consequences, in *Aging in the 1980's: Psychological Issues*, Poon, L.W., Ed., American Psychological Association, Washington, D.C., 1980.
8. Birren, J. E. and Schaie, K.W., *Handbook of the Psychology of Aging*, Van Nostrand Reinhold, New York, 1985.
9. Borkan, G.A. and Norris, A.H., Assessment of biological age using a profile of physical parameters, *J. Gerontol.*, 35, 177, 1980.
10. Botwinick, J., *Aging and Behavior: A Comprehensive Integration of Research Findings*, Springer-Verlag, New York, 1985.
11. Buskirk, E.R., Health maintenance and longevity: exercise, in *Handbook of the Biology of Aging*, Finch, C.E. and Schneider, E.L., Eds., Van Nostrand Reinhold, New York, 1985.
12. Busse, E.W. and Pfeiffer, E., *Mental Illness in Later Life*, American Psychological Association, Washington, D.C., 1973.
13. Chodzko-Zajko, W.J. and Ismail, A.H., MMPI interscale relationships before and after an eight month fitness program, *J. Clin. Psychol.*, 40, 163, 1984.
14. Chodzko-Zajko, W.J. and O'Connor, P.J., Plasma cortisol, the dexamethasone suppression test and depression in normal adult males, *J. Psychosom. Res.*, 30(3), 313, 1986.
15. Chodzko-Zajko, W.J. and Ismail, A.H., The discrimination power of the MMPI and selected physiological and biochemical variables to differentiate between high and low fit males, in *Exercise Physiology*, Vol. 2, Humphrey, J.H. and Dotson, C.O., Eds., AMS Press, New York, 1986, 99.
16. Chodzko-Zajko, W.J. and Ringel, R.L., Physical fitness measures and sensory and motor performance in aging, *Exp. Gerontol.*, 22, 317, 1987.
17. Chodzko-Zajko, W.J. and Solomon, J.L., Individual Differences in Cognitive Decline in Old Age: The Role of Physiological Health Status, paper presented at the 22nd Gatlinburg Conference on Research and Theory in Mental Retardation, Gatlinburg, TN, March 1989.
18. Costa, P.T. and McCrae, R.R., Functional age: a conceptual and empirical critique, in *Epidemiology of Aging*, NIH Publ. No. 80-969, Haynes, S.G. and Feinleib, M., Eds., Bethesda, MD, 1980.
19. Corson, J.F., Age and sex differences in pure tone thresholds, *Arch. Otolaryngol.*, 77, 385, 1963.
20. Costa, P.T., Zonderman, A.B., McCrae, R.R., Coroni-Huntley, J., Locke, B.Z., and Barbano, H.E., Longitudinal analyses of psychological well-being in a national sample, stability of mean levels, *J. Gerontol.*, 42(1), 50, 1987.
21. Darby, J. K., *Speech Evaluation in Medicine*, Grune and Stratton, New York, 1981.
22. Dean, W., *Biological Aging Measurement: Clinical Applications*, Center for Bio-Gerontology, Los Angeles, 1988.
23. Dirken, J.M., *Functional Age of Industrial Workers*, Woolters-Noordhoff, Grönigen, 1972.
24. Dovenmuehle, R.H., Recklass, J.B., and Newman, G., Depressive reactions in the elderly, in *Normal Aging*, Shock, N.W., Ed., Duke University Press, Durham, NC, 1970.
25. Dustman, R.E., Ruhling, R.O., Russell, E.M., Shearer, D.E., Bonekat, H.W., Shigeoka, J.W., Wood, J.S., and Bradford, D.C., Aerobic exercise training and improved neuropsychological function of older individuals, *Neurobiol. Aging*, 5, 35, 1984.
26. Finch, C. E. and Schneider, E.L., *Handbook of the Biology of Aging*, Van Nostrand Reinhold, New York, 1985.
27. Fries, J.F. and Crapo, M., *Vitality and Aging*, W. Freeman & Co., San Francisco, 1981.
28. Gellis, M. and Pool, R., Two-point discrimination distances in the normal hand and forearm, *Plastic Reconstr. Surg.*, 59(1), 57, 1977.
29. Greist, J.H., Klein, M.H., Eischens, R.R., Farris, J., Gurman, A.S. and Morgan, W.P., Running as a treatment for depression, *Comp. Psych.*, 20(1), 41, 1979.
30. Harford, E.A., Hearing aid amplification for adults, *Monogr. Contemp. Audiol.*, 4, 1, 1980.
31. Hasher, L. and Zacks, R.T., Automatic and effortful processes in memory, *J. Exp. Psychol. Gen.*, 108(3), 356, 1979.
32. Heron, A. and Chown, S., *Age and Function*, Little, Brown, Boston, 1976.

33. Hofecker, G., Skalicky, M., Kment, A., and Niedermuller, H., Models of the biological age of the rat. A factor model of age parameters, *Mech. Age. Dev.*, 14, 345, 1986.
34. Ingram, D. K., Towards the behavioral assessment of biological aging in the laboratory mouse: concepts terminology and objectives, *Exp. Aging Res.*, 9(4), 225, 1983.
35. Ismail, A.H., Corrigan, D.L., McLeod, D.F., Anderson, V.L., Kasten, R.N., and Elliot, P.N., Biophysiological and audiological variables in adults, *Arch. Otolaryngol.*, 97, 447, 1973.
36. Jackson, A.S. and Pollock, M.L., Generalized equations for predicting body density of men, *Br. J. Nutr.*, 40, 497, 1978.
37. Jalavisto, E., The role of a simple test measuring speed of performance in the assessment of biological vigor: a factorial study of elder women, in *Behavior Aging and the Nervous System*, Welford, A.T. and Birren, J.E., Eds., Charles C Thomas, Springfield, IL, 1965.
38. Jerger, J., Neely, J., and Jerger, S., Speech impedance and auditory brainstem response audiometry in brainstem tumors. Importance of multiple test strategy, *Arch. Otolaryngol.*, 106, 218, 1980.
39. Kaiser, H.F., The varimax criterion for factor rotation in factor analysis, *Psychometrika*, 23, 187, 1963.
40. Katzman, R. and Terry, R., *The Neurology of Aging*, F.A. Davis, Philadelphia, 1983.
41. Larson, R., Thirty years of research on the subjective well-being of older Americans, *J. Gerontol.*, 33, 109, 1978.
42. LaRue, A., Dessonville, C., and Jarvik, L.F., Aging and mental disorders, in *Handbook of the Psychology of Aging*, Birren, J.E. and Schaie, K.W., Eds., Van Nostrand Reinhold, New York, 1985.
43. Lichtman, S. and Poser, E.G., The effects of exercise on mood and cognitive functioning, *J. Psychosom. Res.*, 27(1), 43, 1983.
44. Ludwig, F.C. and Smoke, M.E., The measurement of biological age, *Exp. Aging Res.*, 6, 497, 1980.
45. McNair, D.M., Lorr, M., and Droppleman, L.F., *Manual for the Profile of Mood States*, Educational and Industrial Testing Service, San Diego, 1981.
46. Michaels, D.M., *Visual Optics and Refraction: A Clinical Approach*, C.V. Mosby, St. Louis, 1980.
47. Morgan, W.P., The test of champions, *Psychol. Today*, July, 92, 1980.
48. Morgan, R.F. and Fevens, S.K., Reliability of the adult growth examination: a standardized test of individual aging, *Percep. Motor Skills*, 34, 415, 1972.
49. Parent, C.J. and Whall, A.L., Are physical activity, self-esteem and depression related?, *J. Gerontol. Nursing*, 10(9), 8, 1986.
50. Ramig, L.A., Effects of physiological aging on vowel spectral noise, *J. Gerontol.*, 38, 223, 1983.
51. Ramig, L.A. and Ringel, R.L., Effect of physiological aging on selected acoustic characteristics of voice, *J. Speech Hear. Res.*, 26, 22, 1983.
52. Ringel, R.L. and Ewanowski, S.J., Oral perception: two point discrimination, *J. Speech Hear. Res.*, 8(4), 389, 1965.
53. Salthouse, T.A., Speed of behavior and its implications for cognition, in *Handbook of the Psychology of Aging*, Birren, J.E. and Schaie, K.W., Eds., Van Nostrand Reinhold, New York, 1985.
54. Shephard, R.J., *Physical Activity and Aging*, Croom Helm, Chicago, 1978.
55. Shock, N.W., Greulich, R.C., Andres, R., Arenberg, D., Costa, P.T., Lakatta, E.G., and Tobin, J.D., *Normal Human Aging: The Baltimore Longitudinal Study of Aging*, National Institutes of Health, Bethesda, MD, 1984.
56. Sidney, K.H. and Shephard, R.J., Maximum and submaximum exercise tests in men and women in the seventh, eighth and ninth decades of life, *J. Appl. Physiol.*, 43, 280, 1977.
57. Spirduso, W.W., Reaction and movement time as a function of age and physical activity level, *J. Gerontol.*, 30, 435, 1975.
58. Spirduso, W.W. and Clifford, P., Neuromuscular speed and consistency of performance as a function of age, physical activity level and type of physical activity, *J. Gerontol.*, 33, 26, 1978.
59. Titze, I.R., Parametrization of the glottal area, glottal flow and vocal fold contact area, *J. Acoust. Soc. Am.*, 75, 570, 1984.
60. Welford, A.T., Motor skills and aging, in *The Aging Motor System*, Mortimar, J.A., Pirozzolo, F.J., and Maletta, G.J., Eds., Praeger, New York, 1982.

CHAPTER 11

DETERMINATION OF HUMAN BIOLOGICAL AGE

WERNER RIES

TABLE OF CONTENTS

I. INTRODUCTION

As early as 1963, a seminar held by the European Bureau of the World Health Organization (WHO) in Kiev, Ukraine called on gerontologists to seek methods to determine biological age. For a long time thereafter this appeal met with little response and only occasionally did papers appear on the subject. The situation has changed completely, and a multitude of research teams are at work in all parts of the world trying to measure biological age and dealing, from different angles, with the terminological, philosophical, methodological, mathematical, clinical, and organizational problems involved.[2,4,5,8,13,14]

II. TERMINOLOGY

While the chronological age of an individual is the period that has elapsed from birth to date of examination, the biological age describes a person's general condition at a particular time of the chronological age. The characteristics used to determine it are physical, psychological, and social, and allowance must be made not only for orthological (normal), but also for pathological findings. This integrated approach has been summarized by Beier[1] as the vitality of a biological system. The chronological and biological age of a person may, but need not, coincide.

0-8493-0129-7/94/$0.00+$.50

III. METHODS

Biological age is determined via "test batteries". The first studies of this kind were made by Hollingsworth et al.[7] on radiation-exposed inhabitants of Hiroshima and Nagasaki. The most extensive test battery with a total of 60 parameters was proposed by Comfort.[3] Apart from physical tests, it included psychometric and bioptic procedures but, as far as we know, has never been practiced on a larger scale.

The selection of methods depends both on the subjective approach of the researcher in question and the objective ways of action open to him. Any parameters chosen must permit quantitative evaluation and numerical expression of the results. Findings must be recorded independent of the examiner's judgment, whether they are pathological or not, and the test battery itself should be feasible and reasonable. Great physical and psychological stress should be avoided, particularly in mass screening. Most importantly, the test battery must concern itself with those organic characteristics that are essential in assessing biological age. For example, it is doubtful whether the color or density of a person's hair can serve as reliable indicators of biological substance.

A test battery has been developed[10,11] that takes physical, psychological, and social markers into account. The physical parameters include blood pressure, circulatory efficiency data, vital capacity, partial oxygen pressure in the arteries, hand grip strength, articular mobility, visual acuity, audiometry, and the condition of the teeth.

Psychometry uses the following procedures: the concentration time test, visiomotor coordination, acoustic and visual reaction time, maze test, and psychomotor tempo tapping. To perform all of these with one instrument, a unit known as the Geromat has been developed which has proven its worth at laboratories in Leipzig and Halberstadt, Germany (Figure 1).

Social indicators included the complaints questionnaire according to Höck and Hess,[6] the ENR (extraversion, neuroticism, rigidity) questionnaire, the Leningrad cluster, and the Giessen test.

A total of 47 indicators were obtained for a variety of functions. Methodical details and references to the literature are given by Pöthig.[9]

IV. CALCULATION

Calculation for biological age is made in three steps.

A. PARTIAL INDEX (PI)

The best (G) and worst (V) data is recorded for each method, and the partial index is determined with the help of the measured data (W) as follows:

$$\mathrm{PI} = \frac{G - W}{G - V}$$

Examples: systolic blood pressure, $G = 100$ Torr, $V = 240$ Torr, $W = 130$ Torr

$$\mathrm{PI} = \frac{100 - 130}{100 - 240} = \frac{30}{140} = 0,21$$

This type of calculation in effect represents normalization and invariably gives results between 0 and 1.

B. BIOLOGICAL INDEX (BI)

This is the arithmetic mean of all the partial index values which results from the summation of the individual values and division of the sum by the number of values (in this case 47):

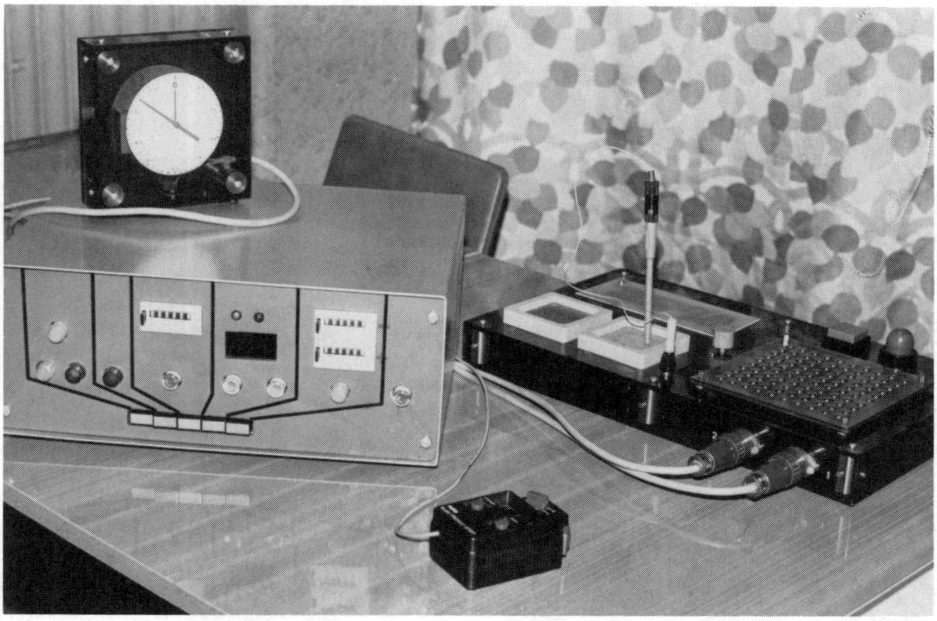

Figure 1 Geromat for psychological testing.

$$BI = \frac{1}{47}\left(\sum_{i=1}^{47} PI_i\right)$$

In the same way, biological indices can be obtained for particular groups of parameters, i.e., physical, psychological, or social.

C. BIOLOGICAL AGE (BA)

When it is assumed that biological and chronological age (A) coincide for the "average person", then the following regression statement can be made:

$$A = b_0 + b_1 \cdot \ln BI$$

A logarithmic approach is preferred here, and the biological age results from the sum of the constants (b_0) and the natural logarithm of the biological index multiplied by b_1.

V. RESULTS

In order to obtain a "normal curve", a defined reference population was studied. This consisted of residents of the city of Leipzig showing an almost homogeneous age and sex distribution. The study was randomized with regard to medical and social risk factors, while the reference population was established with these two aims in mind:

1. To check the extent to which the proposed test battery yields meaningful results when allowance is made for the premises listed
2. To find reference values of comparative studies of specific groups

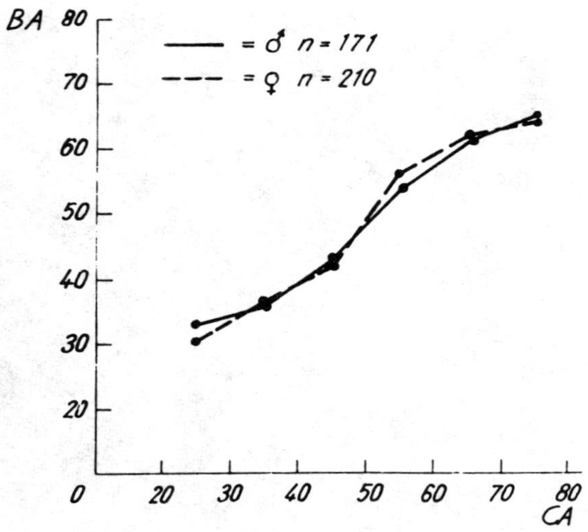

Figure 2 Biological (BA) and chronological (CA) age of a reference population.

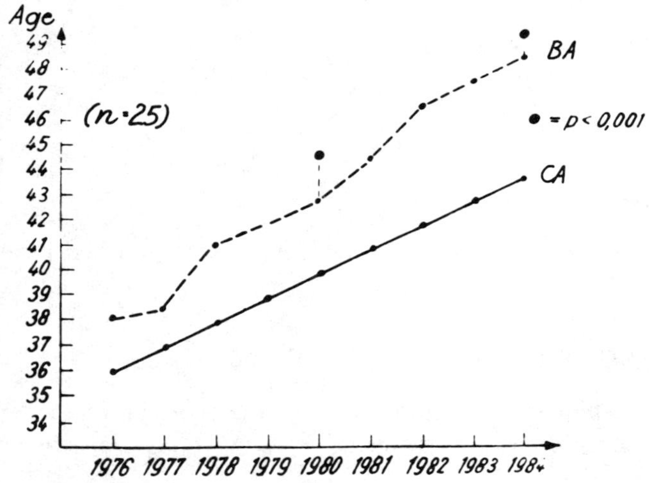

Figure 3 Biological (BA) and chronological (CA) age of overweight men in a longitudinal study.

The age- and sex-related averages shown for the biological age in Figure 2 are sufficiently correlated with the chronological age of the test persons and show the test battery to be practical. No major differences were found between sexes.

Previous studies of particular groups of diseases have concentrated on patients exposed to cardiac risks. In these studies premature aging was repeatedly found in overweight persons, as borne out particularly by a longitudinal study begun by Ingrid Hunecke in 1976 (Figure 3). After a clinical weight reduction, these patients showed a marked improvement in biological age, especially as regards the mental aspect (Figure 4).

Another study concerned itself with the biological age of patients suffering from arteriosclerotic, peripheral circulatory disturbances, and Figure 5 clearly shows premature aging in most cases when a comparison is made with the male reference population.

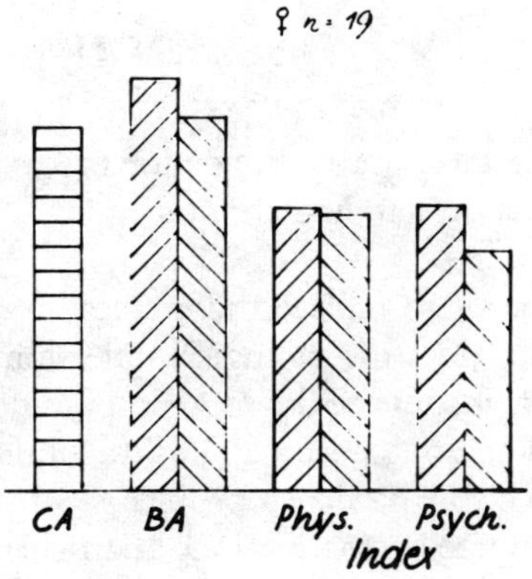

Figure 4 Biological age (BA), physical and psychological index of overweight women before (left) and after (right) weight reduction.

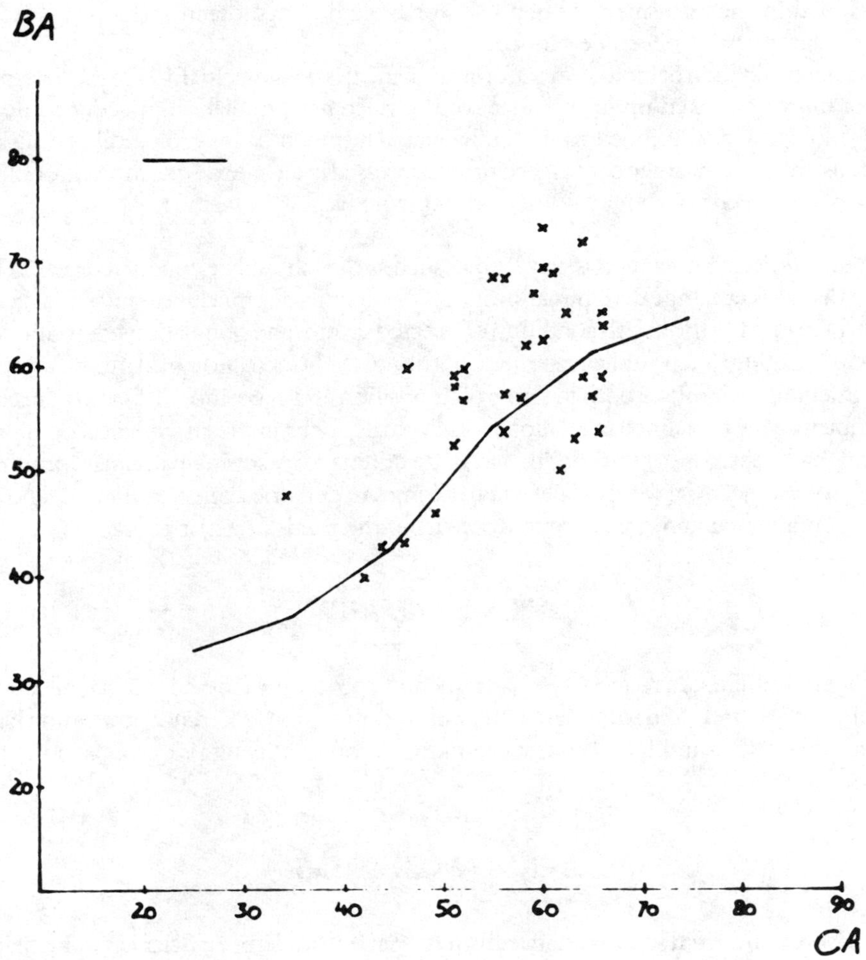

Figure 5 Biological age (BA) of 32 male patients with arteriosclerotic peripheral circulatory disturbances compared with a reference population.

VI. DISCUSSION

The test battery developed for biological age determination has proven its worth, but a few comments are in place to avoid possible misunderstanding about its role:

1. The test battery is not meant to replace the medical examination of a patient, which remains indispensable. Nor does the biological index cover all human functions, even though an integrated look at some of the more important functions can provide useful pointers to the biological age of a person. Thus, the index is merely a specific facet of examination employed to clarify particular problems.
2. The biological index does not tell us for how long a particular finding has existed, although this would be of great interest from a pathological point of view. More thought should be given to the question of how the time factor can be integrated with the individual data and how it can be calculated.
3. No conclusions can be drawn naturally from the results as to the remaining life span of a person, even though premature aging is actually found in individuals and groups. While theoretical approaches taken by Tokar and Parkin[12] suggest that mortality might be included in the assessment of methods for biological age determination, no practical procedures have yet been developed.
4. The determination of biological age of an individual is possible. In this case the determined data must be looked up in the table for the reference population in order to find the chronological age assigned to the individual. This, then, is his biological age. In other words, the biological age of a test person, as expressed in an index, equals the chronological age of a test person from a "normal" group who has the same index.

The one question that remains is why studies such as ours should be conducted at all. The answer can only be that biological age determination is of great significance for clinical and social gerontology alike. It can help identify the health condition of selected groups and populations, as well as risk factors in the process of aging. Such studies can then contribute to the detection of alarming symptoms and to the treatment of their causes both in terms of disposition and exposition. It is also conceivable that specific problems may be defined in relation to individuals, for example, in a medical opinion or at the workplace. Finally, there is hope of finding accurate criteria for assessing particular forms of therapy which can also be objectivized, especially when it comes to geriatric agents, as they are known. Thus, the principal motives behind our research derive from the needs of geriatric practice.

VII. SUMMARY

Biological age determination requires test batteries, and a procedure is described that makes allowance for physical, psychological, and social parameters. Studies involving a reference population have shown the method to be useful and have laid the groundwork for identifying risk groups in the process of aging.

ACKNOWLEDGMENT

The studies were conducted with assistance from the Saxon Academy of Sciences in Leipzig, and we are grateful for the help given by Erika Koch and Erika Schmidt, who served as medical and laboratory assistants.

REFERENCES

1. Beier, W., Vitalitätskonzept und biologischer Index nach Ries, *Z. Gerontol.,* 18, 353, 1985.
2. Borkan, C.A., *The Assessment of Biological Age during Adulthood*, Ph.D. dissertation, Michigan University, Michigan, 1978.
3. Comfort, A., Test battery to measure ageing-rate in man, *Lancet,* 27, 1411, 1969.
4. Furukawa, T., Inoue, M., Kajiya, F., Inada, H., Takasugi, S., Fukui, S., Takeda, H., and Abe, H., Assessment of biological age by multiple regression analysis, *J. Gerontol.,* 30, 422, 1975.
5. Heikkinnen, E., Suominen, H., Pohjolainen, P., Parkatti, T., and Kiiskinen, A., Assessment of biological age, in *5th Eur. Symp. Basic Research in Gerontology*, Schmidt, U.J., Bruschke, G., Lang, E., Viidik, A., Platt, D., Frolkis, V.V., and Schulz, F.H., Eds., Straube, Erlangen, 1976, 524.
6. Höck, K. and Hess, H., *Der Beschwerdefragebogen*, VEB Deutscher Verlag der Wissenschaften, Berlin, 1975.
7. Hollingsworth, J.W., Hashizume, A., and Jablon, S., Correlations between tests of aging in Hiroshima subjects. An attempt to define "physiological age", *Yale J. Biol. Med.,* 38, 11, 1965.
8. Nakamura, E., Kimura, M., Nagata, H., Miyao, K., and Ozeki, T., Evaluation of the progress of aging based on specific biological age as estimated by various physiological functions, *Jpn. J. Hyg.,* 36, 853, 1982.
9. Pöthig, D., Experimentelle Entwicklung eines klinischen Diagnostikmodells zur Objektivierung des biologischen Alters des Menschen, Ph.D. dissertation, University of Leipzig, Leipzig, 1984.
10. Ries, W., *Studien zum biologischen Alter,* Sitzungsberichte der Sächsischen Akademie der Wissenschaften, Math.-Nat. Klasse 116, Heft 1, Akademie-Verlag, Berlin, 1982.
11. Ries, W. and Sauer, I., Studien über das biologische Alter, in *Prozesse des Alterns,* Beier, W., Laue, R., Leutert, G., Rotzsch, W., and Schmidt, U.J., Eds., Akademie-Verlag, Berlin, 1988, 1.
12. Tokar, A.V. and Parkin, J.U., Mortalität und biologisches Alter beim Menschen, *Z. Alternsforsch.,* 40, 323, 1985.
13. Voitenko, V.P. and Tokar, A.V., The assessment of biological age and sex differences of human aging, *Exp. Age Res.,* 9, 239, 1983.
14. Webster, J.W. and Logie, A.R., A relationship between functional age and health status in female subjects, *J. Gerontol.,* 31, 548, 1976.

CHAPTER 12

TWO DECADES OF RESEARCH AND PRACTICE WITH THE ADULT GROWTH EXAMINATION. A BRIEF STANDARDIZED TEST OF ADULT AGING: THE 20TH YEAR PROGRESS REPORT

ROBERT F. MORGAN

TABLE OF CONTENTS

I. THE HISTORIC ALTERNATIVE: DEATH AS YARDSTICK

Death is the end of the aging process, but not its only measure. Effective conquest of aging will produce health as well as survival.

The termination of existence has long obsessed mankind. We have chosen to deny it, fear it, covet it, and count on it. Some of the more philosophical tell us that death is nature's way of telling us to slow down. Others view a person's death as a kind of permanent sabbatical, with some real benefit for those of us left behind. As far back as Mechnikov in the early 1900s some have viewed

0-8493-0129-7/94/$0.00+$.50

death as the triumph of the unnecessary disease of aging.[86] Today, death remains the most prevalent method of marking the end of the aging process.

Human and animal studies of attempts to slow the aging process typically measure success by how long life has been extended. The advantages:

1. Death is usually a clearly observed, consensually agreed upon event. There is, it is true, some continuing contemporary conflict on whether death is a state defined by "irreversible" cessation of brain function (EEG determined) or instead by the much later occurring cessation of heartbeat and respiration. The Presidential Commission for the Study of Ethical Problems in Medicine and Biomedical and Behavioral Research has been unable to decide which of these is the better definition.
2. Postponing death is usually, though not always, an applauded objective for science. It is a much desired personal goal of most members of our culture to delay their death.
3. By working with short-lived animals and using death as the terminal measure of their aging, we can assess the effect of life-extending interventions on survival itself.

The disadvantages:

1. There is more to aging than death; there is more to living than survival. The true goal of gerontology is to prevent the degenerative processes of aging and not just to maintain existence. Death is an inadequate measure of this: we need to measure aging long before mortality occurs.
2. While extending the maximum survival of a species is a convincing way to demonstrate the potency of an antiaging intervention,[128,129] we are limited to how much time in our own life span is available for such studies. If we pick animals too distant on the evolutionary scale from humans (rotifer, fruit flies) we are hindered in our ability to generalize to our own species. Even mammals cannot be equated — a rat is not a man — and good research with mammals takes quite a while. A few scientists have used a very short-lived strain of mice (average life span <1 year), but their effective interventions have been written off by many as only focusing on the anomaly that made them short-lived in the first place. Longevity measures for humans can be used in controlled studies only when the experimenter is likely to outlive the subjects: usually this means work with senescent adults. Waiting for the deaths of human experimental and control subjects is a little too depressing for many researchers. This problem is usually in evidence at gerontology conventions and conferences: "Throughout all the papers and discussions there appeared a certain feeling of frustration related to one of the basic problems of the researcher concerned with life span oriented functions in the human organism...the pervasive call for longitudinal studies sounds hollow when...the professional life span of a given investigator can encompass only a portion of the problem."[117]

There are some limited solutions to this problem. For one, several generations of experimenters may systematically follow a group of adults. Such longitudinal studies were begun in a few gerontology programs here in North America including one at Duke University[91-94] and one in Boston.[109-112] Another approach is to take the animal studies, limited generalizability or not, as the best methods available for "educated guessing". Or we might look at demographic vital statistics on human mortality to look for a pattern in post-dictive rather than predictive studies. None of these approaches, however, will tell us much about our own personal individual aging.

A better measuring system than survival is presented in this chapter. However, given the preceding reservations about death as a yardstick, there are some important leads such data can give us.

The basic vital statistics on human mortality are available from several well-known sources. These would include the World Health Organization, the Metropolitan Life Insurance Company, the National Center for Health Statistics, the U.S. Public Health Service, and the American Heart Association. Here, we can investigate comparative survival on the basis of chronological age, geographical residence, sex, race, and cause of death. Some basic patterns do emerge:

- Prominent men over 45, as listed in *Who's Who* had a mortality rate 30% below that of the general population.[98]
- Largest cause of human mortality (50% of all deaths) is now due to diseases of the heart and blood vessels.[1]
- Celibacy and lack of companionship increase mortality probabilities significantly.[24,74]
- Competitive athletics can be as much a disadvantage as having no exercise at all: moderate exercise for fun seems the best path.[96]
- Counties with the highest death rates tend to be on the Atlantic or Gulf Coasts and at low altitudes while counties with lowest death rates tend to be at higher elevations.[116] The low death rate counties had more residents over 65 than the high death rate counties, so their greater survival was not due to a younger population.
- There is some evidence that certain blood types are associated with greater longevity.[120]
- Mortality from lung cancer has increased tremendously since 1950, with the greatest risk at the younger adult decades; chronic bronchitis has doubled. Also showing a significant increase are cirrhosis of the liver, emphysema, and arteriosclerotic heart disease. From 1950 to 1966 lung cancer mortality per 100,000 males went from 19.9 to 41.4 (108% increase); for females it went from 4.5 to 7.1 (58% increase). Later data[54] confirmed a continuation of this pattern with increasing mortality rates for malignant neoplasms, diabetes mellitus, bronchitis, emphysema, asthma, cirrhosis of the liver, suicide, and homicide. Per 100,000 people, motor vehicle accidents accounted for 27.6 deaths while heart disease and stroke accounted for 468.7 and cancer for 160.0.

The gloomy picture reflected in the latter pattern would seem to go against the commonly held belief that our life span has increased through medical advances over the last few decades. Let us look closer:

- In 1975 the National Center for Health Statistics gave the average life expectancy from birth as 71.3 years (75.3 for females; 67.6 for males). In this analysis of vital statistics we also saw a continuing increase in cirrhosis of the liver (up 2% from 1972) and homicide (up 4% from 1972) as causes of death; infant mortality decreased 2% from 1972. Perhaps the latter is the clue: it in fact turns out that decreased infant mortality is responsible for the majority of the variance leading to longer average life span today. On the other hand, probability of survival for mature adults has not improved greatly and is apparently dropping. This means that nowadays babies have a better chance to live to be an adult while adults have a poorer chance of living much past retirement.
- For those biostatisticians interested in demonstrating the superiority of our medical technology, this can be frustrating. The turning point was about 1950, when the negative aspects of our environment equaled medical progress and began to surpass it. In a 1964 analysis, Moriyama[84] announced:

> "After a long period of decline, the trend of the crude death rate now appears to have leveled off. In the United States, the crude death rate has been more or less stationary during the period 1950 to 1960. The failure to experience a decline in mortality during this period is unexpected in view of the intensified attack on medical problems in the postwar years...at no time in the history of the country have conditions appeared so favorable for health progress."

How did he explain it?

> "Radioactive fall-out, air pollution, and other manmade hazards cannot be completely ignored...(but) it is obviously impossible for the death rate to decline indefinitely. At some point in time the mortality rate must level off as it reaches the irreducible minimum."

Invoking an "irreducible minimum" of progress in combating death was typical of the official optimism of the Public Health Service at the time. If we were making no more progress against mortality, perhaps it was because we have done everything that can be done. The "manmade hazards" were minimized and alcohol and tobacco unmentioned. Passwater[95] told us that cancer, for example, will kill one in four; 1 million are treated for it in the U.S. every year and more than one third die from it. While it is true that the average life span has gone from 47 in 1900 to 71 in 1975, this is so much a product of infants' greater survival that the years remaining to a 55-year-old are only 2 years more on the average than in 1900. There have been medical advances. Where is all this increased mortality coming from? Passwater blamed malnutrition at all economic levels. He cited Jean Meyer of Harvard's Department of Nutrition as locating fully 30 nations with citizens of greater life expectancies on the average than in North America since 1950.

What predictions can we make about longevity based on the vital statistics we have accumulated? Bender et al. in 1970 told us that we have finally added 50 years of life expectancy to the 22 years the ancient Romans expected, and we will add another 50 in the fairly near future. Rand scientists predicted in 1964 that we would achieve our next 50 by the year 2020; 5 years later scientists from Smith, Kline, and French upped this target year to the early 1990s.

We also know that given our present institutions for the aged, we have a high probability of mortality for anyone so committed (see Goldfarb's 1969 7-year follow-up study, for example), particularly in the first 3 months.

Going to the several strong longitudinal studies now available, the best predictors for long life seem to be

- Work satisfaction[89,91-94]
- No cigarette smoking[89,90,92,93]
- No cardiovascular disease[89,90,92,93]
- High personal happiness[89,90,92,93]
- Good health and basic physical functioning[89,90,92,93]
- High intelligence[89,93]
- A positive view of life[90]
- A useful and satisfying role in society[90]
- Sound financial status[93]
- Intact marriages[93]
- Rarely worried[112]
- Older than spouse[112]
- A conserver of personal energy[112]
- Up to the age of 40 looked young for chronological age[112]
- Not easily aggravated[112]
- Older sibling[110]
- Fewer children[110]
- Continued work activity after retirement age[110]
- Long-lived parents[110]
- Raised by a young mother[5-7,88,110]

Pfeiffer summarized many of these:

> "...there is no single factor which determines longevity but rather a constellation of biological, psychological, and social factors, amounting to what may be best described as elite status. Persons

with high intelligence, sound financial status, well-maintained health, and intact marriages, may be expected to live significantly longer than their less intelligent and poorer brothers and sisters whose health is also declining and whose marriages are no longer intact."[93]

The measurement of aging for normal adults has an immediate conceptual history. For myself, the real beginning was with an engaging and catalytic lecture in general psychology by Professor Stanley C. Ratner in 1960. After completing a review of the theory and practice of standardized testing, he went on to a new unit: the physiological effects of aging (with special emphasis on presbyopia). After the lecture I suggested a combination of these two areas... a standardized test of physiological aging. Ratner was most encouraging. In subsequent discussions with other psychology professors then at Michigan State University (Paul Bakan, Abram Barch, S. Howard Bartley, M. Ray Denny, Robert L. Green, John King, Hans Toch), I received further encouragement and suggestions.

Other life events intervened: marriage, graduate school, children, degrees. Finally, while a clinical psychologist at Hawaii State Hospital in 1966, I was able to accumulate enough of my own time to develop a prototype set of age measures. These were called the Hawaii Age Test (HAT). The licensed beverages industries were given a research proposal offering to assess the effect of alcohol on aging.[65] Ultimately they declined, expressing a preference for research on alcoholism and not on the ordinary intake of alcohol.

In 1967, I began work as an associate professor of psychology at Saint Bonaventure University in Olean, NY. The climate there was congenial to research and innovation. Soon the HAT metamorphosed into a better structured five-item form called the Adult Growth Examination (AGE). The first article on the AGE, published in 1968, was primarily a showcase for the concept and its potential.

While in Nova Scotia, Stan Fevens and other students from Acadia University did some useful work with body age measurement and factors leading to differential aging. MacPherson and Schofield[59] found chronic happiness, among lesser factors, to contribute to a low body age.

The basic work, however, was the routine labor of building norms, field testing procedures, determining reliabilities and validities. A basic study of this kind, and the first with the final form of the AGE, was published 3 years later after my move to California. By then the first formal test manual had been printed and was being distributed to other researchers.[71] The reliability article follows.[73]

Reliability of the Adult Growth Examination: A Standardized Test of Individual Aging

Robert F. Morgan and Stanley K. Fevens

Summary — 50 male residents of Nova Scotia from 20 to 70 chronological years old were paid volunteers in a test-retest study of the Adult Growth Examination (AGE) test of bodily aging. With test-retest intervals of from 1 to 8 wk., the product-moment correlations of reliability were .88 full test, .75 systolic blood pressure subtest, .92 hearing level subtest, .93 near vision subtest; the standard error of measurement of body age was 4.98 yr. AGE full-test Body-age scores correlated .81 with chronological age. Additional subtest correlations and inter-correlations are made and comparisons with results from other samples and related research are included. All correlations were high and significant ($p = .01$).

People age at different rates. Benjamin in 1949 was among the first to suggest a reliable test of aging as an individual difference. Subsequent suggestions for items and procedures in such a test were offered by Murray in 1951. Although Murray suggested an age test would greatly benefit science, medicine, and insurance companies, there followed no further papers on the subject for nearly a decade. In the early 1960s several authors renewed the search for systematic indices of biological or physiological aging (Clarke, 1960; Bourliere, 1963; Jalavisto and Makkonen, 1963a, 1963b; Jalavisto, 1965). In 1968 Morgan revived the concept of a brief standardized age test by using data from a 1962 United States National Health Survey (Linder, 1964) to illustrate the utility of his 'Adult Growth Examination.' There was some suggestive evidence that race and sex were characterized by different patterns of aging. Adult Growth Examination (AGE) uses and items were discussed subsequently in the United States (*Science Digest,* 1969), Great Britain (Morgan, 1969), and Canada (Morgan, 1970). On the basis of professional feedback and further research the AGE test was standardized* and validated (Morgan, 1971). While the manual included age norms in years for optional supplementary measures (glucose tolerance, cholesterol level, finger dexterity, peridontal index, dental decay) the basic test consisted of three short painless subtests in the areas of hearing, vision, and blood pressure. All three subtest areas changed systematically with adult aging and, therefore, age norms in years were associated with subtest raw scores. The full-test Body-age was considered to be the median age score of the three subtests. At this stage it was considered useful to evaluate the reliability of the full test and its subtests.

METHOD

Measurement Instrument

The Adult Growth Examination is presently based on norms derived from a carefully collected cross sample of several thousand United States adults tested in the 1962 National Health Survey (Linder, 1964) as well as subsequent norms from hundreds of adults examined in New York state in 1969 and then in Nova Scotia in 1970.*

The first subtest, systolic blood pressure, was the average of three readings made at rest separated by intervening activity (the other two subtests). Measurements were made with the middle of the cuff over the bulge in the upper left arm, with the cuff remaining loose on the arm between measurements. Only the systolic blood pressure was recorded. Procedures derive from Gordon (1964) and Florey and Acheson (1969).*

The second subtest, hearing loss at high frequency, was recorded at 6000 cycles per second for the better ear after a rehearsal at 1000 cycles per second for both ears. An audiometer with comfortable air-conduction earphones was used to communicate standard pure tones at varying decibel intensities (range 0 to 110 db). *S* faced the audiometer with his back to the tester and signaled by a raised hand on the side of the ear stimulated that the tone had been heard. Beginning with an intensity large enough for the tone to be heard, usually 50 db, intensity was decreased until a level was reached at which *S* missed the tone about half the time. Once this level was confirmed by retesting at 5-db intervals above and below it, it was recorded. Procedures derive from Glorig and Roberts (1965) and Roberts (1968a).*

The third subtest measure, lens accommodation tested by near vision threshold, was the closest measured distance for uncorrected binocular vision that a printed target (pica: 11 letters per inch) sentence would begin to blur at. *S* with his chin on a rest sighted down a ruled slide at the white printed target card at the far end of the

* R. F. Morgan. The Adult Growth Examination (AGE), manual for a compact standardized test of individual aging. (Unpublished manual, California School of Professional Psychology, 1971.)

slide. The tester moved the slide closer until blurring was reported. The tester continued to move the target somewhat closer and then gradually returned to the point of blurring, eventually recording the point at which blurring was seen to commence from either direction. Procedures derive from Chapanis, *et al.* (1949, 1956), Hofstetter (1954), Roberts (1968b) and Roberts and Cohrssen (1968).*

Subjects

Fifty adult male volunteers answered an advertisement for short-term employment in the only major Nova Scotia newspaper. Since past research had indicated sex differences probable on the AGE (Morgan, 1968), it was decided to test one sex at a time rather than maintain the same number of *S*s subdivided into two separate sex groups (a limited budget precluded increasing the number of *S*s). It was agreed to replicate the present study with both sexes at a later date presuming greater financial affluence. The male volunteers in the present study agreed to be examined at two sessions separated by at least a week in time with payment following the second session. They ranged in age from 20 to 70 yr., with a mean age of 38. The age distribution generally followed the Province-wide pattern (by decade: 20s– 18 *S*s, 30s– 8 *S*s, 40s– 6 *S*s, 50s– 7 *S*s, 60s– 7 *S*s, 70s– 4 *S*s). Income level, marital status, family size, and education (except at the 20s where college students were a majority) reflected Province-wide patterns.

Procedure

The male volunteers were tested on the AGE on a test-retest basis, with a range of 1 to 8 wk. and a median of 1.6 wk. between sessions. None were told at the end of the first session that the second session was to involve the same procedure. All those tested at the first session returned for the second session and their remuneration.

RESULTS

All test-retest product-moment correlations were significant (p = .01). Raw-score reliabilities for the three subtest measures ranged from .79 for systolic blood pressure to .93 for near vision and .95 for hearing level. When subtest raw scores were converted to Body-age scores, test-retest reliability correlations ranged from .75 for systolic blood pressure to .92 for hearing level and .93 for near vision. The total Body-age score of the AGE, median of the three subtest age scores, showed a test-retest reliability correlation of .88. The standard error of measurement was 4.98 yr.

Occasionally one of the AGE subtests may be inappropriate for some *S* (e.g., deaf or blind *S*s). It was therefore decided to determine the effect on the reliability of the total Body-age score of dropping each of the subtests, one at a time. The three resulting combinations yielded acceptably high correlations which ranged from .81 (near vision missing) and .83 (hearing level subtest missing) to .95 (systolic blood pressure subtest missing). These data are found in Table 1.

Other correlational analyses are depicted in Table 2. The reliability sample of this study was compared with a validation sample of Nova Scotians presented in another study (Morgan, 1971). Correlations with chronological age across subtests and total Body-age score are high, significant, and similar for both groups. Clarke in 1960, also testing Nova Scotians, found similar correlations with age for his 102 *S*s (hearing loss .57, systolic blood pressure .65, near vision .67). Florey and Acheson in 1969, examining more than 3000 *S*s from 18 to 79 yr., also reported significant correlations with age for AGE subtest measures (.62 white females, .59 black females, .47 black males, .43 white males) of systolic blood pressure.

TABLE 1

ADULT GROWTH EXAMINATION (AGE) TEST-RETEST CORRELATIONS FOR 50 MALES WITH CHRONOLOGICAL AGES OF 20 TO 70 YEARS

AGE Variables	Raw score *t*	Age score *t*
Subtest 1: Hearing loss	.95*	.92*
Subtest 2: Near vision	.93*	.93*
Subtest 3: Systolic blood pressure	.79*	.75*
Mdn of Subtests 1 + 2		.95*
Mdn of Subtests 1 + 3		.81*
Mdn of Subtests 2 + 3		.83*
AGE total scores: *Mdn* of all subtests		.88*

* $p < .01$.

TABLE 2

SELECTED ADULT GROWTH EXAMINATION (AGE) CORRELATIONS AND COMPARISONS

AGE Variables	Raw score *t**		Age score *t**	
A. With chronological age				
Subtest 1: Hearing loss	.68	(.66)	.76	(.69)
Subtest 2: Near vision	.73	(.57)	.84	(.78)
Subtest 3: Blood pressure	.55	(.69)	.51	(.67)
AGE total score				
B. Subtest intercorrelations				
Subtests 1 + 2	.66	(.46)	.73	(.63)
Subtests 1 + 3	.38	(.47)	.43	(.52)
Subtests 2 + 3	.59	(.43)	.60	(.53)
C. Subtests with AGE total score				
Subtest 1: Hearing loss	.67	(.65)	.73	(.74)
Subtest 2: Near vision	.84	(.64)	.89	(.81)
Subtest 3: Blood pressure	.81	(.84)	.82	(.85)

Note —All correlations in parennthesis are based on a validation sample of 107 male and female Nova Scotians in the chronological age range of 20 to 70 yr. They are included for comparison with the correlations derived from data collected from the 50 male Nova Scotians aged 20 to 70 yr. and rested in the present study. Validation sample correlations derive from Morgan (1971).

* $p < .01$ for every product-moment correlation in the table.

The total Body-age score of the AGE correlated .81 with chronological age for the reliability sample in the present study and .82 with chronological age for the validation sample (Morgan, 1971).

Across both samples, subtest intercorrelations ranged from .38 to .73. The hearing-loss subtest was less effective at predicing the total Body-age score than the other two subtests.

In summary, the total Body-age score of the Adult Growth Examination was highly correlated with chronological age (.81) and highly reliable on a test-retest basis (.88).

Reprinted with permission of author from Morgan, R. F. and Fevens, S. K., Reliability of the adult growth examination: a standardized test of individual aging, *Percept. Mot. Skills*, 34, 415–419, 1972.

In California, most of my time was devoted to a new professional school of psychologists. By then, the AGE was receiving attention from other psychologists and gerontologists. The pioneer hypnotic work of Leonard Elkind in 1972 (group body age of middle-aged women averaged a drop of 11 years) is one case in point. The use of AGE to assess long-term meditation effects[79,126] is another. The time I was able to devote to the measurement of aging focused primarily on library research and data retrieval analyses.

I was soon able to find out who had thought of the same approach long before I had. Some ideas went as far back as Helmholtz. Apparently, however, no one had developed an applied test to the extent of the AGE. In the process of data retrieval, I accumulated 50 more references relevant to the measurement of body age. It seemed time (1976) to bring the 1971 manual up to date.

II. ADULT GROWTH EXAMINATION TEST MANUAL

A. PART I: DIRECTIONS FOR ADMINISTRATION AND SCORING

You do not have to be a psychologist or a physician to give the Adult Growth Examination (AGE). On the other hand, you may well wish to consult with such professionals to interpret any results significantly different from normal or the calendar age. What you do need to give this test effectively is highly practiced familiarity with the test materials and careful adherence to the test instructions. Courses in psychological testing, assessment of adult aging, and gerontology would also be helpful. After sufficient supervised practice, the AGE may be used by any intelligent adult to monitor his or her body age and the relative aging of friends and family. The test may also be used professionally by psychologists, physicians, mental health workers, nurses, researchers, and other specialists within the health or life sciences.

1. Test Materials

A complete test kit includes manual, portable electronic blood pressure monitor, portable audiometric monitor, portable visual near point indicator and cards, a pack of 100 score sheets, and a carrying case for the equipment.

Battery operated, with solid-state circuitry, the portable electronic blood pressure monitor allows accurate, rapid measurement without a stethoscope. Cuff microphone and digital readout models are now quite inexpensive.

The portable audiometric monitor operates on normal AC wall current, has solid-state circuitry, stereo earphones, microphone, variable volume dial (up to 59 dB by increments of 1 dB), two frequencies of 1000 cps and 6000 cps. Hearing level is tested.

The portable visual near point indicator contains visual target cards with pica type sentence (three different sentences for three different cards) and card insert on graded measurement ruler expandable up to 65 in. Near point of clear focus tested.

2. Time Requirements

Most people can be tested in 10 to 15 min on this untimed test. Relaxed accuracy is much more important than speed with AGE.

3. Administering the Test (General Suggestions)

1. Set up the test equipment in a quiet, well-illuminated room with ample movement space.
2. The examiner should be relaxed, positive, encouraging, and postpone irrelevant discussion until all measures are completed. Discussions of the test's background, meaning, or purpose also should not be done during the actual testing.

3. Direction to the person being examined should be read aloud rather than given from free memory. It is useful to have the persons being examined follow the reading of the directions on their own copy.
4. Never rush the person being examined.
5. It is often useful to give the test several times to the same person, say, a few days apart and at varying hours. This will determine the individual stability or reliability of the body age score.
6. Significantly high or unusual age results should be referred to a health professional. Persons tested should be told that this test, like all tests, is subject to error. Results should be carefully double-checked before any serious personal or research decisions are made in consequence. The most frequent use of the test will be for personal knowledge and, as such, it can lead to a greater enjoyment of life if properly used.
7. Before examining subjects for this test, they should know its purpose and should provide their clear approval to be tested. In addition to this informed consent, the examinee is always entitled to the results of the test, transmitted in a clear, comprehensible form. Because confidentiality is promised, it must be honored. Also, no test result is irreversible.
8. Ethical standards, federal and professional, for testing or research with humans all apply to this test.

4. *Test Procedure*

1. The person to be tested (examinee) is seated on a comfortable chair next to a table. On the table is the score sheet. The basic background information is completed at this time.
2. The examiner reads: "*You are about to have a short, painless series of tests of health measures associated with aging. You may let the examiner know if the directions are not clear, but otherwise please hold all questions until the test series is over. Do I have your consent to begin?*"
3. With consent, the first blood pressure measurement is made. The examiner reads: "*This will be the first of three blood pressure readings to be taken in the test series.*" The blood pressure measurement is made with the subject wearing the blood pressure monitor cuff over the bulge in the upper left arm. This places the cuff microphone directly over the brachial artery. The cuff is then plugged into the instrument case, the instrument switched on, and the air valve closed by rotating the cap clockwise with thumb and forefinger. The cuff is then inflated by pumping the hand bulb. The light may flash on the control panel while the cuff is moved or inflated. This is caused by noise picked up by the sensitive microphone in the cuff. The red flashing will cease when the inflation is stopped and pressure is above systolic pressure (inflate to about the systolic pressure you would expect at 20 calendar years above the age of the person being tested up to a maximum pressure of 160 mmHg). The cuff is then slowly deflated by gradually opening the air valve, turning the cap counterclockwise. The first flash or readout on the dial occurs at systolic pressure (the maximum pressure in the arteries when heart is not at rest) and the pressure must be read at exactly that instant. When the reading has been made, let out all the pressure. Leave the cuff loose and uninflated on the left arm. Record the first systolic blood pressure reading on the score sheet. (*Note:* Corday and Vyden[16] have shown that blood pressure will go up 10 to 30 mmHg up to 45 min after eating; they also found excessively warm rooms to lower blood pressure while excessively cold rooms raise it. It therefore makes sense to test only in a comfortably temperate room and not after the examinee has just finished eating.)
4. The examiner reads for the hearing test. "*Next is a hearing test. Please put on the earphones. Make sure they are firmly on your ears, but are not so tight as to be painful.*" When this is done, the examiner speaks through the portable audiometric monitor's (PAM) microphone and continues: "*Nod if you can hear me. All right. Now I would like*

you to turn so that your back is to me. This will help you concentrate on the sound in the earphones without the distraction of seeing the tones turned on. It also helps me keep from letting you know when I am sounding a tone." Tune PAM to 1000 cps at 40 dB for the right ear. "*When you hear a tone in your right ear, raise your right hand all the way up...like this*" (sound tone). "*When you hear a tone in your left ear, raise your left hand all the way up...like this*" (switch the left ear and sound tone). "*Good. Be sure to raise your hand all the way up on the side you hear the tone when you can hear the tone. We are now ready to start the test.*" The frequency is still set at 1000 cps. This is a normal conversation frequency and is not an age measure. It is used to warm up the examinee to the test and to get a rough indication of the quality of normal hearing. It is also a chance to make sure the equipment is in good order. Test the right ear and then the left. Use 1-s tones. Begin testing each ear at 50 dB. If no hand goes up at that level, raise to 59. If at 59 dB, the hand still has not gone up, cut in with the microphone and reread the directions. If still no success, check PAM and see if the examinee has fallen asleep. Most people will raise their arm at 50 dB. If so, decrease the volume by gradual steps until you find the volume level so low that the examinee hears it only about half the time. Record that as the hearing level score for each ear. Now do the same for each ear at the age-related high frequency of 6000 cps. The "better ear" score is the lowest volume in decibels scored at 6000 cps, whether it is the right or the left ear. Turn off PAM.

5. Time for another blood pressure test. After removing the earphones, the examinee turns in the chair to again face the examiner. When comfortable, examinee is told: "*This is the second of three blood pressure readings to be taken in this test series.*" Inflate the cuff to about 20 mmHg higher than the first systolic reading (up to 160 maximum). Take and record the second systolic blood pressure reading. Then, leaving the cuff loose on the left arm, go to the vision test.
6. The examiner reads: "*This is a test of near vision or how closely you can see printed material without any blurring.*" One of the three target cards is inserted in the near point indicator (NPI) at the far end from the examinee. Lighting should be excellent without glare. "*Look down the ruler to the far end where you see a white card. I am going to move this card toward you until you can see the printed letters clearly. Say when. Good. Now I am going to keep moving it toward you very slowly. Tell me when it begins to blur in any way. All right. Now I am going to move the card away from you. Tell me when it stops blurring.*" In this manner, the distance at which the sentence on the card blurs is recorded. No glasses are allowed. Record distance to the nearest tenth of an inch if at all possible. Any one of the three target cards may be used; alternatives are for retesting. When done, the examinee is again made comfortable in the chair.
7. The examiner reads: "*This is the third of three blood pressure readings to be taken in this test series.*" Again, inflate the cuff to about 20 mmHg higher than the last reading (up to 160 maximum). Take and record the third systolic blood pressure reading. Then, remove the cuff from the examinee's arm and turn off the machine. Make sure all equipment is off. Compute the average of the three systolic blood pressure readings and record that on the score sheet. Thank the examinee for their time and cooperation. Present and explain the results, once they are determined by converting raw scores to body age scores.

5. Scoring the Test

Using conversion tables (Tables 1 to 3) convert the raw score for each subtest into the equivalent age score. Then rank order the three scores. The middle one, or median (neither the highest nor the lowest), is the tested body age of the examinee. It is the best estimate of the body age at the time of testing. Additional measures, listed in the decade charts (Tables 4 and 5) may be used as supplementary indicators of aging if available from professional medical, dental, or psychological

Table 1 Conversion table: hearing loss raw scores to body age scores

Hearing loss (dB)	Men: body age (years)	Women: body age (years)
0	19–	20
1	19–	23
2	19–	25
3	19–	27
4	20	29
5	21	32
6	22	35
7	24	39
8	25	41
9	27	44
10	28	45
11	29	48
12	31	50
13	34	51
14	35	52
15	38	53
16	39	54
17	41	56
18	43	58
19	45	58
20	46	59
21	48	60
22	50	61
23	50	63
24	51	65
25	52	66
26	52	68
27	53	70
28	54	71+
29	54	71+
30	55	71+
31	55	71+
32	56	71+
33	57	71+
34	57	71+
35	58	71+
36–37	59	71+
38	60	71+
39–40	61	71+
41	62	71+

Table 1 Conversion table: hearing loss raw scores to body age scores (continued)

Hearing loss (dB)	Men: body age (years)	Women: body age (years)
42–43	63	71+
44	64	71+
45	65	71+
46–47	66	71+
48	67	71+
49–50	68	71+
51	69	71+
52	70	71+
53+	71+	71

Table 2 Conversion table: near vision raw scores to body age scores

Near vision (in.)	Men and women: body age (years)
0.0–3.9	19
4.0–4.1	20
4.2	21
4.3	22
4.4–4.5	23
4.6–4.76	24
4.8	25
4.9–5.0	26
5.1	27
5.2–5.3	28
5.4	29
5.5–5.7	30
5.8–6.1	31
6.2–6.5	32
6.6–6.8	33
6.9–7.1	34
7.2–7.5	35
7.6–7.9	36
8.0–8.2	37
8.3–8.5	38
8.6–8.9	39
9.0–9.5	40
9.6–10.1	41
10.2–10.7	42
10.8–11.3	43

Table 2 Conversion table: near vision raw scores to body age scores (continued)

Near vision (in.)	Men and women: body age (years)
11.4–11.9	44
12.0–12.5	45
12.6–13.1	46
13.2–13.7	47
13.8–14.3	48
14.4–14.9	49
15.0–17.3	50
17.4–19.7	51
19.8–22.1	52
22.2–24.5	53
24.6–26.9	54
27.0–29.3	55
29.4–31.7	56
31.8–34.1	57
34.2–36.5	58
36.6–38.9	59
39.0–41.3	60
41.4–43.7	61
43.8–46.1	62
46.2–48.5	63
48.6–50.9	64
51.0–53.3	65
53.4–55.7	66
55.8–58.1	67
58.2–60.5	68
60.6–62.9	69
63.0–65.3	70
65.3+	71+

Table 3 Conversion table: systolic blood pressure raw scores to body age scores

Systolic blood pressure (mmHg%)	Men: body age (years)	Women: body age (years)
0–110	19–	19–
111	19–	20
112	19–	21
113	19–	23
114	19–	25
115	19–	28
116	19–	30
117	19–	32

Table 3 Conversion table: systolic blood pressure raw scores to body age scores (continued)

Systolic blood pressure (mmHg%)	Men: body age (years)	Women: body age (years)
118	19–	33
119	19–	35
120	19–	36
121	20	37
122	21	39
123	24	40
124	27	41
125	30	42
126	32	43
127	35	44
128	38	45
129	40	46
130	42	46
131	44	47
132	46	48
133	48	49
134	50	50
135	51	52
136	52	53
137	53	55
138	54	56
139	55	58
140	56	59
141	57	59
142	58	61
143	59	61
144	60	62
145	63	62
146	65	63
147	67	63
148	69	64
149	71	64
150	72	65
151	73	65
152	74	66
153	76	66
154	77	67
155	78+	67
156–157	78+	68
158–159	78+	69
160	78+	70
161+	78+	71+

Table 4 Decade chart of aging for men: three basic measures and five supplementary measures

	Body age decade (years)						
Measure	**20+**	**30+**	**40+**	**50+**	**60+**	**70+**	**Units**
Basic							
Hearing, loss (HL)[33]	+4	+12	+17	+22	+38	+52	Decibels
Vision, near (NPV)	4.0	5.5	9.0	15.0	39.0	63.0	Inches
Blood, systolic pressure (SBP)	121	125	129	134	144	149	mmHg%
Supplementary							
Dexterity (FD)	48	48	45	42	37	34	Filled holes 4 min
Glucose (GT)	95	102	115	118	130	140	mg%
Cholesterol (CL)	178	206	227	231	233	[a]	mg%
Periodontal (PI)	0.62	0.92	1.27	1.62	2.15	2.50	Periodontal index
Tooth decay (DMF)	14	16	18	21	24	27	No. of teeth DMF

Note: *These norms and the procedures used to derive them may be found in their original sources as follows.*

HL: *Glorig and Roberts, 1965; Roberts, 1968; Morgan, 1966–1972; Corso, 1959; Rosen et al., 1964; Spoor, 1967*
NPV: *Chapanis, 1949, 1956; Roberts 1964–1968; Morgan, 1966–1972; Heidemann, 1932; Steinhaus, 1932; Bernstein, 1945; Friedenwald, 1952; Bruckner, 1959*
SBP: *Gordon, 1964; Morgan, 1966–1972. Roberts, 1975*
FD: *Walk, 1965; Gavurin, 1963; Morgan, 1971*
GT: *Garst, 1966; Florey, 1969; Morgan, 1968, 1971*
CL: *Moore, 1967; Florey, 1969; Morgan, 1968, 1971*
PI: *Kelly, 1965; Morgan, 1968, 1971; Johnson et al., 1965*
DMF: *Kelly, 1967; Morgan, 1968, 1971; Johnson et al., 1965*

[a] *No further increase with age.*

testing. If for any reason one of the three basic subtests is unusable, average the two body age scores measured as the best estimate available of bodily aging (e.g., as with a blind or deaf examinee).

6. Interpreting the Test

1. Read the entire manual before interpreting body age scores.
2. No test score is the final word. Even if totally accurate, there are always many ways to change it for better or worse.
3. The body age scale goes from 19 to 71 years. Those with body ages under 19 or over 71 will be off the scale and not precisely assessed. As such, the test is most likely to capture exact body ages for the 30 to 60 chronological age set. Until norms for older people are available, it will not be useful for some over 70 unless they are very youthful for their age. Many, of course, are and such feedback is great for morale.
4. There is little fluctuation in body age from one test to the next. However, an age score that is consistently at least 10 years above or below the calendar age may be viewed as significantly older or younger in body age than the generation born the same year (2 S.D. away).
5. In addition to the overall body age score, if a subtest score is 10 or more years beyond what the calendar age indicates it should be, a confirming visit to a relevant medical specialist is indicated. With systolic blood pressure raw scores, 140 mmHg is borderline hypertension and 160 mmHg (at any age) is definite hypertension.[37] The American Heart Association.[1] (AHA) considers normal systolic blood pressure to be under 120 mmHg; over 150 mmHg heart attack risk has doubled and stroke risk has quadrupled. The AHA also defines a normal cholesterol level as below 194 mg% with any excess milligram percent tripling the risk of heart attack or stroke.

Table 5 Decade chart of aging for women: three basic measures and five supplementary measures

Measure	Body age decade (years) 20+	30+	40+	50+	60+	70+	Units
Basic							
Hearing, loss (HL)	+0	+5	+8	+12	+21	+27	Decibels
Vision, near (NPV)	4.0	5.5	9.0	15.0	39.0	63.0	Inches
Blood, systolic pressure (SBP)	111	116	123	134	142	160	mmHg%
Supplementary							
Dexterity (FD)	48	47	45	42	37	34	Filled holes 4 min
Glucose (GT)	104	110	118	133	145	160	mg%
Cholesterol (CL)	185	198	214	237	262	266	mg%
Periodontal (PI)	0.48	0.60	1.82	1.23	2.56	1.62	Periodontal index
Tooth decay (DMF) DMF	14	18	20	20	26	28	No. of teeth

Note: *These norms and the procedures used to derive them may be found in their original sources as listed in Table 4. The conversion tables of pages 192 to 195 also derive from primary sources as listed by subtest measure in Table 4.*

6. Those who are involved in reversing the aging processes generally choose 19-year subtest levels as their objective.
7. As with any test, the norms will need regular updating and expansion. It is meant primarily for information, enjoyment, and self-awareness. It is a test of aging and as such is no substitute for a comprehensive health examination.

Table 6 is a sample score sheet.

B. PART II: GENERAL INFORMATION AND BACKGROUND

In 1856 Hermann von Helmholtz wrote a handbook on the physiology of optics, which included the observation that there are individual differences in the optical physiology of aging.[41] His specific focus was on "presbyopia", or the increasing difficulty of seeing things clearly at close range experienced by most people as they age. Helmholtz noted that "persons with early progressing presbyopia die early and persons with late progressing presbyopia die late".[4] Several decades later, the grand champion of individual differences (and the philosophical precursor of clinical psychology) Sir Francis Galton,[30] confirmed both vision and hearing decrements with age after systemically testing more than 9000 people aged 5 to 80 years.

Following on the early work of Helmholtz and Galton, Steinhaus and his doctoral student, Heidemann, began a careful combing of 5000 patients who had been seen for eye difficulties over a long period of time. They published their results in 1932 in both dissertation[40] and journal[119] form. Although their sample was much narrower in nature than Galton's 1884 survey, they did confirm, based on 1000 death records, the very high correlation between presbyopia and mortality. They found presbyopia to be primarily (at least with their sample) a predictor of death by heart disease. They found presbyopia to be so potent an aging characteristic that it was unaffected in its progress by social class, rural/urban living, or sex differences. In 1945 mathematician Felix Bernstein[4] suggested these studies justified the use of presbyopia as the basis for an index of physiological aging. It was an intelligent and well-documented recommendation, which went ignored by the scientific community. Bernstein did not standardize a test based on his insight.

In 1949, a test of body age was recommended by Benjamin[3] to be based on sexual function. In 1951, Murray[85] suggested a more practical approach based on vision, strength, and other indices.

Table 6 Adult Growth Examination score sheet

Name____________________ Date of Birth ____________________

Identifying Number______________________________

Address __________________________________

Telephone__________________ Sex ____________________

Occupation__________________ Education ____________________

Marital Status_______________ Referred by ____________________

Medical Problems ______________________________

I know the purpose of this test and consent to take it of my own free will. I understand the results will be handled in a professional and ethical manner.

____

Signature Date

The Examiner: ______________________________

Time test begun ______________________________

Measurements Body Temperature __________

SBP-1 Systolic blood pressure ________ mmHg

HL Hearing loss at 1000 cps: Right ear ________ dB Left ear________ dB

HL Hearing loss at 6000 cps: Right ear ________ dB Left ear________ dB

*HL Hearing loss at 6000 cps: Better ear ________ dB

SBP-2 Systolic blood pressure __________ mmHg

*NPV Near point vision ________________ in.

SBP-3 Systolic blood pressure __________ mmHg

*SBP Average of three readings __________ mmHg

Time test concluded ____________________Total testing time ______________minutes

Results

*HL raw score	________	HL age score	________	Body age	________
*NPV raw score	________	NPV age score	________	Birth age	________
*SBP raw score	________	SBP age score	________	Difference	________

Monitor Record — Adult Growth Examination

Name ______________________________

Date of testing	Body age:	NPV	HL	SBP	Total	Birth age	Difference

Every other space may be left to record intervening activity.

The Adult Growth Examination was developed by Dr. Robert Morgan, Department of Psychology, Antioch University at Santa Barbara, 801 Garden Street, Santa Barbara, CA, 93101. Research results and individual score sheets are welcome.

He predicted body age would be as important a concept to the last half of the 20th century as mental age was to the first half. He recommended insurance companies take a close look at this approach. They did not. Benjamin and Murray were not heard from again on this subject.

Also in 1951, H.B. Jones and colleagues[49] promoted the "lipo-protein index" as an index of aging. By basic blood test technique it has often since been used to assess the risk of vascular disease. While the "lipo-protein index" (see also Reference 5) is too gross an index to yield year by year body age scores, it was still a step forward in that it called attention to the circulatory system as another fruitful direction for assessing body age. As we have seen, vision had been noticed since Helmholtz in 1856[4] and hearing since Galton in 1907.[30]

In 1959, James Birren[5] edited what is still one of the finest handbooks of aging extant: *Handbook of Aging and the Individual: Psychological and Biological Aspects.* Birren called for the recognition of "functional age" because individuals age at different rates. Body age was compared conceptually to mental age as an age-specific variable worth tracking. For the next 15 years, a distinguished variety of gerontologists would call for a test of functional age, without following through to standardize one themselves (and without giving Birren or his historical antecedents credit).

In 1960, Burgess presented a valuable interdisciplinary collection of objective measures of aging.[9] 1960 was also the year this chapter's author first began planning a body age test. The most valuable contributors of the early 1960s, in my opinion however, were Linder and colleagues from the U.S. Public Health Service. More interested in health than aging, their systematic health measures survey of 1962 collected essential data on adults of all ages, several thousand, carefully selected as a representative sample of Americans.[57,58] These confirmed, on a normative American sample, the sensitive age indices of near vision, hearing level at high frequency, systolic blood pressure, and other measures. The early development of my own AGE relied heavily on these norms. Subsequent publications by public health analysts provided key data for developing age charts for hearing level,[33,103] near vision,[99-103] and systolic blood pressure.[35,36,107] The vision work was also facilitated by the data collection of Friedenwald,[28] Bruckner,[8] Rosen et al.,[114] and Spoor.[118] The early vision work of Chapanis,[11,12] as communicated through many general texts in the early 1960s was also of great value. By the end of the 1960s my own test was standardized and in practice.[65-72]

In the 1960s Hollingsworth and colleagues[42,43] did some groundwork on body age testing by defining physiologic age with correlations of health measures on Hiroshima subjects. Again, the results, published in the *Yale Journal of Biological Medicine,* were potentially fruitful as step one in the evolution of body age test. No step two emerged from these authors.

In 1968 Dirken[20,21] attempted to develop a functional age test based on the abilities of industrial workers. However, he found his approach poor in differentiating rapidly aging workers from slowly aging workers.

In 1969 and again in 1972, Comfort pooled an exhaustive 59 measures of aging ranging from biopsies to gray hairs and including systolic blood pressure (he found the latter to correlate 0.519 with calendar age).[14,15] Comfort's battery was much more comprehensive than the one I developed several years earlier (AGE), but it was this comprehensiveness that limited its application. To be evaluated was time consuming, occasionally painful, and required expensive and sophisticated equipment and personnel.

Burr[10] suggested an even more imaginative measure of well being and aging in 1972: the monitoring of the electric patterns of life. It was in this year that the call for applied measures of functional age became most frequently expressed. Rose[111] suggested we use it to quantify social age; Robert Kastenbaum and colleagues[50] called for a functional age of the self concept; J.L. Fozard[27] illustrated ways for functional age to be derived from measured abilities and personality; Nuttall[87] called for a functional age based on life expectancy (years from death rather than years from birth). It was Nuttall who was subsequently credited by several gerontology publications as originating the concept of functional age.

Correlational analysis of age-sensitive factors remains in high gear, ranging from Clarke's factorial analysis in 1960[13] to Furukawa and associates' multiple regression analysis in 1975.[29] The results follow the same pattern: blood pressure, near vision, hearing loss at high frequency, and other measures (see Tables 4 and 5) correlate significantly with calendar age and may be used to predict aging for specific populations by specific formulas.

1. New Directions

Despite the periodic published work of Comfort[14,15] and Morgan,[67-80] the concept of standardized tests for body age continues to be rediscovered. The late Benjamin Schloss eloquently regaled life extension gatherings in the late 1970s to develop such a measure, adding creative innovations of his own (such as "Sanar cabinets").[23] The Linus Pauling Institute has collected urine samples from 235 volunteers at a California Veterans Administration Hospital: a computer analysis suggested 30 separate promising age-related constituents.[108] Eventual age scores, based on urine samples, would be used to evaluate the effects of vitamins on aging. More recently, Richard Hochschild, at the University of California at Irvine, School of Medicine, has been developing a 12-test battery to determine the effects of deanol and lecithin on aging.[53] The Hochschild battery included reaction time, decision time, short-term memory, picture recognition, movement speed, vital capacity of the lungs, forced expiratory volume, fingertip vibration acuity, near vision, and high frequency hearing level. The last two, of course, overlap the AGE. However, Hochschild omits blood pressure or any other blood measures.

Computerized urine analysis and 12-item test batteries lose the simplicity and speed of the AGE, but may yet be the wave of a less populist-oriented future. Both approaches have the potential for higher reliability and validity; both should be encouraged. The main advantage of reinventing the wheel is that sometimes it can be a better wheel.

A complete history of the progress and development of the concept of the AGE was given in preceding material. To summarize, a wide variety of physiological measures that correlate with age were evaluated for their effectiveness as subtest measures for brief, painless, reliable, and valid tests of adult body age. Dark adaptation was discarded because of the high cost of reliable measurement equipment and the great length of time needed to measure it (although it remains an extremely sensitive indicator of aging). Vital capacity was discarded because of equipment costs and weight. Strength and speed tasks were often insufficiently sensitive to pinpoint a body age to the nearest year (as was the lipoprotein index). Blood measures and urine measures that involved costly, painful, or time-consuming analysis were discarded. Dental measures lacked sufficient year-specific sensitivity. In the end, the three basic subtests of near vision, hearing loss, and systolic blood pressure were adopted when they were found to be both reliable and valid as well as brief, relatively inexpensive, and comfortable for an examinee to undergo. Extensive and representative norms were available for all of them and, as reported, their history was long and respectable.

For those who wish to explore additional promising measures, several are given in the decade charts of Tables 4 and 5. Dark adaptation techniques, for those with enough time and money, seem potentially of superior effectiveness.[22,127] Vibration sensitivity continues to hold promise,[18] but the most age-sensitive spot is the big toe, and many examinees resent vibrating this ticklish digit.

2. Test Standardization

Subtests were standardized by Morgan and colleagues from 1966 to 1972 in Hawaii, New York State, and Nova Scotia. Where applicable, the standardized procedures of the Public Health Service examiners[57,58] were continued. The present examination procedure has been field tested in a variety of settings for the last decade with apparent success. More than 1000 people have been tested at each decade of life.

Table 7 Adult Growth Examination (AGE) test-retest correlations for 50 males with chronological ages of 20 to 70 years[72]

AGE variables	Raw score *r*	Age score *r*
Subtest 1: hearing loss	0.95[a]	0.92[a]
Subtest 2: near vision	0.93[a]	0.93[a]
Subtest 3: systolic blood pressure	0.79[a]	0.75[a]
Median of subtests 1, 2	—	0.95[a]
Median of subtests 1, 3	—	0.81[a]
Median of subtests 2, 3	—	0.83[a]
AGE total score: median of all subtests	—	0.88[a]

[a] $p < 0.01$.

Table 8 Selected Adult Growth Examination (AGE) correlation comparisons[72]

AGE variables	Raw score *r*[a]	Age score *r*[a]
Correlation with chronological age		
Subtest 1: hearing loss	0.68 (0.66)	0.76 (0.69)
Subtest 2: near vision	0.73 (0.57)	0.84 (0.78)
Subtest 3: systolic blood pressure	0.55 (0.69)	0.81 (0.82)
AGE total score (median 1, 2, 3)	—	0.81 (0.82)
Subtest intercorrelations		
Subtests 1, 2	0.66 (0.46)	0.73 (0.63)
Subtests 1, 3	0.38 (0.47)	0.43 (0.52)
Subtests 2, 3	0.59 (0.43)	0.60 (0.53)
Correlation of subtests with AGE total score		
Subtest 1: hearing loss	0.67 (0.65)	0.73 (0.74)
Subtest 2: near vision	0.84 (0.64)	0.89 (0.81)
Subtest 3: systolic blood pressure	0.81 (0.84)	0.82 (0.85)

Note: All correlations in parentheses are based on a validation sample of 107 Nova Scotia male and female volunteers aged 20 to 70 years. They are presented above for comparison with correlations based exclusively on the 50 Nova Scotia male volunteers aged 20 to 70 years who were tested and retested for the present reliability study. The former sample's data derive from Morgan 1970.

[a] $p < 0.01$ *for every product-moment correlation on the table.*

3. Establishment of Norms

Original sources are listed below the decade chart in Table 4. Local norms may at times be more appropriate, but the nationally representative norms of the tables remain viable for normal usage.

4. Reliability

To be reliable, a test should give approximately the same results at different times, different places, and in a wide variety of test conditions. The AGE was found to be reliable. In a study of 50 male volunteer Nova Scotians, the test-retest coefficient was 0.88 with subtest reliability of 0.93 (NPV), 0.92 (HL), and 0.75 (SBP). The results of this study[73] are tabled in Tables 7 and 8. While the results

Table 9 Selected analyses of Adult Growth Examination (AGE) scores of nova scotians of both sexes aged 20 to 70 years[71]

Selected analyses	Raw scores	Age scores	*n*
Correlation with chronological age			
AGE total score for both sexes	—	*r* is 0.82[a]	107
AGE total score for females only	—	*r* is 0.83[a]	56
AGE total score for males only	—	*r* is 0.81[a]	51
Subtest 1 — hearing loss	*r* is 0.66[a]	*r* is 0.69[a]	107
Subtest 2 — near vision	*r* is 0.57[a]	*r* is 0.78[a]	101
Subtest 3 — systolic blood pressure	*r* is 0.69[a]	*r* is 0.67[a]	105
Median subtests 1, 2	—	*r* is 0.69[a]	101
Median subtests 1, 3	—	*r* is 0.78[a]	106
Median subtests 2, 3	—	*r* is 0.66[a]	101
Subtest intercorrelations			
Subtests 1, 2	*r* is 0.46[a]	*r* is 0.63[a]	101
Subtests 1, 3	*r* is 0.47[a]	*r* is 0.52[a]	106
Subtests 2, 3	*r* is 0.43[a]	*r* is 0.53[a]	101
Correlation with AGE total score			
Subtest 1 — hearing loss	*r* is 0.65[a]	*r* is 0.74[a]M/I	107
Subtest 2 — near vision	*r* is 0.64[a]	*r* is 0.81[a]M/I	101
Subtest 3 — systolic blood pressure	*r* is 0.84[a]	*r* is 0.85[a]M/I	106
Median subtests 1, 2	—	*r* is 0.85[a]	101
Median subtests 1, 3	—	*r* is 0.89[a]	106
Median subtests 2, 3	—	*r* is 0.93[a]	101

[a] p *<0.01 for every product-moment correlation in the table.*

were highly satisfying, it is still recommended that individual body age scores be reassessed several times if reliability is essential. The standard error of measurement was found to be about 5 years; therefore body age scores <5 years from the calendar age may be due to measurement fluctuation and the person may be considered to be in the normal range for their age. For research purposes, significantly rapid or slow agers are considered to be those who vary ±10 years from their calendar age.

In 1975 Roberts published the results of a new Public Health Service study involving the examination of >6000 persons considered to be representative of the American population. Although the sample tested ranged in age from 18 to 59 and was a more contemporary group than the 1962 sample, the norms were not appropriate to our standardized test. The percentage of the representative probability sample drawn that was actually tested was too low at many age levels to be truly representative.

Further, the systolic blood pressure measures were based on only one reading (as opposed to three in 1962), with subsequently poor reliability. Yet, Roberts reports the mean values of this 1972 study to differ by a negligible amount from the 1962 study. Systolic blood pressure in 1962 was 121.2 for people 18 to 44 and 136.5 for people 45 to 49; in 1972 it was an average 121.3 for those who were 45 to 49. The standard error of the mean SBP for the total group was 1 mmHg or less, depending on the decade.

It can be concluded that the AGE has solid reliability for testing purposes.

Table 10 Further analyses of Adult Growth Examination scores (AGE) of Nova Scotians of both sexes aged 20 to 70 years[71]

Analysis	**Results**
Standard error (S.E.) is estimate (in years) of chronological age	
AGE total score for both sexes	S.E. is 9.30 years, n = 107
Subtest 1 — hearing loss	S.E. is 11.23 years, n = 107
Subtest 2 — near vision	S.E. is 8.11 years, n = 101
Subtest 3 — systolic blood pressure	S.E. is 14.33 years, n = 106
Median subtests 1, 2	S.E. is 7.61 years, n = 101
Median subtests 1, 3	S.E. is 10.05 years, n = 105
Median subtests 2, 3	S.E. is 8.87 years, n = 101
Medians per item (M/I) frequencies (Morgan, 1964) by subtest	
Subtest 1 — hearing loss	M/I is 21[a] n = 101
Subtest 2 — near vision	M/I is 44[a] n = 101
Subtest 3 — systolic blood pressure	M/I is 36[a] n = 101
Distribution of AGE scores in relation to chronological age	
BA[b] = CA 7% sample; BA older than CA: 50% sample; BA younger than CA: 43%; BA within ±5 years of CA: 47% of samples; BA within ±10 years CA: 67% sample; average difference in years between BA and CA: 8 years	
Individual estimates of body age (EBA)	
For full sample (n = 107) median EBA is 35 years; median BA and median CA: 40 years	
Average difference in years between EBA and BA is 7½ years, correct EBAs: 7%	
Sex differences: none of the above analyses demonstrated significant sex differences	

[a] $p < 0.05$.[62]

[b] *BA is body age (total AGE score).*

5. *Validity*

A valid test of body age would naturally have a strong sensitivity to chronological age. As a predictor of an examinee's calendar age, the full test and all three subtests correlated well: 0.82 for the full test (subtests in 0.60 and 0.70s).[72] Complete results are presented in Tables 9 and 10. From Helmholtz[41] and Galton[30] to Clarke,[13] Comfort,[14,15] and Furukawa,[29] we have strong correlational confirmation that our subtests can predict and characterize chronological age.

In longitudinal studies, it has been demonstrated that the scores on subtests continue to decrease at similar rates right through the 70s and, more important, are good predictors of longevity.[93,109-111] Predictive validity is long documented for some of the subtests (e.g., Helmholtz and presbyopia) when it is longevity that is to be predicted. This is described for our vision test by Bernstein,[4] for systolic blood pressure (SBP) by Lew,[56] and the 11-year longitudinal study of Granick and Patterson[38] (nonsmoking and low SBP best survival predictors).

It seems clear that the three measures comprising the overall test of body age have good predictive validity in their individual use. They can be used to predict chronological age or

Table 11 Analyses of slow, normal, and rapid age rate groups of Nova Scotians of both sexes: age in years by birth (CA), by measurement (BA), by self-estimate (EA)[76]

	Age rate group		
	"Young" slow agers	Normal agers	"Older" rapid agers
Number of people	9	18	10
Average CA	53	52	46
Average BA	38	52	61
Average EA	47	52	47
CA range	40–60	40–60	40–60
BA range	19–49	35–65	53–71+
EA range	30–60	32–60	35–55
Mean difference from CA			
BA-CA	–15	0	+15
EA-CA	–6	0	+1
Mean difference from BA			
CA-BA	+15	0	–15
EA-BA	+9	0	+14

Note: On EA, using CA as a reference point, 0% of the "young" slow agers estimated themselves older than their birth age (normal agers estimated themselves older 17% group), while "older" rapid agers estimated themselves younger than their birth age in only 20% of the group (normal agers estimated themselves younger 44% group). Thus, incidence of mistaken direction of aging was low in both slow and rapid age rate groups.

differential survival. With time, the entire test as an entity can also be used for these predictive purposes. In theory, AGE should be a better survival predictor for an individual than insurance company actuarial tables.

People who score 10 or more years over their calendar age almost always can be discerned from those scoring 10 years or less — the cosmetic differences are obvious. Further, the examinees know their rapid or slow aging status themselves, although they may understate its magnitude. Comparing such extreme groups is another approach to test validation.[75] Such comparisons are often dramatic examples of the promise of gerontology. I clearly remember examining two Nova Scotian women, both born 40 years before, where one had a body age of 19 and the other a body age of 60. They both looked their body ages.

6. Uses

A test of individual body aging may be used for information, enjoyment, self-awareness, research, and social change. Often, local norms will be needed to maximize its effectiveness. For example, a test corporation is considering the addition of this test to its health multiphasic battery as used for the workers in a giant corporation. Norms for workers in that corporation, at each year of chronological age, initially would be gathered and computerized as a database for individual comparison. Norms would also be needed for cultures much different from ours: Rosen et al.[114] found hearing loss at 6000 cps to decline much more gradually with age for Mabaans than has been found to be true for American and European cultures. In American culture, the subtests seem fairly

Table 12 Analyses of slow, normal, and rapid age rate groups of Nova Scotians of both sexes: selected differentiating factors from questionnaire data[76]

	Age rate group		
	"Young" slow agers	Normal agers	"Older" rapid agers
No. of people	9	18	10
% Females	44	56	80
Median annual income	$6000.00	$6000.00	$3881.00[a]
Maximum annual income	$20,000.00	$15,000.00	$6000.00
Lifetime happiness	78%	67%	40%
Present happiness	44%	56%	50%
First born	22%	22%	56%
Median no. of cigarette packs smoked/week over lifetime	0	0	2

Note: Undifferentiating factors— marital status, marital satisfaction, number of children, number of occupants in house, religion, church attendance, present health, lifetime health, physical appearance, personal adjustment, punctuality, job satisfaction, present happiness, alcohol consumption, intercourse frequency.

[a] $p < 0.05$; *efficiency percentage[67] for differentiating rapid agers from normal group is 90% and from slow agers is also 90%.*

Table 13 Expected relationship between birth age and body age[71]

I. Birth age the same as body age: about 7% (1 in every 14) of those tested
II. Birth age within 10 years of body age: about 67% (2 of every 3) of those tested
III. Birth age within 5 years of body age: about 47% (1 of every 2) of those tested
IV. Body age >10 years older than birth age: about 16.5 (1 of every 6) of those tested
V. Body age >10 years younger than birth age: about 16.5 (1 of every 6) of those tested

hardy and widely applicable. As a research tool, it has already suggested some important rate of aging differences between ethnic groups of sexes.[68] Many will use this test to evaluate the effects of special diets, health programs, occupations, and even marriages. One can choose to isolate the many factors leading to premature aging or exceptional youth. Why do women age most rapidly in their 40s? Why do black males average an age jump 5 years higher than white males in their first decade of adult life? These findings must be confirmed and explained before they can be changed. Explorers such as MacPherson and Schofield[59] follow the effect of chronic happiness on aging and determine that lifelong happiness retards the aging process. Wallace et al.[126] used the AGE test to assess the impact of habitual meditation on aging: of 47 meditators averaging 53 chronological years, those meditating for more than 5 years (24 people) averaged 15 years younger than their birth certificate would predict; the 23 meditators of less than 5 years' experience showed half that advantage (7 years younger). As with "chronic" happiness, a fairly consistent block of intervention, 5 years or more, seems to make a substantial difference.

Elkind[25] investigated the effects of hypnosis on aging, using this test as the index, and found that in fact age yields to hypnosis. Comparisons from test-identified groups of prematurely aged and extremely youthful people are now possible,[77] and Tables 11 and 12 illustrate this. Following these tables is a chart you may wish to use for monitoring your own body age scores over time or in response to changes in your lifestyle.

The era of self-determination is with us, and that self-determination includes a decision as to how fast you will allow yourself to age. The AGE is an important first step. It lets you know where you stand and it gauges your success when you attempt improvement.

BIBLIOGRAPHIES

Dean, W., *Biological Aging Measurement: Clinical Applications,* Center for Bio-Gerontology, Los Angeles, CA, 1988.

Kent, W., *The Life Extension Revolution,* Morrow, New York, 1980.

Poon, L.W., *Aging in the 80's: Psychological Issues,* American Psychological Association, Washington, D.C., 1980.

Walford, R., *Maximum Life Span,* Norton, New York, 1983.

Walford, R., *Maximum Life Span,* Avon, New York, 1984.

Wolman, B.J., *Handbook of General Psychology, Developmental Psychology,* Chapter 42 on aging. Prentice-Hall, Englewood Cliffs, NJ, 1973, chap. 42.

The author suggests the following readings on applied gerontology and the measurement of human aging:

Morgan, R.F., *Conquest of Aging: Modern Measurement & Intervention,* 2nd ed., Applied Gerontology Communications, Pueblo, CO 1977. (This edition is now sold out, but copies are available in many university libraries or through the author.)

Morgan, R.F., The Adult Growth Examination: follow-up note on comparisons between rapidly aging adults and slowly aging adults as defined by body age, *Inter-Am. J. Psychol.,* 11, 10, 1977.

Morgan, R.F., An introduction to applied gerontology, *Longer Term Care & Health Services Administration Q.,* 1, 168, 1977.

Morgan, R.F., *Measurement of Human Aging in Applied Gerontology,* Kendall & Hunt, Dubuque, IA, 1981.

Morgan, R.F., *Interventions in Applied Gerontology,* Kendall & Hunt, Dubuque, IA, 1981.

Morgan, R.F., *Growing Younger: Measuring and Controlling Body Age,* Methuen, Toronto, 1982.

Poon's book was an excellent summary of research on aging from the psychological point of view with one significant omission: no chapters focus on the systematic measurement of human aging as a general process. The mystery of this blind spot may be explained by Welford's summarizing chapter which states "Functional age of individuals can, therefore, be assessed only for particular tasks: One individual may be functionally older than another for one task but functionally younger for a different task. No meaningful overall index of functional age is possible" (p. 618). The strong significant correlations between measures, and with subsequent mortality for each measure, used in body age measurement batteries suggests a much more optimistic picture than Welford portrays. Maybe aging in the 21st century will be more up to date.

REFERENCES

1. American Heart Association, Major risk factors in heart disease, *World Almanac & Book of Facts 1976,* Newspaper Enterprise Association, New York, 1976.
2. Bender, L., Alpha and omega of childhood schizophrenia, *J. Autism Childh.,* 1, 115, 1971.
3. Benjamin, H., Outline of a method to estimate the biological age with special reference to the role of sexual functions, *Int. J. Sexol.,* 3, 34, 1949.
4. Bernstein, F., Law of physiologic aging as derived from long range data in refraction of the human eye, *Arch. Ophthalmol.,* 34, 378, 1945.
5. Birren, J.E., Ed., *Handbook of Aging and the Individual: Psychological and Biological*

Aspects, University of Chicago Press, Chicago, 1959.
6. Birren, J.E., *The Psychology of Aging,* Prentice-Hall, Englewood Cliffs, NJ, 1964.
7. Botwinick, J., *Aging and Behavior,* Springer-Verlag, New York, 1973.
8. Bruckner, R., Uber Method Longitudinaler Alternsforschung Am Auge, *Opthalmologica,* 138, 59, 1959.
9. Burgess, E.W., A comparison of the interdisciplinary findings of the study of objective criteria of aging, in *Social and Psychological Aspects of Aging — Around the World: Proceedings of the Fifth Congress of the International Association of Gerontology in San Francisco,* Tibbits, C. and Donahue, W., Eds., Columbia University Press, New York, 1962.
10. Burr, H.S., *Blueprint for Immortality: The Electric Patterns of Life,* Neville Spearman, Ltd., London, 1972.
11. Chapanis, A., Garver, W., and Morgan, C.T., Applied experimental psychology, in *Introduction to Psychology,* Morgan, C.T., Ed., McGraw Hill, New York, 1949.
12. Chapanis, A., Garver, W. and Morgan, C.T., *Applied Experimental Psychology,* John Wiley & Sons, New York, 1956; cf. Chapanis, A., in *Introduction to Psychology,* Morgan, C.T., Ed., McGraw-Hill, New York, 1956, 449.
13. Clarke, J., The aging dimension: a factorial analysis of individual differences with age on psychological and physiological measurements, *J. Gerontol.,* 15, 183, 1960.
14. Comfort, A., Test-battery to measure ageing-rate in men, *Lancet,* 2, 1411, 1969.
15. Comfort, A., Measuring the human aging rate, *Mech. Age. Dev.,* 1, 101, 1972.
16. Corday, E. and Vyden, K., Electronic monitors in medicine, *J. Am. Assoc. Med. Instrum.,* 7, 1966.
17. Corso, J.F., Age and sex differences in pure-tone thresholds, *J. Acoust. Soc. Am.,* 31, 498, 1959.
18. Cosh, J.A., Studies on the nature of the vibrations sense, *Clin. Sci.,* 12, 131, 1953.
19. Dean, W., *Biological Aging Measurement: Clinical Applications,* Center for Bio-Gerontology, Los Angeles, CA, 1988.
20. Dirken, J.M., The functional age of industrial workers, *Mens Ondernem* 22, 226, 1968.
21. Dirken, J.M., A tentative judgment about the "yardstick" for functional age, *Mens Ondernem,* 22, 342, 1968.
22. Domey, R., McFarland, R., and Chadwock, E., Threshold and rate of dark adaptation as a function of age and time, *Hum. Factors,* 2, 109, 1960.
23. Donaldson, T.K., Books: manual for the Adult Growth Examination, *Long Life,* 4(2), 17, 1980.
24. Dunker, T. and Tippit, R., *Live Longer Through Sex,* Concord House, Hermosa Beach, CA, 1973.
25. Elkind, L., Effects of Hypnosis on the Process of Aging, unpublished doctoral dissertation, California School of Professional Psychology, San Francisco, 1972.
26. Florey, C. and Acheson, R.M., Blood Pressure as it Relates to Physique, Blood Glucose, and Serum Cholesterol, PHS Publ. No. 100, Ser. 11, No. 34, U.S. Public Health Service, Washington, D.C., 1969.
27. Fozard, J.L., Predicting age in the adult years from psychological assessments of abilities and personality, *Aging Hum. Dev.,* 3, 175, 1972.
28. Friedenwald, J.S., The eye, in *Cowdry's Problems of Aging,* 3rd ed., Lansing, A.I., Ed., Williams & Wilkins, Baltimore, 1952.
29. Furukawa, T., Inoue, M., Kajiya, F., Inada, H., Takasugi, S., Fukui, S., Takeda, H., and Abe, H., Assessment of biological age by multiple regression analysis, *J. Gerontol.,* 30, 422, 1975.
30. Galton, F., *Inquiries Into Human Faculty and Its Development,* 2nd ed., Dutton, New York, 1907.
31. Garst, C.C., Blood Glucose Levels in Adults, PHS Publ. No. 1000, Ser. 11, No. 18, U.S. Public Health Service, Washington, D.C., 1966.
32. Gavurin, E.I. and Pockell, N.E., Comparison of bare handed and glove handed finger dexterity, *Perceptual Mot. Skills,* 16, 246, 1963.
33. Glorig, A. and Roberts, J., Hearing Levels of Adults by Age and Sex, PHS Publ. No. 1000, Ser. 11, No. 11, U.S. Public Health Service, Washington, D.C., 1965.
34. Goldfarb, A.I., Predicting mortality in the institutionalized aged, a seven year follow-up, *Arch. Gen. Psych.,* 21, 172, 1969.
35. Gordon, T., Blood Pressure of Adults by Age and Sex, PHS Publ. No. 1000, Ser. 11, No. 4, U.S. Public Health Service, Washington, D.C., 1964.
36. Gordon, T., Blood Pressure of Adults by Race and Area, PHS Publ. No. 1000, Ser. 11, No. 5, U.S. Public Health Service, Washington, D.C., 1964.

37. Gordon, T. and Devine, B., Hypertension and Hypertensive Heart Disease in Adults, PHS Publ. No. 1000, Ser. 11, No. 13, U.S. Public Health Service, Washington, D.C., 1966.
38. Granick, S. and Patterson, R.D., Human Age II: An Eleven Year Follow-Up Biomedical and Behavioral Study, USDHEW Publ. (HSM) 71-9037, National Institute of Mental Health, Washington, D.C., 1971.
39. Hardin, L., Effects of Behavioral Modification Skills of Dietary Change and Aerobic Exercise on Cardiovascular Functioning, Physical Fitness Measures, Personal Appearance, and Self-Concept, Doctoral dissertation, California School of Professional Psychology, Fresno, 1986.
40. Heidemann, R., Presbyopie Und Lebensdauer, Inaugural Dissertation, Göttingen, 1932.
41. Helmholtz, H.V., *Handbook of Physiological Optics,* University of Heidelberg, Germany, 1856.
42. Hollingsworth, D.R., Hollingsworth, J.W., and Bogitch, S., Neuromuscular tests of aging in Hiroshima survivors, *J. Gerontol.,* 24, 276, 1969.
43. Hollingsworth, J.S., Hashizume, A. and Jabon, S., Correlations between tests of aging in Hiroshima subjects — an attempt to define physiological age, *Yale J. Biol. Med.,* 38, 11, 1965.
44. Hudson, D.W., Asserti-Care Assertion Training for the Elderly Client, Peter Lang Publishers, New York, 1983.
45. Jalavisto, E. and Makkonen, T., On the assessment of biological age. I. Factor analysis of physiological measurements in old and young women, *Ann. Acad. Fenn. Sci.,* 100, 1, 1963.
46. Jalavisto, E. and Makkonen, T., On the assessment of biological age: II. A factorial study of aging in postmenopausal women, *Ann. Acad. Fenn. Sci.,* 101, 1, 1963.
47. Jalavisto, E., The role of simple tests measuring speed and performance in the assessment of biological vigor: a factorial study of elderly women, in *Behavior, Aging, and the Nervous System,* Welford, A. and Birren, J., Eds., Charles C Thomas, Springfield, IL, 1965.
48. Johnson, E.S., Kelly, J.E., and Van Kirk, L.D., Selected Dental Findings for Adults, PHS Publ. No. 1000, Ser. 11, No. 7, U.S. Public Health Service, Washington, D.C., 1965.
49. Jones, H.B., Gofman, J.W., Lindgren, F.T., Lyon. T.P., and Strisower, B., Lipoproteins in atherosclerosis, *Am. J. Med.,* 11, 358, 1951.
50. Kastenbaum, R., Derbin, V., Sabatini, P., and Artt, S., "The ages of me": toward personal and interpersonal definitions of functional aging, *Aging Hum. Dev.,* 3, 197, 1972.
51. Kelly, J.E. and Van Kirk. L.E., Periodontal Disease in Adults, PHS Publ. No. 1000, Ser. 11, No. 12, U.S. Public Health Service, Washington, D.C., 1965.
52. Kelly, J.E., Van Kirk, L.E., and Garst, C.C., Decayed, Missing, and Filled Teeth in Adults, PHS Publ. No. 1000, Ser. 11, No. 23, U.S. Public Health Service, Washington, D.C., 1967.
53. Kent, S., *The Life Extension Revolution,* Morrow, New York, 1980.
54. Klebba, A.J., Maurer, J.D., and Glass, E.J., Mortality Trends for Leading Causes of Death: United States 1950–1969, USDHEW (HRA-74-1853) Ser. 20, No. 16, U.S. Department of Health, Education and Welfare, Rockville, MD, 1974.
55. Kohn, H.T. and Guttman, P.H., Age at exposure and the late effects of X-rays: survival and tumor increase in CAF mice irradiated at one to two years of age, *Radiation,* 18, 348, 1963.
56. Lew, E.A., High blood pressure, other risk factors, and longevity: the insurance viewpoint, *Am. J. Med.,* 55, 281, 1973.
57. Linder, F.E., Cycle I of the Health Examination Surgery: Sample and Response, PHS Publ. No. 1000, Ser. 11, No. 1, U.S. Public Health Service, Washington, D.C., 1964.
58. Linder, F.E., The health of the American people, *Sci. Am.,* 214(6), 21, 1966.
59. MacPherson, K. and Schofield, M., Happiness is a Warm Bed, unpublished research at Acadia University, Wolfville, Nova Scotia, Canada, 1971.
60. Marsey, C.A., Personality and Attitude Change in Psychiatric Nursing As a Function of Nursing Experience, unpublished doctoral dissertation, California School of Professional Psychology, Fresno, 1988.
61. Moore, F.E. and Gordon, T., Serum Cholesterol Levels in Adults, PHS Publ. No. 1000, Ser. 11, No. 22, U.S. Public Health Service, Washington, D.C., 1967.
62. Morgan, R.F., The M/I frequencies: a quick and computation-free nonparametric method of test item evaluation, *Psychol. Rep.,* 14, 723, 1965.

63. Morgan, R.F., Note on the psychopathology of senility: senescent defense against the threat of death, *Psychol. Rep.*, 16, 305, 1965.
64. Morgan, R.F., The Hawaii Age Tests (HAT) for Bodily Aging in Adults: Standardization and Reliability of Measures. (Alias: The Effects of Rate and Duration of Consumption of Alcoholic Beverages on Bodily Aging.), Unpublished research proposal at Hawaii State Hospital, Kaneohe, 1966.
65. Morgan, R.F., Memory and senile psychosis: a follow-up note, *Psychol. Rep.*, 20, 733, 1967.
66. Morgan, R.F., The need for greater use of efficiency percentages to supplement reports of statistical significance, *Perceptual Mot. Skills.*, 27, 338, 1968.
67. Morgan, R.F., Are your older than you think? *Sci. Dig.*, 66, 20, 1969.
68. Morgan, R.F., The Adult Growth Examination: Standardization and Normative Data for Male and Female Adults in New York and Nova Scotia, unpublished study at Acadia University, Wolfville, Nova Scotia, Canada, 1969.
69. Morgan, R.F., How old are you really: techniques for assessing differential aging, *Can. Mag.*, February 28, p. 2, 1970.
70. Morgan, R.F., The Adult Growth Examination (AGE): Manual for a Compact Standardized Test of Individual Aging, unpublished manual, 1st ed., California School of Professional Psychology, San Francisco, 1971.
71. Morgan, R.F., The Adult Growth Examination: validation, analysis, and cross-cultural utility of a brief compact test of individual aging, *Inter-Am. J. Psychol.*, 6, 245, 1972.
72. Morgan, R.F. and Fevens, S.K., Reliability of the Adult Growth Examination: a standardized test of individual aging, *Perceptual Mot. Skills.*, 34, 415, 1972.
73. Morgan, R.F., Revision of the Diagnostic and Statistical Manual (DSM-II) by the addition of iatrogenic disorders and the listing of celibacy as a sexual deviation, *J. Irreproducible Results*, 21(2), 21, 1975.
74. Morgan, R.F., The Adult Growth Examination (AGE): Manual for a Compact Standardized Test of Individual Aging, 2nd ed. (revised), Psychology Department, University of Southern Colorado, Pueblo, 1976.
75. Morgan, R.F., *Conquest of Aging: Modern Measurement & Intervention*, 2nd ed., Applied Gerontology Communications, Pueblo, CO, 1977.
76. Morgan, R.F., The Adult Growth Examination, follow-up note on comparisons between rapidly aging adults and slowly aging adults as defined by body age, *Inter-Am. J. Psychol.*, 11, 10, 1977.
77. Morgan, R.F., An introduction to applied gerontology, *Longer Term Care & Health Services Administration Q.*, 1, 168, 1977.
78. Morgan, R.F., *Measurement of Human Aging in Applied Gerontology*, Kendall & Hunt, Dubuque, IA, 1981, 85.
79. Morgan, R.F., *Interventions in Applied Gerontology*, Kendall & Hunt, Dubuque, IA, 1981.
80. Morgan, R.F., *The Iatrogenics Handbook: A Critical Look at Research and Practice in the Helping Professions*, IPI Publishing, Toronto, 1983.
81. Morgan, R.F. and Wilson, J., *Growing Younger: Measuring and Controlling Body Age*, Methuen, Toronto, 1982.
82. Morgan, R.F. and Wilson, J., *Growing Younger: Measuring and Controlling Body Age*, Stein & Day, New York, 1983.
83. Moriyama, I.M., The Change in the Mortality Trend in the United States, PHS Publ. 1000, Ser. 3, No. 1, U.S. Public Health Service, Washington, D.C., 1964.
84. Murray, I.M., Assessment of physiological age by combination of several criteria: vision, hearing, blood pressure, and muscle force, *J. Gerontol.*, 6, 120, 1951.
85. Nikitin, V.N., Russian Studies on Age-Associated Physiology, Biochemistry, and Morphology: Historic Description with Bibliography, PHS Publ. No. 857, Public Health Service, Bethesda, MD, 1961.
86. Nuttall, R.L., The strategy of functional age research, *Aging Hum. Dev.*, 3, 149, 1972.
87. Ostfeld, A.M. and Gibson, D.C., Summary Report and Selected Papers from a Research Conference on the Epidemiology of Aging, PHS Publ. No. 75-711, U.S. Public Health Service, Bethesda, MD, Washington, D.C., 1972.
88. Palmore, E., Physical, mental, and social factors in predicting longevity, *Gerontologist*, 9, 103, 1969.
89. Palmore, E., Predicting longevity: a follow-up controlling for age, *Gerontologist*, 9, 247, 1969.

90. Palmore, E., Ed., *Normal Aging: Reports from the Duke Longitudinal Study 1955-1969,* Duke University Press, Durham, NC, 1970.
91. Palmore, E., Predicting longevity: a new method, in *Normal Aging II: Reports from the Duke Longitudinal Studies 1970-1973,* Palmore E., Ed., Duke University Press, Durham, NC, 1974.
92. Palmore, E., *Normal Aging II: Report from the Duke Longitudinal Study, 1970-1973,* Duke University Press, Durham, NC, 1974.
93. Palmore, E. and Jeffers, F., Eds., *Prediction of Life Span,* Heath, Lexington, MA, 1971.
94. Passwater, R., *Supernutrition: Megavitamin Revolution,* Dial Press, New York, 1975.
95. Polednak, A.P. and Damon, A., College athletics, longevity, and cause of death, *Hum. Biol.,* 42, 28, 1970.
96. Poon, L.W., *Aging in the 80's: Psychological Issues,* American Psychological Association, Washington, D.C., 1980.
97. Quint, J. and Cody, B., Pre-Eminence and Mortality: Longevity of Prominent Men, Statistical Bulletin of the Metropolitan Life Insurance Company, January, 1968, 2.
98. Roberts, J., Binocular Visual Acuity of Adults, PHS Publ. No. 1000, Ser. 11, No. 3, U.S. Public Health Service, Washington, D.C., 1964.
99. Roberts, J., Weight By Height and Age of Adults, PHS Publ. No. 1000, Ser. 11, No. 14, U.S. Public Health Service, Washington, D.C., 1966.
100. Roberts, J., Binocular Visual Acuity of Adults By Region and Selected Demographic Characteristics, PHS Publ. No. 1000, Ser. 11, No. 25, U.S. Public Health Service, Washington, D.C., 1967.
101. Roberts, J., Hearing Status and Ear Examination Findings Among Adults, PHS Publ. No. 1000, Ser. 11, No. 32, U.S. Public Health Service, Washington, D.C., 1968.
102. Roberts, J., Monocular-Binocular Visual Acuity of Adults, PHS Publ. No. 1000, Ser. 11, No. 30, U.S. Public Health Service, Washington, D.C., 1968.
103. Roberts, J. and Bayliss, D., Hearing Levels of Adults by Race, Region, and Area of Residence, PHS Publ. No. 1000, Ser. 11, No. 31, U.S. Public Health Service, Washington, D.C., 1968.
104. Roberts, J. and Cohrssen, J., Hearing Levels of Adults by Education, Income, and Occupation, PHS Publ. No. 1000, Ser. 11, No. 31, U.S. Public Health Service, Washington, D.C., 1968.
105. Roberts, J. and Cohrssen, J., History and Examination Findings Related to Visual Acuity Among Adults, PHS Publ. No. 1000, Ser. 11, No. 28, U.S. Public Health Service, Washington, D.C., 1968.
106. Roberts, J., Blood Pressure of Persons 18-74 Years in the United States 1971-1972, Publ. HRA 75-1632, U.S. Public Health Service, Washington, D.C., 1975.
107. Robinson, A.B., Why do we age? Can we diminish the rate and debilitating effect of aging? *Linus Pauling Inst. Newsl.,* 1, 3, 1978.
108. Rose, C.L., Social factors in longevity, *Gerontologist,* 4, 27, 1964.
109. Rose, C.L. and Bell, B., *Predicting Longevity: Methodology and Critique,* Heath, Lexington, MA, 1971.
110. Rose, C.L., Measurement of social age, *Aging Hum. Dev.,* 3, 153, 1972.
111. Rose, C.L., Enslein, K. and Nuttall, R.L., Univariate and Multivariate findings from a longevity study, *Proc. 20th Annu. Meet. Gerontological Society,* 196, 42, 1967.
112. Rosee, B.G., Untersuchungen uber das normale Harvermogen in der verscheidenen Lebensaltern unter besonderer Herucksichtigung der Prufung mit dem Audiometer, *Z. Laryngol., Rhinol., Otol. Grenzgebiete,* 32, 414, 1953.
113. Rosen, S., Plester, D., El-Mofty, E., and Rosen, H.V., High frequency audiometry in presbycusis: a comparative study of the Mabaan tribe in the Sudan with urban populations, *Arch. Otolaryngol.,* 70, 18, 1964.
114. Rossi, E.L. and Cheek, D.B., *Mind-Body Therapy: Methods of Ideodynamic Healing in Hypnosis,* Norton, New York, 1988.
115. Sauer, H.I. and Parke, D.W., Counties with extreme death rates and associated factors, *Am. J. Epidemiol.,* 99, 258, 1974.
116. Schaie, K.W., *Theory and Methods of Research on Aging,* West Virginia University, Morgantown, WV, 1968.
117. Spoor, A., Presbycusis values in relations to noise induced hearing loss, *Int. Audiol.,* 6, 48, 1967.
118. Steinhaus, H., Untersuchungen uber den Zusammenhang von Presbyopie und Lebensdauer, unter Berucksichtigung der Todesursachen, *Arch. Augenkd.,* 105, 731, 1932.

119. Sturgeon, P., Beller, S., and Bates, E., Study of blood group factors in longevity, *J. Gerontology,* 24, 90, 1969.
120. Sweetland, R.C. and Keyser, D.J., Tests — A Comprehensive Reference for Assessment in Psychology, Education, and Business, 2nd ed., Test Corporation of America, Kansas City, MO, 1986.
121. Walford, R., *Maximum Life Span,* Avon, New York, 1983.
122. Walford, R., *Maximum Life Span,* Norton, New York, 1984.
123. Walford, R., *The 120 Year Diet,* Simon & Schuster, New York, 1986.
124. Walk, D.E., Finger Dexterity of the pressure suited subjected on the Purdue Pegboard Dexterity Test, U.S. Air Force AMRC-TDR No. 64-41, USAF, Washington, D.C., 1965.
125. Wallace, R.K., Jacobs, D.E., and Harrington, B., Reversal of Biological Aging in Subjects Practicing the Transcendental Meditation Technique, paper delivered to the 36th Annu. Meet. American Geriatrics Society, 1979.
126. Weale, R.A., The eye and measurement of aging rate, *Lancet,* 1, 147, 1970.
127. Wolman, B.J., Ed., *Handbook of General Psychology, Developmental Psychology,* Buhler, Keith-Speigel and Thomas, Eds., Prentice Hall, Englewood Cliffs, NJ, 1973.
128. Kohn, R.R., *Principles of Mammalian Aging,* Prentice Hall, Englewood Cliffs, NJ, 1971.
129. Kohn, R.R., Effects of anti-oxidants on life span of C57BL mice, *J. Gerontol.,* 26, 378, 1971.

CHAPTER 13

BIOLOGICAL AGE AS A TOOL FOR THE DETERMINATION OF THE RATE OF AGING

TAMARA L. DUBINA

TABLE OF CONTENTS

I. INTRODUCTION

Aging may be defined most generally as the changes that take place in living organisms under the influence of time. Because a major property of any process occurring with time is its rate, the ability to measure the rate of aging is one of the most important problems of gerontology.

Although aging of different species and different individuals of the same species is extremely diversified in its form, two major manifestations of aging may be distinguished: (1) an age-related decrease of the organism's adaptability to the environment and (2) an age-related increase of the probability of death during each subsequent period of time. Evidently, the age-related increase of an individual's probability of death results from a reduction of the ability to withstand the environmental pressure, and the two manifestations of aging can, in principle, be expressed in terms of each other. In reality a detailed description of their relation is, however, far from easy and has been the objective of several mathematical theories of aging.[4,31,34] It seems important to this discussion that the two basic manifestations of aging can be used for determination of level and rate of aging.

In spite of numerous attempts to find some predictors of death,[2,25] the probability of death of a living organism can only be expressed in terms of a statistically estimated mortality of the population to which the individual belongs. On the other hand, adaptabilities of particular physiological systems and functions making up viability of the whole organism can be easily measured in every individual with the aid of some well-known tests. This essential difference marks the

0-8493-0129-7/94/$0.00+$.50

boundary between the domain of the validity of the two methods for estimating the level of aging. The way of expressing the level (and the rate) of aging in terms of the organism's adaptability is directly concerned with the problem of biological age (BA).

II. IS THERE SUCH A THING AS BIOLOGICAL AGE?

Estimation of human or animal chronological age (CA) is often needed in medicine and biology[23,35] when there are no certified data on an individual's age. Whatever parameter is taken as a basis for the determination, the resultant estimate would inevitably contain an error. This fact can be shown easily by comparing the estimated ages with the actual data from birth certificates of the individuals to whom the method was applied for checking the accuracy of the estimates. The statement may be illustrated by Table 1, which contains the ages of rats estimated from the simple linear regression equation from one of two parameters. The data show that the calculated ages of the animals were either overestimated or underestimated with regard to their real age of 24 months at the moment of determination.

Another implication of Table 1 is that the age estimation error depends on the method used: the variance appeared smaller when the age was estimated on the basis of blood oxidized glutathione than it was when relative musculus gastrocnemius weight was taken for the age assessment. Does this mean that the age determination error is purely methodical?

In our everyday life we consciously or unconsciously try to determine the age of persons we meet. Estimation of the age of people we deal with is an essential component of our consciousness just as perception of time and space. It may happen that after having learned the birthdate of a person we are amazed by a discrepancy between our estimate and the person's real age. It should be noted, however, that we do not have the slightest doubt in our ability to determine the age of people at first sight. We explain our mistake by a certain specific feature inherent in that particular individual, i.e., we admit that something exists which has led us to misestimation of the person's age. The

Table 1 Age of rats (females) calculated[a] on the basis of blood oxidized glutathione (OG) and the relative weight of musculus gastrocnemius (RWMG)[10]

Rats[b]	Age (months) calculated on the basis of	
no.	OG	RWMG
1	26.1	31.1
2	22.3	17.0
3	22.9	14.2
4	19.1	31.1
5	25.5	36.8
6	20.7	—
7	23.9	32.5
8	24.5	25.5
9	21.3	15.6
$M \pm \sigma$	22.9 ± 2.31	25.5 ± 8.76

[a] *The age (y) was calculated from the following equations: $OG = 2.50 + 0.188y$; $RWMG = 0.631 - 0.0071y$. The regression equations were obtained with indices measured in 50 animals in the age range of 5 to 24 months.*

[b] *The actual certified age of all 9 rats was 24 months.*

"something" is a set of signs, both physical and mental, the manifestation of which contradicts our idea of what they are normally in a person of that age. In other words, we have to admit that our error in estimation of the individual's age implies that apart from CA, there is also a BA, and they do not always coincide.

While visually estimating a person's age we estimate the level of aging, comparing some signs such as skin state, a capacity for work, mobility, acuteness of vision and hearing, memory, hair graying, etc., with some general ideas of these indicators, corresponding to each age range, that we have developed from our experience; i.e., using "a standard of normal aging", the term suggested by Skalicky et al.[30] Then we infer the age of a person of interest from the level of aging.

At least three conclusions can be drawn from the above discussion. The first is that in our subjective estimation of a person's age we actually determine the level of aging, i.e., a BA rather than a CA. Consequently, the idea of a BA extends in the human mind irrespective of the level of knowledge, intellect, culture, and education. Even if one cannot explain what a BA means or hears this word combination for the first time, he or she operates with this concept, while mentally determining the age of another person. This was tacitly implied in the earliest publication concerned with a BA, and it was the reason that their authors could do without its strict definition.[3,16,18,19] Criticism of the recent decade[5,17] associated with the difficulties of objective estimation of a BA and its use as a diagnostic and prognostic tool has buried in oblivion the above fundamental statement and has eventually given rise to the question whether there is such a thing as a BA.

The second conclusion is that our idea of a BA becomes especially distinct in the case of a discrepancy between estimated and real age of a person. If our estimate coincides with the certified age (which is most often the case), the idea of a BA would remain in our subconscious. This may be the reason that in the pioneer studies, instead of a strict definition, the concept of a BA was explained in terms of great deviation of the "apparent" age from the true one; e.g., "One, at fifty, may be young in body and soul, while another exhibits numerous signs of premature senescence."[3]

The third conclusion is that the term "individual BA" means that physiological and mental functions of a person suit a certain statistical "norm", i.e., it expresses the level of aging of the individual as compared to population to which the individual belongs. Without comparison of an individual with the population the concept of "BA" is senseless.

BA of the whole organism may be expressed as some weighted average sum of BAs of particular systems and functions. The BA of a person determined on the basis of a single index corresponds to the CA of such a representative of the population in whom the value of the index is most typical. Similarly, the BA of an individual based on all measured indices is expressed by the CA of a hypothetical averaged representative of this population that possesses the same combination of indices.

III. WHY ARE OBJECTIVE METHODS OF DETERMINING THE BIOLOGICAL AGE NEEDED?

The interest that gerontologists have in the concept of BA may be ascribed to its distinctive feature: unlike a CA which indicates the number of years lived, a BA expresses the level of aging and can be used, therefore, for measuring the rate of aging. However, to be useful it is necessary to be able to measure BA with a more objective method than that estimation "at first sight" we make in everyday life. Moreover, whereas it is possible to estimate the CA (and biological, too!) of humans from individual external signs, this "procedure" does not accurately apply to laboratory animals. Meanwhile, rapid progress in densing techniques or agents which can retard aging largely depends on the availability of objective methods for the determination of the BA of animals.

The lack of reliable methods for assessment of the age status is a serious obstacle in geriatricians' work. As far back as 1960, in a review analyzing the usefulness of procaine therapy, it was noted

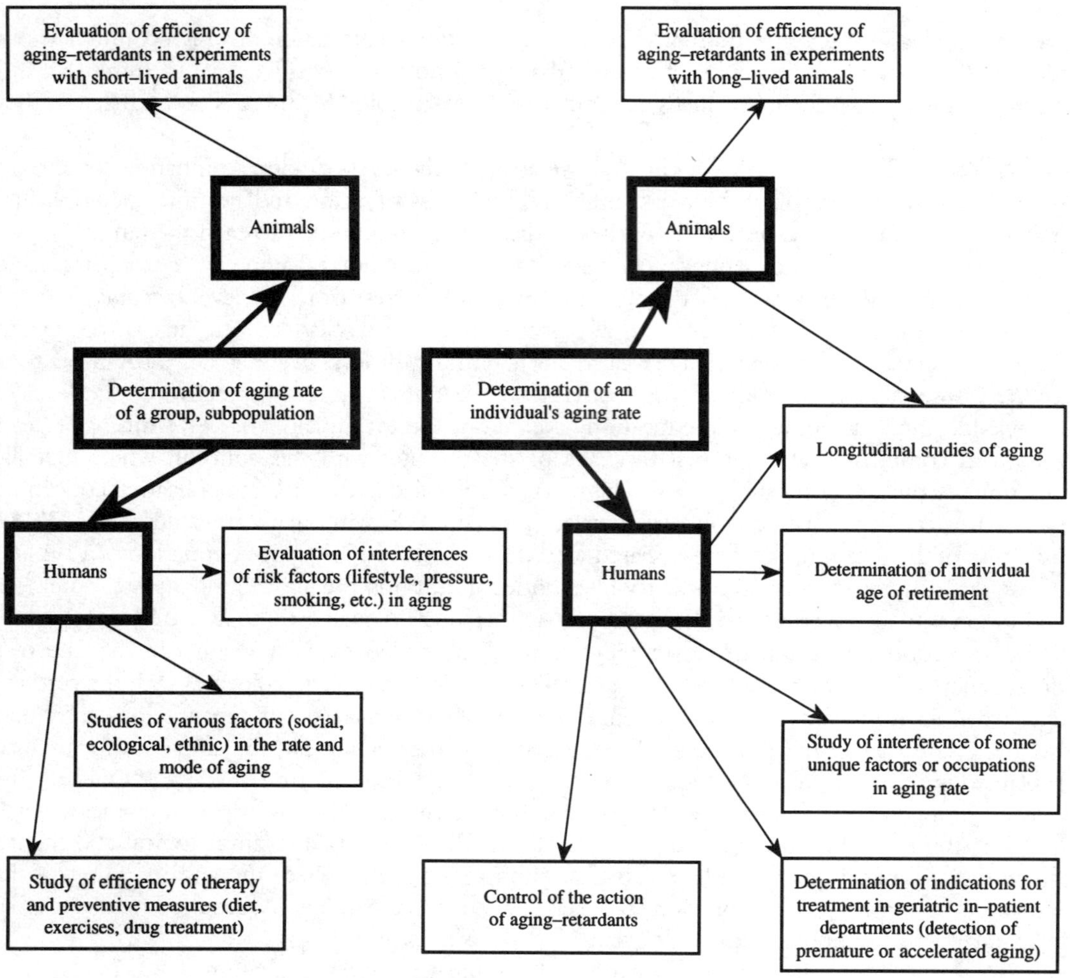

Figure 1 The problems to be solved with the aid of BA estimation.

that although the preparation had a favorable effect on the severity of disease in senescent patients, the investigators had no criteria to judge its efficacy when it was given to healthy elderly persons.[21]

The development of objective methods for the determination of a BA seems important for the solution of some problems of gerontology both in humans and in animals.

In the studies in which of primary concern is the rate of aging of some special group or subpopulation, determination of a BA may be useful as a source of additional information, the mortality data being the main tool.

When survivability- and mortality-based methods for determining the rate of aging appear inapplicable because of ethical or other reasons (such as the time it will take to do the study), and when it is an individual's rate and level of aging that is to be estimated, calculation of BA is the only way to solve the problems of which the following can be enumerated: evaluation of the aging-retardants in humans or in experimental long-lived mammals, studies of the influences of some unique factors such as longtime zero-gravity conditions on aging, determination of an individual date of retirement, and determination of the indications for hospitalization in a gerontological clinic.

Figure 1 schematically shows the problems in which determination of a BA is the only or an additional method to measure the rate of aging.

IV. HOW TO MEASURE BIOLOGICAL AGE

If we return in our imagination to the age estimation procedures we mentally performed with regard to different people, we will note that the procedure consists of the following operations: assessment of the extent of manifestation of each index important for aging in the person of interest, comparison of the extent of manifestation of each sign with the standard in the aging scale we developed in our mind from our experience, and integral estimation of the person's age as an average of all separate estimates.

The same algorithm is used in all studies concerned with objective determination of BA. The differences in the studies of different workers are as follows: (1) they use different sets of indices considered important for characterization of aging; (2) they may fully or partly follow the above algorithm. In either case, the initial steps always involve selection of the indices and examination of a normal population (or a sufficiently representative sample from it) in order to develop "a standard of normal aging" for the indices selected.

If the algorithm is followed completely, an individual's BA has integral quantitative expression (in time units); when algorithmization is partial, the authors restrict themselves to semiquantitative estimation of the age: "The age index is 'larger' or 'smaller' than its standard of normal aging, that is, the individual observed is 'older' or 'younger' than his (her) chronological age." There may also be an intermediate evaluation of BA when the estimates obtained for each index separately are not integrated into a total quantity. The order of steps in the objective determination of BA is shown in Figure 2. The following discusses two steps of the algorithm: the selection of parameters for developing the standard of normal aging and the methods for obtaining an integrated estimate of BA.

A. SELECTION OF INDICES

As was stated by Strehler,[31] the main problem of the biology of aging is, undoubtedly, to find the relation between the age, on the one hand, and morphological and functional specificities, on the other. At present, a vast amount of information has been accumulated on age-related changes, both of particular physiological functions and of whole systems with their complicated regulatory mechanisms. Which of the indices can and must be used for determination of BA? How many parameters are needed for the determination?

Any selection requires certain criteria, and such criteria have been developed.[3,6,27] They may be classified as formal ones, which, irrespective of the essence of parameter, only characterize its relation with time, and criteria which are concerned with the essence of aging processes.

The formal suitability criteria can be briefly enumerated as follows: a one-way direction with sufficient intensity of the age-dependent changes during the period from mature to old ages, with a linear relation between the index and the age, which is reflected in the magnitude of the coefficient of correlation.

As related to the formal criteria, all of the indices are suitable for the determination of BA, which closely correlate with the CA. However, a too-high correlation (about 1.0) implies that the parameter considered depends on time alone and does not concern the processes of biological aging; therefore, it cannot be used for characterization of biological aging.[5,27,32]

Our experience[9,10,12] suggests that if only one parameter is used for estimation of BA, its correlation with CA should be at least 0.7, otherwise the estimation error may be ridiculous. If the BA is determined on the basis of several parameters, it is possible to use those with a medium correlation of 0.4 to 0.7. It is especially helpful if the parameters under consideration are of great value in meaning, i.e., if they meet the essentiality criterion (a parameter is regarded as important to the aging processes it reflects).

As was mentioned above, the BA of organism as a whole may be expressed as a quantity made up of many components, each representing the BA of a particular physiological system or function:

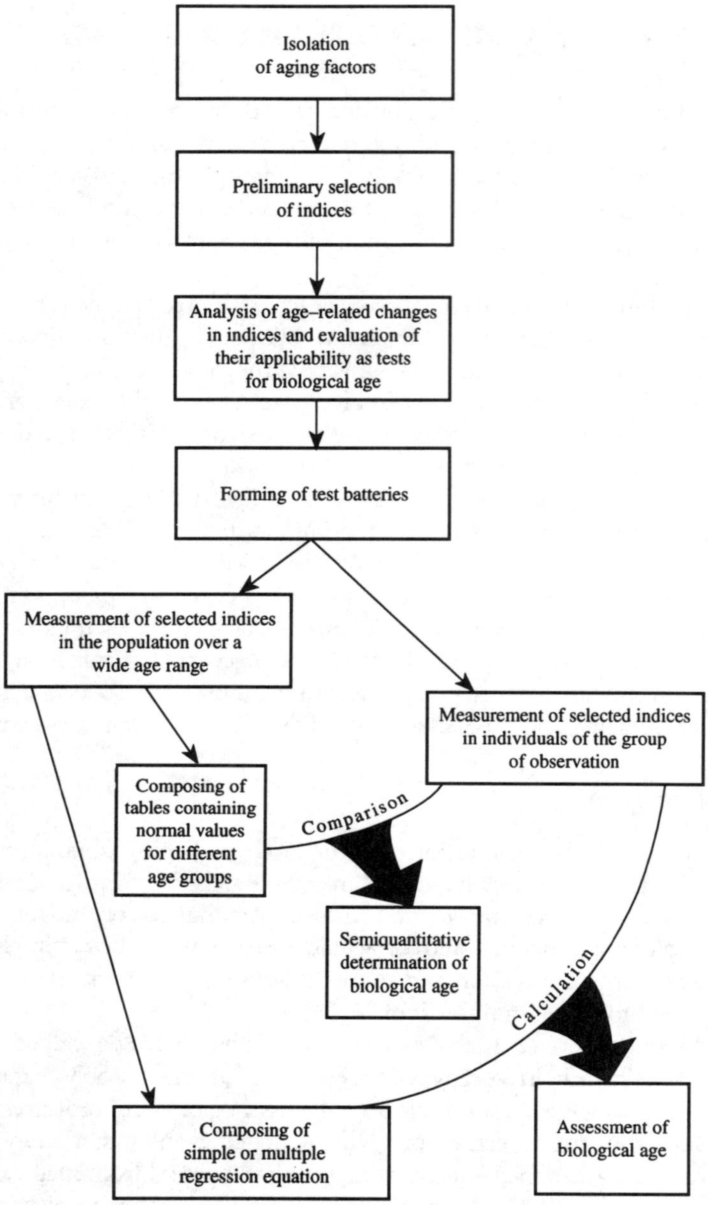

Figure 2 Determination of BA (succession of steps).

$$BA_i = K_1Y_1 + K_2Y_2 + \ldots K_jY_j + \ldots K_nY_n \qquad (1)$$

where BA_i is the individual's BA; $Y_1, Y_2, \ldots, Y_j, \ldots, Y_n$ are the BAs of particular systems; $K_1, K_2, \ldots K_j, \ldots, K_n$ are the coefficients which indicate the contribution of the system or the function to aging of the whole organism and take into account all the various relations between the systems.

A perfectly complete characterization of BA would require investigation of the status of all systems, i.e., a test battery consisting of an infinite number of parameters. As this is impossible, from the infinite number of physiological functions and systems one should select a limited number of parameters essentially important for aging.

Consequently, the question: which functions and systems are essential for aging, is of key importance for selection of tests for the determination of BA. It seems prudent to emphasize that the search for reliable indices of BA ("biomarkers of aging") does not proceed independent from the basic research of the aging mechanisms but is supported by and encourages that research. Contraposition of these approaches to aging research to give one preference over the other[1] may result from the lack of a well-developed theory of BA and from underestimation of the close relation between these approaches.

The signs essential for aging may be subdivided into two large classes. The first class comprises indices showing the intensity of primary aging at a molecular level or those that follow directly from them at the level of organelles or a cell. The second class embraces the signs in which deterioration with aging manifests itself in some systems most important for survivability. Selection of such systems and processes is certainly performed by each researcher in accordance with their understanding of aging mechanisms. Because no generally recognized theory of aging exists, the list of major aging processes and systems affected by aging can vary markedly in studies by different investigators.

B. INTEGRAL ESTIMATION OF BIOLOGICAL AGE: THE MULTIPLE REGRESSION MODEL

When an investigator uses many measured indices and operates with a large number of different estimates of BA for every system or function studied, the general idea of the whole organism's BA is lost. This is the reason that a general integral estimate obtained on the basis of many measured indices is extremely important for the development of a standard method for determination of BA.

One of the principles of the concept of biological age states that the organism's biological age is a weighted average of several estimates for particular systems and physiological functions (see Equation 1). Obtaining a general integral estimate is a matter of calculating the coefficients of the summands. Different methods can be used to calculate these coefficients, but the multiple regression analysis is most popular. Extensive studies of its applicability to estimate BA were started in the 1970s,[7,11,16,33] although the analysis had been used earlier.[19]

The BA of a certain individual (BA_i) estimated on the basis of several (k) measured parameters using multiple regression analysis is the sum whose components are a product of the value of parameter X_j in the i-th individual and the coefficient b_j:

$$BA_i = b_0 + b_1 X_{1(i)} + b_2 X_{2(i)} + b_j X_{j(i)} + \ldots b_k X_{k(i)} \qquad (2)$$

The coefficients b are calculated from the correlations between the CA and each of the parameters and between all the parameters. The calculations are complicated and require a computer.

The multiple regression model is consistent with the two main principles of the concept of a BA: (1) an individual's BA is the sum of several quantities, and the summands reflect the status of particular biological systems and functions in the individuals; (2) an individual's BA can only be estimated in comparison with the status of the population to which the individual belongs. Equation 2 clearly shows that BA_i is really the sum whose components $X_1, X_2, \ldots, X_j, \ldots, X_k$ are the values of physiological parameters measured in the individual of study. The coefficients at each of the summands express the relation between the aging of the person considered and other members of the population because they are calculated with measured $X_1, X_2, \ldots, X_j, \ldots, X_k$ in the whole population (or in a representative sample) over a wide age range.

Moreover, linearity of this model is consistent with a linear rate of age-related decline of vital function. This empirical fact reported in many earlier[28,31] and more recent studies[18,20,26] underlies both our everyday ideas of aging and some mathematical theories.

The advantages of an integral estimation of BA based on the multiple regression model are illustrated by Table 2, which compares BA estimates obtained with each of the three measured parameters (hand grip strength, short-term memory, and vibrotactile sensitivity) and those calculated from the multiple regression equation comprised of the three parameters. As can be seen from the table, the estimates obtained with one parameter appear so diverse that they are of limited use

Table 2 Biological age of women in the Kiev elderly population[14] calculated on the basis of particular indices[a] and from the multiple regression equation including all three indices[b]

Individual BA (years) calculated on the basis of			
Hand grip dynamometry (*D*)	**Short-term memory (*M*)**	**Vibrotactile sensitivity (*V*)**	**All 3 indices**
	Group 63–64 Years Old		
53.3	50.3	61.4	63.9
78.2	88.9	52.5	73.2
78.2	73.0	68.1	76.4
57.1	75.3	65.9	68.3
64.1	58.2	90.3	76.6
62.4	61.6	68.1	69.8
50.1	63.9	52.5	61.0
	Group 93 Years Old		
93.8	80.9	90.3	88.6
86.3	91.8	90.7	86.9
96.8	85.0	110.8	96.0
100.3	101.9	81.8	90.2
100.3	111.0	95.2	94.7
93.3	106.5	84.0	88.6
89.8	99.7	88.5	88.1

[a] *BA (y) was calculated in terms of one index from the simple linear regression equation obtained for the population of study:*

$$D = 65.46 - 57y$$
$$M = 126.23 - 0.88y$$
$$V = -14.64 + 0.45y$$

[b] *Integral BA (BA_i) was calculated from the equation*
$$BA_i = 84.30 - 0.639;\ D - 0.086;\ M + 0.641\ V.$$

when trying to determine the aging level of the whole organism rather than of a particular function. In this sense, an integral estimate seems more advantageous. The question may, however, arise: can this integral estimate be considered reliable? In other words, in order for multiple regression methods to be a really useful tool for assessing the level and rate of aging, one should be aware of its accuracy.

An approach to the accuracy of BA estimates may be comparisons of BA average for a group of individuals at the same age with their CA. The concept of a BA assumes that in a normal population the age of individuals with a normal (moderate) rate of aging is close to their CA, whereas individuals with higher or lower rates should be biologically "older" or "younger" than their CA. The mean BA of all individuals at the same age in a normal population should be equal to their CA. Consequently, coincidence of the mean BA in a group of persons with the CA may be a measure of accuracy of BA estimates.

When the individual BA is calculated from the multiple regression model, the theoretically predicted coincidence of mean BA in a group of individuals at the same age with their CA may only be found in the regression center. At the regression edges the effect of "narrowing" is observed, i.e., underestimated BA averages for the upper edge and overestimated mean BA for the lower edge of the regression. The "narrowing" effect was shown both for human[14,23,33] and animal[12] populations[33] The values in the left-hand column of Table 3 ("conventional" estimates) are a good illustration of the effect.

Table 3 Mean BA (years) of groups of individuals at the same age calculated by different methods[14]

CA of a group (years)[a]	*n*	BA (years) estimated: Conventional method[b] (M ± S.E.)	BA (years) estimated: With correction[c] (M ± S.E.)
		Women	
64 – 65 (64.4 ± 0.18)	9	69.6[d] ± 1.85	64.7 ± 1.83
80 – 81 (80.5 ± 0.19)	8	80.9 ± 1.20	80.8 ± 1.23
93 – 94 (93.4 ± 0.15)	11	90.6[d] ± 1.02	94.5 ± 1.02
		Men	
65	13	70.4[e] ± 1.34	66.3 ± 1.33
78	13	76.5 ± 1.55	76.9 ± 1.55
94	8	88.6[f] ± 2.40	94.7 ± 2.40

[a] *Bracketed figures are mean ± standard error.*
[b] *Individual BA was calculated from the multiple regression equation: for women see Table 2; for men* $BA_i = 93.02 - 0.561\,D - 0.096\,M + 0.435\,V$.
[c] *The correction was calculated from Equation 4 with the following values: for women* $\bar{Y} = 80.8$ *years,* $b = 0.699$*; for men* $\bar{Y} = 76.6$ *years,* $b - 0.646$.
[d] *Statistically significant difference between mean BA and CA of the group is* $p < 0.02$
[e] *Statistically significant difference between mean BA and CA of the group is* $p < 0.001$.
[f] *Statistically significant difference between mean BA and CA of the group is* $p < 0.05$.
From Dubina, T.L. et al., Exp. Gerontol., *19, 133, 1984. With permission.*

The deviation of mean BA at the regression edges from the CA implies that the individual estimates are wrong as well. Figure 3 shows that the individual BA estimates for women based on the multiple regression model are concentrated at the line crossing the coordinate origin only in the center of the plot. Most of the points for younger representatives of the population studied fall above the line, while those corresponding to older individuals lie largely under it.

Thus, a persistent error is inherent in BA estimates obtained by multiple regression. This may be ascribed to the fact that the age in this model is a dependent variable. It should be noted that the magnitude of error depends on the two factors: (1) on the distance of an individual's CA (or that of a group of individuals at the same age) from the regression center, and (2) on the consistency of the regression under study with the linear model, i.e., on the magnitude of the coefficient of multiple correlation.[12,14]

The above-mentioned facts impose certain limitations upon the method. When the author and co-workers used it to evaluate the effect of 3-d periodic fasting on the aging of rats,[11] we found that the mean BA of the rats fasted was higher than that of the control animals (19.6 ± 1.55 and 12.8 ± 0.95, respectively), which indicates that fasting is unfavorable for aging of rats. However, the mean BA of the control rats, which according to the concept of BA should be equal to CA, was also higher (the age of experimental animals at the moment of killing was 11.5 months). This discrepancy, caused by an error of multiple regression analysis, requires additional explanations while interpreting the results.

In studies which compare the BAs of human subpopulations having some differences this discrepancy is avoided by comparing mean BA of all (over a wide age range) representatives of subpopulations studied followed by calculation of the deviation from mean BA of all the representatives in the main population.[16,33] In this approach the error persistent in the multiple regression method used for assessing BA appears nonessential.

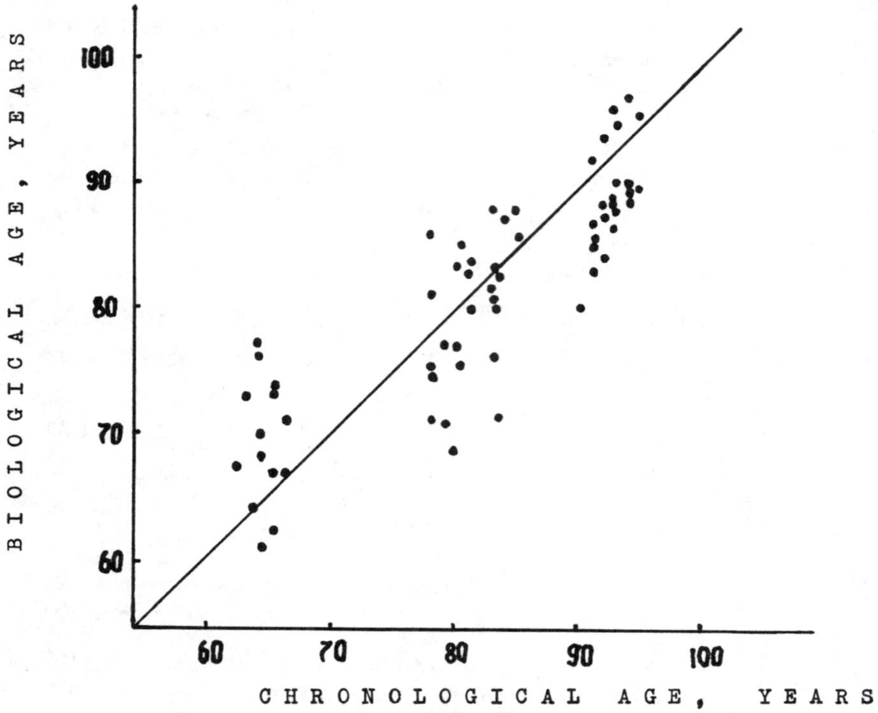

Figure 3 Individual BA of women in three age groups estimated with the multiple regression method. The calculating equation is given in the footnotes to Table 2.

When an individual's exact estimate of BA is required, and especially when it should regularly be estimated in longitudinal studies, the distortions in the BA estimates become a serious obstacle for using multiple regression.

In order to overcome the obstacle, a method was suggested, which is based on comparing BA estimates with certain ranges of a possible statistical variation of the normal BA value for every group of individuals at the same age in the population studied.[23]

When this approach is used, a 93-year-old woman should be assumed to age at a normal rate if her BA is within the range of 87.8 to 92.4 years. If her BA is more than 92.4 years, she may be said to age at a higher rate, whereas the estimated BA younger than 87.8 years suggests a favorable aging rate.

The approach described above is based, first, on the assumption that BA which generally reflects such a species parameter as an aging rate obeys the normal law of distribution. The second point to be discussed is the choice of the "normal" range of BA. We have chosen the range $\pm 0.67\sigma$, because at normal distribution the range of $x + 0.67\sigma$ to $x - 0.67\sigma$ includes 50% of all variables in a population. A similar procedure based on comparison of BA estimates with the "realistic" values was used in a study by Voitenko et al.[32]

Because neither of these methods allows a direct comparison between an individual's BA and their CA in order to arrive at a conclusion as to their rate of aging, we decided to introduce a correction into the multiple regression model to bring it to conformity with the concept of BA and to avoid the distortion of BA estimation at the regression edges.

The derivation of the correction is described in Reference 14 and is omitted here. With the correction factor suggested the corrected BA (Y_i) is the sum:

$$Y_i = BA_i + z \quad (3)$$

where BA_i is the BA of the individual calculated from the multiple regression equation, and z is the correction. The correction z is defined by the equation

$$z = (Y_i - \bar{Y})\ (1 - b) \tag{4}$$

where Y_i is an individual's CA; $\bar{Y}$ is the average CA of the whole sample (the regression center); b is the coefficients of simple linear regression which expresses the relation between biological and chronological age in the sample.

If an individual is at CA in the older part of the population ($Y_i > \bar{Y}$), it follows from Equation 4 that $z > 0$. In this case the correction should be added to underestimated BA. On the other hand, when $Y_i < \bar{Y}$ (i.e., the individual is in the younger part of the population) $z < 0$, then the correction is subtracted from overestimated BA value.

As follows from Equation 4, the absolute value of z depends on the magnitude of two factors: one expresses the distance of the individual's CA from the regression center, the other is a function of the degree of consistence of the multiple regression considered with the linear model. The longer the distance of Y_i from the regression center, the larger the absolute value of the factor ($Y_i - \bar{Y}$), and consequently, the larger is z. When $Y_i = \bar{Y}$, z is zero. Thus, when an individual is at a CA near the regression center, that is, in the region of the most accurate BA estimates, z is close to zero.

The role of the second factor in Equation 4 is associated with the fact that b can vary between 0 and 1. At low b, which is the case at a moderated coefficient of multiple correlation between the measured parameters and the age, the factor ($1 - b$) approaches 1 (its maximum). At high b (i.e., at a large coefficient of multiple correlation), the factor and the correction z tend to zero.

Thus, the magnitude of the correction is larger the more an individual's CA differs from the regression center and the poorer the agreement of the regression with the linear model. Consequently, the correction introduced allows the persistent error inherent in the multiple regression model of BA to be ameliorated.

The data in the right-hand column of Table 3 present average BAs for groups of elderly persons calculated from the multiple regression equation with the correction z. As can be seen from the comparison with the left-hand column of the table, the group averages in this case are much closer to the CA than are they when calculated without the correction. In some groups (women aged 93 to 94 years and men of 65 and 78 years) the difference between the corrected group average BA and CA exceeds 1 year, but remains, however, statistically insignificant.

Table 4 illustrates how the correction z improves individual BA estimates.

V. HOW ESTIMATION OF BIOLOGICAL AGE CAN BE USEFUL IN SOLVING SOME THEORETICAL PROBLEMS OF GERONTOLOGY

In gerontological research estimation of the BA is most often considered an applied task, as a method useful for the solution of other problems, such as control of the efficiency of some treatment or environmental or social interference in aging, etc. The determination of BA is, in the author's opinion, a method that may be very useful also in solving many theoretical problems pertinent to basic gerontological research. Some examples are illustrated below.

Our everyday experience shows that BA of most people either coincides with their CA or slightly deviates from the latter in one or the other direction, while considerable differences ("he or she looks 10 years younger or older") are less frequent. And what about objective estimation of BA?

In Figure 4 a frequency distribution curve for deviation of BA from CA is given for 310 normal men, ages 60 to 100 years, whose BA was estimated with three parameters. As can be seen, the distribution curve is close to normal. In a little over half of the persons examined (55%) the difference of BA from CA lies in the range from +3 to -3 years. Deviations in either direction exceeding 8 years

Table 4 Individual BA of women in two groups calculated from the multiple regression equation with and without correction

CA (years)	BA (years) calculated	
	By conventional method[a]	With correction[b]
	Group 63–65 Years Old	
63	63.9	58.5
	73.2	67.8
64	76.4	71.4
	68.3	63.3
	76.6	71.6
	69.8	64.8
	61.0	56.0
65	73.1	68.4
	62.8	58.0
	66.6	61.8
	72.6	67.8
	Group of 93–94 Years Old	
93	88.6	92.2
	86.9	90.6
	96.0	99.6
	90.2	93.9
	94.7	98.4
	88.6	92.3
	88.1	91.8
94	89.7	93.7
	88.8	92.8
	89.4	93.4
	96.6	100.5

[a] *See Table 2.*
[b] *See Table 3.*

are not very frequent and amount to 7%. Larger deviations are very rare, one example being a 14-year delay (in a man of 78) and another being an excess of 12 years (in a man, aged 91).

Thus, an objective estimation of BA seldom involves substantial deviations of BA from CA.

We have analyzed the frequency of coincidence and essential deviations of BA from the respective CA in a group of men, aged 90 to 100, and made a comparison with the whole examined group of 60 to 100 years.[13] The results are given in Table 5. The BA in this study was estimated using five indices. The percentage of patients whose BA coincided with their CA at the moment of study was the same in the long-lived group and in the whole group examined (28 and 29%, respectively). The percentage of men whose BA was younger than their CA was the same, too (7%, by 8 years or more). In the long-lived group, however, the percentage of individuals with their BA exceeding their CA by 8 years or more appeared higher (23 vs. 7% in the whole group examined). Because the probability of an individual's death in the subsequent period of time in individuals aged 90 to 100 is greater, such a relatively high number of individuals whose BA is older than their CA in that group may render support to the statement that an individual's BA is indeed an objective indicator of the aging level and the distance from death.

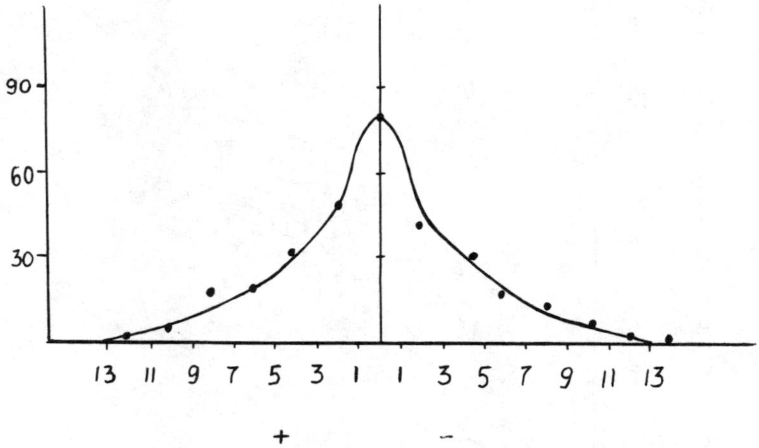

Figure 4 The frequency distribution of the differences between BA and CA in men, aged 60 to 100 years. The vertical axis is the frequency of cases, the horizontal axis is the difference between BA and CA (years). To the left of the central axis are shown cases in which the BA is older than the CA (the difference is positive); to the right of it are cases in which the BA is younger that the chronological age (a negative difference). The individual BA was calculated with three parameters using the multiple regression method with a correction (see the footnote to Table 3).

Table 5 Frequencies of coincidence of individual BA[a] and CA and of considerable differences between them in men of the Kiev population[13]

		Frequency of					
	Total no. examined	**Coincidence (BA differs from CA by at most +1.5 yr)**		**Large excess of BA over CA (over 8 years)**		**Large delay of BA from CA (over 8 years)**	
	(n)	***(n)***	**(%)**	***(n)***	**(%)**	***(n)***	**(%)**
All examined (60–100 years)	208	61	29.3	14	6.7	15	7.2
Long-lived group (90–100 years)	43	12	27.9	10	23.3	3	7.0

[a] *BA was calculated from the multiple regression equation including 5 indices: hand grip strength dynamometry* (D), *short-term memory* (M), *vibrotactile sensitivity* (V), *rate of pulse wave propagation through vessels of muscular* (P_m) *and elastic* (P_e) *type:*

$BA_i = 64.000 - 0.385\ D - 0.044\ M + 0.390\ V + 0.003\ P_m + .200\ P_e$

R = *0.841.*

The correction was calculated with $\overline{Y} = 77.54$; b − *0.707.*

On the other hand, similar frequencies both of concordance between BA and the CA and of individuals with a younger BA than CA in the whole group examined and among persons of 90 to 100 years may suggest that the oldest group in the study does not belong to a unique long-lived subpopulation. Rather, this represents the tail of the life span probability distribution in an ordinary population which consists of individuals with long, medium, and short life spans.

Figure 5[14] gives typical examples of BA changes of the same individual under longitudinal study. The rate of change of BA estimated in terms of three parameters is shown as plots of BA vs. CA.

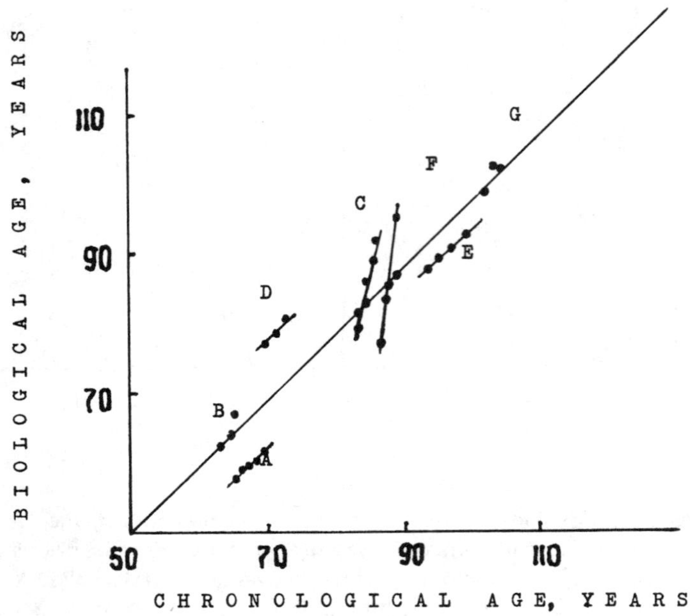

Figure 5 Examples of typical changes in individual BA. A, Men examined at age 64 to 69 years; B, women examined at 62 to 66 years; C, men examined at 76 to 82 years; D, men examined at 69 to 72 years; E, men examined at 92 to 97 years; F, men examined at 79 to 85 years; G, men examined at 100 to 102 years. The BA values were calculated from equations for women and for men using the correction suggested (see Table 3). (From Dubina, T.L. et al., *Exp. Gerontol.*, 19, 133, 1984. With permission.)

The BA of some individuals is younger than their CA during the whole period of observation (E, a delay of 4 to 5 years; A, an 8- or 9-year delay), in the others the two values coincide (B; G). Plot D shows BA 7 years older than the CA at all three points. In all these cases the rate of BA change was nearly the same and approximately equaled a 1-year increase per calendar year ("the normal aging rate"). It should be noted that the plots either coincide with the axis crossing the coordinate origin at 45° or are parallel to it.

Plots C and F in Figure 5 demonstrate a different mode of aging when the rate of BA change is higher than the normal one (the plots cross the axis) and vary from 2 to 7 years of BA per calendar year. At the time of the first examination both individuals were biologically satisfactory (for C, BA was 4 years younger than his CA, F was biologically 10 years younger than his CA). In subsequent years BA caught up to the CA, and then surpassed it. In these people the rate of BA change was nonuniform, and on average it was 3 years per calendar year for C, and nearly 4 years per calendar year for F.

The analysis of BA change in 65 men and women, aged 60 to 100 years, examined three times or more in succession in a longitudinal program, has revealed that the percentage of individuals with a "normal rate of aging" is 44.6%. The percentage of individuals with a high rate of BA change ("accelerated aging") was 52.3%. There were some cases of dramatically rapid senescence, e.g. a 20-year increase of BA during 2 calendar years. In two cases we observed a short-term decrease of BA, which in subsequent examinations returned to the normal mode. This reduction of the aging rate may be due to inaccuracy in measurement of the parameters, but because all of the individuals examined were patients of the Kiev Institute of Gerontology, it cannot be excluded that the temporary improvement in BA resulted from a favorable effect of the treatment.

Thus, more than half of the cases observed in the longitudinal studies of normal individuals older than 60 years exhibit an increasing rise of BA that eventually leads to a considerable gap

Table 6 Characteristics of three test-programs used for BA estimation in men of the Kiev population

Systems and functions involved in test programs	Test program and sample size: 3 Indices $n = 310$ ($R = 0.804$)	5 Indices $n = 208$ ($R = 0.841$)	10 Indices $n = 98$ ($R = 0.882$)
Neurophysical sphere			
Vibrotactile sensitivity	+	+	+
Short-term memory	+	+	+
Capacity for mental work			+
Rheoencephalography			+
Muscular strength			
Right-hand grip strength dynamometry	+	+	+
Cardiovascular system			
Rate of pulse wave propagation through vessels of			
Muscular type		+	+
Elastic type		+	+
Lipid metabolism			
Blood plasma levels of			
Cholesterol			+
Triglycerides			+
Lipoproteins			+

between BA and CA. In a smaller group of apparently healthy persons observed over 3 to 8 years, BA was either the same as CA or a few years younger during the entire observation period. However, in those people as well, the rate of BA change was year to year or higher. Evidently, the hypothesis suggesting that at old age there are periods when all parameters remain unchanged for a long time and, consequently, BA remains at the same level, is a myth.

Unfortunately, we could not complete our work to compare the data of our longitudinal studies with the time of death. If we could find that an accelerated increase of BA is a precursor of death, it would show that estimation of BA may be an important predictor of death and convince all who doubt the validity of this technique.

Estimation of BA may be extremely helpful in studying qualitative diversity of aging, which is still inadequately investigated. The longitudinal studies described above were carried out at the Kiev Institute of Gerontology by a group directed by Mints. The observations on men and women at the age of 60 to 100 years followed a general program comprising 21 physiological, biochemical and psychological indices.[22] The BA of men in the Kiev population was estimated in terms of three[14] and five[13] indices. In addition the estimation of BA was performed following a test program that included ten parameters. The characteristics of all three test programs are given in Table 6. The first program is based on three parameters characterizing the status of the neuromuscular system; the second consists of five tests which represent the neuromuscular and the cardiovascular systems; the third program consisted of ten tests characterizing both systems involved in the first two programs and, in addition, lipid metabolism status. Thus, the BA estimates following each of the three test programs are based on a different number of physiologic functions tested.

Comparison of BA values estimated for the same individuals from the three different equations shows that for some individuals all of the three BA estimates coincided, whereas for other individuals there were distinct differences.[15,24]

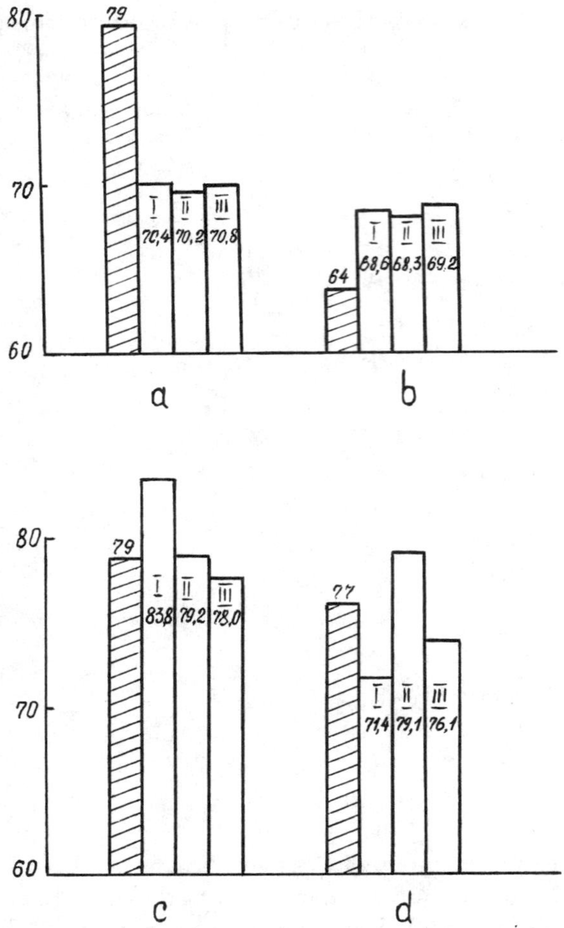

Figure 6 Examples of coincident (a, b) and noncoincident (c, d) estimates of BA calculated under test programs I, II, and III (see the explanation in the text). The vertical axis is the age (years). Dashed columns are chronological age, light columns are BA.

In the upper part of Figure 6 two cases are presented (a, CA of 79 years; b, 64 years) in which the BAs calculated from all three test programs were the same. It should be noted that in one case the BA was younger than the CA (a), while in the other BA was older than the CA (b). The two examples illustrate relatively harmonious aging as regards its quality, i.e., if a person is 8 or 9 years "younger" than his CA, all the parameters are "younger"; if an individual is 4 or 5 years "older", then all the studied functions of the organism are "older".

In the lower part of Figure 6 there are several examples in which the BAs estimated under the three test programs are different. In case (c) following test programs II and III BA is, in general, close to the CA; however, the BA, based on test program I, which tested muscular and nervous abilities, is approximately 4 years "older" than the CA. This indicates some deficiency in the neuromuscular functions, although the function of the whole organism was satisfactory. On the other hand, case (d) points to excellent condition of the neuromuscular functions, but to unsatisfactory performance in the cardiovascular parameters included in test program II. In general, however, the BA of the man suggested a normal mode of aging.

Thus, comparison of the three BA estimates allows a researcher to ascertain whether there is harmonic or disharmonic aging of each individual and to identify the impaired functional systems when the aging is disharmonic. Detection of an impaired system before a respective pathology arises may be of importance in preventing age-related disease. Additionally, theoretically, this approach may be extremely helpful for developing a classification system of aging types.[15]

ACKNOWLEDGMENT

This work is based on the research performed at the Sector of Gerontology, Academy of Science of Bielorussia, Minsk, and at the Institute of Gerontology, Academy of Medical Sciences of Ukraine, Kiev.

I want to express my gratitude to my former co-worker from Minsk, Dr. V. Levdanskaya-Dyundikova, and to the participants of the Kiev Longitudinal Observation Program, directed by Dr. A. Mints.

REFERENCES

1. Adelman, R.C., Editorial: biomarkers of aging, *Exp. Gerontol.,* 22, 227, 1987.
2. Arking, R., Successful selection for increased longevity in Drosophila: analysis of the survival data and presentation of a hypothesis on the genetic regulation of longevity, *Exp. Gerontol.,* 22, 199, 1987.
3. Bourliere, F., The assessment of biological age in man, *Publ. Health Pap.*, No. 37, 1970.
4. Brown, K.S. and Forbes, W.F., A mathematical model of aging processes, *J. Gerontol.,* 29, 46, 1974.
5. Brown, K.S. and Forbes, W.F., Concerning the estimates of biological age, *Gerontology,* 22, 428, 1976.
6. Comfort, A., Test-battery to measure ageing-rate in man, *Lancet*, 7635, 1411, 1969.
7. Dirken, J.M., Ed., *Functional Age of Industrial Workers*, Wolters-Noordhoff, Gröningen, 1982.
8. Dubina, T.L., On biochemical methods for estimating biological age of experimental animals, in *The Metabolism and Functions of Aging Organism*, Mikhailova-Lukashova, V.D., Gatsko, G.G., and Razumovich, A.N., Eds., Nauka i Tekhnika, Minsk, 1969, 97 (in Russian).
9. Dubina, T.L., On the accuracy of estimating the biological age, in *Demographic, Physiological and Biochemical Aspect of Aging*, Gatsko, G.G., Ed., Nauka i Tekhnika, Minsk, 1976, 79 (in Russian).
10. Dubina, T.L. and Razumovich, A.N., *Introduction to Experimental Gerontology*, Nauka i Tekhnika, Minsk, 1975 (in Russian).
11. Dubina, T.L., Dyundikova, V.A., and Zhuk, E.V., Evaluation of the efficiency of some factors on aging with the use of biological age estimates, in *Lifespan Prolongation: Prognoses, Mechanisms, Control, Gerontology and Geriatrics 1979 Year Book,* Chebotarev, D.F. and Frolkis, V.V., Eds., Institute of Gerontology of the Academy of Medical Science, Kiev, 1979, 111 (in Russian).
12. Dubina, T.L., Dyundikova, V.A., and Zhuk, E.V., Biological age and its estimation. II. Assessment of biological age of albino rats by multiple regression analysis, *Exp. Gerontol.,* 18, 5, 1983.
13. Dubina, T.L., Mints, A.Ya., and Korkushko, O.V., The biological age of long-lived persons, in *Long-Lived Persons. 11th Sci. Conf., Materials,* October 29-30, 1984, 28.
14. Dubina, T.L., Mints, A. Ya., and Zhuk, E.V., Biological age and its estimation. III. Introduction of a correction to the multiple regression model of biological age and assessment of biological age in cross-sectional and longitudinal studies, *Exp. Gerontol.,* 19, 133, 1984.
15. Dubina, T.L. and Orlov, M.M., The relationships underlying the age-related changes of physiological parameters and aging types, in *Advances in Science and Technology, General Problems of Biology (Populational Gerontology)*, Burlakova, E.B. and Gavrilov, L.A., Eds., Vol. 6, VINITI, Moscow, 1987, 6 (in Russian).
16. Furukawa, T., Inoue, M., Kajiya, F., Inada, H., Takasugi, S., Fukui, S., Takeda, H., and Abe, H., Assessment of biological age by multiple regression analysis, *J. Gerontol.,* 30, 422, 1975.

17. Gavrilov, L.A., The critical analysis of mathematical models of aging, mortality and longevity, in *Advances in Science and Technology, General Problems of Biology (Populational Gerontology)*, Burlakova, E.B. and Gavrilov, L.A., Eds., Vol. 6, VINITI, Moscow, 1987, 155 (in Russian).
18. Goyal, V.K., Lipofuscin pigment accumulation in the central nervous system of the mouse during aging, *Exp. Gerontol.*, 17, 89, 1982.
19. Hollingsworth, J.W., Hashizume, A., and Jablon, S., Correlations between tests of aging in Hiroshima subjects — an attempt to define "physiologic age", *Yale J. Biol. Med.*, 38, 11, 1965.
20. Hubbard, B.M. and Anderson, J.M., Sex differences in age-related brain atrophy, *Lancet*, 8339, 1447, 1983.
21. Luth, P., A review of procaine therapy in elderly individuals, *J. Gerontol.*, 15, 395, 1960.
22. Mints, A. Ya., Longitudinal studies of aging (methodological approaches, organization and general results), in *Problems of Gerontology, Transactions of the Coordinating Committee on Gerontological Research in the East-European Socialist Countries*, No. 2, Chebotarev, D.F., Ed., Institute of Gerontology of the Academy of Medical Science, Kiev, 1980, 52 (in Russian).
23. Mints, A. Ya., Dubina, T.L., Lysenyuk, V.P., and Zhuk, E.V., Determination of individual biological age and estimation of the aging level, *Fiziol. Zh.*, 30, 39, 1984 (in Russian).
24. Mints, A. Ya., Dubina, T.L., Korkushko, O.V., and Bogatskaya, L.N., The determination of human biological age in longitudinal studies, in *Symposium on Biological Age as a Problem of Theoretical and Practical Medicine*, October 22-24, Kiev, October 22-24, 1985 (in Russian).
25. Palmore, E.B. and Stone, V., Predicators of longevity: a follow-up of the aged patients in Chapel Hill, *Gerontologist*, 13, 88, 1973.
26. Rowe, J.W., Anders, R., Tobin, J.D., Norris, A.H., and Shock, N.W., The effect of age on creatinine clearance in man: a cross-sectional and longitudinal study, *J. Gerontol.*, 31, 155, 1976.
27. Schneider, E.L., Reff, M.E., Finch, C.E., and Weksler, M., Potential application of biological markers for assessing interventions of physiological aging, in *Biological Markers of Aging, Proc. Conf. Nonlethal Biological Markers of Physiological Aging*, NIH Publ. No. 82-2221, Reff, M.E. and Schneider, E.L., Eds., National Institutes of Health, Bethesda, MD, 1982, 237.
28. Shock, N.W., The physiology of aging, *Sci. Am.*, 206, 100, 1962.
29. Schwendeman, M., Cummins, L.B., Moore, G.T., and McMahan, C.A., Age estimation in baboons *(Papio cynocephalus)* using dental characteristics, *Lab. Anim. Sci.*, 30, 860, 1980.
30. Skalicky, M., Hofecker, G., Kment, A., and Niedermuller, H., Models of the biological age of the rat. II. Multiple regression models in the study of influencing aging, *Mech. Age. Dev.*, 14, 361, 1980.
31. Strehler, B.L., *Time, Cells and Aging*, Academic Press, New York, 1962.
32. Voitenko, V.P. Polyukov, A.M., Barbaruk, L.G., Kolodchenko, V.P., and Khodzinskii, A.N., The biological age as the key problem of gerontology, in *Biological Age, Heredity and Aging, Gerontology and Geriatrics 1989 Year Book,* Mints, A. Ya. and Voitenko, V.P., Eds., Institute of Gerontology of the Academy of Medical Science, Kiev, 1984, 5 (in Russian).
33. Webster, W. and Logie, A.R., A relationship between functional age and health status in female subjects, *J. Gerontol.*, 31, 546, 1976.
34. Woodbury, M.A. and Manton, K.G., Mathematical model of the physiological dynamics of aging and correlated mortality selection. I. Theoretical development and critiques, *J. Gerontol.*, 38, 398, 1983.
35. Young, J.C. and Rickert, W.T., Concerning the precision of age estimates based on biological parameters, *Exp. Gerontol.*, 8, 337, 1973.

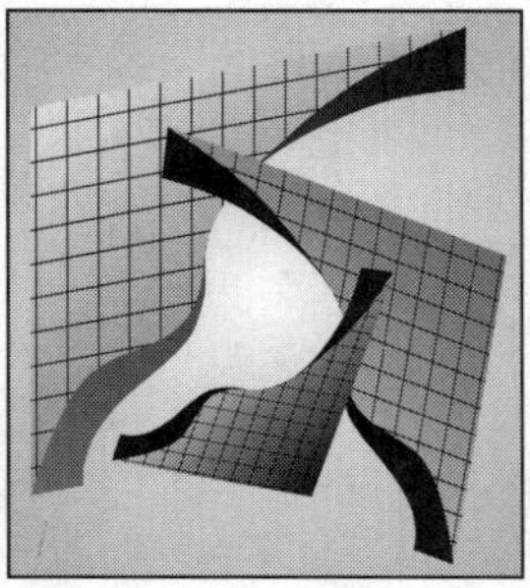

METABOLIC PROFILES

CHAPTER 14

ENTROPY AS A BIOLOGICAL MARKER IN HUMAN AGING

DANIEL HERSHEY AND WILLIAM E. LEE, III

TABLE OF CONTENTS

0-8493-0129-7/94/$0.00+$.50

I. ENTROPY AND AGING

Entropy is not something tangible, nor anything capable of being seen or touched. Hence, entropy is a very difficult concept to grasp. It is not a solid, it is not hot or cold, and does not have a physical consequence, such as temperature. We can say that entropy is a measure of the disorder of a system and can show that more disorder means higher entropy content. For example, a container is divided in two, with molecules A on one side and molecules B on the other. This system has a certain entropy content and is ordered in its own way. Remove the partition that divides the container and after a while molecules A and B will mix thoroughly. This mixed state has a higher entropy content and we say it is more disordered.

Automobile engine pistons, before ignition, contain mixtures of gasoline and air under pressure, a relatively ordered system compared to the exhausted gases after ignition coming out of the tailpipe of this automobile. We say the process of combustion has proceeded from a state of low entropy (in the pistons) to one of high entropy (out of the tailpipe). Real processes tend to go in the direction of increasing entropy. Aging can be envisioned as an irreversible process of entropy accumulation. Getting older means having less control of body functions, being more disordered. Death is the ultimate disorder, a state of maximum entropy. This point has been speculated upon by other scientists, including Jones[7] and Von Bertalanffy.[13]

Entropy as a concept originated during the development of the scientific field of thermodynamics, the study of how heat is converted into work. It was defined by the German physicist, Clasusius, in 1868.[3] Earlier, in his studies on the efficiency of heat engines, Carnot in 1824 introduced the second law of thermodynamics, which essentially says that systems will run down of their own volition if left to themselves. In other words, the entropy content tends toward a maximum. Thus, increasing entropy could be an indication of the direction the system is inclined to go. Unless there is outside intervention, the second law of thermodynamics codifies the one-sidedness of time, or time's arrow. We can only move forward, i.e., time is irreversible.

Everything we know is tending toward chaos (unless there is outside intervention), toward an equilibrium with the environment. To quote Von Bertanlanffy:[13]

> "The significance of the second law can be expressed in another way. It states that the general trend of events is directed toward states of maximum disorder, the higher forms of energy such as mechanical, chemical, and light energy being irreversibly degraded to heat, and heat gradients continually disappearing. Therefore, the universe approaches entropy death when all energy is converted into heat of low temperature, and the world process comes to an end."

It was not until the 1950s that entropy started to seriously emerge in discussions of living phenomena. Complicated biological processes such as cell differentiation, growth, aging, etc., were now analyzed from the second law of thermodynamics and entropy calculations made. Bailey[1] wrote, "Entropy is a very viable concept for the biological and social sciences. It applies to both open and closed systems. It can be discussed in terms of organization or order." Jones[7] said, "One common feature of biological processes is their unidirectionality in time, that is, they are not reversible, except under special circumstances. Since entropy is the only physical variable in nature which generally seems to parallel the direction and irreversibility of time, these should be fertile areas for the effective use of entropy models."

Much of the historical development of entropy has dealt with isolated or closed systems. A closed system is one that can exchange energy but not matter with the surrounding environment. The second law of thermodynamics states that a closed system must evolve to a state in equilibrium with its environment, a condition of maximum entropy. Open systems are those which can exchange both matter and energy with the surroundings. Obviously we, the living, are examples of open systems. Open systems must maintain the exchange of energy and matter in order to sustain themselves, or slow the approach to the final state, death.

II. OPEN SYSTEM ANALYSIS

A. OPEN SYSTEM ENERGY BALANCE

Given the volume element shown here, and flows, J, in and out, an energy balance is written as

$$J \rightleftarrows \begin{matrix} \text{Volume}, V \\ \text{Surface}, \Omega \end{matrix}$$

$$\sum_{\text{in}}^{\text{Flow}} - \sum_{\text{out}}^{\text{Flow}} + \left\{ \begin{matrix} \text{Production} \\ \text{or} \\ \text{Depletion} \end{matrix} \right\} = \text{Rate of accumulation} \tag{1}$$

or

$$P(E) + \phi(E) = \frac{\partial E}{\partial t} \tag{2}$$

where $P(E)$ is internal energy production and $\phi(E)$ is energy flow through the surface.

We can write

$$P(E) = \int \sigma(E) dV \tag{3}$$

where $\sigma(E)$ is internal energy production per unit time and volume and

$$\phi(E) = \int_{\Omega} \mathbf{J} d\Omega \tag{4}$$

or

$$\phi(E) = \int_{\Omega} \mathbf{J} \cdot \mathbf{n} d\Omega \tag{5}$$

where $\mathbf{n}$ is the normal unit vector.

Using the Gauss divergence theorem, Equation 5 becomes

$$\phi(E) = \int_{v} \operatorname{div} \mathbf{J}\, dV \tag{6}$$

where div signifies the divergence vector operation. From Equations 2, 3, and 6, we get

$$\frac{\partial E}{\partial t} = \int_{v} \sigma(E)\, dV + \int_{v} \operatorname{div} \mathbf{J}\, dV \tag{7}$$

where $\sigma(E)$ deals with internal (i) phenomena and $\mathbf{J}$ relates to external (e) flow phenomena. Another way of writing Equation 7 is

$$\frac{dE}{dt} = \frac{d_i E}{dt} + \frac{d_e E}{dt} \tag{8}$$

A "local" form of Equation 7 is

$$\frac{d\overline{E}}{dt} = \sigma(E) + \operatorname{div} \mathbf{J} \qquad (9)$$

where

$$\overline{E} = \frac{dE}{dV} \qquad (10)$$

B. OPEN SYSTEM MASS BALANCE

In an analogous fashion, we get from Equation

$$\frac{dm_j}{dt} = \frac{d_i m_j}{dt} + \frac{d_e m_j}{dt} \qquad (11)$$

for component *j*. The flow term $d_e m_j/dt$ can be written from Equations 5 and 6:

$$\frac{d_e m_j}{dt} = \int_{\Omega} \mathbf{J}_j \cdot \mathbf{n}\, d\Omega = \int_{v} \operatorname{div} \mathbf{J}_j\, dV \qquad (12)$$

where $\mathbf{J}_j$ is flux of species *j* at the surface, Ω.

The internal mass production is

$$\frac{d_i m_j}{dt} = \sum_{k=1}^{l} \nu_{jk} r_k \qquad (13)$$

where the mass of component *j* is being produced or consumed by chemical reaction within volume, *V*. There are *l* chemical reactions involving component, *j*, and ν_{jk} is the stoichiometric coefficient of species, *j*, in the *k*th reaction, and r_k is the reaction rate of the *k*th reaction.

With Equations 11, 12, and 13, we get

$$\frac{dm_j}{dt} = \int_{v} \Sigma \nu_{jk} r_k\, dV + \int_{v} \operatorname{div} \mathbf{J}_j\, dV \qquad (14)$$

The local or per volume form of Equation 14 is

$$\frac{d\rho_j}{dt} \sum_{k=1}^{l} \nu_{jk} r_k + \operatorname{div} \mathbf{J}_j \qquad (15)$$

where ρ_j is the density of component *j*.

C. OPEN SYSTEM ENTROPY BALANCE

The classical Gibbs entropy equation for an open system is

$$TdS = dU + PdV - \sum_{j=1}^{n} \mu_j dm_j \qquad (16)$$

where μ_j is chemical potential (energy per unit mass) of component *j*, *T* is temperature, *S* is entropy, *U* is internal energy, and *P* is pressure. This can be rewritten as

$$dS = \frac{dU + PdV}{T} - \sum_{j=1}^{n} \frac{\mu_j}{T} dm_j \tag{17}$$

From an energy balance (Equation 17; the first law of thermodynamics) we can write

$$dU = d\overline{Q} - PdV \tag{18}$$

where $\overline{Q}$ is heat transfer by conduction and convection (mass flows).

With Equations 17 and 18 we can write

$$dS = \frac{d\overline{Q}}{T} - \sum_{j=1}^{n} \frac{\mu_j}{T} dm_j \tag{19}$$

or

$$\frac{dS}{dt} = \frac{1}{T}\frac{d\overline{Q}}{dt} - \sum_{j=1}^{n} \frac{\mu_j}{T}\frac{dm_j}{dt} \tag{20}$$

where *dS/dt* is entropy production (with respect to time). From Equations 15 and 20 we get for a unit volume element

$$\frac{dS}{dt} = \frac{1}{T}\frac{d\overline{Q}}{dt} - \sum_{j=1}^{n} \frac{\mu_j}{T} \sum_{k=1}^{l} \nu_{jk} r_k - \sum_{j=1}^{n} \frac{\mu_j}{T} \operatorname{div} J_j \tag{21}$$

From vector calculus, with *f* a scalar and **F** a vector field, we can write Equation 18

$$\operatorname{div}(f\mathbf{F}) = f \operatorname{div}\mathbf{F} + \mathbf{F} \cdot \nabla f \tag{22}$$

where ∇ is vector gradient operation.

From Equation 22 we can show

$$\sum_{j=1}^{n} \frac{\mu_j}{T} \operatorname{div} J_j = \operatorname{div}\left(\sum_{j=1}^{n} \frac{\mu_j}{T} J_j\right) - \sum_{j=1}^{n} \left(J_j \cdot \frac{\nabla \mu_j}{T}\right) \tag{23}$$

and this substituted into Equation 21 gives

$$\frac{dS}{dt} = \frac{1}{T}\frac{d\overline{Q}}{dt} - \sum_{j=1}^{n} \frac{\mu_j}{T} \sum_{k=1}^{l} \nu_{jk} r_k - \operatorname{div}\left(\sum_{j=1}^{n} \frac{\mu_j}{T} J_j\right) + \sum_{j=1}^{n} \left(J_j \frac{\nabla \mu_j}{\overline{T}}\right) \tag{24}$$

From Equation 24 we can collect these terms

$$\frac{1}{T}\frac{d\overline{Q}}{dt} - \operatorname{div}\left(\sum_{j=1}^{n} \frac{\mu_j}{T} J_j\right) \tag{25}$$

and note that they relate to exchanges with the surroundings. Also, from Equation 24 we can collect the rest of the terms on the right-hand side of the equation, i.e.,

$$-\sum_{j=1}^{n} \frac{\mu_j}{T} \sum_{k=1}^{l} \nu_{jk} r_k + \sum_{j=1}^{n} \left(J_j \frac{\nabla \mu_j}{T} \right) \tag{26}$$

and infer that they relate to internal phenomena (chemical reactions and diffusion). Therefore, Equation 24 has the form

$$\frac{dS}{dt} = \frac{d_i S}{dt} + \frac{d_e S}{dt} \tag{27}$$

The second law of thermodynamics requires

$$\frac{d_i S}{dt} \geq 0 \tag{28}$$

where the equality holds for reversible processes and the inequality applies to irreversible processes. For an adiabatic, closed system (both heat and mass transfer to the surroundings are not possible), $d_eS/dt = 0$ and Equation 27 becomes

$$\frac{dS}{dt} = \frac{d_i S}{dt} \geq 0 \tag{29}$$

For a closed system (heat transfer is possible but not mass transfer),

$$\frac{d_e S}{dt} = \frac{d\bar{Q}}{T}$$

and Equation 27 becomes

$$\frac{dS}{dt} \geq \frac{d\bar{Q}}{T} \quad \text{closed system} \tag{30}$$

where $\bar{Q}$ is heat supplied to the system. For open systems, d_eS/dt can be positive or negative and greater or lesser than d_iS/dt. Therefore dS/dt can be positive or negative or equal to zero at steady state.

III. ENTROPY PRODUCTION

We can say that entropy accumulation within the living system is composed of two parts. The first is the internal entropy production based on the myriad of irreversible chemical reactions which constitute the chemistry of life. Second, there is the entropy flow through our boundaries, such as in the food consumed, air inhaled and exhaled, biological waste products, heat loss from the skin, etc. The internal entropy production derived from our chemical reactions always proceeds in the direction of increasing our entropy content, as the chemistry of life is inherently irreversible. However, the food in, air in and out, waste products out, and heat out may in total contribute positive or negative entropy flows through our boundaries, which then affects the rate of accumulation of entropy in our living body.

For a closed system with chemical reactions, Equation 20 can be rewritten for mole fractions, n_j

$$dS = \frac{d\bar{Q}}{T} - \sum_{j=1}^{m} \frac{\mu_j}{T} dn_j \tag{31}$$

We can write for the change in the concentration of component *j*,

$$dn_j = \nu_j \, d\xi \tag{32}$$

where ν_j is the stoichiometric coefficient and $d\xi$ is the extent of the chemical reaction. Also,

$$r = \frac{d\xi}{dt} \tag{33}$$

where *r* is reaction velocity. From Equations 32 and 33 we can obtain

$$\frac{dn_j}{dt} = \nu_j r \tag{34}$$

and thus Equation 31 becomes

$$dS = \frac{d\overline{Q}}{T} - \sum_{j=1}^{m} \frac{\mu_j}{T} \nu_j \, d\xi$$

or

$$\frac{dS}{dt} = \frac{d}{dt}\left(\frac{d\overline{Q}}{T}\right) - \sum_{j=1}^{m} \frac{\mu_j}{T} \nu_j \frac{d\xi}{dt}$$

$$= \frac{1}{T}\frac{d\overline{Q}}{dt} - \sum_{j=1}^{m} \frac{\mu_j}{T} \nu_j r \tag{35}$$

With the definition of chemical affinity, *A*,

$$A = -\sum_{j=1}^{m} \nu_j \mu_j \tag{36}$$

Equation 35 becomes

$$\frac{dS}{dt} = \frac{1}{T}\frac{d\overline{Q}}{dt} + \frac{Ar}{T} \tag{37}$$

or

$$\frac{dS}{dt} = \frac{d_iS}{dt} + \frac{d_eS}{dt} \tag{38}$$

where

$$\frac{d_eS}{dt} = \frac{1}{T}\frac{d\overline{Q}}{dt} = \text{external entropy flow through the boundary}$$

and

$$\frac{d_iS}{dt} = \frac{Ar}{T} = \text{internal entropy production.} \tag{39}$$

From Equation 39 we note that d_iS/dt is composed of a flow term (r, the rate of reaction) and a driving force (A, the chemical affinity). In general, the internal entropy production can be written as

$$\frac{d_iS}{dt} = \frac{1}{T}\sum_{j=1}^{m} (\text{flow})_j \cdot (\text{driving force})_j \tag{40}$$

or

$$\frac{d_iS}{dt} = \frac{1}{T}\sum_{j=1}^{m} J_j X_j = \sigma(s) \tag{41}$$

where J_j is the flow term and X_j is the driving force.

Flow is proportional to a coefficient multiplied by a gradient, or

$$\text{Flow } \alpha \text{ (Coefficient)} \cdot \text{(Gradient)} \tag{42}$$

which becomes

$$J_\alpha = \sum_{\beta=1}^{m} L_{\alpha\beta} x_\beta . \tag{43}$$

For example, an electric current flowing in a wire requires these equations

$$J_1 = L_{11}X_1 + L_{12}X_2 \tag{44}$$

$$J_2 = L_{21}X_1 + L_{22}X_2 \tag{45}$$

where L_{11} is the wire resistance, L_{22} is the thermal resistance, J_1 is the electric current, J_2 is the heat flow, X_1 is the voltage potential, and X_2 is the temperature gradient.

The Onsager reciprocity relationship, $L_{12} = L_{21}$ applies here. These relationships, especially Equation 43, are applicable in the linear domain, close to equilibrium. At equilibrium, the X_β is equal to zero which implies $J_\alpha = 0$.

We can define a dissipative function, ϕ, from Equation 41:

$$\phi = T\sigma(s) = \sum_{j=1}^{m} J_j X_j \tag{46}$$

which relates entropy production, $\sigma(s)$, to energy flows and forces.

IV. AN ENTROPY THEORY OF AGING

Old age or senescence may be the decline in our ability to produce free energy. Less free energy means diminished cell function. Vitality might be defined as our biological and thermodynamic strength, the ability to expend energy to restore ourselves to near original conditions. In other words, aging can be thought of as the process of loss of vitality.

Zotin[15] proposed that we evolve toward a final state, death, by a series of changes, each change called a stationary state. We settle into a stationary state, stay for a while, until pushed to the next stage, and the next. This is clearly seen in the transformation of butterfly larvae and pupae, dramatic physical changes. Balmer[2] applied entropy concepts to the study of an aging annual fish. This species displays

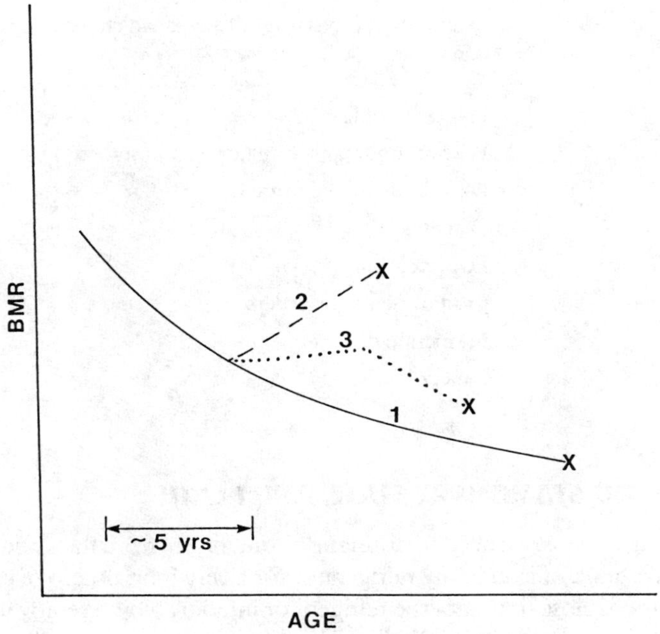

Figure 1 Generalized plots of BMR vs. age, which illustrates types I, II, and III behavior. "X" indicates the occurrence of death.

all the characteristics of birth, growth, aging, and senile death, over a short 12-month period. Balmer identified entropy flows into and out of the fish, such as food, excrement, and body heat dissipation.

A. BASAL METABOLIC RATE AND AGING

The major influence on life span, assuming we are reasonably healthy, is internal chemistry. These chemical reactions give off heat (much as an atomic bomb does, but of much less magnitude, of course). It is this heat transfer that gives us a clue as to the vitality of our living system. It is this heat evolution, under prescribed resting conditions, that we call the basal metabolic rate (BMR), a quantity known to decrease with age. We can convert this BMR into entropy units.[5] Most people show what we call type I BMR behavior, as shown in Figure 1. People who display type I history are living "normal" lives, which means being free from significant medical stresses such as prolonged illness. Another BMR pattern observed is called type II, where a subject begins in a type I mode, but then shows a BMR which increases steadily (also indicated in Figure 1). The subject may die while tracing out a type II line, whose duration may be 1 to 5 years. (The stress causing this aberrant behavior is defined as a "killing stress".) Obviously the virulence of this killing stress depends on the age of onset and its intensity. Table 1 suggests some causes of these killing stresses. The subject may recover from type II behavior, through the natural healing powers of the body or by medical intervention, and resume the more normal pattern we originally called type I. Figure 1 also illustrates the recovery phase, type III. This person has recovered from the type II stress, so obviously it was not a killing stress. The life spans for type III subjects tend to be less than type I, but there are a variety of possibilities. For example, the stress might have been promptly diagnosed and successfully treated, suggesting perhaps an extended longevity potential. The efficacy of the treatment is reflected in the resumption of the normal downward slant of the BMR. Factored into this history, in additon to the promptness of the diagnosis, is the severity of the stress and the natureof the treatment (some obese patients might initiate weight loss and exercise programs). Obviously diagnosis does not guarantee recovery; for example, some of the type II cases might arise from untreatable cancer.[9]

Table 1 Examples of physiological states which may constitute a "killing stress"[a]

Hyperthyroidism
Physical trauma (severe burns, injuries, etc.)
Deep body temperature rise
Diabetes
Hypertension
Cardiovascular disorders
Endocrine disorders
Cancer

[a] *For more details, see Reference 9.*

B. EQUILIBRIUM, THE STATIONARY STATE, AND DEATH

In describing the aging process, we need to distinguish equilibrium from the stationary (steady) state. Suppose I have kept a hunk of iron in my refrigerator for a very long time. We can assume that the temperature of the iron is close to that of the refrigerator interior. Now I remove the metal from the refrigerator and place it on a table in my kitchen. We know that the metal will begin to warm, heat flowing into the iron from the surrounding, warmer air. The driving force for heat flow is the temperature difference between the ambient air and the iron. In the beginning, with the greatest temperature driving force, a relatively large amount of heat enters the iron, warming it quickly. The warming iron receives less and less quantities of heat, because the temperature driving force between the metal and the air is diminishing. After a few hours, the temperature of the iron is almost that of the room, the temperature driving force is approaching zero, and the heat flow to the iron is negligibly small. If we wait long enough, we can say that the iron is now in equilibrium with its environment; the temperature driving force is approaching zero, as is the heat flow. Nothing is changing as there are no driving forces to cause change.

On the other hand, suppose I have a tank half-filled with water. There is a pipe attached which will allow new water to enter the tank and we have a drain at the bottom through which water exits. If the amount of water entering is constant and equal to the exiting water, then the liquid level in the tank remains constant. To the observer, things look steady. Though there are driving forces available, these forces are balanced and nothing changes. We say we are at a stationary (steady) state. This is not to be confused with equilibrium, where the driving forces are zero. Thus, there are important differences between equilibrium and the stationary state.

C. AGING AS AN ENTROPY-DRIVEN PROCESS

We can consider the aging process as a series of steps, proceeding from one stationary state to the next and the next. We can talk of entropy driving forces, causing the evolution from one stationary state to the next. Each time we achieve a stationary state, we "rest" for a "moment", and then go on to the next. In each stationary state, we hunker down, collect ourselves, minimize our entropy production, smooth out our chemistry, and await the next push. And so we age. Thus, the stationary state can be characterized as an entropy- (disorder) producing state, where this entropy production is drawn down to a minimum, before going on to the next stationary state where a new minimum is established. The theorem of minimum entropy production is a fundamental concept of the stationary state, first developed by Prigogine and co-workers.[10,11] Death is the final state to which we are drawn, where there no longer exists a tension for life; the driving forces have been reduced to nothing or some minimum level, below which life cannot be supported.

D. STATIONARY STATES AND MINIMUM ENTROPY PRODUCTION

At a nonequilibrium stationary state, from Equation 27 we can write

$$\frac{dS}{dt} = 0, \text{ or } \frac{d_jS}{dt} = \frac{d_eS}{dt} \tag{47}$$

Minimum entropy production implies a minimum value of d_iS/dt, or $\sigma(S)$ from Equation 41 or ϕ from Equation 46. equilibrium requires $X_i = 0$ (the forces are zero) and $J_i = 0$ (flows are zero), and hence, $\phi = \sigma = 0$ from Equations 41 and 46. This is demonstrated below. In the stationary state, where the X_i are not zero, we can show that in this stationary state, the system seeks to minimize ϕ, but ϕ does not necessarily go to zero.

From Equation 46,

$$\phi = T\sigma(S) = \sum_{j=1}^{n} J_i X_j \tag{48}$$

and with Equation 43 in Equation 48 we get

$$\begin{aligned} \phi = T\sigma(S) &= \sum_{j=1}^{n} \left[\sum_{k} L_{jk} X_k \right] X_j \\ &= \left(L_{11}X_1 + L_{12}X_2\right)X_1 + \left(L_{21}X_1 + L_{22}X_2\right)X_2 \end{aligned} \tag{49}$$

for $j = 1, 2$ and $k = 1, 2$. Multiplying the terms in Equation 49 we get

$$\phi = T\sigma(S) = L_{11}X_1^2 + L_{12}X_2X_1 + L_{21}X_1X_2 + L_{22}X_2^2. \tag{50}$$

Using the Onsager identity, $L_{12} = L_{21}$, we get

$$\phi = T\sigma(S) = L_{11}X_1^2 + 2L_{12}X_1X_2 + L_{22}X_2^2. \tag{51}$$

Now we look for critical points, extrema of ϕ, maxima or minima. These critical points are found from (52) through (54):

$$\frac{\partial\sigma}{\partial X_1} = \frac{\partial\sigma}{\partial X_2} = 0 \tag{52}$$

and for a minimum point,

$$\frac{\partial^2\sigma}{\partial X_1^2} > 0 \quad \frac{\partial^2\sigma}{\partial X_2^2} > 0 \tag{53}$$

and

$$\frac{\partial^2\sigma}{\partial X_1^2} \cdot \frac{\partial^2\sigma}{\partial X_2^2} - 4\frac{\partial^2\sigma}{\partial X_1 \partial X_2} > 0 \tag{54}$$

evaluated at the critical point, (X_1^c, X_2^c). A maximum satisfies (52) through (54), but the inequalities are reversed, i.e., they are less than zero. The analysis is indeterminate if (54) is equal to zero.

From (49), rearranged, we have

$$T\sigma(s) = \Sigma X_j \, \Sigma L_{jk} X_k \tag{55}$$

and hence (without T),

$$\frac{d\sigma}{\partial X_j} = 2L_{jj}X_j + 2\sum_{\substack{j=1 \\ j\neq k}}^{n} L_{jk}X_k = 2\sum_{k=1}^{n} L_{jk}X_k = 2J_j \tag{56}$$

where Equation 43 was used to get the final result. These operations can be demonstrated by a concrete example from (51):

$$\frac{\partial\sigma}{\partial X_1} = 2L_{11}X_1 + 2L_{12}X_2 = 2\sum_{k=1}^{2} L_{1k}X_k$$

or

$$\frac{\partial\sigma}{\partial X_j} = 2\sum_{k=1}^{n} L_{jk}X_k = 2J_j$$

We can also get from Equation 56

$$\frac{d^2\sigma}{dX_j} = 2L_{jj} \tag{57}$$

and

$$\frac{\partial^2\sigma}{\partial X_j \partial X_k} = 2L_{jk} \tag{58}$$

from (51). Now from (52) set

$$\frac{\partial\sigma}{\partial X_1} = \frac{\partial\sigma}{\partial X_2} = 0 \tag{59}$$

This requires from (56)

$$\frac{\partial\sigma}{\partial X_1} = 0 = 2J_1$$

or

$$J_1 = 0$$

and

$$\frac{\partial\sigma}{\partial X_2} = 0 = 2J_2$$

or

$$J_2 = 0$$

This implies no flows and from (48), $\phi = T\sigma(S) = 0$. To determine whether the extremum is a minimum, use (53) and (57)

$$\frac{\partial^2 \sigma}{\partial X_1} = 2L_{11} > 0 \tag{60}$$

and

$$\frac{\partial^2 \sigma}{\partial X_2} = L_{22} > 0 \tag{61}$$

since L_{jj} are always positive. From (54), (57), (58), (60), and (61) we get

$$\frac{\partial^2 \sigma}{\partial X_1^2} \cdot \frac{\partial^2 \sigma}{\partial X_2^2} - \frac{\partial^2 \sigma}{\partial X_1 \partial X_2} = 4L_{11}L_{22} - 2L_{12}. \tag{62}$$

Prigogine[11] states that $4L_{11}L_{22} - 2L_{12}$ is usually greater than zero. Therefore, with (62) positive, we have found that the critical point is a minimum. From (59) through (62) we can conclude that $\sigma(S) = 0$ is a minimum. At equilibrium, no flows are present ($J_i = 0$) and $\sigma(S) = 0$ (no entropy production) and this critical point is a minimum.

Now consider a system that has external influences imposed on it. A constant temperature difference is created and maintained between two vessels. Thus, there are two gradients, X_m and X_T, corresponding to a mass flow (driven by the chemical potential) and a heat flow (caused by the temperature gradient). These two gradients give rise to a mass flow J_m and a heat flow, J_T. From Equation 43 we can write

$$J_m = L_{mm}X_m + L_{mT}X_T \tag{63}$$

and

$$J_T = L_{Tm}X_m + L_{TT}X_T \tag{64}$$

where L_{mm} is the diffusion coefficient, L_{TT} is the thermal conductivity, and $L_{mT} = L_{Tm}$ is the thermal diffusivity. We can write from Equations 43, 63 and 64 the entropy production

$$\begin{aligned} T\sigma(S) &= J_m X_m + J_T X_T \\ &= \left(L_{mm}X_m + L_{Tm}X_T\right)X_m + \left(L_{Tm}X_m + L_{TT}X_T\right)X_T \\ &= L_{mm}X_m^2 + 2L_{Tm}X_T X_m + L_{TT}X_T^2 \end{aligned} \tag{65}$$

With the external temperature gradient maintained, the flow of mass will eventually cease ($J_m \to 0$). A stationary state will be established and from (65)

$$T\sigma(S) = J_T X_T = L_{TT}X_T^2. \tag{66}$$

The question is whether this is the minimum level of $T\sigma(S)$ under the given constraints. Under the above constraints $T\sigma(S)$ is a minimum, given by the Lagrangian multiplier implicit method. We seek the minimum of

$$F = f + \lambda g \tag{67}$$

where f is the system describing equation, g is the equation that describes the system constraints, and λ is the Lagrangian multiplier.

We seek the minimum of

$$f = T\sigma(S) = L_{mm}X_m^2 + 2L_{Tm}X_TX_m + L_{TT}X_T^2 \tag{68}$$

where (65) is used. This is subject to the constraint on the thermal flow, J_T, from (64)

$$J_T = L_{TT}X_T + L_{Tm}X_m = \text{ constant } \neq 0 \tag{69}$$

The constraining equation, g, is given by

$$g = L_{TT}X_T + L_{Tm}X_m - J_T = 0 \tag{70}$$

From (67), (68), and (70), we get

$$\begin{aligned} F &= f + \lambda g \\ &= L_{mm}X_m^2 + 2\,L_{Tm}X_TX_m + L_{TT}X_T^2 + \lambda\left(L_{TT}X_T + L_{Tm}X_m - J_T\right) \end{aligned} \tag{71}$$

From (52), to find the critical points that minimize (71), we need

$$\frac{\partial F}{\partial X_m} = 0 \tag{72}$$

and

$$\frac{\partial F}{\partial X_T} = 0 \tag{73}$$

which yields from (71)

$$\frac{\partial F}{\partial X_T} = 2\,L_{Tm}X_m + 2\,L_{TT}X_T + \lambda\,L_{TT} = 0 \tag{74}$$

$$\frac{\partial F}{\partial X_m} = 2\,L_{mm}X_m + 2\,L_{Tm}X_T + \lambda\,L_{Tm} = 0 \tag{75}$$

Simultaneous solution of (74) and (75) yields for the critical point, (X_T^c, X_m^c) the result $(-\lambda/2, 0)$, where $\lambda = -2X_T$. This minimum critical point, when inserted into (71) yields

$$F = L_{TT}X_T^2 \tag{76}$$

which is equivalent to

$$F = \left(L_{TT}X_C + L_{Tm}X_m\right)X_T = J_TX_T \tag{77}$$

where J_T is obtained from (69) and X_m is zero under the conditions set forth here. Thus, the entropy production $T\sigma(S) = J_TX_T$ is a minimum value, set by the constrained parameters. The unconstrained flow (J_m) goes to zero at the minimum stationary state.

V. EXCESS ENTROPY AND EXCESS ENTROPY PRODUCTION: DRIVING FORCES FOR AGING

Having introduced the idea of longevity as an entropy-driven process involving an evolution through innumerable stationary states, we can now explore the nature of the entropy driving force for life. If death represents the ultimate disorder (and our maximum entropy content) then we can characterize our longevity potential and vitality by the distance we are from the "black hole" of death. We can calculate a difference in entropy content, from the present (where we are) to where we are heading (toward death). This difference is called excess entropy (EE) and is a driving force for life. By tracking EE vs. age, we can see our life unfolding, or winding down, as EE approaches zero, the end of the journey.[6,8]

Not only is EE an important parameter in tracing our life span, but so too is the rate of change of EE. In other words, how quickly EE is diminishing with age is another key marker. We call this second parameter excess entropy production (EEP).

A. EXCESS ENTROPY AND EXCESS ENTROPY PRODUCTION

From (49), we can write for a reference state, entropy production, $\sigma^0(S)$

$$\sigma^0(S) = \frac{1}{T}\sum_{j=1}^{n} J_j^0 X_j^0 \tag{78}$$

A deviation from the reference state is

$$\sigma(S) = \sigma^0(S) + \delta\sigma(S) \tag{79}$$

provided $\delta\sigma(S)$ is small. From (79) we get

$$\delta\sigma(S) = \sigma(S) - \sigma^0(S) \tag{80}$$

or, with (49) and (78)

$$\delta\left[\frac{1}{T}\Sigma J_j X_j\right] = \frac{1}{T}\Sigma J_j X_j - \frac{1}{T}\Sigma J_j^0 X_j^0 \tag{81}$$

Because σ^0 is a minimum in the reference state, then $\delta\sigma(S) > 0$. We define $\delta\sigma(S)$ as EEP, a thermodynamic driving force

$$\text{EEP} = \delta\sigma(s) \tag{82}$$

If EEP is the rate of production of the excess, beyond the reference state, then

$$\text{EE} = \int \delta\sigma(\text{S})\,dt = \int \text{EEP}\,dt \tag{83}$$

or

$$\frac{d}{dt}\text{EE} = \text{EEP} \tag{84}$$

From Equation 41, entropy production is

$$\frac{dS}{dt} = \Sigma J_j X_j \tag{85}$$

The first variation of entropy production is

$$\delta\left(\frac{dS}{dt}\right) = \delta\left[\Sigma J_j X_j\right] = \Sigma J_j \delta X_j + \Sigma X_j \delta J_j \tag{86}$$

However, $\delta(dS/dt) = d(\delta S)/dt$ from the communicative properties of derivatives and differences. The second variation is

$$\delta\left[\delta\left(\frac{dS}{dt}\right)\right] = \delta\left[\frac{d(\delta S)}{dt}\right] = \frac{d\left(\delta^2 S\right)}{dt} \tag{87}$$

where we again interchange the order of operations of derivatives and differences. Thus, from (86)

$$\begin{aligned}\delta\left[\delta\left(\frac{dS}{dt}\right)\right] &= \delta\left[\Sigma J_j \delta X_j + \Sigma X_j \delta J_j\right] \\ &= \left(\Sigma J_j \delta^2 X_j + \Sigma \delta J_j \delta X_j\right) + \left(\Sigma X_j \delta^2 J_j + \Sigma \delta X_j \delta J_j\right) \\ &= \Sigma J_j \delta^2 X_j + 2\Sigma \delta J_j \delta X_j + \Sigma X_j \delta^2 J_j\end{aligned} \tag{88}$$

Assuming $\delta^2 X_j << \delta X_j$ and $\delta^2 J_j << \delta J_j$, then (88) becomes

$$\delta\left[\delta\left(\frac{dS}{dt}\right)\right] = 2\Sigma\, \delta J_j \delta X_j$$

or from (87)

$$\frac{d\left(\delta^2 S\right)}{dt} = 2\Sigma\, \delta J_j \delta J_j \delta X_j \tag{89}$$

Let

$$\delta^2 S = \text{EE}$$

and

$$\frac{d\left(\delta^2 S\right)}{dt} = \text{EEP}$$

where

$$\delta J_j = J_j - J_j^0$$

and

$$\delta X_j = X_j - X_j^0$$

Excess entropy is a second order excess entropy because it is conveniently expressed in terms of fluctuations in flows and forces. Also, $\delta S = 0$ at the reference state (extremum) while $\delta^2 S$ is not.

Another way of showing $\delta^2 S$ is EE is to expand S in a Taylor series about a reference state, S^0,

$$S(X_i) = S(X_i^0) + (X_i - X_i^0)\frac{dS(X_i)}{dX_i}\bigg|_{\substack{\text{reference}\\ \text{state}}} + \frac{1}{2}(X_i - X_i^0)^2 \frac{d^2[S(X_i)]}{dX_i^2}\bigg|_{\substack{\text{reference}\\ \text{state}}} + \cdots \tag{90}$$

For small deviations from the reference state, we can write

$$\delta X_i = (X_i - X_i^0) \cong dX_i \tag{91}$$

$$(\delta X_i)^2 = (X_i - X_i^0)^2 \cong dX_i^2 \tag{92}$$

$$d[S(X_i)] \cong \delta[S(X_i^0)] \tag{93}$$

$$d^2[S(X_i)] \cong \delta^2[S(X_i^0)] \tag{94}$$

With (91) through (94) substituted into (90) we can get

$$S(X_i) = S(X_i^0) + (X_i - X_i^0)\frac{\delta[S(X_i^0)]}{(X_i - X_i^0)} + \frac{1}{2}(X_i - X_i^0)\frac{\delta^2[S(X_i^0)]}{(X_i - X_i^0)^2}$$

or

$$S(X_i) = S(X_i^0) + \delta[S(X_i^0)] + \frac{1}{2}\delta^2[S(X_i^0)] \tag{95}$$

If the reference state is equilibrium, then $\sigma[S(X_i^0)] = 0$ and (95) becomes

$$S(X_i) - S(X_i^0) = \Delta S = \frac{1}{2}\delta^2[S(X_i^0)] \tag{96}$$

which implies

$$\frac{1}{2}\delta^2[S(X_i^0)] = \text{EE} \tag{97}$$

and

$$\text{EE} < 0 \tag{98}$$

because $S(X_i^0)$ is greater than $S(X_i)$.

The Lee-Hershey theory,[6] developed from some of Prigogine's ideas, predicts the behavior of EE and EEP, and is presented in Figures 2 and 3. We can see from Figure 2 that EE is negative because we are subtracting from our entropy content at a given age, the maximum entropy content in the vicinity of death. With time, as we age, our entropy content approaches the maximum, and so EE tends toward zero.

The rate of change of EE is the "slope" of the EE curve and from Figure 2 we find that the slope is positive. Excess entropy production is this slope, producing a positive but decreasing track with age, as shown in Figure 3. In the vicinity of death, Lee and Hershey showed that EEP should approach zero.[6,8] It is easier to conceptualize why EE should go to zero in the vicinity of death because by definition, near death, our entropy content approaches the maximum value. However, Lee and Hershey demonstrated that EEP is easier to calculate than EE. Excess entropy production can be written in terms of the flow (ingestion) of nutrients (such as protein) and driving forces (the chemical potential of the protein metabolism reaction). At death, the equilibrium state, these flows, and forces, and hence EEP, go to zero. Thus, we can say that in the vicinity of death both EEP and EE approach zero.

Our life's course is considered stable so long as the positive-valued EEP descends and the negative-valued EE ascends. From the stability theory developed by Liapunov, we can say that when both EE and EEP are positive, the living system becomes unstable. Thus, we have another criterion for death, when the EE lines passes into the positive-valued domain (it crosses the zero axis). In other words, instability in the life process prevents us from exercising the control required to maintain a proper tension of life, so we die.

B. LIAPUNOV STABILITY

1. Definition One

a. $\left|y(\alpha_i, t_0) - y(\alpha_i, t)\right| < \varepsilon$ for all $t > t_0$ *(99)*
   $y(\alpha_i, t)$ is stable.

b. $\lim_{t \to \infty} \left|y(\alpha_i, t_0) - y(\alpha_i, t)\right| = 0$ *(100)*
   $y(\alpha_i, t)$ is quasi-asymptotically stable.

c. If (a) and (b) are true, $y(\alpha_i, t)$ is asymptotically stable.

d. If (a) is true, but (b) is not $y(\alpha_i, t)$ is weakly stable.

e. If (a) through (d) are not true $y(\alpha_i, t)$ is unstable.

2. Definition Two

Stable function: if V is positive and its derivative is negative, or vice versa. Unstable function: if V and its derivative are of the same sign.

More specific definitions of stability can be given by referring to Figure 4. Curve (a): stable, $|\text{displacement}| <_\varepsilon$ for all $t > t_0$. Curve (b) asymptotically stable, $|\text{displacement}| <_\varepsilon$ for all $t > t_0$ and (b) approaches zero asymptotically. Curve (c): stable, but not asymptotically stable. Curve (d) unstable, $|\text{displacement}| <_\varepsilon$ is not true and in some region $V > 0$ and $\dot{V} > 0$. Curve (e): quasi-asymptotically stable, some regions where $V > 0$ and $\dot{V} > 0$, but $\lim|V - V_0| \to 0$, $t \to \infty$.

C. EXCESS ENTROPY AND STABILITY

From (97), $\delta^2 S$ is EE and is in the negative domain, and increases toward zero with increasing time. The $\delta^2 S$ function is illustrated in Figure 2. Then,

$$\frac{d(\delta^2 S)}{dt} \geq 0 \qquad (101)$$

because the dependent variable ($\delta^2 S$) and the independent variable (t) in (101) are both increasing. The $d(\delta^2 S)/dt$ function is illustrated in Figure 3. Thus, we know from previous results that following an upset at t_0,

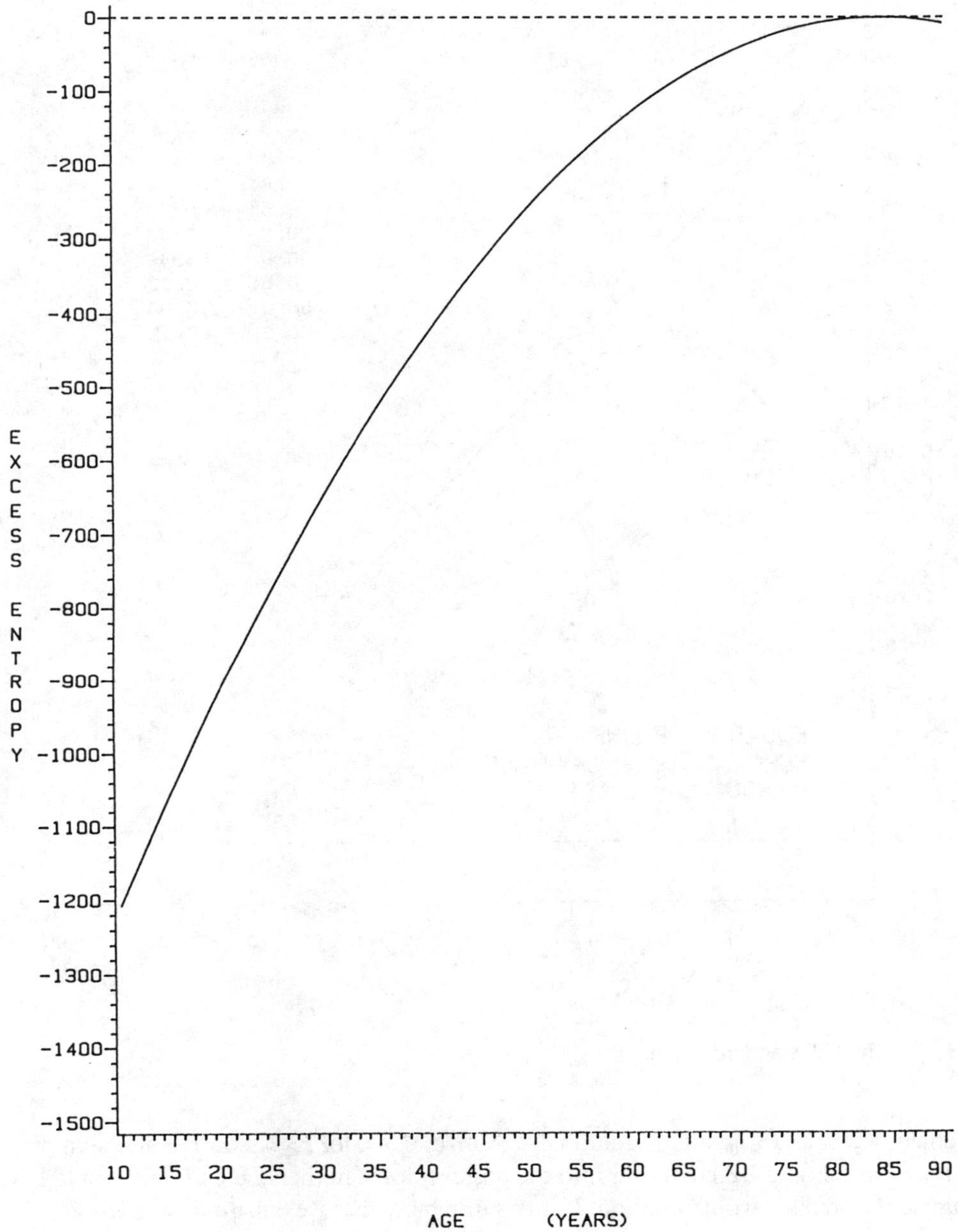

Figure 2 The EE standard curve.

$$\mathrm{EE} = \delta^2 S \rightarrow 0, t \rightarrow \infty$$

and

$$\mathrm{EEP} = \frac{\mathrm{d}\left(\delta^2 S\right)}{dt} \rightarrow 0, t \rightarrow \infty$$

We can say EE = $\delta^2 S$ is a Liapunov function and stable since $\delta^2 S$ and $d\delta^2 S/dt$ are opposite in sign everywhere (Definition Two). Furthermore, using Definition One, there is stability because $|\delta^2 S$

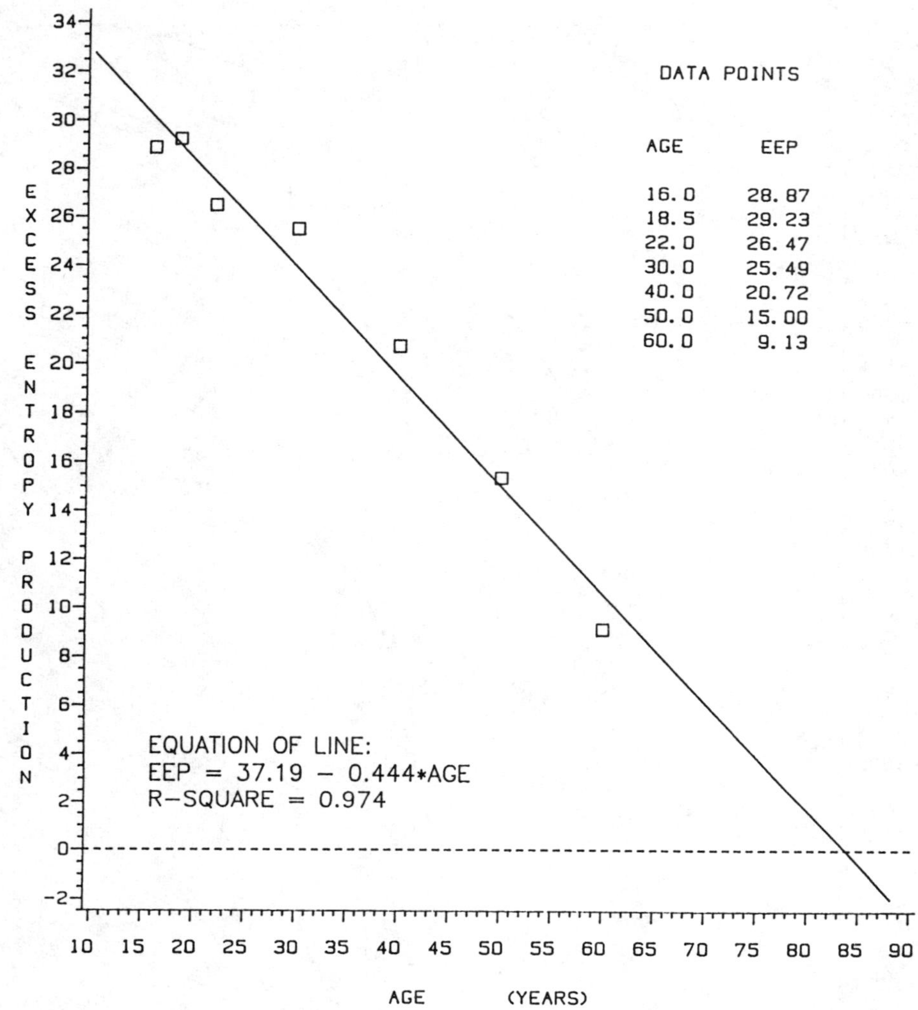

Figure 3 The EEP standard curve.

displacement$| <_{\varepsilon}$ for all $t > t_0$ and in addition $t \rightarrow \infty \lim |\delta^2 S^* = 0$ for $t > t_0$, so EE is also asymptotically stable. However, should EE cross over into the positive domain, then EE and EEP would have the same sign and instability would develop. It is this instability that we equate with death.

D. LONGEVITY PREDICTIONS BASED ON EXCESS ENTROPY PRODUCTION AND EXCESS ENTROPY TRACKS CALCULATION OF EXCESS ENTROPY PRODUCTION

From (89) we can write

$$\text{EEP} = \frac{d(\delta^2 S)}{dt} = \Sigma\,\delta(X)\,\delta(J) \qquad (102)$$

and from (39) we can equate the chemical affinity driving force, A, with X and reaction velocity flow, r, with J. Thus, (102) becomes

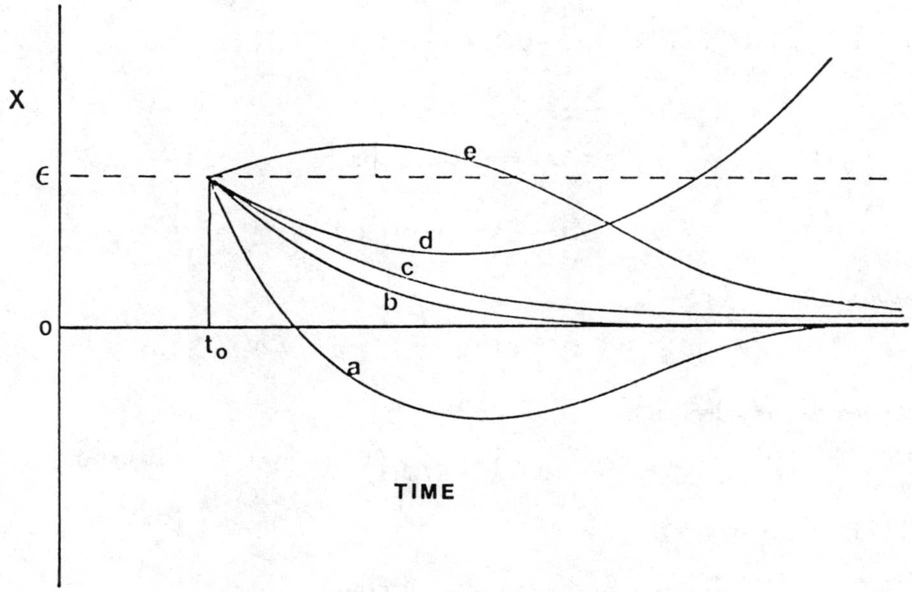

Figure 4 Response curves that illustrate the various types of stability. A system upset is introduced at time t_0. (a) Stable response; (b) asymptotic stability; (c) stable, but not asymptotically stable; (d) unstable response; (e) quasi-asymptotically stable.

$$\text{EEP} = \frac{d(\delta^2 S)}{dt} = \frac{1}{T}\Sigma\,\delta(A)\,\delta(r) \tag{103}$$

For a specific chemical reaction and the definition of affinity, A

$$Z + Y \rightarrow C + D$$

$$A = \log\left[\frac{ZY}{CD}\right] \tag{104}$$

We can write

$$\delta A = \delta \log\left[\frac{ZY}{CD}\right] = \frac{\delta Z}{Z} \tag{105}$$

and

$$\delta r = \delta ZY = Y\delta Z \tag{106}$$

The concentrations Y, C, and D are considered constants and for simplicity we will set the rate constants equal to unity. From (103) through (106) we can write

$$\text{EEP} = \frac{d(\delta^2 S)}{dt} \sim \frac{\delta Z}{Z} \cdot Y\delta Z \sim \frac{(\delta Z)^2}{Z} \tag{107}$$

Applying (107) to the metabolism of protein (leucine) we can write

$$\underset{\text{(leucine)}}{C_6H_{12}O_2N} + 7\frac{1}{2}O_2 \rightarrow 5\frac{1}{2}CO_2 + 5\frac{1}{2}H_2O + \frac{1}{2}\underset{\text{(urea)}}{CO(NH_2)} + 780\text{ cal} \tag{108}$$

$$r = KZY = K[\text{leucine}][O_2]^{7.5} \tag{109}$$

$$A = -\sum \nu_i \mu_i (\text{from (36)}) \tag{110}$$

and for (108)

$$A = \mu_{\text{leucine}} + 7 \cdot 5\mu_{O_2} - 5 \cdot 5\mu_{CO_2} - 5 \cdot 5\mu_{H_2O} - 0 \cdot 5\mu_{\text{urea}} \tag{111}$$

Chemical potential, μ, is defined by

$$\mu = \mu^0 + RT \ln z \tag{112}$$

From (111) and (112) we get

$$\begin{aligned} A = {} & \mu^0_{\text{leucine}} + 7 \cdot 5\mu^0_{O_2} - 5 \cdot 5\mu^0_{CO_2} - 5 \cdot 5\mu^0_{H_2O} - 0 \cdot 5\mu^0_{\text{urea}} \\ & + RT \left\{[\text{leucine}][O_2]^{5.5} / [CO_2]^{5.5} [H_2O]^{5.5} [\text{urea}]^{0.5}\right\} \end{aligned} \tag{113}$$

which yields

$$\delta A = RT\,\delta \left\{ \frac{[\text{leucine}][O_2]^{7.5}}{[CO_2]^{5.5}[H_2O]^{5.5}[\text{urea}]^{0.5}} \right\} \tag{114}$$

and from (109)

$$\delta r = K\delta[\text{leucine}][O_2]^{7.5} \tag{115}$$

where δ defines the perturbation from a reference, minimum state (equilibrium). Focusing only on fluctuations in protein (leucine) metabolism, from (114) and (115) we get

$$\begin{aligned} \delta r\,\delta A & \cong \delta[\text{leucine}]\,\delta \ln[\text{leucine}] \\ & \cong \delta[\text{leucine}] \cdot \delta \frac{[\text{leucine}]}{[\text{leucine}]} \\ & \cong \frac{(\delta[\text{leucine}])^2}{[\text{leucine}]} \end{aligned} \tag{116}$$

From (103), (107), and (116), we get

$$\text{EEP} = \frac{d(\delta^2 S)}{dt} \cong \frac{(\delta[\text{leucine}])^2}{[\text{leucine}]} \tag{117}$$

or, in general,

$$\text{EEP} = \frac{d(\delta^2 S)}{dt} = \frac{(\delta[\text{protein}])^2}{[\text{protein}]} \quad (118)$$

where

$$\delta[\text{protein}] = \begin{matrix}\text{Daily protein}\\ \text{consumption, g/d}\end{matrix} - \begin{matrix}\text{Minimum protein}\\ \text{requirement, g/d}\end{matrix} \quad (119)$$

or

$$\delta[\text{protein}] = [\text{protein}] - 56 \quad (120)$$

where 56 g/d is the minimum protein requirement to sustain life, obtained from data on elderly males in the vicinity of death. Replace 56 by 48 when working with females. It is apparent from (118) that EEP is always positive and approaches zero in the vicinity of death because [protein] approaches 56.

E. CALCULATION OF EXCESS ENTROPY

From (118)

$$\text{EEP} = \frac{\text{d}(\delta^2 S)}{dt} = \frac{(\delta[\text{protein}])^2}{[\text{protein}]} \quad (121)$$

or from (83)

$$\text{EE} = \delta^2 S = \int \text{EEP}\, dt + \text{constant} \quad (122)$$

If

$$\text{EEP} = mt + b \quad (123)$$

then,

$$\text{EE} = \frac{mt^2}{2} + bt + C \quad (124)$$

Because EE and EEP go to zero in the vicinity of death, then

$$\text{EE}\Big|_{t=t_{\text{death}}} = 0 = \frac{mt_{\text{death}}^2}{2} + bt_{\text{death}} + C$$

or, with $t_{\text{death}} = t_d$

$$C = -\frac{mt_d^2}{2} - bt_d \quad (125)$$

where m is the slope of the EEP line, b is the intercept of the EEP line, and t_d is death age, extrapolated from the EEP line, where EEP goes to zero. Thus, EE can be calculated from (124) with m, b, and

t_d determined from the EEP line, (123), and C obtained from (125). There are three patterns of EEP data, types I, II, and III.

1. Type I Behavior

The basic descriptive equation is

$$\mathrm{EEP_I} = m_\mathrm{I} t_\mathrm{I} + b_\mathrm{I} \tag{126}$$

from (123). At death, EEP = 0 and

$$t_d = -b_\mathrm{I} / m_\mathrm{I} \tag{127}$$

From (125)

$$C_\mathrm{I} = -\frac{m_\mathrm{I} t_d^2}{2} - b_\mathrm{I} t_d \tag{128}$$

and from (124)

$$\mathrm{EE_I} = \frac{m_\mathrm{I} t_\mathrm{I}^2}{2} + b_\mathrm{I} t_\mathrm{I} + C_\mathrm{I} \tag{129}$$

2. Type II Behavior

The basic equations are

$$\mathrm{EEP_{II}} = m_\mathrm{II}\, t_\mathrm{II} + b_\mathrm{II} \tag{130}$$

and

$$\mathrm{EE_{II}} = \frac{m_\mathrm{II} t_\mathrm{II}^2}{2} + b_\mathrm{II} t_\mathrm{II} + C_\mathrm{II} \tag{131}$$

At $t_\text{I-II}$

$$\mathrm{EE}\Big|_{t_\text{I-II}} = \text{ obtained from } (5-52)\Big|_{t_\text{I-II}} \tag{132}$$

In track II, $\mathrm{EEP_{II}}$ is calculated from (118), (119), and (130) with m_II and b_II known. Then, C_II is calculated from (131) and (132) at $t_\text{I-II}$. Now, calculate the $\mathrm{EE_{II}}$ track from (131) for $t > t_\text{I-II}$. If EE becomes zero during the type II track, we can find the death age $t_{d\mathrm{II}}$.

3. Type III Behavior

The basic equations are

$$\mathrm{EEP_{III}} = m_\mathrm{III}\, t_\mathrm{III} + b_\mathrm{III} \tag{133}$$

and

$$\mathrm{EE_{III}} = \frac{m_\mathrm{III} t_\mathrm{III}^2}{2} + b_\mathrm{III}\, t_\mathrm{III} + C_\mathrm{III} \tag{134}$$

At $t_{II\text{-}III}$, $EE|_{t_{II\text{-}III}}$ is obtained from (131), and with

$$EE_{II}\Big|_{t_{II\text{-}III}} = EE_{III}\Big|_{t_{II\text{-}III}} \tag{135}$$

EEP_{III} is calculated, and from (133) we can determine m_{III} and b_{III}. From (134), at $t_{II\text{-}III}$, we can calculate C_{III}, using (135). Finally, calculate EE_{III} from (134) for $t > t_{II\text{-}III}$.

F. SUMMARIZING THE EXCESS ENTROPY PRODUCTION AND EXCESS ENTROPY THEORIES OF AGING

In Figure 3, we can see that the EEP track declines steadily with age, in a straight line, ending at zero when the age of about 85 has been attained. For these pooled data,[8] a life span track projects an expected life span of about 85 years for the average male.

Using the same pooled data, the standard EE track constructed in Figure 2 goes to zero, around age 85, as expected. EEP and EE tracks for types I, II, and III individual subjects are represented in Figures 5, 6, and 7. The life span projections for these three subjects are 89 (82, actual, type I), 76 (74, actual, type II), and 89 (92, actual, type III). Our life span predictions for other subjects, based on EEP and EE tracking, are given in Table 2. In summary form, as shown in Table 3, we can see that the EEP track tends to give predictions that are slightly higher than the actual life span (by 3.1 years), while the EE method yields on average predictions less than the actual life span (by 2.6 years). The EEP method is applicable for types I and III. The EE method is most useful for types II and III.

Another way of characterizing the accuracy of the EEP and EE life span predictions is given in Tables 4 and 5. The data show that about 16% of the EEP predictions were within 1 year of the actual life span (8% for EE), 23% of the EEP predictions were accurate within 2 years (21% for EE), 48% within 4 years (37% for EE), and 74% within 7 years (63% for EE).

The EEP and EE theories of longevity tracking yields the following:

1. EEP is positive and decreasing (type I).
2. A stress period can be identified as a time of sustained, increasing EEP (type II). A killing stress is one in which death occurs while in the stress period. A survivable stress is defined by the resumption of a normal, decreasing EEP history after the stress period (type III).
3. Death is impending when the EEP track approaches zero.
4. EE is negative.
5. EE ascends to zero in the vicinity of death.
6. Stability describes the living state. Instability implies death (maximum disorder). Type III behavior implies a stable response to an upset (stress) because the upset is survived and the downward EEP evolution is reestablished. For type II subjects, the upset is severe enough to force the subject from stability (life) to instability (death). Instability is introduced when EE becomes positive.

VI. EXCESS ENTROPY PRODUCTION AND EXCESS ENTROPY TRACK AS MEDICAL DIAGNOSTIC TOOLS

The EEP track parallels the BMR, which also decreases with age. A variety of physiological and pathological factors are known to cause increases in the BMR and hence the EEP. Some of these factors were listed in Table 1. For example, severe hyperthyroidism can increase the BMR by as much as 100%. Gump[4] has recently suggested that BMR measurements may be useful in the treatment of patients who

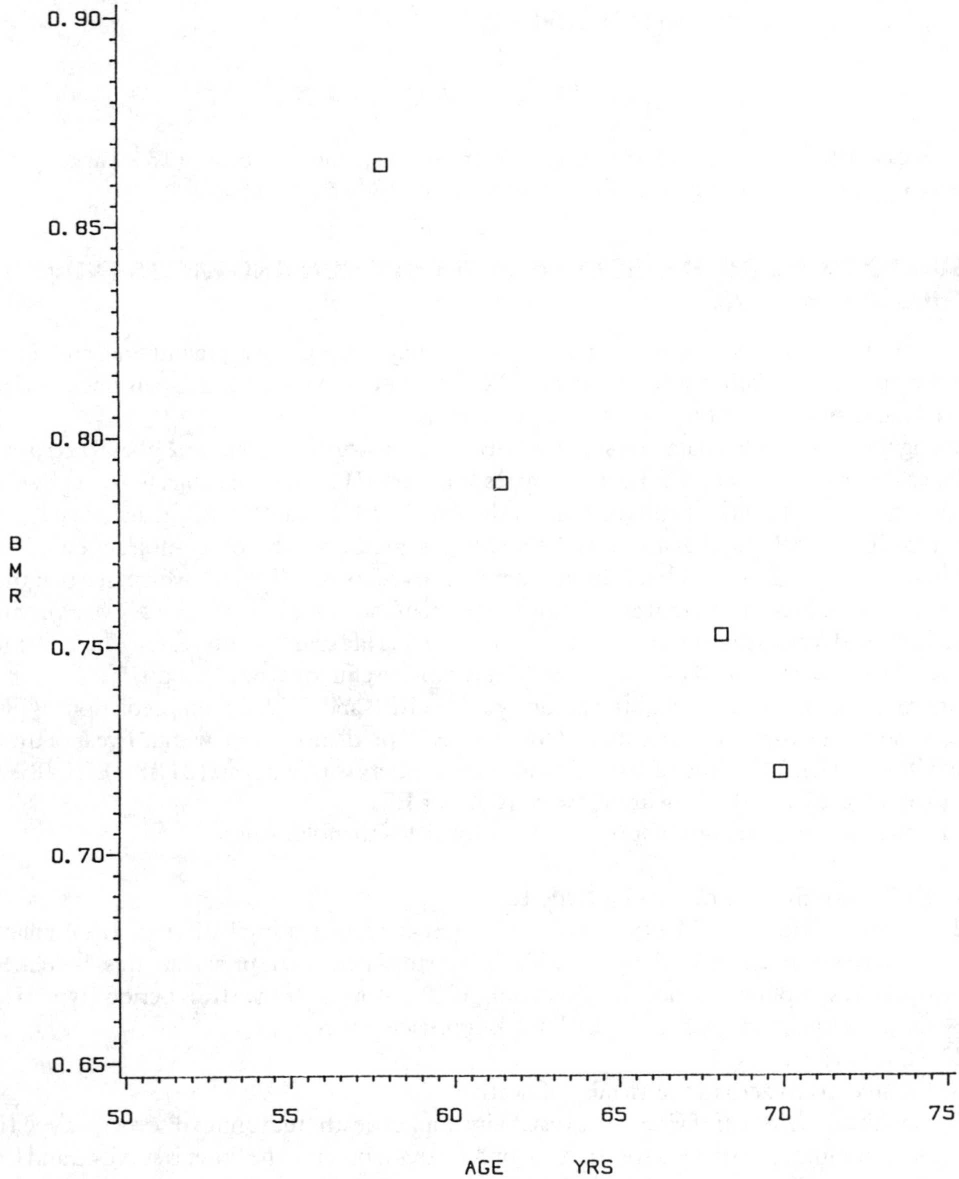

Figure 5 An example of a type I subject.

received serious injury. However, this is an after the fact application. Of more interest is the suggestion that the BMR (and hence EEP) measurements may be useful in the diagnosis of a variety of conditions.

Of particular interest is cancer. Warnold et al.[14] recorded an increase in the metabolic rate of cancer patients. We should, therefore, see an analogous EEP rise (type II behavior). Also, we should find that the magnitude of the increase in BMR and EEP is related to the degree of advancement of the cancer. If the onset of cancer causes an observable rise in EEP, then establishing an EEP track could assist in the diagnosis of the abnormality. This should also be true for other major illnesses. An observed EEP rise (type II) would imply that a potential problem exists. It would then be the responsibility of the patient's physician to determine if in fact this is true and if so, proceed to treat the ailment. If the treatment is effective, it should be possible to flag this by noting the resumption of the downward track of the EEP (type III).

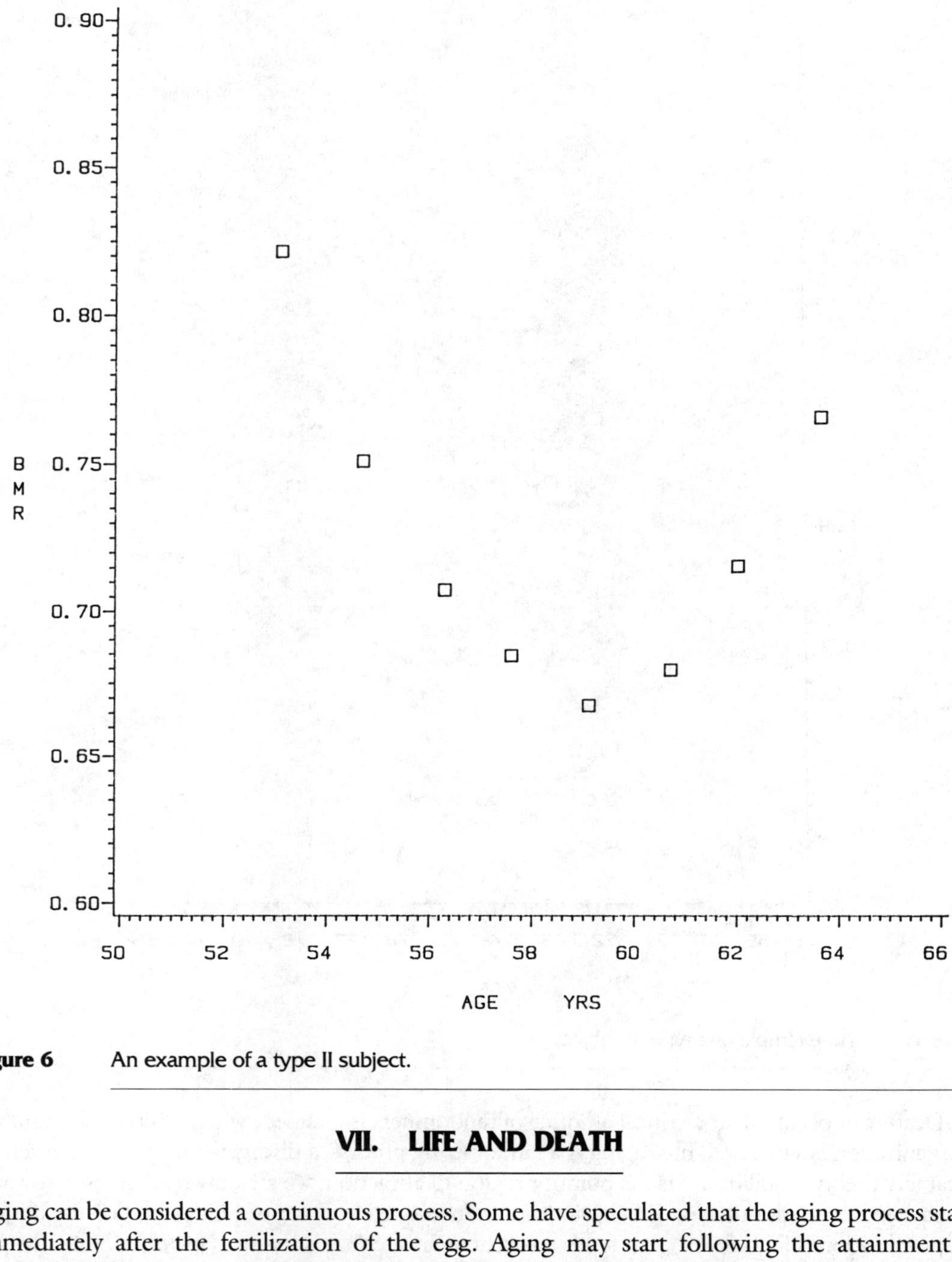

Figure 6 An example of a type II subject.

VII. LIFE AND DEATH

Aging can be considered a continuous process. Some have speculated that the aging process starts immediately after the fertilization of the egg. Aging may start following the attainment of adulthood, after the periods of childhood and adolescence, which are times marked by rapid growth and major body changes. Beyond these phases of life the BMR and EEP steadily decrease with age; the body is slowing down.

Aging may be the evolution toward a more probable state, the equilibrium state. As the body ages (returns to equilibrium) the EE driving force weakens or diminishes. Schrodinger[12] wrote, "Living systems survive by avoiding the rapid decay into the inert state of equilibrium." Jones[7] proposed that "The approach to equilibrium is a sign of death. Death may also be thought of as the attaining of a critical, maximum state of entropy during our journey towards equilibrium." Schrodinger[12] further stated, "Thus a living organism continually increases its entropy... and tends to approach the dangerous state of maximum entropy, which is death."

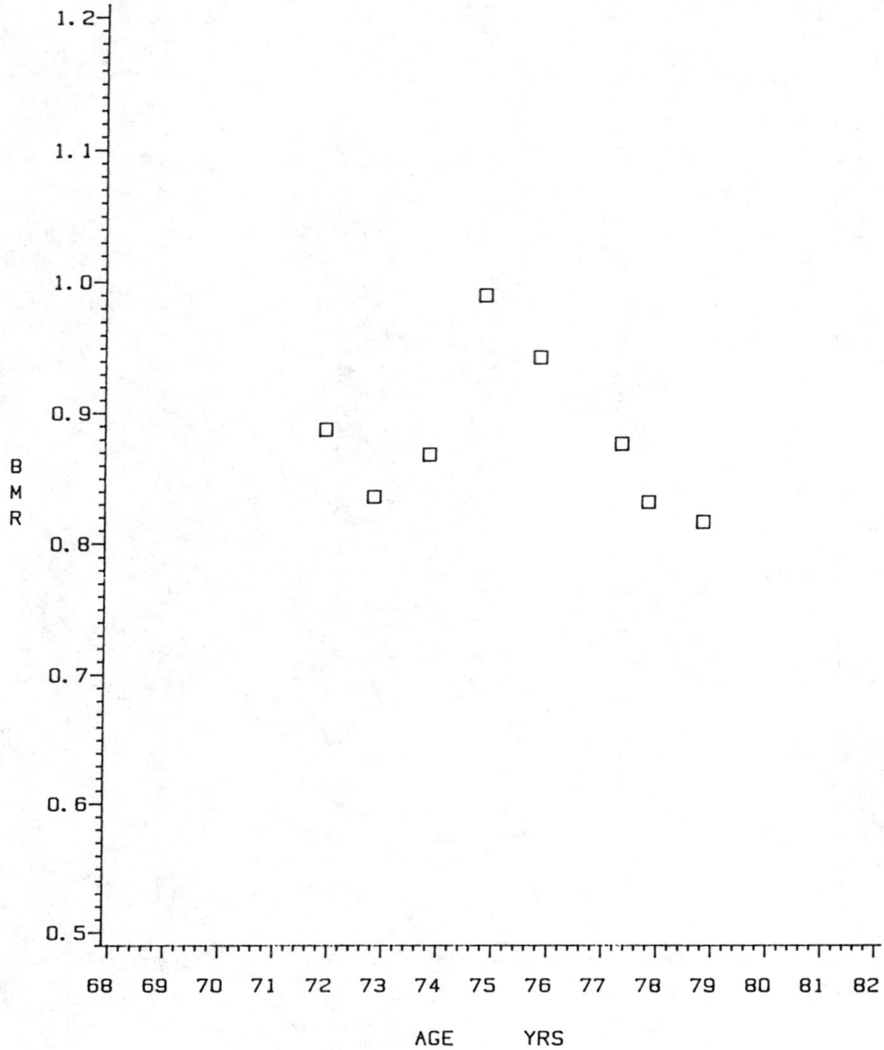

Figure 7 An example of a type III subject.

Death can occur when a critical amount of randomness is attained, when a certain amount of disorganization is suffered. Thus, aging is a randomizing process, a disorganizing process. In terms of stability theory, equilibrium is the point or region of attraction; we are drawn relentlessly toward equilibrium. Death during type II behavior can be envisioned as a catastrophic event because it is an abrupt transition (life to death) that tends to occur at an age that is less than expected. Life may be considered analogous to the spring-wound watch, where the timepiece may stop by one of two possible mechanisms. It can simply wind down (approach equilibrium). This is the watch's version of type I death. The second mechanism is that the internal machinery can somehow fail and the watch "dies" prematurely. This is equivalent to type II death. (Because this is not a self-repairing system, a type III track is probably not possible.) Thus, type I and III deaths can be described as equilibrium deaths, and type II as instability or catastrophic death.

Life may be considered a temporary upset from or perturbation of equilibrium. Equilibrium is absolutely stable, a universal attractor. Equilibrium always wins, as does death. Aging is a spontaneous process, where the body dissipates its EE. The various theories of aging (cross-linking, wear and tear,

Table 2 Summary of the life span predictions based on the EE and EEP methods

Subject no.	Actual life span (years)	Curve type	Pred. life span Hershey-Wang finite pot.	Pred. life span EE production	Pred. life span EE
26	76	2	109.4	—	74.2
31	85	3	97.7	85.7	80.8
36	80	3	84.0	87.8	77.0
51	76	3	79.8	83.8	72.9
53	92	3	97.5	88.5	83.2
69	74	2	91.0	—	76.3
74	79	3	101.1	78.1	—
77	84	3	92.4	83.0	72.7
78	91	3	92.8	90.2	90.5
79	72	2	93.6	—	72.2
81	84	3	92.4	89.2	77.5
82	82	3	97.6	90.0	76.6
92	78	2	74.1	—	73.8
96	64	2	107.5	—	61.1
99	82	1	93.5	88.8	89.0
102	77	1	100.9	79.4	79.0
103	88	1	95.9	103.0	97.3
104	96	3	110.4	92.7	86.6
105	73	3	86.9	84.5	76.1
106	86	3	92.0	82.9	71.8
107	90	3	105.3	88.5	84.9
113	78	1	100.6	86.4	86.0
114	73	2	94.9	—	71.4
117	84	1	100.8	86.4	86.0
120	79	3	103.5	85.4	87.4
121	92	3	104.0	97.5	78.8
127	81	3	81.8	86.5	76.5
128	69	2	86.9	—	70.4
133	95	3	84.5	91.9	86.1
158	58	1	120.1	67.6	68.4
162	69	3	79.3	64.1	59.3
163	85	3	94.3	89.9	76.6
176	69	3	90.4	73.7	64.4
200	79	3	98.8	77.9	72.1
204	79	3	78.2	75.1	75.8
207	84	3	90.7	84.3	75.1
208	78	3	95.2	80.3	77.5
213	74	3	88.8	81.9	81.1
244	76	2	97.3	—	65.6

Table 3 Summary statistics on the accuracy of the life span predictions[a]

	Mean	Standard deviation
Type I subjects ($n = 6$)		
EE	6.5	3.6
EEP	7.4	4.8
Type II subjects ($n = 8$)		
EE	−2.1	4.0
EEP	—[b]	—
Type III subjects ($n = 25$)		
EE	−5.1	5.7
EEP	2.1	4.7
All subjects subjects ($n = 39$)		
EE	−2.6	6.5
EEP	3.1	5.1

[a] *Accuracy = predicted life span − actual life span.*
[b] *EEP calculations cannot be done on type II subjects.*

Table 4 More detailed statistical analysis of the accuracy of the EEP method

Accuracy	Frequency	Cumulative frequency	Percent	Cumulative percent
Within 1 year	5	5	16.13	16.13
1–2 years	2	7	6.45	22.58
2–3 years	3	10	9.68	32.26
3–4 years	5	15	16.13	48.39
4–5 years	3	18	9.68	58.06
5–7.5 years	5	23	16.13	74.19
7.5–10 years	6	29	19.35	93.55
10–15 years	2	31	6.45	100.00

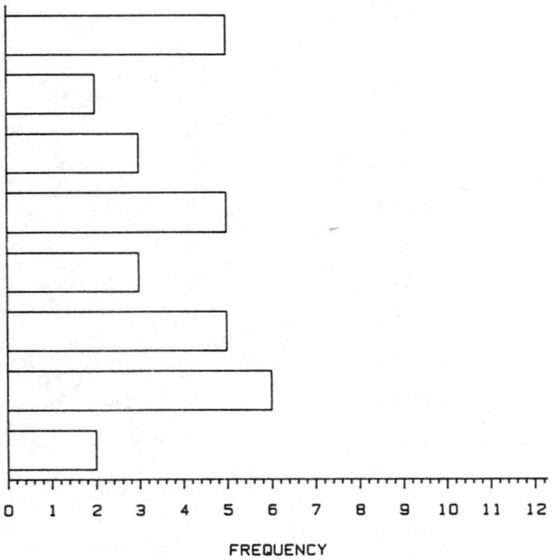

free radical, etc.) all imply a declining metabolic rate with age, and by extension, a diminishing EE and EEP. Evolution may be the natural process of prolonging the time that an organism spends in the far from equilibrium state. Genetics still plays its role in determining longevity potential, but is not in conflict with the ideas presented here. The tendency to return to equilibrium will always be expressed; the entropy laws will always apply. Death will always have a probability of absolute certainty.

Table 5 More detailed statistical analysis of the accuracy of the EE method

Accuracy	Frequency	Cumulative frequency	Percent	Cumulative percent
Within 1 year	3	3	7.89	7.89
1–2 years	5	8	13.16	21.05
2–3 years	3	11	7.89	28.95
3–4 years	3	14	7.89	36.84
4–5 years	4	18	10.53	47.37
5–7.5 years	6	24	15.79	63.16
7.5–10 years	9	33	23.68	86.84
10–15 years	5	38	13.16	100.00

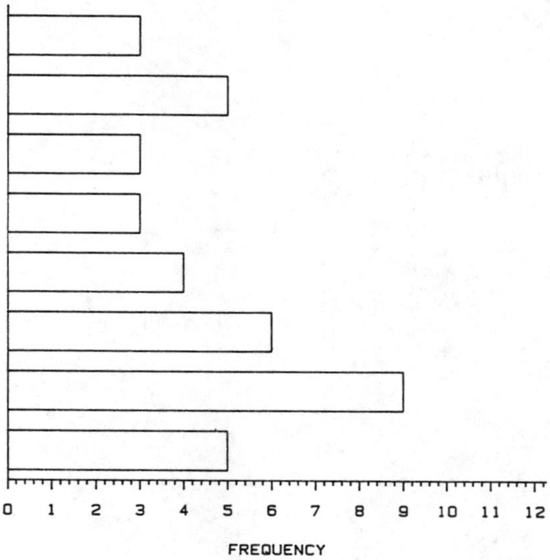

REFERENCES

1. Bailey, K.D., Equilibrium, entropy, and homeostasis: a multidisciplinary legacy, *Syst. Res.,* 1, 25, 1984.
2. Balmer, R.T., Entropy and aging in biological systems, *Eng. Commun.,* 17, 171, 1982.
3. Fast, J.D., *Entropy,* Gordon & Breach, New York, 1968.
4. Gump, F.E., Whole body metabolism, in *Handbook of Shock and Trauma,* Vol. 1, *Basic Sciences,* Altura, S. M. et al., Eds., Raven Press, New York, 1983, 241.
5. Hershey, D. and Wang, H.H., *A New Age-Scale for Humans,* Lexington Books, Lexington, MA, 1980.
6. Hershey, D. and Lee, W.E., III, Entropy, aging and death, *Syst. Res.,* 4, 269, 1987.
7. Jones, D.D., Entropic models in biology: the next scientific revolution?, *Persp. Biol. Med.,* 20, 285, 1977.
8. Lee, W.E., III, Analysis to Understand the Thermodynamics of Living Aging Systems, Ph.D. dissertation, University of Cincinnati, Cincinnati, 1984.
9. Lee, W.E., III and Hershey, D., The utilization of BMR measurements as a routine diagnostic procedure in normal health maintenance, *Med. Hypoth.,* 16, 147, 1985.
10. Nicolis, G. and Prigogine, I., *Self-Organization in Non-Equilibrium Systems,* John Wiley & Sons, New York, 1977.
11. Prigogine, I., *Introduction to Thermodynamics of Irreversible Processes,* Charles C Thomas, Springfield, IL, 1955.
12. Schrodinger, E., *What is Life? The Physical Aspects of the Living Cell,* Cambridge University Press, Cambridge, U.K., 1955.
13. Von Bertalanffy, L., The theory of open systems in physics and biology, *Science,* 111, 23, 1950.
14. Warnold, I., Lundholm, K., and Schersten, T., Energy balance and body composition in cancer patients, *Cancer Res.,* 38, 1801, 1978.
15. Zotin, A.I., *Thermodynamics of Biological Processes,* Walter de Gruyter, Berlin, 1978.

CHAPTER 15

QUANTITATIVE MEASUREMENT OF HUMAN PHYSIOLOGICAL AGE BY PROFILING OF BODY FLUIDS AND PATTERN RECOGNITION

Arthur B. Robinson and Laurelee R. Robinson*

TABLE OF CONTENTS

I. INTRODUCTION

There are many hypotheses regarding the primary cause of the observed intrinsic life span of organisms.[1-10] It is to be expected that the eventual resolution of this unsolved problem in molecular biology will lead to methods of altering the primary causes of aging and thereby the life span of organisms, including humans.

These alterations may be expected to be of the two types illustrated in Figures 1 through 3.[11] First, the death rate of humans during the years much earlier than their intrinsic life span will be reduced. Second, the intrinsic life span itself will be increased.

It should, however, be possible to extend human life spans by means of empirical experimentation even prior to the advent of a thorough understanding of the molecular biology of human aging. Observations of animals and humans suggest that substantial progress of the type illustrated in Figure 2 and modest progress of the type illustrated in Figure 3 should be possible.

The principal impediment to this empirical progress is the fact that the humans carrying out the experiments have life spans of comparable length to those of the human subjects whom they are studying. If carried to completion, a single rigorous experiment on human life span as a function of, for example, diet or environment could require as much as 50 to 80 years. Even if this is reduced to 10 to 20 years by clever experimental design, a complete series of experiments will still proceed too slowly to be of benefit to humans who are now living. In the absence of real progress and as a result of the understandably high human interest in this subject, many sensible but unproved aging hypotheses have given rise to fads and cults, especially as pertain to diet.

* Laurelee Robinson died on November 12, 1988. She saw and approved all of the figures and tables in this chapter, but did not read the final manuscript.

0-8493-0129-7/94/$0.00+$.50

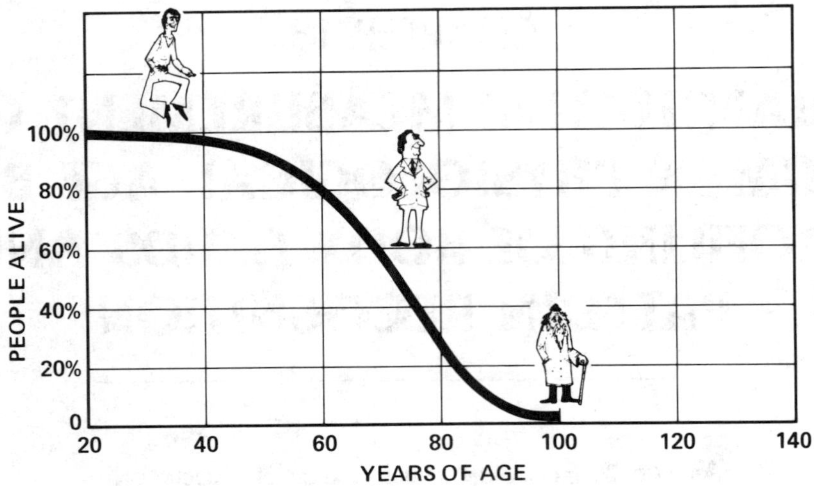

Figure 1 Aging curve for a population comprised of American males as calculated from life expectancy compilations of the U.S. Public Health Service. (From Robinson, A.B., *Mech. Age. Dev.*, 9, 225, 1979. With permission.)

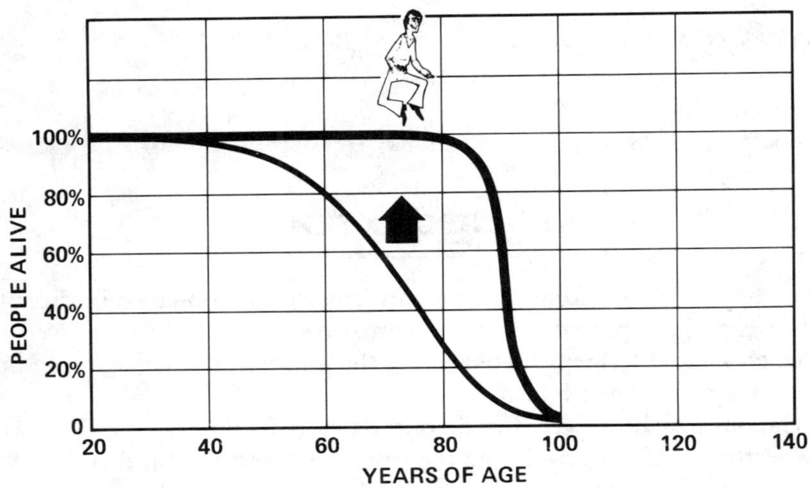

Figure 2 Example of a change in the human aging curve through improvements in diet and other living conditions, but with no change in intrinsic life span. (From Robinson, A.B., *Mech. Age. Dev.*, 9, 225, 1979. With permission.).

The impediment to human aging research of long experiment times would be removed if an objective and quantitative means for determining human physiological age with reasonable accuracy could be developed. This would allow empirical experiments on aging rate to be carried out with experiment times in groups of humans of a few months per experiment or less.

Moreover, quantitative analysis of human age would allow the monitoring of the rate of aging in single individuals, so that biochemical individuality and individuality of particular environmental circumstances could be taken into account in devising conditions that minimize the rate of aging in each individual.

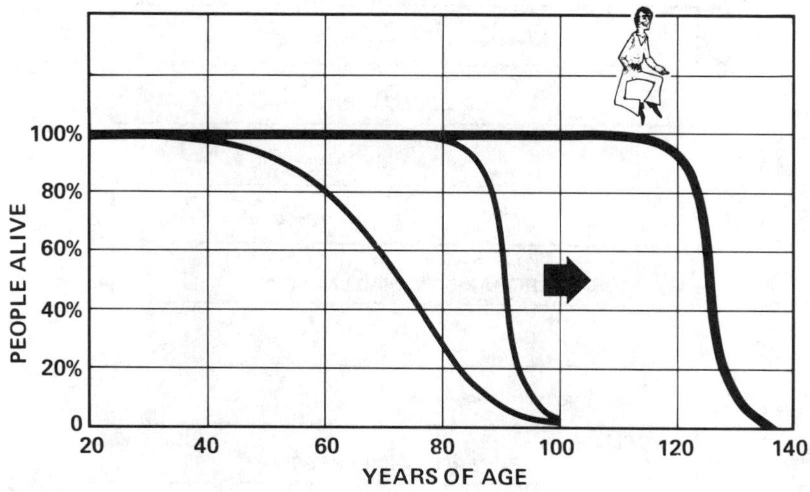

Figure 3 Example of a change in the human aging curve through improvements in diet and other living conditions and through an increase in the intrinsic life span. (From Robinson, A.B., *Mech. Age. Dev.*, 9, 225, 1979. With permission.).

The authors have long been interested in the development of a procedure for the quantitative measurement of human physiological age.[11-14] This interest has been a part of our general interest in the quantitative measurement of human health, especially with respect to degenerative disease. If by means of inexpensive quantitative analysis the state of each person could be determined on quantitative axes, as illustrated in Figure 4, then their productive and actual life spans could be extended; their illnesses could be more effectively cured; and their health could be guarded by preventive measures that combat the probability of disease rather than disease itself.

It is an essential obligation of scientists to do all that they can to optimize the quality of all human life. This optimization requires, in part, the minimization of disease and the maximization of life span for the entire human population. Techniques of the sort illustrated in Figure 5 and discussed below have substantial potential to meet these parts of that obligation.

The authors have limited themselves to those techniques that have potential, in mass application, to quantitatively measure the amounts of a large number of substances in human body fluids at a cost of about $20 or less for an entire analysis including its computerized interpretation. This limitation assures that the techniques developed will be available to most people rather than a wealthy few. Having measured within this restriction as many parameters as possible, we then have attempted to extract as much information from these measurements as possible by simple computerized pattern recognition techniques.

This is a departure from the usual approach of developing observational techniques for those substances thought to be of importance to a particular hypothesis or theory. Fundamental science is more entertaining. In work on deamidation and molecular clocks,[10,11,20] the authors have enjoyed this as well. In fact, an added benefit of the profiling work has been the discovery of a few correlations which happen by chance to be relevant to basic research. Nevertheless, choice of substances by economics and simplicity of analysis rather than by hypothesis is an essential part of rapid progress in the practical profiling of human health.

The authors' work has comprised the use of ion exchange chromatography (IEC), gas-liquid chromatography (GLC), and direct mass spectrometry (MS), including chemical ionization and field ion mass spectrometry (FIMS; without chromatographic separation), of samples

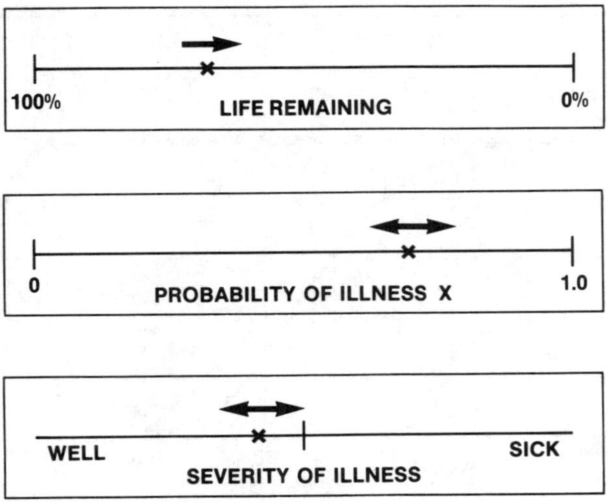

Figure 4 Representative axes of physiological age, probability of a specific illness, and the severity of a specific illness. It is the quantitative determination of the positions on these axes of specific individual humans, by means that are low in cost and generally applicable to all well individuals at frequent intervals, that is the goal of the authors' work on the physiological profiling of human body fluids.

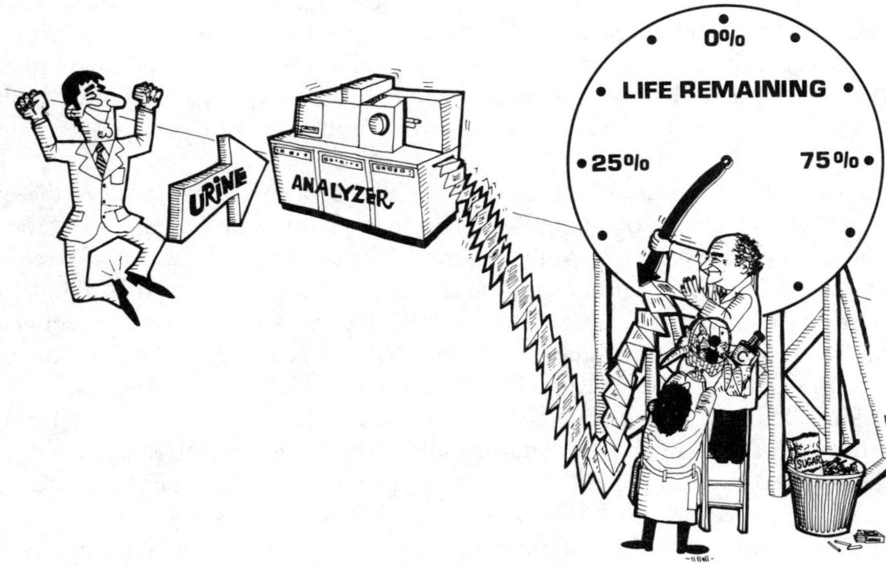

Figure 5 One aspect of the optimization of the quality of human life.

of urine, blood, and breath from humans and mice. Some work has also been carried out on the whole body compositions of fruit flies.[12]

For the most part, however, this work has been restricted to humans. Because this approach is empirical in nature and has an immediate practical objective, the authors prefer to avoid extrapolations between animals and humans in the interpretations of results. In a highly automated laboratory,[15] about 20,000 analyses of human body fluids, including the quantitative analysis of over 2 million amounts of substances, have been carried out by us and under our supervision.[12,13,15,16] The primary focus of this work has been on states of disease. A small part was devoted to the measurement of organismic age[12,14] in mice and fruit flies. We report herein a few experiments that were carried out to test the measurement of chronological and physiological age in humans by urinalysis.

II. URINALYSIS

Figures 6 and 7 illustrate the analytical techniques used in these urinalysis experiments. Graphs of this sort were not used in the experiments, however. The detector voltages as a function of time from the analytical machines were sampled by multiplex, collected on magnetic tape, and transferred to a calculation computer. There, by means of automatic computer programs that we developed, a baseline was fitted and subtracted; the peaks were integrated; retention time variation was eliminated and the peaks were matched within the entire experimental set; the peak areas were normalized in order to remove systematic variations in kidney function or water elimination; the experiments were evaluated by nonparametric statistics and by diagnostic power calculations; the diagrams shown in Figures 8, 9, and 13 through 17 were automatically drawn; and the values given in Tables 1 and 2 were automatically calculated. "Diagnostic powers", D_A, were calculated according to the method of Robinson and Westall[17] and the "diagnostic coefficients", R_A, were calculated as described in Reference 14.

Casual urine samples and chronological ages of 205 men were obtained from Dr. A. Cherkin of the Veterans Administration hospital in Sepulvida, CA. In addition, casual urines for 30 men were obtained from the same source wherein the ages of individuals were kept at Sepulvida and not communicated to us until after the calculations shown in Table 3 had been completed. Casual urine without dietary or other controls was used, so that the results would reflect those to be expected from mass, simple sampling of the population at large. One sex was used because our earlier experiments had shown strong sex-dependent patterns in humans which were not the subject of these experiments.

A staggered alternation procedure for order of analysis of these samples was used to avoid possible systematic errors from machine drift. In addition, extensive experience with the analytical techniques assured their stability and reliability. Urinary amines, amides, and amino acids were determined by application of urine directly to the high pressure liquid chromatography (HPLC) column of an automated Durrum amino acid analyzer with a ninhydrin detector. Volatile urine compounds were analyzed as described in Reference 15.

After integration and peak matching a unique normalization procedure was applied to the peak areas. Each peak area was normalized by division by the sum of most of the matched peak areas in its individual chromatogram. Peaks with large areas were weighted less so as not to dominate the normalization. In this way systematic variations in kidney function and water excretion are far more effectively eliminated than with the usual procedures of timed samples or normalization to creatinine or other single substances.

The authors previously developed a graphical method for determination of the existence and extent of patterns that distinguish paired sets of samples. This method was used in these aging experiments. First, the nonparametric probability, *P*, of the null hypothesis that there is no quantitative difference between the young and old groups was calculated by means of a two-tailed Wilcoxon test[18] for each substance. The Wilcoxon test statistic was assumed to be asymptotically normal, corrected for ties and by a continuity correction of 0.5, according to Verdooren and Lehman, and corrected by the first term of the Fix and Hodges correction. All of the statistical and experimental procedures were selected so that any errors in the estimated values of *P* would always tend to make these values higher and too pessimistic rather than lower

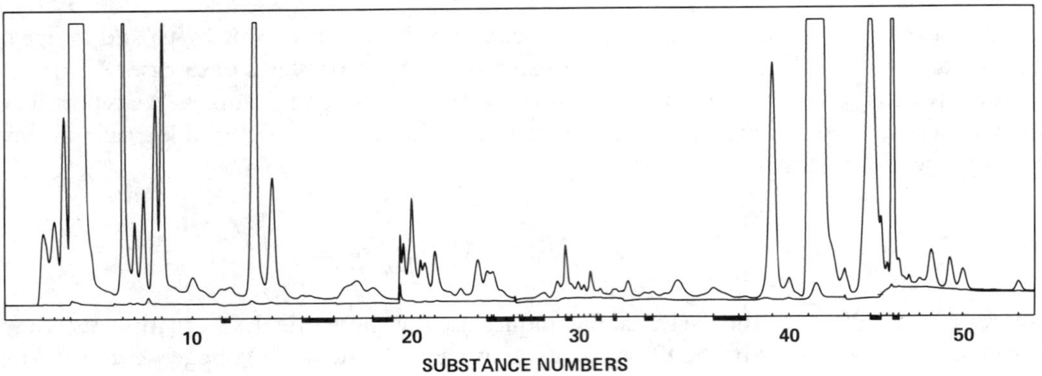

Figure 6 An example chromatogram of the amines, amides, and amino acids in human urine as used in these experiments. The baseline is computer drawn. The darkened strips along the bottom axis show peaks which the computerized procedure has decided to combine for computational analysis.

and too optimistic. Second, the cumulative distribution functions of these calculated values of *P* were plotted as shown in Figures 8 and 9. For the purposes of this calculation the men were divided into two age groups as shown in Figure 10.

If no aging pattern existed, the values of *P* would fall on the straight diagonal line shown in the figures. This has been the case in some other types of experiments we have performed. In the case of age, however, these values show a very strong pattern. The asymptotes of the curved data lines indicate that about 30 urine amines, amides, and amino acids and about 30 urine volatile compounds show such strong age correlation that they can be experimentally demonstrated with fewer than 40 men in each group.

These age correlations are shown in Tables 1 and 2. These tables give the substance identity where known, the direction of the correlation, (P_{AGE}), expected and found numbers of substances at various values of *P*, normalized area, and age diagnostic powers (DP_{AGE}) for each substance. The values of DP_{AGE} were calculated as described in Reference 17 and illustrated in Figures 13 through 17. DP_{AGE} is underestimated in these groups because the overlap in life expectancies makes a perfect separation improbable. For this reason a corrected value, DP_C, was also calculated as shown in Figures 13 through 17.

Figure 10 shows linear regression lines for the 15 most strongly age diagnostic substances. Of these 15 substances, 7 decrease with age, while 8 of them increase with age. The diagnostic strength of these correlations is not only a function of age dependence, but also a function of contributions to the substance distribution functions from diet and the many other uncontrolled variables in this real-world sampling. A substance may be very strongly age dependent and yet have a low diagnostic power because its distribution function is broadened by other variables. Also, some of the chromatogram peaks contain two or more substances in comparable amounts, which usually weakens their correlations.

Life expectancy distribution functions for the two groups of men of known ages are shown in Figure 11. These were calculated from U.S. Public Health Service statistics as applied to the age of each individual. The expectation values of the years of remaining life were then used to construct Figure 11. Figure 12 shows, for example, a graph of the fourth most diagnostic peak as a function of years of remaining life for these men.

The two curves in Figure 11 overlap significantly. We are measuring physiological parameters which are expected to correlate best with physiological age rather than chronological age, and we have only chronological ages available for the human subjects of the experiment.

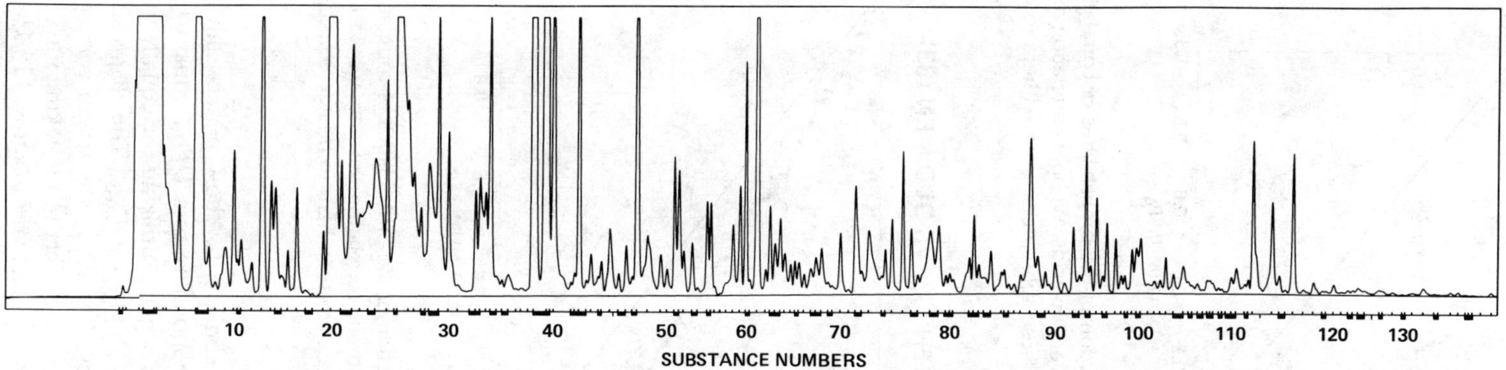

Figure 7 An example chromatogram of the volatile compounds in human urine as used in these experiments. This analytical technique is described in detail in Reference 15. The baseline is computer drawn. The darkened strips along the bottom axis show peaks which the computerized procedure has decided to combine for computational analysis.

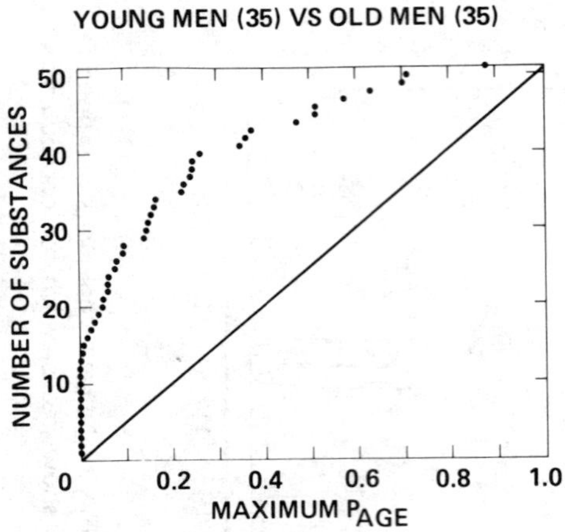

Figure 8 Cumulative distribution function of the probabilities of correlation with human age of 51 urinary amines, amides, and amino acids. Without correlation the dots would fall along the diagonal line. About 30 of these substances are seen here to be age correlated.

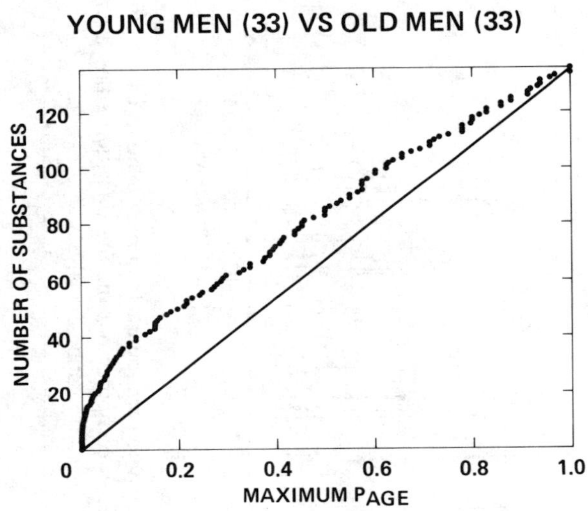

Figure 9 Cumulative distribution function of the probabilities of correlation with human age of 135 urine vapor substances. Without correlation the dots would fall along the diagonal line. About 30 of these substances are seen here to be age correlated.

Therefore, we cannot expect this technique to show perfect chronological age separation between the two groups of men corresponding to a DP_{AGE} equal to 1.00.

Figure 13 shows a diagnostic power graph utilizing the equally weighted five urine amines that decrease with age and show the highest DP_{AGE}. The diagonal straight line is the line expected with uncorrelated substances. A point in the origin corresponds to DP_{AGE} equal to 1.00. The smooth, curved line represents a perfect result, taking into account the overlap of the distribution functions of life expectancy as shown in Figure 11. The stepped function is the experimental result. DP and DP_C are the fractions of separation achieved experimentally compared to a point in the origin and to the curved line, respectively.

The computerized calculation determines R_{AGE}[14] for each sample and thereby places each individual on a linear axis between young and old patterns. It then separates the individuals at all possible points along this axis and tabulates and graphs the errors as shown. To avoid bias, the average patterns were recalculated for each individual excluding that individual from the averages. Where two experiments are available (as in the blind experiment described below and in Table 3), none of the test samples are included in the average patterns.

The series of Figures 13 through 17 shows the gradual increase of reliability of this technique as more substances are added to the calculation. The five decreasing amines have DP_C of 0.69 (Figure 13). This is increased to 0.91 when the seven increasing amines are included (Figure 15) and to 0.93 when the three most diagnostic urine vapor compounds are included (Figure 17). Figures 14 and 16 show DP_C for the increasing amines and for the urine vapor substances alone.

A pattern for aging was calculated for these 15 substances and evaluated by means of the diagnostic coefficient, R_{AGE}, as described in Reference 14. By this method the individuals can be positioned along a linear axis of the type illustrated in Figure 4. R_{AGE} values for the 66 men after separation into five groups with similar life expectancies are shown in Figure 18.

Finally, each of the 30 men whose ages had not been given to us were placed on the linear aging axis by means of their individual R_{AGE} as determined from urinalysis, the 15 substances, and calculations identical to those described above. The successful results of this blind experiment, along with the subsequently revealed ages of 15 of the men, are given in Table 3. These 15 included, according to Cherkin, the seven youngest and eight oldest members of the group of 30.

It must be emphasized that these are results from the analysis of substances picked only by ease of analysis, not by interest to aging researchers, and samples obtained casually from humans without special controls. Sample controls can narrow the distribution functions substantially as can sampling of genetically homogeneous populations and other precautions.

For example, in Figure 19[12] the R_{AGE} for six sets of 24 enzymatically digested *Drosophila melanogaster*, four each from each day of six consecutive 6-day periods, are given for only two correlations: the increase in glutamic acid and decrease in glutamine that occur with age. This experimental result is remarkably exact, but it is also of little immediate applicability to the quantitative measurement of physiological age in large populations of humans.

About 60 substances or about one third of the substances measured in these human experiments were found to be age correlated, but only 15 of these have been included in the calculations reported here. Inclusion of the next few most diagnostic substances has no significant effect on the results. Thereafter, the DP_{AGE} decreases when additional substances are included in the calculation. These additional substances include some independent age information, but their distribution functions also contain so much noise from other effects such as diet that they do not make a positive contribution to these calculations.

III. STANDARDIZED HUMAN SAMPLES

The principal limitation of these experiments and of advances in clinical chemistry in general is the lack of standardized human samples with which to test and calibrate the techniques.

Here, for example, the authors have used samples characterized as to chronological age, although our interest is in physiological age. We do not know of the existence anywhere of a set of human urine samples that have been carefully and quantitatively characterized as to the physiological age of the subjects.

The authors have previously proposed[11] that a national sample bank of human blood, urine, breath, and other tissues be established. This should be done by the sampling of about 50,000 healthy Americans at least at 6-month intervals with the samples stored at –76°C or lower in a bank of small freezers with appropriate equipment duplication and sample redundancy.

Table 1 Aging pattern for men as determined by 51 ninhydrin-positive urinary amines, amides, and amino acids

Substance no.	Standard substance with identical elution time	Higher group	p_{AGE}	No. substances expected with $p \leq p_{AGE}$	No. substances found with $p \leq p_{AGE}$	Av. normalized area for 35 young men	Av. normalized area for 35 old men	AGE diagnostic power
6	Aspartic acid	Old	$<10^{-8}$	$<10^{-6}$	1	4.78 ± 0.19	6.23 ± 0.16	0.68
1	Phosphoserine	Old	4.8×10^{-7}	0.000025	2	7.45 ± 0.27	9.44 ± 0.27	0.55
45	Histidine	Young	2.9×10^{-6}	0.00015	3	58.2 ± 1.8	43.6 ± 2.3	0.45
9	Asparagine + Glutamine	Young	4.1×10^{-6}	0.00021	4	40.0 ± 2.0	27.3 ± 1.6	0.47
8	Serine	Young	1.2×10^{-5}	0.00061	5	28.4 ± 2.1	19.5 ± 0.9	0.39
12	Glycine	Young	1.3×10^{-5}	0.00068	6	97.0 ± 7.4	59.2 ± 4.8	0.35
22	—	Old	2.2×10^{-5}	0.0011	7	3.16 ± 0.11	3.67 ± 0.11	0.47
7	Threonine	Young	2.4×10^{-5}	0.0012	8	15.43 ± 1.21	9.88 ± 0.62	0.41
5	Glutathione	Old	8.3×10^{-5}	0.0042	9	26.1 ± 0.9	30.2 ± 0.8	0.39
20	Methionine	Old	3.0×10^{-4}	0.015	10	6.65 ± 0.30	7.60 ± 0.21	0.28
19	Cystathione	Old	4.8×10^{-4}	0.025	11	2.82 ± 0.10	3.48 ± 0.17	0.18
24	—	Old	9.3×10^{-4}	0.047	12	1.50 ± 0.08	1.91 ± 0.10	0.24
28	—	Old	2.8×10^{-3}	0.14	13	1.74 ± 0.09	2.15 ± 0.11	0.10
18	—	Old	7.1×10^{-3}	0.36	14	1.43 ± 0.06	1.74 ± 0.08	—
10	—	Old	8.9×10^{-3}	0.45	15	4.69 ± 0.21	5.63 ± 0.32	—
34	—	Old	1.8×10^{-2}	0.90	16	1.58 ± 0.29	1.59 ± 0.10	—

44	—	Young	2.5×10^{-2}	1.3	17	1.64 ± 0.15	1.16 ± 0.12	—
30	—	Old	3.4×10^{-2}	1.7	18	1.16 ± 0.06	1.49 ± 0.09	—
36	—	Old	4.2×10^{-2}	2.1	19	1.47 ± 0.07	1.71 ± 0.11	—
16	Cystine	Old	5.1×10^{-2}	2.6	20	3.76 ± 0.21	4.66 ± 0.33	—
14	α-Aminobutyric acid	Young	5.2×10^{-2}	2.7	21	4.09 ± 0.11	3.63 ± 0.18	—
13	Alanine	Young	6.3×10^{-2}	3.2	22	28.2 ± 1.7	24.9 ± 2.2	—
42	Lysine	Young	6.3×10^{-2}	3.2	23	10.49 ± 1.19	8.43 ± 1.03	—
2	Phosphoethanolamine	Old	6.5×10^{-2}	3.3	24	9.79 ± 0.42	11.10 ± 0.42	—
15	Valine	Young	7.8×10^{-2}	4.0	25	3.91 ± 0.11	3.49 ± 0.24	—
33	α-Aminobutyric acid	Old	8.2×10^{-2}	4.2	26	0.93 ± 0.04	1.00 ± 0.06	—
39	Ethanolamine	Young	9.5×10^{-2}	4.9	27	40.3 ± 1.9	35.9 ± 2.2	—
21	—	Young	9.8×10^{-2}	5.0	28	2.92 ± 0.27	2.34 ± 0.16	—
48	—	Young	1.4×10^{-1}	7.2	29	3.42 ± 0.71	1.71 ± 0.31	—
3	Taurine	Young	1.5×10^{-1}	7.4	30	52.8 ± 4.9	44.0 ± 5.3	—
11	Glutamic acid	Old	1.5×10^{-1}	7.6	31	5.93 ± 0.23	6.21 ± 0.27	—
40	Ornithine	Old	1.6×10^{-1}	8.0	32	2.75 ± 0.12	3.12 ± 0.28	—
17	—	Old	1.6×10^{-1}	8.3	33	3.77 ± 0.19	4.08 ± 0.24	—
23	Leucine	Old	1.7×10^{-1}	8.5	34	6.62 ± 0.16	6.90 ± 0.19	—

Note: *The substances are listed in order of decreasing probability of correlation with age.*

Table 2 Aging pattern for men as determined by 135 urine vapor substances[15]

Substance no.	Standard substance with identical elution time	Higher group	P_{AGE}	No. substances expected with $P \leq P_{AGE}$	No. substances found with $P \leq P_{AGE}$	Av. normalized area for 33 young men	Av. normalized area for 33 old men	AGE diagnostic power
87	—	Young	2.0×10^{-6}	0.00027	1	0.323 ± 0.038	0.104 ± 0.012	0.62
8	2-Butanone, 2-methylfuran, 3-methylfuran	Young	1.4×10^{-4}	0.019	2	41.9 ± 7.5	15.9 ± 2.4	0.48
14	2-Pentanone	Young	2.4×10^{-4}	0.032	3	16.4 ± 2.6	9.5 ± 2.8	0.47
77	—	Old	4.4×10^{-4}	0.059	4	0.400 ± 0.027	0.875 ± 0.123	0.48
12	3-Methyl-2-butanone, benzene, 2-methyltetrahydrofuran	Young	1.3×10^{-3}	0.18	5	1.77 ± 0.11	1.24 ± 0.11	0.39
44	—	Young	2.2×10^{-3}	0.30	6	0.626 ± 0.073	0.416 ± 0.036	—
15	3-Pentanone	Young	2.4×10^{-3}	0.33	7	1.59 ± 0.11	1.06 ± 0.09	—
91	2-Nonen-4-one	Young	2.4×10^{-4}	0.33	8	0.223 ± 0.018	0.152 ± 0.010	—
41	3-Heptanone	Old	3.5×10^{-3}	0.47	9	1.14 ± 0.12	2.55 ± 0.74	—
83	2-Nonanone	Young	4.1×10^{-3}	0.56	10	0.746 ± 0.088	0.586 ± 0.099	—
117	Carvone	Young	5.5×10^{-3}	0.75	11	8.99 ± 2.69	3.86 ± 1.66	—
38	—	Young	7.0×10^{-3}	0.94	12	0.155 ± 0.014	0.105 ± 0.017	—
124	—	Old	9.0×10^{-3}	1.2	13	0.128 ± 0.013	0.168 ± 0.012	—
42	Allyl isothiocyanate, 2-heptanone	Young	1.0×10^{-2}	1.4	14	5.26 ± 0.96	3.04 ± 0.46	—
109	—	Old	1.0×10^{-2}	1.4	15	0.246 ± 0.094	0.210 ± 0.017	—
134	—	Old	1.7×10^{-2}	2.3	16	0.037 ± 0.005	0.057 ± 0.006	—
97	—	Young	1.9×10^{-2}	2.6	17	0.431 ± 0.052	0.266 ± 0.037	—

Note: *The substances are listed in order of decreasing probability of correlation with age.*

Table 3 Predicted years of life remaining for 30 men of ages unknown to the investigators at time of prediction

Person no.	R_{AGE}	Predicted years life remaining	Actual age
64	35.4	68	26
75	32.1	64	25
80	29.2	59	24
97	24.3	52	26
70	24.3	52	24
67	21.0	48	24
85	19.7	46	
51	19.3	45	
93	19.2	45	
58	18.5	44	
56	16.4	41	
46	12.6	35	
87	12.0	34	24
26	11.7	34	
77	11.2	33	
90	10.9	33	
21	8.2	29	
15	6.4	26	
61	6.2	26	
29	6.0	26	57
44	5.7	25	
40	1.3	19	
12	−2.7	13	62
3	−3.2	12	50
59	−3.7	12	
54	−5.1	10	63
23	−13.6	0	55
35	−13.9	0	52
10	−15.8	0	52
48	−39.9	0	60

Note: The ages of the seven youngest and eight oldest men were subsequently revealed and are listed above.

Over the course of a 5-year period a statistically useful number of these 50,000 people will fall ill of various disease down to and including the incidence of multiple sclerosis. The bank will then contain prospective samples for the individuals and for the group that can be used to calibrate machines which may be able to detect disease before the individuals fall ill. Medicine could then combat the probability of illness, rather than illness itself. This bank would also allow the use of individuals as their own controls, thereby improving the resolution of clinical techniques.

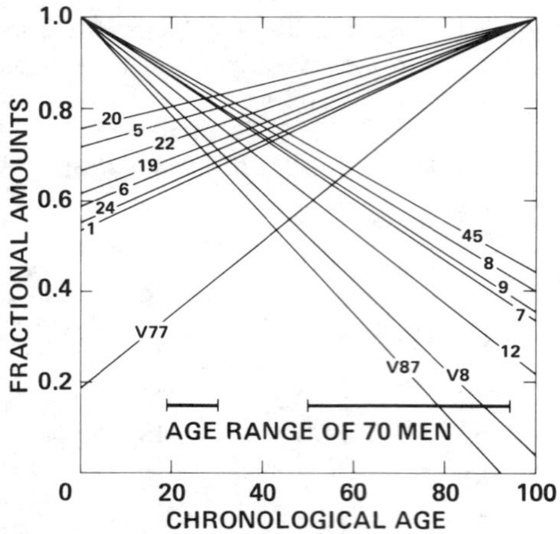

Figure 10 Linear regression lines for the 15 substances with strongest diagnostic power for age in these experiments. The substance numbers on the lines correspond to those in Tables 1 and 2. Seven of the substances decrease with age and eight of the substances increase with age. The regression lines were extrapolated to ages 0 and 100 years and then plotted to pass through those years at 1.0 solely for the purposes of this illustration. All data were accumulated for men in the age ranges shown in the figure.

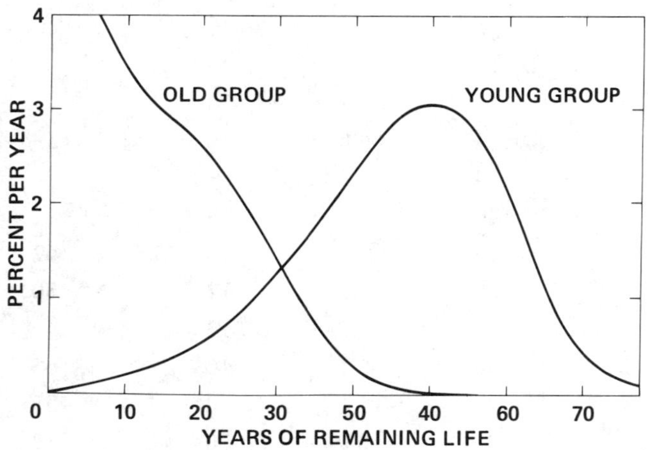

Figure 11 Life expectancy distributions for the young and old groups of men used for the calculations illustrated in Figures 13 through 17. The life expectancy of each man was tabulated from his chronological age and U.S. Public Health Service compilations. The smooth, curved lines were then drawn by interpolation.

This advance in preventive medicine would itself have a positive effect on human longevity. However, direct effects on aging research would be even more pronounced.

As the years pass and the 50,000 individuals gradually die, the bank of samples would contain an increasingly valuable set of samples from individuals whose years of life remaining would then be known. Subdivided with respect to cause of death, these samples, characterized as to true individual physiological age, would be valuable.

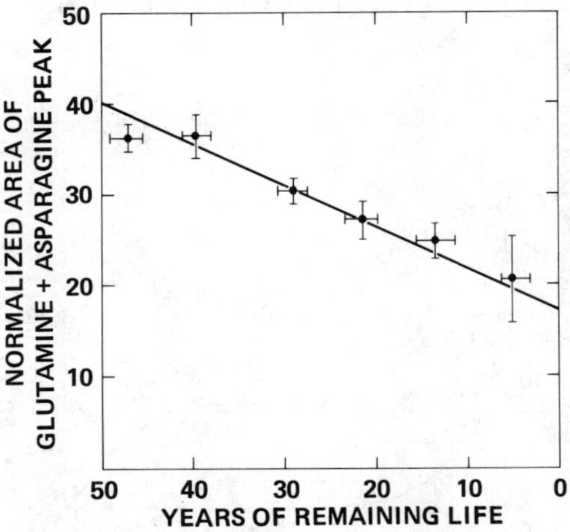

Figure 12 Normalized urine amide values for the 205 men grouped and averaged in six groups of similar age. The groups contained 38, 60, 53, 32, 13, and 9 men from young to old, respectively. The years of remaining life were calculated from actual ages of the men and U.S. Public Health Service compilations. The error bars are drawn for 1 S.D. of the means.

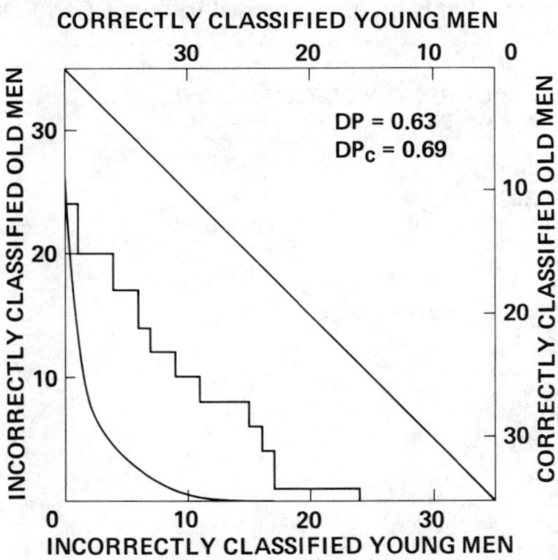

Figure 13 Age classification with five ninhydrin-positive urine compounds which decrease with age. Those with the highest diagnostic powers from Table 1 have been used. By means of their diagnostic coefficients, R_{AGE}, the men have been placed on a one-dimensional axis extending from young to old aging patterns. They have then been divided into two groups at all possible division points along that axis, and the errors of division between young and old tabulated. No individual has been compared to a pattern which included his own values in its determination. The diagonal line is the random expectation, a point in the origin would be perfect separation, the curved line represents the theoretically perfect result given the overlap in life expectancies, and the stepped function is the experimental results. *DP* and DP_C are explained in the text.

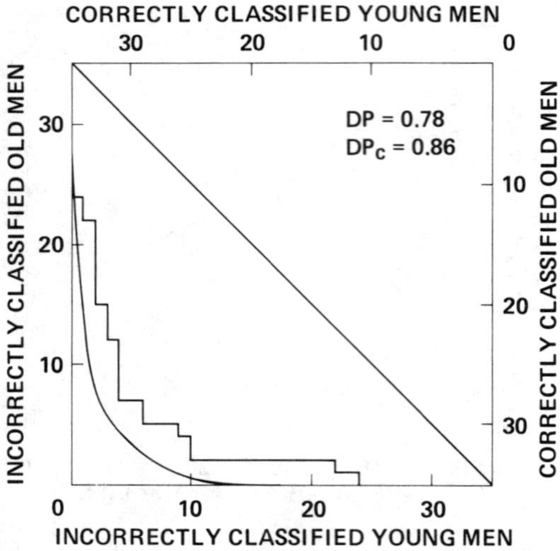

Figure 14 Age classification with seven ninhydrin-positive urine compounds which increase with age. Those with the highest diagnostic powers from Table 1 have been used. By means of their diagnostic coefficients, R_{AGE}, the men have been placed on a one-dimensional axis extending from young to old aging patterns. They have then been divided into two groups at all possible division points along that axis, and the errors of division between young and old tabulated. No individual has been compared to a pattern which included his own values in its determination. The diagonal line is the random expectation, a point in the origin would be perfect separation, the curved line represents the theoretically perfect result given the overlap in life expectancies, and the stepped function is the experimental results. *DP* and DP_C are explained in the text.

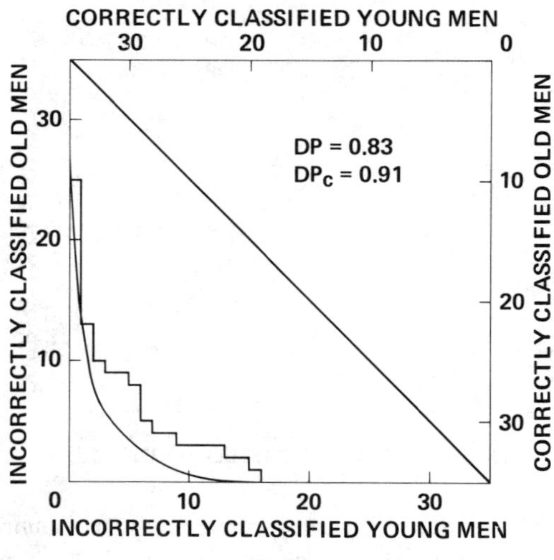

Figure 15 Age classification with 12 ninhydrin-positive urine compounds which increase and decrease with age. Those with the highest diagnostic powers from Table 1 have been used. By means of their diagnostic coefficients, R_{AGE}, the men have been placed on a one-dimensional axis extending from young to old aging patterns. They have then been divided into two groups at all possible division points along that axis, and the errors of division between young and old tabulated. No individual has been compared to a pattern which included his own values in its determination. The diagonal line is the random expectation, a point in the origin would be perfect separation, the curved line represents the theoretically perfect result given the overlap in life expectancies, and the stepped function is the experimental result. *DP* and DP_C are explained in the text.

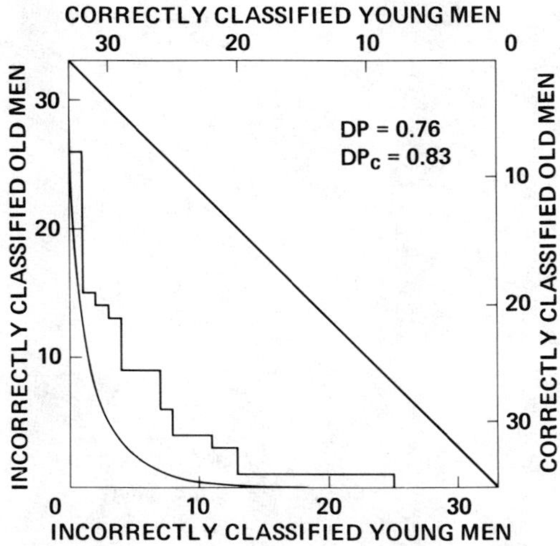

Figure 16 Age classification with three urine vapor substances. Those with the highest diagnostic powers from Table 2 have been used. By means of their diagnostic coefficients, R_{AGE}, the men have been placed on a one-dimensional axis extending from young to old aging patterns. They have then been divided into two groups at all possible division points along that axis, and the errors of division between young and old tabulated. No individual has been compared to a pattern which included his own values in its determination. The diagonal line is the random expectation, a point in the origin would be perfect separation, the curved line represents the theoretically perfect result given the overlap in life expectancies, and the stepped function is the experimental result. *DP* and DP_C are explained in the text.

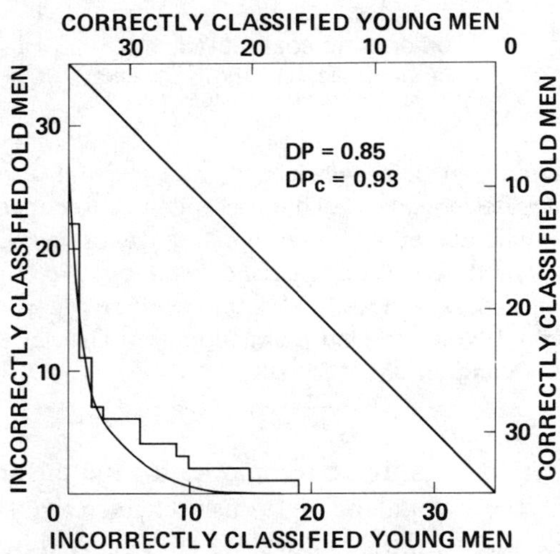

Figure 17 Age classification with 15 urine compounds: 5 ninhydrin-positive compounds that decrease with age; 7 ninhydrin-positive compounds that increase with age, and 3 urine vapor compounds. Those with the highest diagnostic powers from Tables 1 and 2 have been used. By means of their diagnostic coefficients, R_{AGE}, the men have been placed on a one dimensional axis extending from young to old aging patterns. They have then been divided into two groups at all possible division points along that axis, and the errors of division between young and old tabulated. No individual has been compared to a pattern which included his own values in its determination. The diagonal line is the random expectation, a point in the origin would be perfect separation, the curved line represents the theoretically perfect result given the overlap in life expectancies, and the stepped function is the experimental result. *DP* and DP_C are explained in the text.

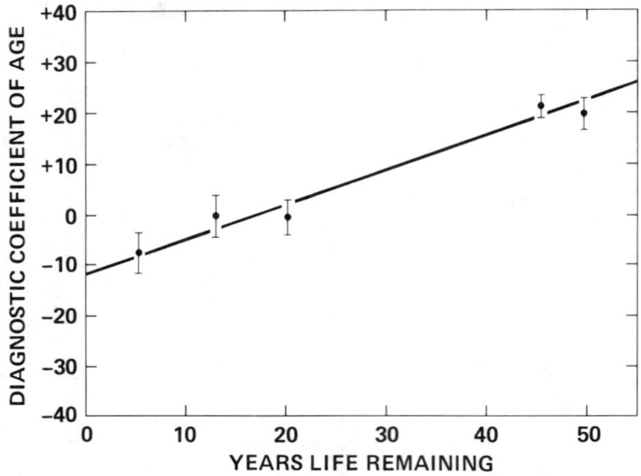

Figure 18 The diagnostic coefficients, R_{AGE}, for the 15 substances of the 66 men used in the calculations shown in Figures 13 through 17. The men have been grouped into five groups of similar age. The ages and diagnostic coefficients were then averaged to give the points shown on this figure. The error bars are drawn for 1 S.D. of the means.

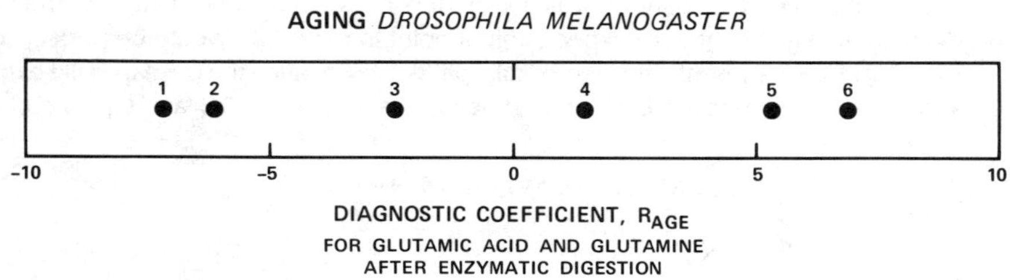

Figure 19 Values of the age diagnostic coefficient, R_{AGE}, of glutamic acid and glutamine for six sets of 24 *Drosophila melanogaster*, each representing consecutive 6-day periods. The groups are consecutively numbered with 1 designating days 1 to 6, 2 designating days 7 to 12, and so on. (Reprinted from *Experimental Gerontology,* Volume 11, Robinson, A.B. et al., Age dependent amines, amides, and amino acids residues in *Drosophila melanogaster,* p. 113, copyright 1976, with kind permission from Elsevier Science Ltd, The Boulevard, Langford Lane, Kidlington OX5 1GB, UK.)

The samples could be used to calibrate techniques for the quantitative analysis of human physiological age. Because they would be rigorously characterized and available to various experimenters from a single source, the samples also could be used in comparative experiments to determine which techniques are most useful for the measurement of age.

This sample bank should be started uniquely for this purpose and should be of the highest possible quality. Efforts to salvage old sample sets from other projects would probably lead to expensive, yet suboptimum results.

It is important to emphasize that the bank must contain *samples*, not the results of analyses. It would be tragic to undertake this project with limitation to one or more particular analytical techniques which happen to now be available and popular. Surely those techniques would be obsolete by the time results were obtained. If, however, the samples had not been retained, no further advance would be possible.

If the authors could make only one contribution to the advancement of the use of modern technology for the improvement of human health, the creation of this sample bank of body fluids from well individuals would be our choice. If this bank had been created when we first formally proposed it 18 years ago, substantial improvements in clinical medicine and in empirical aging research already would be in evidence.

IV. CONCLUSION

We conclude that a very strong systematic metabolic pattern exists for human age, and we estimate that these techniques should be able to be refined with relative ease to measure the physiological age of individual human subjects to an accuracy level of ±3 years. This would permit the measurement of physiological age in a group of 300 individuals to an accuracy within 2 months or 1300 individuals to an accuracy within 1 month. Rate of aging experiments could then be performed to an accuracy of about 10% over a period of 1 year. As experience is gained, this should be improved by about one additional order of magnitude, which would permit smaller, shorter, or more accurate experiments.

Improvements can also be expected from the separation of individuals into types. We observed, for example, in an experiment in which we measured 60 urinary amines, amides, and amino acids in the urine of 1000 newborn infants,[19] that the human distribution functions of amounts of many of these substances were not unimodal. Instead, they were bi- and multimodal. We expect this to be generally true, so that discrete typing of individuals will eventually markedly increase the resolution of these techniques.

Improvements can also be made by particular constraints such as dietary control. We have already demonstrated that with strict dietary control the urinary patterns become so unique that computerized fingerprinting of single individuals with a high degree of accuracy can be carried out. Strict dietary control, however, sharply limits the utility and breadth of applicability of these techniques.

Refinement need not make use of these particular analytical techniques. Any method that measures about 200 metabolic substances quantitatively should be sufficient. (Some methods such as unfragmented ion mass spectrometry have the potential to measure 2000 or more substances within a few minutes or less.)

Refinement, however, absolutely requires that a sample set be available in order to calibrate the technique. Until this sample set is carefully gathered, stored, and made generally available, this technique and many other potential analytical advances in human health will probably remain research curiosities rather than proper contributors to the quality of human life.

We emphasize the following:

1. About one third or more of the metabolic constituents of human body fluids correlate systematically with age, as do the constituents of flies and mice. For practical, empirical purposes, therefore, analytical techniques for profiling should emphasize those substances that are easy and inexpensive to measure quantitatively. Any sufficiently large set of casually selected metabolic substances contain within their amounts the necessary information as to individual physiological age.
2. Simple computerized techniques exist for the test and utilization of data from these profiling experiments. We have also used more sophisticated pattern recognition techniques, but have generally found them cumbersome and without concomitant additional utility. "Eyeballing" chromatograms or mass spectra is, however, essentially without value. Proper nonparametric tests of reliability on statistically useful sets of analyses must be performed. A simple procedure for doing this is illustrated herein.

3. The principal limitation to this work is in sampling, not in analysis or computation. Although other analytical techniques can be utilized and many interesting reports written regarding the analytical profiling of age, further real advances in this effort probably will not be possible until a proper prospective sample bank is established.

REFERENCES

1. Minot, C.S., The problem of age, growth, and death, *Pop. Sci. Monthly*, 71, 481, 1907.
2. Harman, D., Aging: a theory based on free radical and radiation chemistry, *J. Gerontol.*, 11, 298,1956.
3. Bjorksten, J., A common molecular basis for the aging syndrome, *J. Am. Geriatr. Soc.*, 6, 740,1958.
4. Orgel, L., The maintenance of the accuracy of protein synthesis and its relevance to ageing, *Proc. Natl. Acad. Sci. U.S.A.*, 49, 517,1963.
5. Medvedev, Z.A., The nucleic acids in development and aging, *Adv. Gerontol. Res.*, 1, 181,1964.
6. Strehler, B.L., Code degeneracy and the ageing process: a molecular genetic theory of aging, *Proc. 7th Congr. Gerontol. Vienna*, 177, 1966.
7. Walford, L., *The Immunological Theory of Aging*, Williams & Wilkins, Baltimore, 1969, 70.
8. Hart, R.W. and Setlow, R.V., Correlation between DNA excision repair and life span in a number of mammalian species, *Proc. Natl. Acad. Sci. U.S.A.*, 71, 2169,1974.
9. Bada, J.L., Aspartic acid racemization in tooth enamel from living humans, *Proc. Natl. Acad. Sci. U.S.A.*, 72, 2891,1975.
10. Robinson, A.B., McKerrow, J.H., and Cary, P., Controlled deamidation of peptides and proteins: an experimental hazard and a possible biological timer, *Proc. Natl. Acad. Sci. U.S.A.*, 66, 753, 1970; see also Robinson, A.B., *Proc. Natl. Acad. Sci. U.S.A.*, 71, 885, 1974 and Robinson, A.B. and Rudd, C., Deamidation of glutaminyl and asparaginyl residues in peptides and proteins, *Curr. Top. Cell. Reg.*, 8, 247,1974.
11. Robinson, A.B., Molecular clocks, molecular profiles, and optimum diets; three approaches to the problem of aging, *Mech. Age. Dev.*, 9, 225, 1979.
12. Robinson, A.B., Willoughby, R., and Robinson, L.R., Age dependent amines, amides, and amino acids residues in *Drosophila melanogaster, Exp. Gerontol.*, 11, 113, 1976.
13. Robinson, A.B., Weiss, M., Reynolds, W.E., and Robinson, L.R., Use of mass spectrometry for orthomolecular diagnosis, *23rd Annu. Conf. Mass Spectrom.*, Houston, 1975, 182.
14. Robinson, A.B., Dirren, H., Sheets, A., and Lundgren, R., Quantitative aging pattern in mouse urine vapor as measured by gas-liquid chromatography, *Exp. Gerontol.*, 11, 11, 1976.
15. Robinson, A.B., Partridge, D., Turner, M., Teranishi, R., and Pauling, L., An apparatus for the quantitative analysis of volatile compounds in urine, *J. Chromatogr.*, 85, 19, 1973.
16. Robinson, A.B., *Antioch Rev.*, 383, 1981.
17. Robinson, A.B. and Westall, F.C., The use of urinary amine measurement for orthomolecular diagnosis of multiple sclerosis, *J. Orth. Psych.*, 3, 1, 1974.
18. Wilcoxon, F., *Biometrics*, 1, 80, 1945; Lehman, S.Y., *J. Am. Stat. Assoc.*, 56, 293, 1961; Verdooren, L.R., *Biometrika*, 50, 177, 1963; Fix, E. and Hodges, J.L., *Ann. Math. Stat.*, 26, 301, 1955.
19. Robinson, A.B., Robinson, L.R., and Mann, J., unpublished results.
20. Robinson, A.B. and Robinson, L.R., *Proc. Natl. Acad. Sci. U.S.A.*, 88, 8880, 1991.

CHAPTER 16

AGE-DEPENDENT EXCRETION PATTERN OF FREE AMINO ACIDS AND PEPTIDES IN HUMAN URINE

JOZEF ADAM, ANDREJ NICÁK, AND ANDREJ MOLNÁR

TABLE OF CONTENTS

I. INTRODUCTION

Utilization of proteins in organisms is altered during postnatal development.[10] Proteins from food are predominantly utilized for the maintenance of growth in the youth and for the regeneration of tissues and organs in the adult.[17]

Altered protein utilization is reflected in a changed content of free amino acids and peptides, representing terminal metabolites of protein metabolism, in organs and body fluids.

Based on the above findings, the present study focused on monitoring age-dependent changes in the content of free amino acids and peptides in the urine of humans. The urine has been considered a material of choice for the study of amino acids and peptides because it is easily available and it represents a kind of collecting system for a variety of metabolites produced in physiological and pathological conditions in an organism.

II. MATERIAL AND METHODS

The study was performed on urine from healthy individuals aged 1, 9, 20, 32, 40, 50, 60, 69, 85, and 97 years, and also from a prematurely born child. The children were healthy individuals from child care institutions, the adults were clinically healthy male volunteers under standard dietary conditions. The urine was collected for 24 h and was treated with thymol as a preservative during collection.

For analyses, the urine was passed through a column of Dowex® 50x8 ion exchanger in the H^+ form. Washing the column with distilled water removed salts and other undesirable compounds from the urine that might disturb the migration of substances in the electrical field.

0-8493-0129-7/94/$0.00+$.50

Urine samples treated in this way were then separated by high-voltage electrophoresis according to Michl[11] for 2 h in a pyridine-acetate buffer, pH 3.5, at a potential gradient of 60 V/cm on Whatman® No. 1 paper. Reference samples were acid, neutral, and basic amino acid. Electrophoretograms were detected by 0.5% ninhydrin solution in acetone.

Tentative analyses were performed in all cases, with urine amounts corresponding to 1/1500 vol of 24-h diuresis.[4] Preparative high-voltage electrophoresis was carried out in a way similar to basic fractionation. The difference was that aliquots of the urine were applied to 12-cm strips of chromatographic paper. Detection was done on a 1-cm margin of the paper strips. The fractions were stained by 0.5% ninhydrin solution in acetone. Elution of separated zones was carried out with 5% acetic acid.

Electrophoretic fractions that exhibited a mobility different from that of amino acids of the standard mixture were hydrolyzed by HCl (C = 6 mol/l) at 105°C for 18 h. The amino acids released by the hydrolysis were identified by two-dimensional chromatoelectrophoresis. The first direction was performed as chromatography in butanol:acetic acid:water (4:1:5), the other was high-voltage electrophoresis in 2.5% formic acid at 3000 V for 40 min.

III. ASSESSMENT OF ANTIBACTERIAL ACTIVITY OF PEPTIDES

Antibacterial activity of peptides occurring in the human urine was tested using a modified plate method by Grow and Rendall.[7] The meat-peptone agar medium, pH 6.6, was used for cultivation of bacteria *Staphylococcus aureus* as well as for casting the basal layer of the plates. Individual fractions of peptides were evaporated to dryness, weighed, and redissolved in demineralized distilled water.

Aliquots of fractions in concentrations corresponding to 1 mg/ml, and in some cases also to 0.01 mg/ml, were used for testing antibacterial activity. Samples of fractions (80 µl) were pipetted in two series into sterilized cylinders. Following prediffusion of peptides at 4°C for 3 h, bacteria *S. aureus* were incubated at 37°C for 18 h and diameters of inhibition zones were measured.

IV. RESULTS AND DISCUSSION

Results from analysis of ninhydrine positive substances in the urine of humans from various age groups are shown in Figure 1. Present data indicate marked individual differences in excretion patterns of these substances. The highest number of fractions has been recorded in children and in adult individuals; however, a temporary decrease in number of excreted ninhydrine positive substances could be observed in both age groups. The least number of fractions was found in the urine of a 97-year-old individual in which fractions were absent in the acid region and partly also in the weakly basic and basic region, in contrast to other individuals. Differences were observed mainly in the regions of peptide separation, i.e., in the area between aspartic acid and glutamic acid, neutral amino acids (*n*), and basic amino acids (histidine, arginine, lysine).

A comparison of the occurrence of fractions that gave a positive reaction with Pauly reagent for detection of histidine (hatched spots) showed an age-dependent reduction in their number.

In conjunction with changes observed in the excretion pattern of peptides in the urine of humans belonging to different age groups it has been interesting to examine whether there are variations in the peptide excretion pattern in humans of the same age group. For this purpose two age groups were selected, the first comprising 1-year-old children, and the second comprising 20-year-old adult males.

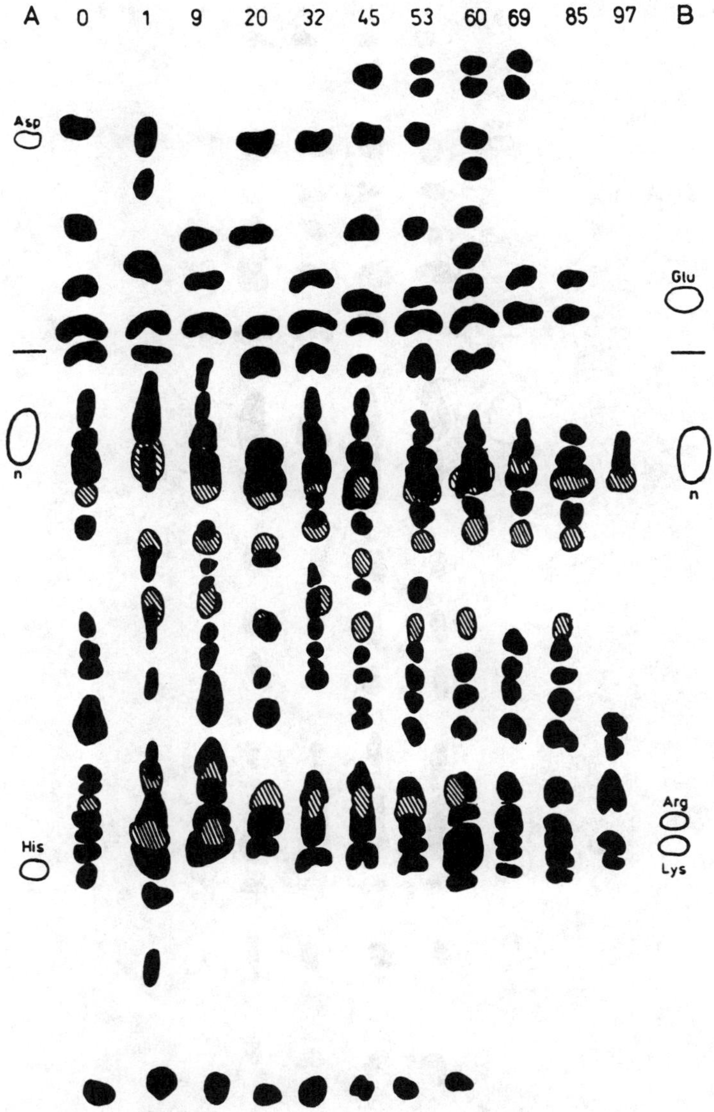

Figure 1 Electrophoretogram of the urine of healthy persons of variousage groups. Electrophoresis was performed in pyridine-acetate buffer, pH 3.5, at a potential gradient of 60 V/cm for 2 h. (A, B) Reference amino acid mixture. (0) Urine of prematurely born child. (1–97) Samples of urine of healthy individuals.

Electrophoretic analysis of infant urine (Figure 2) showed 16 ninhydrin-positive fractions and 15 separate fractions were found in the urine of adult males (Figure 3). A comparison of numbers of fractions and their R_f values inside the two groups revealed no differences in the excretion pattern of ninhydrin-reactive substances among individuals within the same age group.

A mutual comparison of electrophoretic patterns of infant urines and those of adults showed several differences in excretion of ninhydrin-positive substances. The differences were present in acidic (fractions 1 to 5), weakly basic (fractions 9 and 12), and strongly basic (fraction 15) regions.

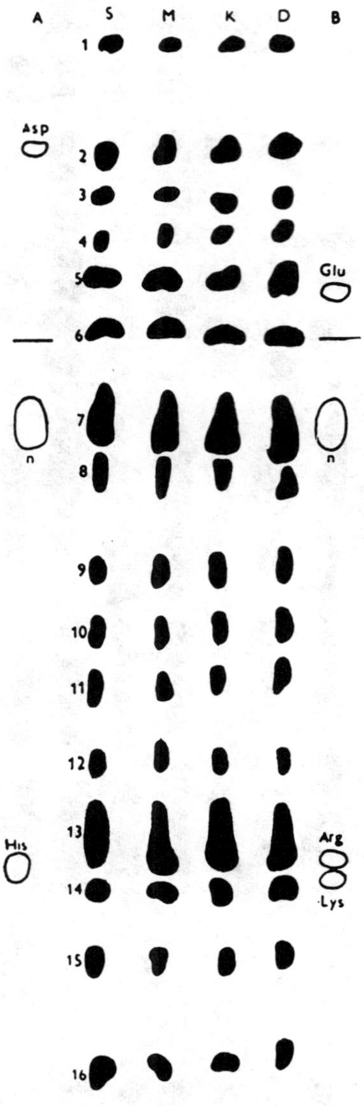

Figure 2 Electrophoregram of urine of healthy children 1 year old. Conditions of electrophoresis as in Figure 1. (A, B) Reference amino acid mixture. (S–D) samples of urine of different individuals; (1–16) numbers of identified fractions.

Observed variability in peptide excretion pattern at different stages of ontogenesis may be conditional on various factors, e.g., changes in metabolism of peptides participating significantly in neuroendocrine regulation[20] or the change in secretion of hormones participating in the regulation of protein metabolism.[5,8,9,13,15,16]

Milne[12] reported that peptides present in the urine belong with those that resisted a hydrolytic action of the tissue and plasmatic peptidases. Difficulties in interpreting changes presented herein arise from insufficient information on the importance of diet on peptide spectra in the urine. Nasset and Tully[14] showed that in healthy humans aged 20 to 30 years, the species

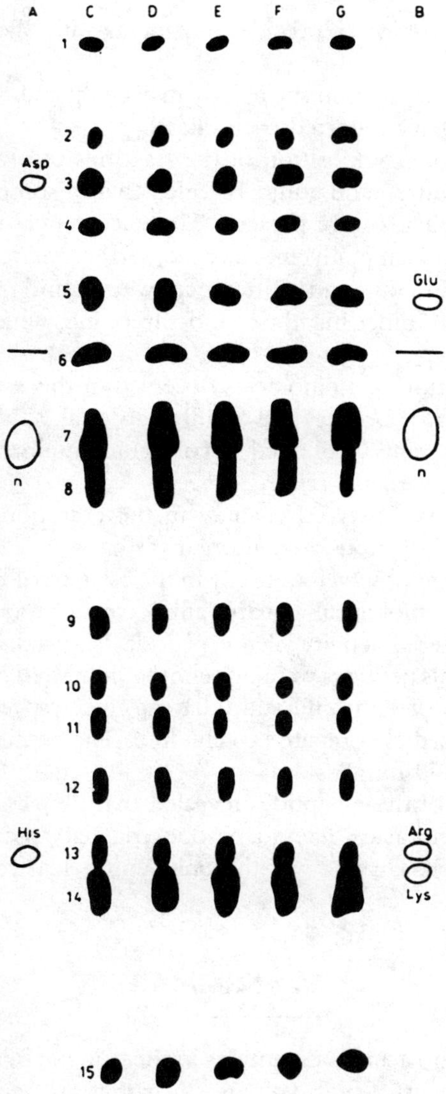

Figure 3 Electrophoretogram of the urine of healthy 20-year-old persons. Conditions of electrophoresis as in Figure 1. (A,B) Reference amino acid mixture; (C–G) samples of urine of different individuals; (1–15) numbers of identified fractions.

of ingested protein has no effect on peptiduria. Similarly, Berman and Kench[3] contradicted the possibility of alimentary modification of the peptiduria.

The above statements were supported by the present results because no differences in the excretion of peptides were found among individuals in the group of 1-year-old children as well as in the group of 20-year-old males (Figures 2 and 3) that consumed various types of rations.

The increased occurrence of peptides in infant urine as compared to adults (Figures 2 and 3) indicates intensive proteosynthesis in the period of growth, which is reflected also in dynamic steady-state in the processes of protein synthesis and protein degradation accompanied by elevated excretion of peptide fragments. This statement also is in accordance with a generally accepted explanation for increased excretion of peptides in patients with Sheehan syndrome after administration of proteinoanabolics.[1]

Decreased excretion of peptides in the elderly may be related to decreased incorporation of labeled amino acids in proteins reported by Frolkis.[6]

The study of amino acid composition of the fractions resolved by high voltage electrophoresis of the urine of children and adults revealed that in some fractions (fractions 2, 5, 7, 8, 13, and 14) free amino acids were present. The occurrence of free amino acids in adults and children was similar for lysine, glycine, alanine, serine, valine, leucine, tyrosine, phenylalanine, aspartic acid, and glutamic acid. Differences were found in proline, which was present only in infant urine and arginine, histidine, and threonine, which were present only in the urine of adults.

Variability in the excretion of amino acids observed in this study in adults and children is in accordance with the data of Berger[2] and Stambaugh et al.,[19] who reported that samples of the urine from healthy humans contained a constant amount of amino acids. They thus concluded that all changes were age related.

Other investigations have observed changes in the excretion of free amino acids during ontogenesis in urine[22] and in various animal organs.[18,21]

Age-related changes were observed not only in the content of free amino acids and peptides in human urine, but also in biological activity (antibacterial properties) of the peptides.

Assessment of antibacterial activity of the peptides showed that in the urine of healthy children and adult individuals peptides were present that inhibited growth of *Escherichia coli* and *S. aureus* in concentrations of 1 mg/ml and 0.01 mg/ml, respectively. The number of these peptides in adults is decreased as compared to children. The peptides with antibacterial activity are absent in the urine of old humans.

More detailed analysis of these peptides revealed that they contain amino acids present in proteins and modified amino acids, like L-aminobutyric acid, β-aminobutyric acid, ornithine, hydroxylysine, and β-alanine. Glycine was the only amino acid regularly present in all of the peptides.

V. SUMMARY

The occurrence of free amino acids and peptides in the urine of healthy individuals was studied as a function of age by means of high-voltage electrophoresis and chromatoelectrophoresis.

Both free and peptidically bound amino acids were found to be present in the urine of healthy humans. Their spectrum varies between different age groups. The highest number of fractions was found in children and in middle-aged adults. The urine of aged individuals was found to contain a reduced number of peptide fractions.

Age-related changes were observed not only in the content of free amino acids and peptides in human urine but also in biological activity (antibacterial properties) of the peptides. Assessment of antibacterial activity of the peptides showed that in the urine of healthy children and adult individuals peptides were present that inhibited growth of *E. coli* and *S. aureus* in concentrations of 1 mg/ml and 0.01 mg/ml, respectively. The number of these peptides in adults is decreased as compared to children. The peptides with antibacterial activity are absent in the urine of old humans.

Experimental results are discussed in relation to factors affecting the excretion of peptides in urine in different stages of ontogenetical development and to the intensity of protein synthesis or protein degradation.

REFERENCES

1. Adam, J., Mäsiar, P., and Moscovic, F., Changes in the excretion of amino acids and other ninhydrin positive substances in the urine of a patient with the Sheehan syndrome before and after dianabol treatment, *Bratisl. Lek. Listy,* 46/II(5), 289, 1966.
2. Berger, H., Determination of amino acids excreted in the urine and their significance in the clinic, *Schweiz. Med. Wochenschr.,* 86, 711,1956.
3. Berman, M. C. and Kench, J. E., Role of peptides in protein metabolism, peptiduria in protein-depleted children, *Clin. Sci.,* 34, 111, 1968.
4. Blauth-Opienska, J., Critical evaluation of methods used in aminoaciduria investigation, *Clin. Chim. Acta,* 4(6), 841, 1959.
5. Bolla, R. I., Hormonal regulation of molecular events during aging, *Life Sci.,* 31, 615, 1982.
6. Frolkis, V. V. *Aging. Neurohumoral mechanisms,* Naukova Dumka, Kiev, 1981, 2.
7. Grow, D. S. and Rendall, V. S. The guide to the laboratory methods in antibiotic research, *Gos. Izdat. Med. Lit.,* 295, 1958.
8. Harman, S. M., Clinical aspects of aging of the male reproductive system, in *The Aging Reproductive Systems,* Schneider, E. L., Ed., Raven Press, New York, 1978, 29.
9. Hylka, V. W., Sonntag, W. E., and Meistes, J., Reduced ability of old male rats to release ACTH and corticosterone in response to CRF administration, *Proc. Soc. Exp. Biol. Med.,* 175, 1, 1984.
10. Krajcovicová-Kudlácková, M. and Dibák, O., Utilization of proteins in dependence on age, intake of fats and saccharides, *Bratisl. Lek. Listy,* 89(4), 264, 1988.
11. Michl, H., Paper electrophoresis at potential differences of 50 volts per centimeter, *Monatschrft. Chem.,* 82, 489, 1951.
12. Milne, M. D., Transport of amino acids and peptides in the gut and the kidney, in *The Scientific Basis of Medicine,* Gilliland, I. and Francis, J., Eds., Athlone Press, London, 1971, 161.
13. Murono, E. P., Naubin, H. R., Lin, T., and Osterman, J., The aging Leydig cell. VI. Response of testosterone precursors to gonadotrophin in men, *Acta Endocrinol.,* 100, 455, 1982.
14. Nasset, E. F. and Tully, R. H., Urinary excretion of essential amino acids by human subjects fed diets containing proteins of different biological value, *J. Nutr.,* 44, 477, 1951.
15. Parker, L., Gral, T., Perrigo, V., and Skowsky, R., Decreased adrenal androgen sensitivity to ACTH during aging, *Metabolism,* 30, 601, 1981.
16. Printz, P. N., Wietzman, E. D., Cunningham, G. R., and Karacan, J., Plasma growth hormone during sleep in young and aged men, *J. Gerontol.,* 38, 519, 1983.
17. Robson, J. R. K., Larkin, F. A., Sandretto, A. M., and Tadyyon, B., *Malnutrition,* Gordon & Breach, New York, 1972, 813.
18. Ryan, W. L. and Carver, M. J., Free amino acids of human fetal and adult liver, *Nature,* 212, 292, 1966.
19. Stambaugh, R., Davidson, D. T., and Elkinson, J. R., Variation in excretion of certain amino acids with age, *Clin. Chem.,* 9, 210, 1963.
20. Tatár, P., The endocrine system in advanced age, *Cs. Fysiol.,* 35, 1, 1986.
21. Turjanica, J. M., Pascenko, A. Je., Dorogij, M. V., Fedorovic, T. M., and Vasser, Ja. P., The distribution of free amino acids in brain of rats in relation to ontogenesis, *Ukr. Biochim. Z.,* 55, 667, 1983.
22. Zelezinskaja, G. A., The content of free amino acids in relation to the growth, *Dokl. Akad. Nauk,* 8, 741, 1969.

CHAPTER 17

ASSESSMENT OF BIOLOGICAL AGE BY MAXIMUM OXYGEN UPTAKE

Sankar N. Koyal, Adrian J. Williams, Silverio Santiago, Donald Schwartz, and Myrvin H. Ellastad

TABLE OF CONTENTS

I. INTRODUCTION

Although many investigators[1-11] have studied various aspects of aging and have formulated a variety of theories to explain aging, very little attempt has been made to measure aging in multiple systems in the same individual and to determine why, or how often, one system functions well and another poorly. In addition, the effects of exercise on different systems as they relate to aging are not well understood. For example, it is known that isotonic exercise of major magnitude reduces the expected loss in maximal cardiac output with aging, but not the age-related reduction in heart rate. There is some evidence that conditioning improves cognitive function. We do not know, however, if conditioning alters tissue elasticity or joint function. Several studies implicate the immune system in aging. If so, does it affect the neuromuscular system, mental competence, or only resistance to infection and/or cancer? Do diet, smoking, alcohol, food additives, vitamins, and many other factors influence only one part of the body or do they have an overall effect?

II. DEFINITION OF BIOLOGICAL AGE

Timiras[39] defined biological age (BA) as the sum of all changes that occur in a living organism with the passage of time, leading to functional impairment with time, and death. Dean[40] defined human BA as the objective assessment of a person's health status, and substantiated in long-term follow-up studies that "those who scored the oldest biologically or physiologically died soonest".

0-8493-0129-7/94/$0.00+$.50

Theoretically, a person's BA in terms of appearance, performance, and functional capacity should be the same as his or her chronological age (CA). However, it is not uncommon to find a person who does not "look his or her age", instead appearing to be much older or much younger than his or her CA. Looking younger or older than CA may depend on many factors. Some of the important determinants may include (1) proper diet and nutrition, (2) a well-defined and appropriate scientifically based exercise program, and (3) the "genetic loci" that control the aging process. We have studied aging and the function of various body systems and have tried to identify factors that may retard aging.

III. BACKGROUND

As early as 1935, Sokolov[12] published an article on the assessment of biological aging. This study was based on indices reflecting skin elasticity. Voitenko and Tokar[13] later published a prediction equation of BA based upon a number of static physiologic, anthropologic, psychometric, and cytologic measurements. In the 1970s and 1980s, Borkan and Norris,[14] Bruce et al.,[15-17] Dundikova et al.,[18] Furukawa et al.,[19] Nakamura,[20,21] Skalicky et al.,[22] Webster and Logie,[23] Chodzko-Zajko and Ringel[24,25] used measurements obtained during rest and exercise to predict BA or physiological age. Others have used measurements of ocular adaptation and accommodation amplitude as predictors of BA.[21,27-29]

Attempts to measure BA in humans have come from investigators from Harvard University,[26] the Gerontology Research Center (GRC) of the National Institute of Aging,[27,28] and laboratories from The Netherlands,[29] Australia,[30] Japan,[31,32] Finland,[33-35] Germany,[36] and the former USSR.[37,38] Most of these investigators used static measurements such as standard body anthropometry, blood chemistry, and forced vital capacity. Very few investigators used dynamic variables such as physical work capacity, maximum exercise tolerance, and its related cardiorespiratory variables (e.g., oxygen uptake, gas exchange ratio, ventilatory threshold, blood lactate, and cardiovascular efficiency index).

IV. SUBJECTS AND METHODS

We randomly selected 155 male and female subjects from Southern California (Los Angeles, Long Beach, Orange County). Table 1 shows the physical characteristics of our subjects. Their ages ranged from 30 to 82 years.

Each individual subject had a series of tests consisting of body anthropometry; health questionnaire; maximum treadmill stress test; pulmonary function tests; vascular compliance tests, including systolic time interval and pulse transmission time; muscular strength and endurance tests; ophthalmological and psychological evaluation; and blood chemistry.

Oxygen uptake and other cardiorespiratory variables such as minute ventilation, CO_2 production, gas exchange ratio, and ventilatory equivalent for O_2 and CO_2 were measured using a SensorMedics Metabolic Cart (Yorba Linda, CA) at rest and during a maximal exercise stress test using a treadmill. Measurements were made at each incremental workload with different speeds and grades following the Ellestad protocol[41] (Figure 1).

We obtained physiological age or BA by comparing the measured value with a predicted value (ideal)[42-44] and averaging the estimated physiological ages based on all 33 measured variables. Representative examples are shown in Figures 2 to 4. Regression analysis was used for assessing correlations.

Table 1 Physical characteristics of male and female subjects

	Male (*n* = 91)		Female (*n* = 81)	
	Mean	S.D.	Mean	S.D.
Age (years)	51.4	± 12.1	53.3	± 13.1
Height (in.)	70.0	± 2.8	64.5	± 2.4
Weight (lb)	172.3	± 25.7	136.0	± 21.3
BSA (m^2)	1.9	± 0.2	1.7	± 0.2

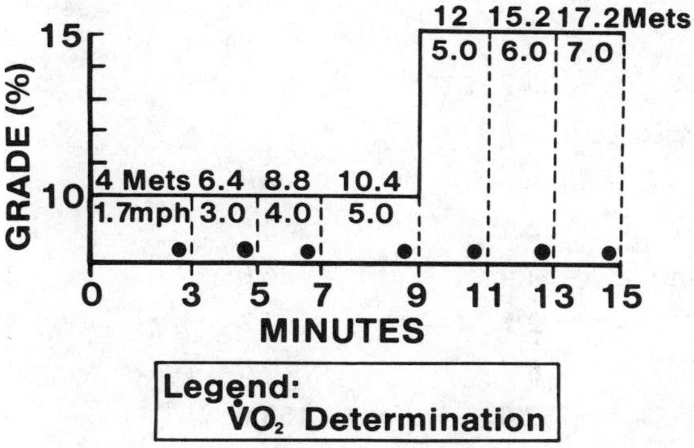

Figure 1 Diagram of work loads used during treadmill stress test. (From Ellestad, M.H., *Stress Testing: Principles and Practice,* 3rd ed., F.A. Davis, Philadelphia, 1986. With permission.)

V. RESULTS

Figure 5 shows the relationship between CA and physiological age or BA in male subjects. The correlation coefficient is +0.97. Figure 6 shows the relationship between chronological and BA of the female subjects with a correlation coefficient of 0.95. Figures 7 and 8 show the relationship between forced vital capacity and maximum O_2 uptake in our male and female subjects (correlation coefficient of +0.87 and 0.71, respectively). Figure 9 depicts the relationship of maximum oxygen uptake and CA of the male subjects with a correlation coefficient of –0.64. The female subjects showed a similar trend with a correlation coefficient of –0.70. When the maximum oxygen uptake was plotted as a function of BA in our male subjects there was a higher correlation coefficient of –0.72 (Figure 10). When $VO_{2\ max}$/kg body weight of our male subjects was plotted against their CA (Figure 11), the correlation coefficient was –0.54). However, when the same data were plotted against the BA, the correlation coefficient was slightly better (Figure 12). Figures 13 and 14 show the relationship of the *difference* between physiologic age or BA and CA and maximum O_2 uptake in our male and female subjects with correlation coefficients of –0.76 and –0.79, respectively.

When $VO_{2\ max}$/kg body weight was plotted against the difference between BA and CA, the correlation coefficient was –0.80 in female subjects (Figure 16). Figure 15 depicts a lower correlation coefficient (–0.72) between $VO_{2\ max}$/kg and the difference between BA and CA in our male subjects.

Figure 2 Aging profile of a subject with a similar physiological age and CA.

A. Physical Characteristics			Age: 67	Sex: M
	Measured	*Ideal*	*% Expected*	*PA*
1. Height (in.)	71.0	71.0	100.0	67.0
2. Weight (lb)	155.0	160.0	96.9	64.9
3. BSA (M^2)	1.9	1.9	99.0	66.3
4. % Body fat	13.3	16.0	83.1	55.7
B. Health Questionnaire				
1. Positive = 6%				
2. Ponderal index	30.7	31.7	96.9	64.9
C. Max. Treadmill Exercise Test				
	Measured	*Ideal*	*% Ideal*	*PA*
1. $VO_{2\ max}$ (l/min)	2.4	2.6	91.2	73.4
2. $VO_{2\ max}$/kg/min (ml)	34.0	36.0	94.4	70.9
3. C.V. efficiency	2.1	2.3	91.7	73.1
4. Exercise time	8.7	9.0	96.7	69.3
5. Max. H.R./min	152.0	153.0	99.3	67.4
6. Max. BP syst.	190.0	192.0	99.0	67.7
7. Max. BP diast.	100.0	81.0	123.5	82.7
8. Mets	9.6	10.5	91.2	73.4
9. Anaerobic threshold	1.4	1.6	91.1	73.6
10. ST changes:	0.0		Time onset:	0.0
11. Rhythm:	Slightly abnormal			
D. Pulmonary Function Test				
	Measured	*Pred. mean*	*% Pred.*	*PA*
1. FVC (l)	4.3	4.6	93.5	71.7
2. FEV1 (l)	3.3	3.1	106.1	63.2
3. %FEV1/FVC	77.4	68.2	113.5	59.0
4. MVV (l/min)	157.7	122.3	128.9	52.0
5. FEF (25–75%)	3.1	2.8	110.2	60.8
E. Vascular Compliance Tests				
1. STI	0.4	0.4	100.0	67.0
2. PTT	55.0	50.0	110.0	73.7

F. Muscular Strength and Endurance Tests							
	RT	*LT*	*RT*	*LT*	*RT*	*LT*	*Mean*
1. Hand grip (kg)	37.0	30.0	37.0	30.0	100.0	100.0	67.0
2. Elbow flexion	4.0	4.0	4.0	4.0	100.0	100.0	67.0
G. Opthalmological Evaluation							
	Measured		*Pred. mean*		*% Pred.*		*PA*
	RT	*LT*	*RT*	*LT*	*RT*	*LT*	*Mean*
1. Pupil size, dark	6.0	6.0	6.0	6.0	100.0	100.0	67.0
2. Pupil size, light	4.0	4.0	4.0	4.0	100.0	100.0	67.0

Figure 2 Aging profile of a subject with a similar physiological age and CA (continued).

	Measured		*Pred. mean*		*% Pred.*		*PA*
	RT	*LT*	*RT*	*LT*	*RT*	*LT*	*Mean*
3. Pupil cyc. time	0.0	0.0	0.0	0.0	100.0	100.0	67.0
4. Accom. amplitude	1.0	1.0	1.0	1.0	100.0	100.0	67.0
5. Arcus senilis	0.0	0.0	0.0	0.0	100.0	100.0	67.0

H. Psychological Evaluation

	Measured	*Ideal*	*%Ideal*
1. Vocabulary age	19.0	21.0	90.5
2. Abstract age	14.2	20.5	69.3
3. Mental age	16.9	20.8	81.3
4. Memory quotient	119.0	130.0	91.5
5. I.Q.	118.0	145.0	81.4

I. Blood Chemistry & HDL

	Measured	*Normal range*
1. Glucose (mg%)	120.0	65–110
2. Uric acid (mg%)	5.9	3.0–6.5
3. Creatine (mg%)	1.2	0.5–1.4
4. SGOT (IU/l)	15.0	5.0–25.0
5. Cholesterol (mg%)	238.0	150–250
6. HDL chol (mg/ml)	66.0	48–84
7. Ratio LDLC/HDLC	3.6	2.9–3.1

Summary:

Mean physiological age:	67.4
Chronological age:	67

Comment: Although the overall performance was good the reduced exercise capacity and oxygen uptake leave room for improvement. There is evidence that regular exercise not only improves fitness, but improves brain function and slows degenerative processes. Attention to an active lifestyle, proper weight, and nutrition would probably reduce physiological age. Based upon your performance your physiological age is 67.4 years. The difference between your chronological and physiological age is –0.4 years.

VI. DISCUSSION

Hypothetical relationships between CA and physiological age or BA have been proposed by Ward.[40] For each yearly increment of CA, the BA increases by 1 year (Figure 17). Persons with sedentary habits, who thrive on unbalanced diets and poor nutrition might "score older biologically than chronological age and thus would probably age faster than one year for each additional year of CA"[40] as in Figure 18. Figure 19 shows that age-retarding programs such as proper exercise, diet, and nutrition might hypothetically reverse the biological or physiological aging process. It is possible that some may attain a BA lower than their CA, as in Figure 20. Only 21 (30%) of the 71 male subjects in our study showed a lower physiological age or BA than their CA. The mean values of CA and BA were 54.15 ± 15.35 (S.D.) and 52.45 ± 4.12 (S.D.) years, respectively, in these 21 male subjects. Interestingly, all 21 subjects had a higher $VO_{2\ max}$ and lower body weight (i.e., higher $VO_{2\ max}$/kg) and all of them were nonsmokers, exercised regularly, and had an active lifestyle with a good diet and good nutrition.

Figure 3 Aging profile of a subject with a lower BA compared to CA.

A. Physical Characteristics						Age: 72		Sex: M
	Measured		*Ideal*		*% Expected*			*PA*
1. Height (in.)	71.0		71.0		100.0			72.0
2. Weight (lb)	158.0		164.8		95.9			69.0
3. BSA (M^2)	1.9		1.9		98.5			70.9
4. % Body fat	12.4		16.0		77.5			55.8
B. Health Questionnaire								
1. Positive = 12%								
2. Ponderal index	31.3		32.7		95.9			69.0
C. Max. Treadmill Exercise Test								
	Measured		*Ideal*		*% Expected*			*PA*
1. $VO_{2\ max}$ (l/min)	2.9		2.2		132.3			54.4
2. $VO_{2\ max}$/kg/min (ml)	40.0		29.0		137.9			52.2
3. C.V. efficiency	2.4		1.2		190.3			37.8
4. Exercise time	13.8		11.0		125.5			57.4
5. Max. hr/min	146.0		148.0		98.6			73.0
6. Max. BP syst.	220.0		190.0		115.8			83.4
7. Max. BP diast.	105.0		100.0		105.0			75.6
8. Mets	11.5		8.7		132.3			54.4
9. Anaerobic threshold	1.7		1.3		132.3			54.4
10. ST changes:	1.0				Time onset:			4.0
11. Rhythm:	Slightly abnormal							
D. Pulmonary Function Test								
	Measured		*Pred. mean*		*% Pred.*			*PA*
1. FVC (l)	4.6		4.5		103.8			69.4
2. FEV1 (l)	3.7		3.0		126.3			57.0
3. %FEV1/FVC	80.8		66.4		121.6			59.2
4. MVV (l/min)	170.1		118.3		143.9			50.0
5. FEF (25–75%)	4.3		2.6		163.6			44.0
E. Vascular Compliance Tests								
1. STI	0.3		0.3		100.0			72.0
2. PTT	40.0		40.0		100.0			72.0
F. Muscular Strength and Endurance Tests								
	RT	*LT*	*RT*	*LT*	*RT*	*LT*		*Mean*
1. Hand grip (kg)	36.0	20.0	36.0	20.0	100.0	100.0		72.0
2. Elbow flexion	35.0	32.0	35.0	32.0	100.0	100.0		72.0
G. Opthalmological Evaluation								
	Measured		*Pred. mean*		*% Pred.*			*PA*
	RT	*LT*	*RT*	*LT*	*RT*	*LT*		*Mean*
1. Pupil size, dark	4.5	4.5	4.5	4.5	100.0	100.0		72.0
2. Pupil size, light	3.0	3.0	3.0	3.0	100.0	100.0		72.0

Figure 3 Aging profile of a subject with a lower BA compared to CA (continued).

	Measured		*Pred. mean*		*% Pred.*		*PA*
	RT	*LT*	*RT*	*LT*	*RT*	*LT*	*Mean*
3. Pupil cyc. time	0.0	0.0	0.0	0.0	100.0	100.0	72.0
4. Accom. amplitude	0.9	0.7	0.9	0.7	100.0	100.0	72.0
5. Arcus senilis	0.0	0.0	0.0	0.0	100.0	100.0	72.0

H. Psychological Evaluation

	Measured	*Ideal*	*%Ideal*
1. Vocabulary age	19.4	21.0	92.4
2. Abstract age	15.7	20.5	76.6
3. Mental age	17.1	20.8	82.2
4. Memory quotient	103.0	130.0	79.2
5. I.Q.	120.0	145.0	82.8

I. Blood Chemistry & HDL

	Measured	*Normal range*
1. Glucose (mg%)	102.0	65–110
2. Uric acid (mg%)	5.0	3.0–6.5
3. Creatine (mg%)	0.8	0.5–1.4
4. SGOT (IU/l)	20.0	5.0–25.0
5. Cholesterol (mg%)	249.0	150–250
6. HDL chol (mg/ml)	67.0	48–84
7. Ratio LDLC/HDLC	3.7	2.9–3.1

Summary:

Mean physiological age: 64.5

Chronological age: 72

Comment: The overall performance was excellent. The good scores in the exercise and pulmonary function tests reduced your physiological age. This is associated with an active life style which reduces degenerative disease and atrophy of disuse. Based on your performance, your physiological age is 64.5 years. The difference between your chronological and physiological age is 7.5 years.

Only 9 (11%) of our 84 female subjects showed a lower physiological age than their CA. Their mean CA was 59.55 years ± 13.08 (S.D.) and their BA was 53.85 years ± 5.23 (S.D.). These subjects were enrolled in an aerobic exercise training program and had a higher $VO_{2\ max}$ than our other female subjects.

Our findings suggest that regularly prescribed exercise, non-smoking, an active lifestyle, and good diet and nutrition are associated with physiological ages lower than CAs. It is well known that a defined exercise training program with proper diet and nutrition significantly increases maximum oxygen uptake and this may explain the relationship we found between $VO_{2\ max}$ and BA–CA. A total of 70% of our male subjects and 89% of our female subjects had higher physiological ages than their CAs. These subjects had sedentary lifestyles which may have contributed to these findings.

There is little evidence that elderly persons are less physically active than younger persons. The Framingham Heart Study supports the view that customary daily physical activity decreases with aging. Interpretation of studies seeking to relate age and physical condition is difficult. Prevalent social attitudes mitigate against even moderate physical activity in the elderly because of vague fears that too much exercise will precipitate injury, exhaustion, or overt illness. It might

Figure 4 Aging profile of a subject with a higher BA than CA.

A. Physical Characteristics					Age: 58		Sex: F
	Measured		*Ideal*		*% Expected*		*PA*
1. Height (in.)	65.0		65.0		100.0		58.0
2. Weight (lb)	160.0		137.0		116.8		67.7
3. BSA (M^2)	1.8		1.7		107.1		62.1
4. % Body fat	34.0		23.0		147.8		85.7
B. Health Questionnaire							
1. Positive = 12%							
2. Ponderal index	38.0		33.0		115.2		66.8
C. Max. Treadmill Exercise Test							
	Measured		*Ideal*		*% Expected*		*PA*
1. $VO_{2\ max}$ (l/min)	1.3		2.1		61.4		94.5
2. $VO_{2\ max}$/kg/min (ml)	17.2		33.0		52.1		111.3
3. C.V. efficiency	0.9		1.9		45.0		128.8
4. Exercise time	4.8		10.0		48.0		120.8
5. Max. hr/min	138.0		168.0		82.1		70.6
6. Max. BP syst.	220.0		177.0		124.3		72.1
7. Max. BP diast.	100.0		81.0		123.5		71.6
8. Mets	5.0		9.0		55.6		104.4
9. Anaerobic threshold	0.7		1.2		54.0		107.3
10. ST changes:	0.0				Time onset:		0.0
11. Rhythm:	None						
D. Pulmonary Function Test							
	Measured		*Pred. mean*		*% Pred.*		*PA*
1. FVC (l)	2.7		3.2		84.4		68.7
2. FEV1 (l)	1.6		2.4		66.7		87.0
3. %FEV1/FVC	59.3		75.0		79.0		45.8
4. MVV (l/min)	61.0		95.0		64.2		90.3
5. FEF (25–75%)	0.9		2.7		33.3		174.0
E. Vascular Compliance Tests							
1. STI	0.3		0.3		100.0		58.0
2. PTT	45.0		45.0		100.0		58.0
F. Muscular Strength and Endurance Tests							
	RT	*LT*	*RT*	*LT*	*RT*	*LT*	*Mean*
1. Hand grip (kg)	26.0	20.0	26.0	20.0	100.0	100.0	58.0
2. Elbow flexion	40.0	37.0	40.0	37.0	100.0	100.0	58.0
G. Opthalmological Evaluation							
	Measured		*Pred. mean*		*% Pred.*		*PA*
	RT	*LT*	*RT*	*LT*	*RT*	*LT*	*Mean*
1. Pupil size, dark	6.5	6.5	6.5	6.5	100.0	100.0	58.0
2. Pupil size, light	3.0	3.0	3.0	3.0	100.0	100.0	58.0

Figure 4 Aging profile of a subject with a higher BA than CA (continued).

	Measured		*Pred. mean*		*% Pred.*		*PA*
	RT	*LT*	*RT*	*LT*	*RT*	*LT*	*Mean*
3. Pupil cyc. time	0.8	0.9	0.8	0.9	100.0	100.0	58.0
4. Accom. amplitude	0.6	0.7	0.6	0.7	100.0	100.0	58.0
5. Arcus senilis	1.0	1.0	1.0	1.0	100.0	100.0	58.0

H. Psychological Evaluation

	Measured	*Ideal*	*%Ideal*
1. Vocabulary age	13.5	21.0	64.3
2. Abstract age	12.5	20.5	61.0
3. Mental age	12.9	20.8	62.0
4. Memory quotient	129.0	130.0	99.2
5. I.Q.	129.0	145.0	89.0

I. Blood Chemistry & HDL

	Measured	*Normal range*
1. Glucose (mg%)	107.0	65–110
2. Uric acid (mg%)	4.6	3.0–6.5
3. Creatine (mg%)	0.8	0.5–1.4
4. SGOT (IU/l)	20.0	5.0–25.0
5. Cholesterol (mg%)	220.0	150–250
6. HDL chol (mg/ml)	66.0	48–84
7. Ratio LDLC/HDLC	3.3	2.9–3.1

Summary:

Mean physiological age:	78.9
Chronological age:	58

Comment: The finding of a significantly higher physiological age than desirable indicates a need for attention to regular activity and a change of lifestyle in the direction of overall health habits. These results should be discussed with your physician, who can use this report to direct your program. Based on your performance, your physiological age is 78.9 years. The difference between your chronological and physiological age is –20.9 years.

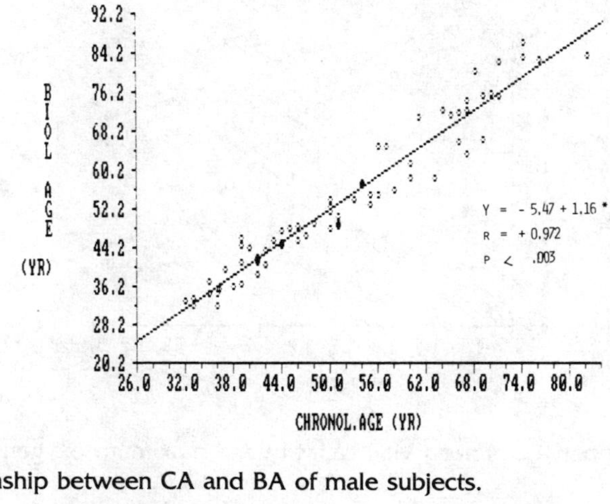

Figure 5 Relationship between CA and BA of male subjects.

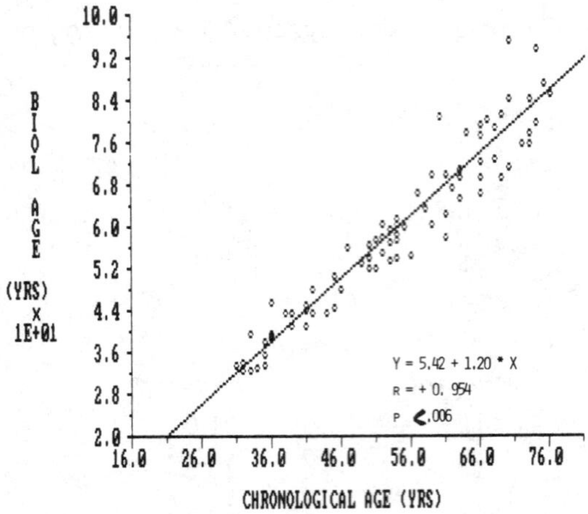

Figure 6 Relationship between CA and BA of female subjects.

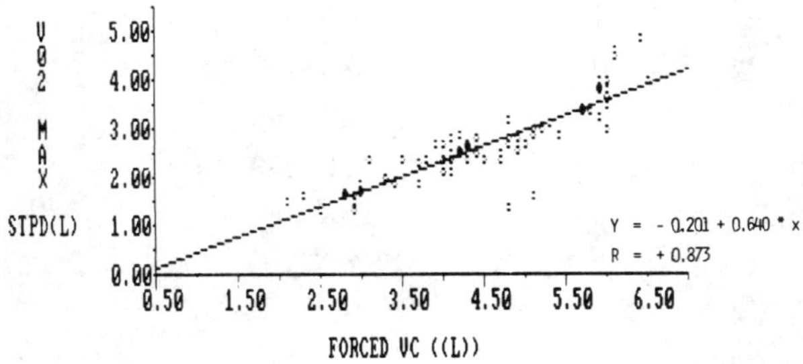

Figure 7 Relationship between forced vital capacity and maximum oxygen uptake in our male volunteers.

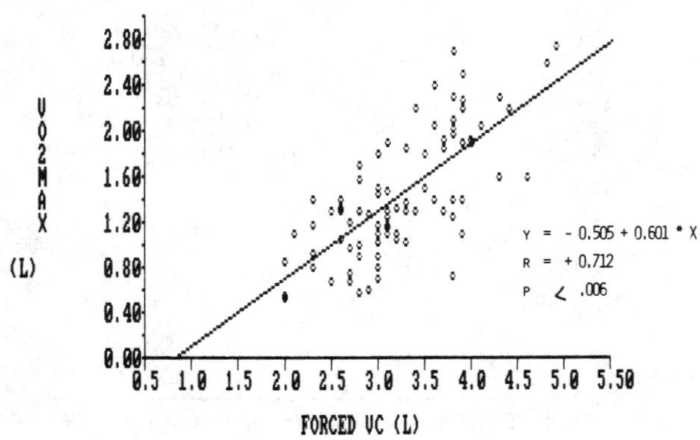

Figure 8 Relationship between forced vital capacity and maximum oxygen uptake in our female volunteers.

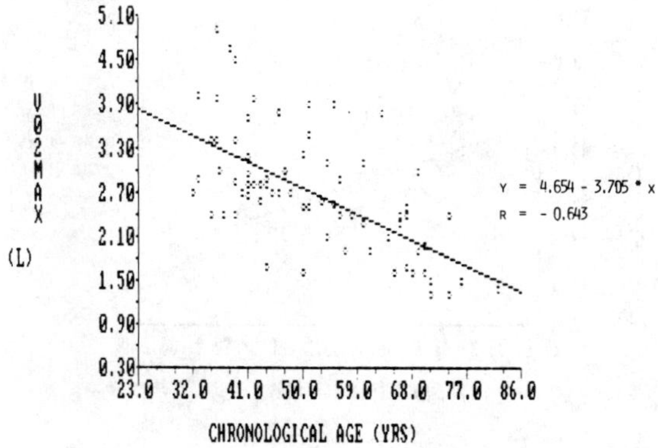

Figure 9 Relationship between maximum oxygen uptake and CA in our male subjects.

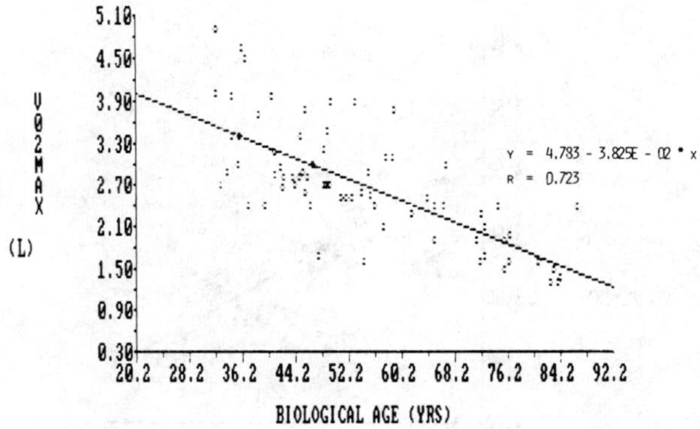

Figure 10 Relationship between maximum oxygen uptake and BA in our male subjects.

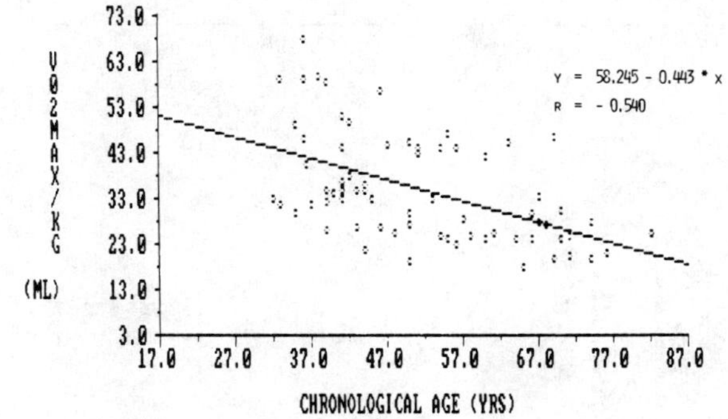

Figure 11 $VO_{2\ max}$/kg body weight of our male subjects plotted against CA.

be possible, however, for elderly persons to arrest or reverse physical deterioration by maintaining their levels of physical activity.

Age-related measurements of physical work capacity indicate a marked decline in maximum oxygen uptake with increasing age.[45,46] A low capacity for physical work in the elderly may be due in part to low levels of customary physical activity. Increased activity levels through training

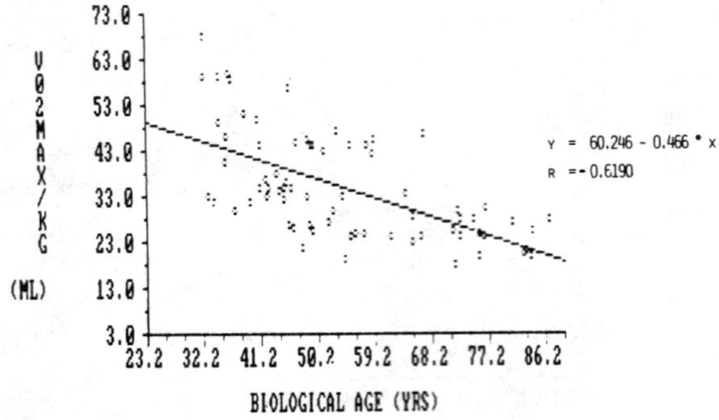

Figure 12 Relationship between BA and $VO_{2\ max}$/kg body weight in our male subjects.

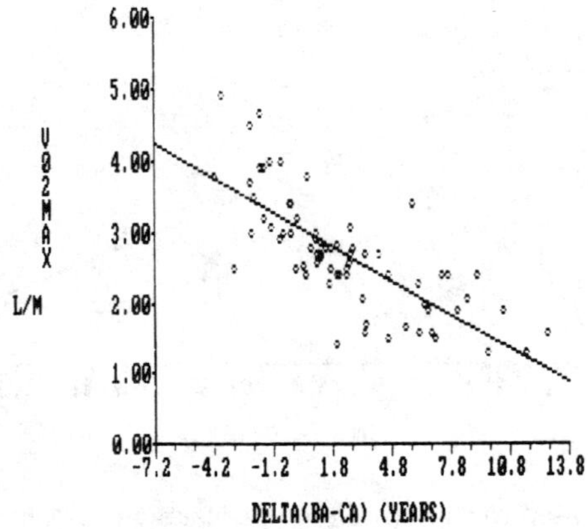

Figure 13 Relationship between maximum oxygen uptake and the difference between BA and CA in our male subjects.

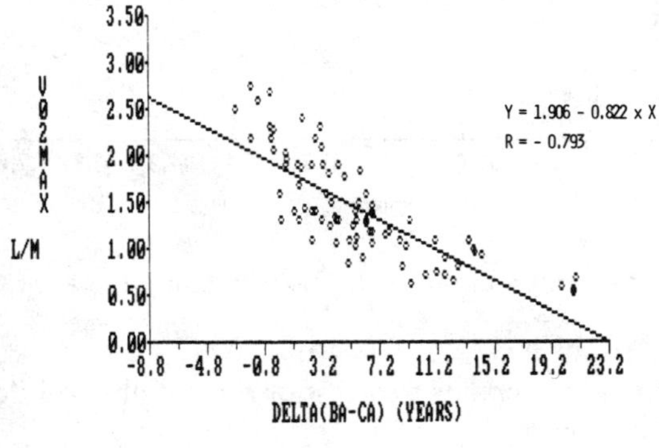

Figure 14 Relationship between maximum oxygen uptake and the difference between BA and CA in our female subjects.

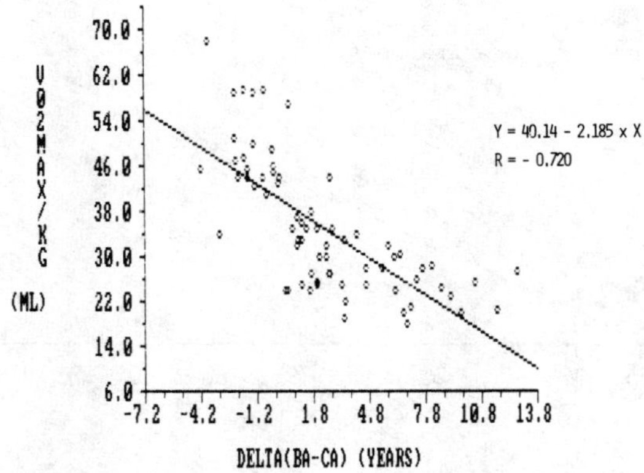

Figure 15 Relationship between $VO_{2\ max}$/kg body weight of our male subjects and the difference between BA and CA.

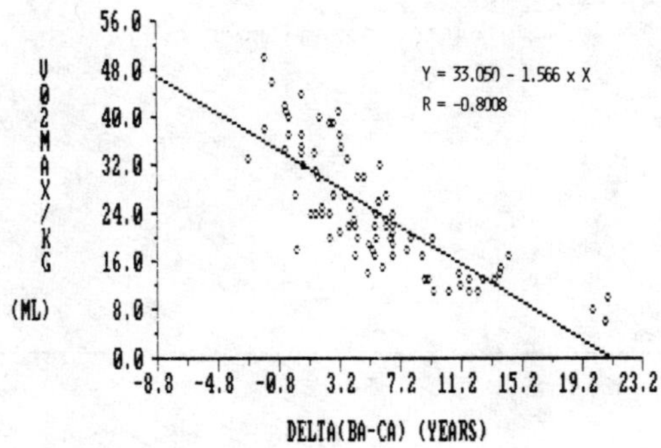

Figure 16 Relationship between $O_{2\ max}$/kg body weight and the difference between BA and CA in our female subjects.

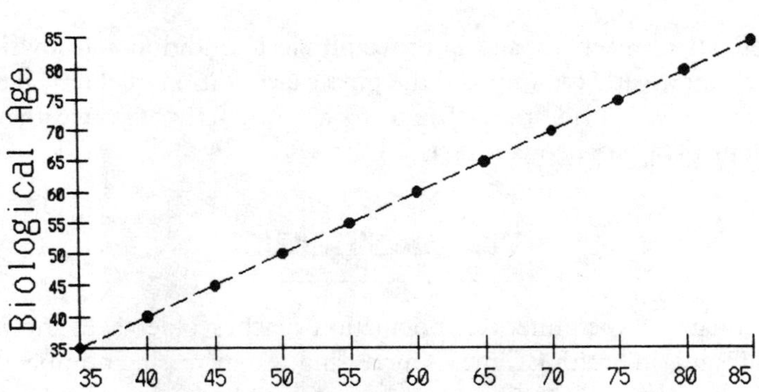

Figure 17 **Normal aging**. Note that the biological age normally increases by 1 year for each year of CA. (From Dean, W., *Biological Aging Measurement-Clinical Application,* 2nd ed., The Center for Bio-Gerontology, Los Angeles, 1988. With permission.)

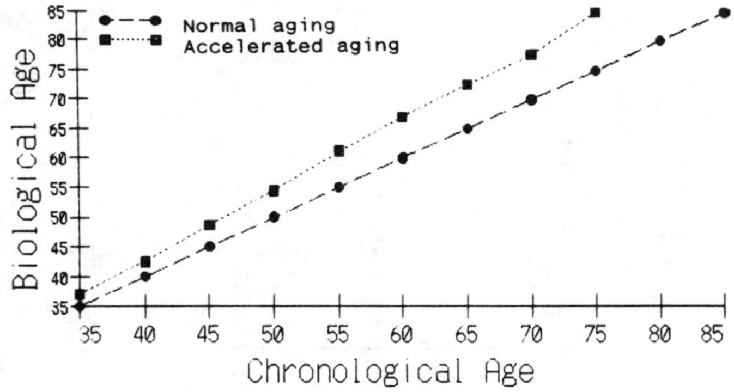

Figure 18 **Accelerated aging**. Accelerated aging may be caused by environmental insults such as poor diet, smoking, excess drinking, or inadequate exercise. Note that BA is increasing more than 1 year for each year of CA. (From Dean, W., *Biological Aging Measurement-Clinical Application,* 2nd ed., The Center for Bio-Gerontology, Los Angeles, 1988. With permission.)

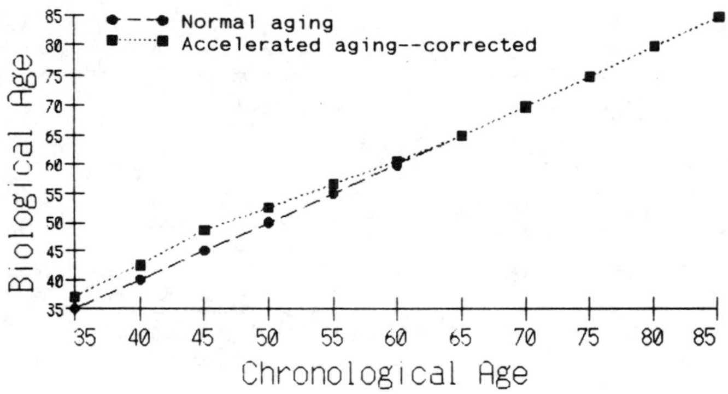

Figure 19 **Corrected accelerated aging**. After the rapidly aging person in Figure 18 improved his lifestyle, the aging rate returned to near "normal" (From Dean, W., *Biological Aging Measurement-Clinical Application,* 2nd ed., The Center for Bio-Gerontology, Los Angeles, 1988. With permission.)

can reverse the effects of inactivity and improve physical condition and physical work capacity in the elderly. Training clearly can improve the physical condition of elderly persons, but it gives no lasting benefit unless it leads to a change to a more active lifestyle that incorporates an appropriate amount of spontaneous exercise.

VII. SIGNIFICANCE

As a larger percentage of the American population reaches older age, the impact of age on American social life and on health facilities is increasing. An increasing number of our subjects are in ages previously thought to be associated with senility and poor function; instead, these people are leading active, productive lives and the understanding of the factors related to their health is vital. The exercise literature is beginning to reflect evidence that certain lifestyle changes will dramatically alter the function of older people. Although this certainly holds true in relationship to cardiac output and aerobic capacity, there are few data to demonstrate what kind of effect this

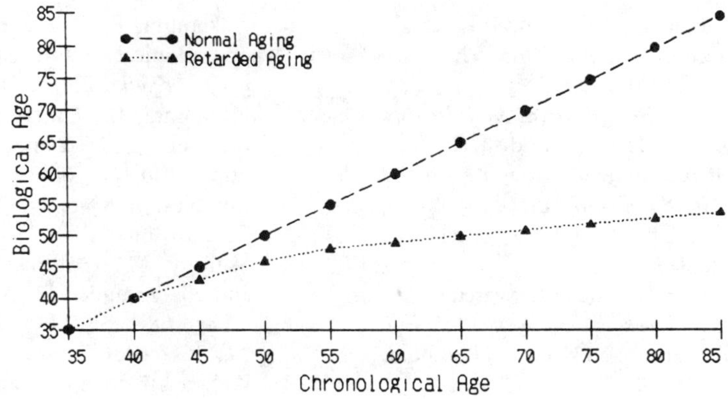

Figure 20 **Highly effective age-retarding program.** There is an almost negligible increase in BA for each year of CA. An extended maximum life span may result. (From Dean, W., *Biological Aging Measurement-Clinical Application,* 2nd ed., The Center for Bio-Gerontology, Los Angeles, 1988. With permission.)

has on brain function. It is believed, however, that it improves self-confidence and promotes better relaxation. It is already known that strenuous exercise causes more rapid deterioration of certain parts of the musculoskeletal system. It therefore appears that regular aerobic exercise is important. Bruce[15] has shown that even mild exercise in older subjects results in conditioning.

We believe that an across the board evaluation of various systems in aging is essential for a better understanding of the changes that are occurring. We also believe this type of testing will be useful, particularly for those people who are entering certain types of programs which they perceive will improve their function, such as special diets, certain types of exercise, transcendental meditation and a myriad of other approaches to health which are now in vogue. Only by obtaining accurate measurements and correlating these with subsequent degenerative processes and illnesses can we advise our subjects as to the best course of action. There is much controversy over the advisability of mandatory retirement at set CAs. Retirement age based on BA might be more meaningful.

VIII. SUMMARY AND CONCLUSIONS

We randomly selected 155 normal male and female volunteers from Los Angeles, Long Beach, and Orange County (mean ages 52.42 and 53.85 years, respectively) to study the effect of aerobic exercise on physiological or biological aging. We measured physiological variables at rest and during maximal exercise. Among 33 variables, maximum oxygen uptake correlated best with biological aging. The greater the difference between BA and CA, the higher the work efficiency. Dynamic testing seems to give the most meaningful results.

REFERENCES

1. Woodruff, D. and Birren, J.E., Eds., *Aging: Scientific Perspectives and Social Issues,* Van Nostrand, New York, 1975.
2. Cole, J.O. and Barret, J.E., Eds., *Psychopathology in the Aged,* Raven Press, New York, 1980.
3. Timiras, P.S., Physiology of aging, in *Medical Physiology,* Mountcastle, V.B., Ed., C.V. Mosby, 1980.
4. Larry, P.P., Prescribing for the elderly, PSG Publishing, Littleton, MA, 1981.

5. Lowenthal, M.F., Berkman, P.L. et al., Eds., *Aging and Mental Disorder,* Jossey Bass, San Francisco, 1967.
6. Shepard, R.J., Ed., *Physical Activity and Aging,* Crohn Helm, London, 1978.
7. Klocke, R.A., Influence of aging on the lung, in *Handbook of the Biology of Aging,* Klocke, R.A., Ed., Van Nostrand Reinhold, New York, 1978.
8. Kohn, R.A., Heart and cardiovascular system, in *Handbook of the Biology of Aging,* Klocke, R.A., Ed., Van Nostrand Reinhold, New York, 1978.
9. Simonson, E., Performance as a function of age and cardiovascular disease, in *Aging and the Nervous System,* Welford, A.T. and Birren, J.E., Eds., Charles C Thomas, Springfield, IL, 1965.
10. Brody, H. and Vijayashaukar, N., Anatomical changes in the nervous system, in *Aging and the Nervous System,* Welford, A.T. and Birren, J.E., Eds., Charles C Thomas, Springfield, IL, 1965.
11. Woodruff, D.S. and Birren, J.E., *Physiology of Exercise and Aging: Aging in Broad Perspective,* Van Nostrand, New York, 1975.
12. Sokolov, P.N., Senile changes of morphological signs in women, *Arkh. Biol. Nauk,* 39(2), 473, 1935.
13. Voitenko, V.P. and Tokar, A.V., The assessment of BA and sex differences of human aging, *Exp. Aging Res.,* 9(4), 1983.
14. Borkan, G. and Norris, A.H., BA in adulthood: comparison of active and inactive U.S. males, *Hum. Biol.,* 52, 787, 1980.
15. Bruce, R.A., Exercise, functional aerobic capacity and aging: another viewpoint, *Med. Sci. Sports Exercise,* 16, 8, 1984.
16. Bruce, R.A., Functional aerobic capacity, exercise and aging, in *Principles of Geriatric Medicine,* Andres, R., Bierman, E.L., and Hazzard, W.R., Eds., McGraw-Hill, New York, 1985, 87.
17. Larson, E.B. and Bruce, R.A., Health benefits of exercise in an aging society, *Arch. Intern. Med.,* 147, 1987.
18. Dundikova, V.A., Silvon, Z.K., and Dubina, T.L., Biological age and its estimation, *Exp. Gerontol.,* 16, 13, 1978.
19. Furukawa, T., Inoue, M., Kajiya, F., and Abe, H., Assessment of biological age by multiple regression analysis, *J. Gerontol.,* 30, 422, 1975.
20. Nakamura, E., The aged people and its physiological ages in relation to work capacity, *Kyoiku Igaku,* 28, 2, ??.
21. Nakamura, E., The assessment of physiological age based upon a principal component analysis of various physiological variables, *J. Kyoto Pref. Univ. Med.,* 94, 757, 1985.
22. Skalicky, M., Hofecker, G., Kment, A., and Niedermuller, H., Models of biological age of the rat (11), *Mech. Aging Dev.,* 14, 361, 1980.
23. Webster, J.W. and Logie, R., A relationship between age and health status in female subjects, *J. Gerontol.,* 31, 546, 1976.
24. Chodzko-Zajko, W.J. and Ringel, R.L., Physiological fitness measures and sensory and motor performance in aging, *Exp. Gerontol.,* 22, 317, 1987.
25. Chodzko-Zajko, W.J., American Aging Association, San Francisco, 1988 (abstract).
26. Damon, A., Predicting age from body measurements and observations, *Aging Hum. Dev.,* 2, 169, 1972.
27. Borkan, G.A. and Norris, A.J., Assessment of BA using a profile of physical parameters, *J. Gerontol.,* 55, 177, 1980.
28. Borkan, G.A. and Bachman, S.S., Comparison of visually estimated age with physiological predicted age as indicators of rates of aging, *Soc. Sci. Med.,* 16, 197, 1982.
29. Dirken, J.M., The Development of a Measuring Device for Determining the Functional Age of Elderly Industrial Workers, Netherlands Institute for Preventive Medicine, Amsterdam, 1963.
30. Wester, I.A. and Logie, A,R., A relationship between functional age and health status in female subjects, *J. Gerontol.,* 31(5), 546, 1976.
31. Furukawa, T., Inoue, M., Kajiya, F., Inada, H., Takasugi, S., Fukui, S., Takeda, H., and Abe, H., Assessment of BA by multiple regression analysis, *J. Gerontol.,* 30(4), 422, 1975.
32. Shimokata, H., Shibata, K., and Kuzuya, F., Assessment of biological aging status, *J. Jpn. Soc. Intern. Med.,* 74, 1344, 1985.
33. Heikkinen, E., Assessment of functional aging, in *Lectures on Gerontology,* Vol. 1, *On Biology of Aging,* Part B, Vidik, A., Ed., Academic Press, New York, 1982.
34. Heikkinen, E., Kiiskinen, A., Kayhty, B., Rimpela, M., and Vuori, I., Assessment of biological age, *Gerontologia,* 20, 33, 1974.

35. Heikkinen, E., Arajarvi, R.L., Era, P., Jylha, M., Klinnunen, V., Liskinen, A.L., Leskinen, E., Masseli, E., Pohjoloainen, P., Rahkila, P., Suominen, H., Turpeinen, P., Vaisanen, M., and Osterback, L., Functional capacity of men born in 1906-10, 1926-50. A basic report, *Scand J. Soc. Med. Suppl.,* 33, 1984.
36. Ries, W. and Pöthig, D., Chronological and biological age, *Exp. Gerontol.,* 19, 211, 1984.
37. Dubina, T.L., Mints, A.Y., and Zhuk, E.V., Biological age and its estimation. III. Introduction of a correlation to the multiple regression mode of biological age and assessment of biological age in cross-sectional and longitudinal studies, *Exp. Gerontol.,* 19, 133, 1984.
38. Mints, A.Y., Dubina, T.L., Lysenyk, V.P., and Zhuk, E.V., Determination of individual Biological age and evaluation of aging degree, *Physiol. Zh.,* 30(1), 39, 1984.
39. Timiras, P., *Developmental Physiology and Aging,* Macmillan, New York, 1972.
40. Dean, W., *Biological Aging Measurement-Clinical Application,* 2nd ed., The Center for Bio-Gerontology, Los Angeles, 1988.
41. Ellestad, M.H., *Stress Testing: Principles and Practice,* 3rd ed., F.A. Davis, Philadelphia, 1986.
42. Masaro, E.J., Adelman, R.C., and Roth, G.S., Eds., *Handbook of Physiology in Aging,* CRC Press, Boca Raton, FL, 1981.
43. Morris, J.F. et al., Spirometric standards for healthy nonsmoking adults, *Am. Rev. Resp. Dis.,* 103, 57, 1971.
44. Morris, J.F., Spirometry in the evaluation of pulmonary function, *West. J. Med.,* 125, 110, 1976.
45. Shock, N.W., Indices of functional age in aging: a challenge to science and society, in *Biology,* Vol. 1, Danen, D. et al., Eds., Oxford University Press, New York, 1981, 270.
46. Astrand, P.O. and Rodahl, K., *Textbook of Work Physiology; Physiological Basis of Exercise,* McGraw-Hill, New York, 1977, 320.

ORGAN SYSTEM APPROACHES

CHAPTER 18

THE MORPHOMETRIC ASSESSMENT OF BIOLOGICAL AGE

Frédéric C. Ludwig

Individuals may be young or old in relation to their number of years.[4] As a result, age-related disease or age-related death may occur at different chronological ages. The reasons for this variability are largely genetic.[17] It follows that the true or practically relevant age of an individual is not adequately defined by the time that has elapsed since birth, but by a figure reflecting the individual's vulnerability to environmental pressure (as long as this vulnerability is not altered by factors unrelated to age). The degree of age-related vulnerability is defined as "biological age". It is relevant to what follows (and implied by what has been stated above) that individuals of different chronological age may yield identical readings of biological age or vice versa. Gerontological research, whether focusing on the patient or on the experimental animal, aims to ascertain (or to achieve) verifiable discrepancies between the biological and the chronological age of organisms.

The age dependence of this vulnerability to environmental pressure is strikingly demonstrated by Table 1, which summarizes data from a clinic specializing in the treatment of severe burns.[1] The data presented are from patients with no lesions other than the burns themselves. While the LD-50 for infants is about 50% area burn, for the age group 15 to 44 it is about 40%, for the middle aged it is 23%, and for the elderly it is about 9%. These observations are of interest for two distinct but closely related reasons: first, they provide empirical evidence of the existence of a biological age (as defined at the outset), and, second, the progression of the changes underlying this biological age and the lethal effect of environmental pressure can be measured in terms of each other.

As long as we limit ourselves to the mere physical appearance of individuals, biological age is a characteristic that can be grasped intuitively, but eludes measurement. The fact that it is indeed a distinct biological entity and amenable to measurement is, as Comfort[5] first emphasized, only revealed by statistical studies of relatively large populations. The question is, therefore, can biological age be actually measured in individuals or small groups of individuals, and how?

What is expected when we talk about measuring biological age is in a sense the opposite of what has been done in Table 1: to quantitate directly the structural changes underlying this time-dependent progression of vulnerability with the purpose of estimating the possible effect of environmental pressure on survival. If environmental pressure were constant or predictable, this would depend solely on the choice of a suitable marker or battery of markers. However, in anything other than a carefully contrived experimental setting, the contribution of environmental pressure to individual life expectancy is uncontrollable and unpredictable regardless of how accurately intrinsic pathogenesis underlying vulnerability is assessed. For this reason I feel that measurement of biological age will be only feasible in the experimental animal, and the possible benefits of preventive manipulation of aging in men will be, in the foreseeable future, always based on generalizations from animal experiments.

0-8493-0129-7/94/$0.00+$.50

Table 1 Amount of area of burn resulting in death of patients of various age groups

Age group	Average age	Area burn resulting in death of 50% of patients	Area burn resulting in death of 25% of patients
0–14	5	51%	42%
15–44	31	43%	34%
45–64	55	23%	18%
65+	71	9%	5%

Measurement of aging, viewed as a target area for research, differs from other areas of gerontology in that conventional benchwork may not be the only and, in many instances, not the most effective way to bring about progress. The laboratory experiment, in focusing on one or two of the manifold expressions of aging, is necessarily limited to a minute aspect of a broad and complex issue. When considering measurement of biological age, analysis of existing data may, at this juncture, be as effective as laboratory experiments in improving our capability of measuring biological age.

In addition to exploration of the genetically conditioned variations in the rate of aging and their distribution in populations, a need exists to ascertain those variations that may result from experimentation with animals or preventive treatment of patients. As we have already pointed out, one obvious goal of gerontological research is to achieve, reproducibly and at will, a verifiable discrepancy between the chronological and biological age of animals and man. To the extent these attempts are successful, naturally occurring discrepancies between chronological and biological age may thus be superseded, complicated, or even offset by artificially induced discrepancies. To discriminate between both forms of discrepancy will cause intricate problems, both conceptually and technically. Genetic discrepancies between chronological and biological age may have structural causes different from those resulting from experimentation or preventive treatment.

At the present time, the approach to measurement of biological age is still predicated by one's definition of aging. If one assents to a biologically definable aging process, occurring in all phyla and in all species, one will be inclined to minimize or to disregard lethal disease when aging alone is assessed. In this perspective, lethal disease occurring from adulthood onward is a mere complication of the aging process. In contrast, if it can be postulated that biological age is the integrated expression of familiar (though not necessarily recognizable) diseases, its measurement would require a complete inventory of lesions detectable by *in vivo* testing and/or postmortem studies. Deceleration of aging would thus express itself by postponement of overall morbidity and acceleration of aging by its earlier than normal occurrence. What is then being measured is not the extent of an age-related change present in all individuals of the population, but the number of discrete diseases that individuals exhibit. This is probably what the Renaissance gerontologist in Lucas Cranach's painting of the Fountain of Youth of 1543 is doing. He is clad in a long red robe and inspects carefully a lady before allowing her to enter the Fountain. Because an individual develops only a fraction of the diseases his species is heir to, this approach entails observation of changes that may or may not be present in a particular individual.

Table 2 Number of lesions in 100 autopsies

Age group	Number of lesions
65–69	517
70–74	639
75–79	759
80–84	842

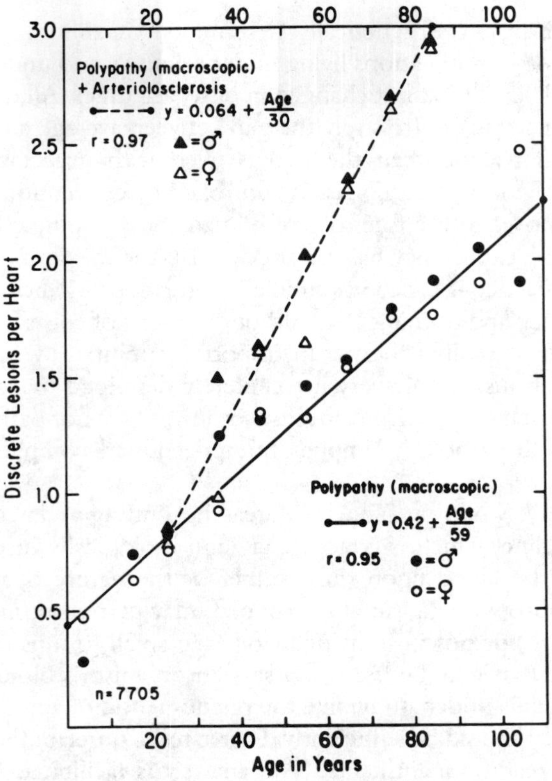

Figure 1 "Multiple pathology" of the human heart, based on 7000 autopsies from men and women.[29-31] Ordinate: number of discrete changes per heart; abscissa: age in years. The straight regression line represents macroscopic changes, the dotted regression line both macroscopic changes and arteriolosclerosis.

Attempts to assess biological age in this manner are on record (Table 2). Howell[21,22] and Howell and Piggot[23,24] have shown that in 100 autopsies of subjects in the age group of 65 to 69 years, 517 discrete lesions are observable; of those in the age group of 70 to 74 years, 639; of those in the age group of 75 to 79 years, 759; and of those in the age group of 80 to 84 years, 842. Linzbach and Akuamoa-Boateng,[29,30] in a remarkable study on 7000 human hearts from subjects newborn to 109 years old (summarized in Figure 1), demonstrated that from the third decade of life on the number of discrete cardiac lesions increases linearly with age. Senescence differs from younger age groups only in that identical diseases increase conspicuously in frequency; no lesion characterizes old age in a qualitative sense. In a later generalization of his work on the pathology of aging, Linzbach[31] postulated that this applies to all organs and to the organism as a whole. Independently emerging lesions interact and potentiate their respective influence on survival. If old age is nothing more than the integrated expression of discrete disease entities, the cure or prevention of one or several of them would amount to a modification of an individual's biological age. An individual demonstrably protected against development of prostatic carcinoma, diabetes, or coronary occlusion could claim to be younger than an individual at risk, even if both were born the same day.[34,35]

It should be noted that most gerontologists favor the existence of a time-dependent, irreversible aging process predisposing to, but not identical with, disease. The increase in life expectancy that medical care has brought is due to prevention of premature death caused by disease; it is not due to manipulation of aging. These diseases are complications but not causes of aging. This view, as Comfort[5,11] has shown, receives strong support from mortality statistics. The more that organisms are protected against disease, the greater and the more uniform their life expectancy. In contrast, the genetically determined maximum life expectancy remains unchanged; it is the same in populations living under primitive and under hygienically advanced conditions, and has in all likelihood not changed in historical times. All that contemporary health care accomplishes is to narrow progressively the gap between average and maximum life expectancy; the remaining interval between the two is filled with intractable, chronic-progressive conditions. As a result, the more that disease is controlled by conventional health care, the more the question of aging moves to the forefront of human and scientific concern.

Once the average life expectancy has caught up with the maximum life expectancy, health care as we define and practice it today has fulfilled its mission. Medicine will then be left with the problem of senescence and nothing else. Although this is, of course, an utopian abstraction, it enables us nonetheless to drive home an important point: old age, whether studied in individuals or in populations, is only very incompletely described by an inventory of diseases. The chronic conditions that emerge from adulthood onward are not pathogenetically unrelated, as the concept of "multiple pathology" implies, but indeed mere complications of an ubiquitous process called aging.

Current gerontology, when probing into areas beyond age-related disease, thus poses a universal process of decline, which is conceptually and biologically distinct from disease. The assessment of this may be based upon the number or the nature of the diseases individuals exhibit. Conventional autopsy data, suitably grouped, may permit estimating the extent of this process in large cohorts, but not in individuals or even small groups of individuals. The first criterion of any change that may be used to assess an organism's biological age is, therefore, occurrence in all individuals under study, like the phenomenon of aging itself. If several lesions are used in a battery, they should be sufficiently diverse to be unrelated to a single process.[7] Any such lesion should be readily quantifiable. The analysis is facilitated if lesions used for age assessment progress at comparable rates. They should furthermore provide significant readings using manageable sample sizes (a condition which is not easily met), and the slope of these readings should allow comparisons between all, or at least a wide variety of age groups. It is also desirable, though not indispensable, that lesions suitable for age assessment do not directly account for mortality. The most important criterion, however, and the most difficult to meet at the present state of the art, is proof that an age-related change does reflect viability and not mere chronological age. This requirement will need more discussion. What lesions might meet the criteria outlined above?

Gerontological literature abounds with reports on quantifiable age-related changes; it almost can be identified as an ever-expanding inventory of such changes. However, among the many changes described, surprisingly few have been evaluated with respect to their usefulness as biomarkers of age. Reports on age-dependent changes often lack the statistical data requisite for their evaluation as suitable measures of age. For instance, in explanted tissue fragments, the first cells emigrate after a latent period, the duration of which is positively correlated with the age of the donor.[41] To estimate the sample size required to determine a given decrement or increment of biological age by means of this technique, one would need raw data not included in the published report. However, in many instances these data are available, and the usefulness of an age-related change as a biomarker can be assessed.

Figure 2 shows a drawing, obtained by means of split beam optics, of thymic tissue coming from a 70-d-old rat. The shaded surfaces represent the cortical portion of a lobule, the open spaces in the center represent the medulla. The occasional dense spots are patches of connective tissue carrying vessels. Between the lobules is fat or connective tissue which is not identified here. Figure 3 shows the same tissue in a 170-d-old rat of the same strain.

At a glance, the tissue looks quite different. A rather complex process of restructuring has taken place which, at first sight, seems to elude quantitative assessment. What aspects may provide a basis for a quantitative comparison between these two different patterns? This parameter is the ratio of cortical over medullar surface, as determined by computerized planimetry.

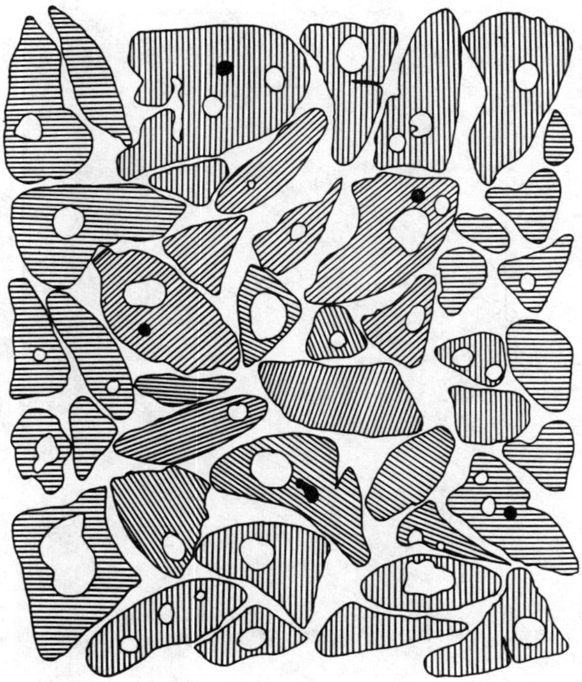

Figure 2 Thymic tissue from a 70-d-old male Buffalo rat. (Original magnification × 40.) The shaded part of a lobule is the cortex, the clear part in the center the medulla. Drawing obtained via split beam optics.

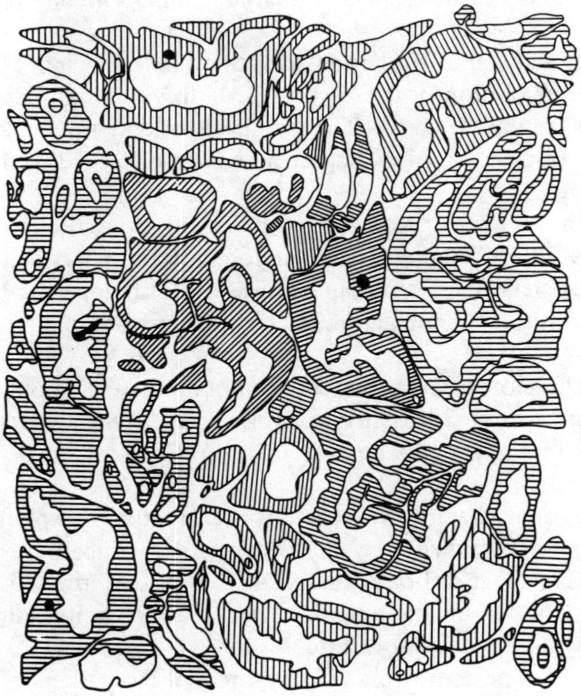

Figure 3 Same material and methods as in Figure 2. The thymus shown is from a 170-d-old male rat of the same strain.

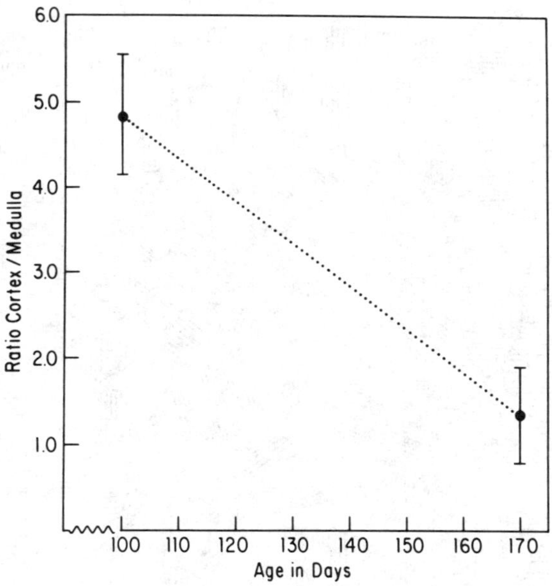

Figure 4 The ratio of cortical over medullar surface in sections of thymic tissue in 70- and 170-d-old male Buffalo rats.

A total of 10 to 12 sections per thymus have been used to assemble the lobules shown in the drawings. Such measurements reveal that during the time period under observation, the total surface of a lobule diminishes, the cortical mass gets smaller, and the medulla exhibits an increase. The most convenient parameter of this rather complex involution process is indeed this ratio (Figure 4).

This technique has allowed us to demonstrate that in syngeneic rat parabionts of different chronological age, the involution of the thymus is slightly but significantly postponed in the older member of the parabiotic pair.[46] The implications and the biological interest of this observation cannot be discussed in this chapter because it is limited to the technical aspects of measuring biological age.

Figure 5 shows an electron micrograph of the renal glomerulus of a 90-d-old rat, at a magnification of about 9000 diameters. Here, a glomerular capillary is hit transversely and the true thickness of its basement membrane can be measured.[10] It appears to be 0.8×10^3 Å in this specimen. Figure 6 shows the same structure, sectioned and magnified as in the previous figure, of a 580-d-old rat.

The thickness of the glomerular basement membrane here is about 2.8×10^3 Å, a nearly fourfold increase. Figure 7 summarizes more complete data on the age dependence of basement membrane thickening in the rat glomerulus, in an independent experiment carried out in Brazil.[40]

The two age-dependent changes we have just seen require morphometric methods to be measured. The first can be studied only in sequentially sacrificed experimental animals. In contrast, capillary basement membrane thickness can be determined not only in kidneys removed at autopsy, but also in muscle biopsies. Thus, it allows longitudinal studies in the same individual, although by an invasive procedure.

Table 3 summarizes some statistical data on potential biomarkers of aging. The thickness of the glomerular basement membrane,[32,33,40] the accumulation of lipofuscin in heart, liver, or nerve cells;[2,3,39,42] the emergence of reactive astrocytes in the hippocampus,[26,27] and the accumulation of chromosomal aberrations in regenerating postmitotic tissues[8,9] all reveal a linear,

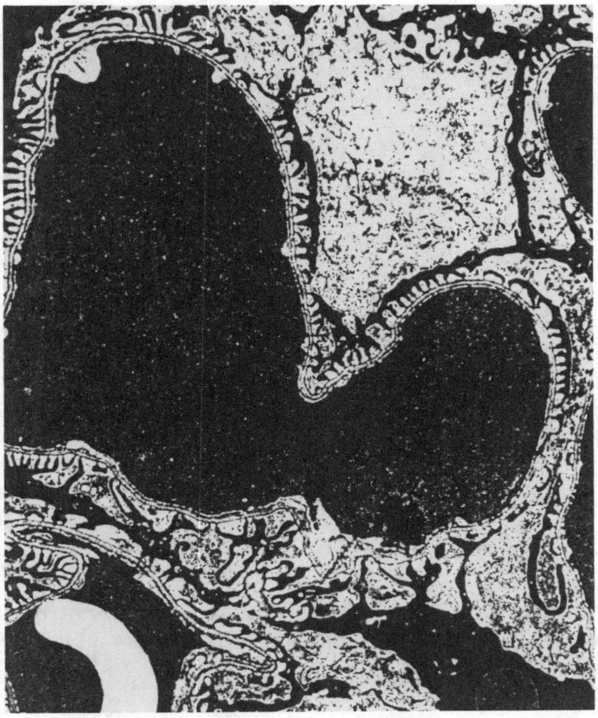

Figure 5 Renal glomerulus of a 90-d-old Buffalo rat. (Electron micrograph, original magnification × 9000. Thickness of capillary basement membrane 0.8 ×10^3 Å.)

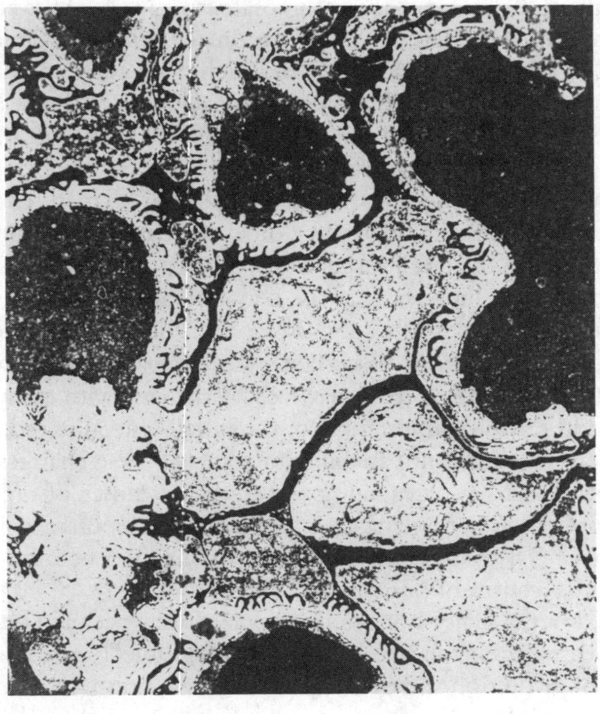

Figure 6 Renal glomerulus of 580-d-old Buffalo rat. Same technique as Figure 5. (Thickness of capillary basement membrane 2.8 × 10^3 Å.)

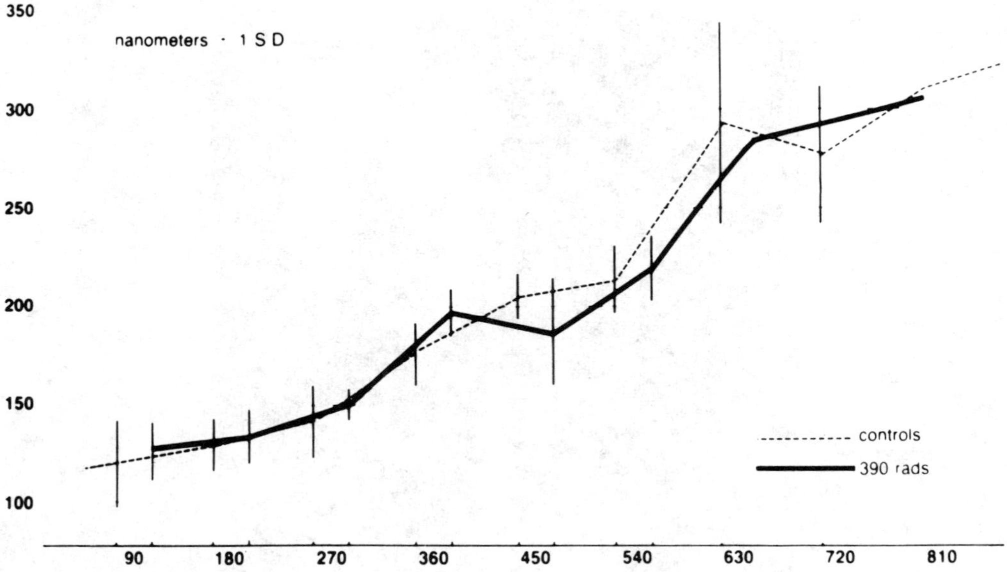

Figure 7 Age-related increase in the thickness of the glomerular basement membrane in male Wistar rats.[40] Whole body exposure to 390 rads of 200 kV X-rays has no recognizable influence on this age-related change.

though individual, rate of increase. In recent publications on positive correlations between oleic acid and linoleic acid absorption by the gut and chronological age,[19,20] one finds all the numerical data required to estimate slope functions and sample size, if one were to use this change for age assessment. Conversely, the count of neuronal cells of the central nervous system, be it in particular areas of the brain or in suspensions of sonicated brains, reveals losses that correlate with the age of the individual.[32,33] Other such decreasing parameters are the thermic contractility of collagen fibers,[43] the physiological capacitance of the stressed organism,[18] the proliferative response of spleen cells to T-cell mitogens,[38] and the cell doubling potential of skin fibroblasts.[12,14-16] To reveal a 10% departure from the assumed life expectancy of a particular species (always assuming the change reflects vulnerability, not mere chronological age), one would need 13 subjects if the thickness of the glomerular basement membrane is observed, 20 if one counts neuronal cells in brain cell suspensions, 39 if lipofuscin accumulation is measured,[42] 64 if reactive astrocytes of the hippocampus are counted, and 220 if the chromosomal aberrations in regenerating postmitotic tissues are assessed.[33] The data on chromosomal aberration suggest that the sample size required to ascertain a given departure from normal life expectancy is not the same in different species.[33] This may well be the case with many of the reported age-dependent changes, and provides an example of the pitfalls encountered in extrapolating from one species to another. The inherent variability of some of these changes is such that they are neither helpful in estimating biological age or likely to be causes of organismic aging.[35] It is surprising that this applies to phenomena such as spleen cell response to T cell mitogens or the regenerative potential of cells transferred into a culture medium because both are regarded by some authors as possible causes of organismic aging.[6,45]

As already pointed out, a major but often unrealized drawback in attempting assessment of biological age by measuring involutive change is a possible lack of correlation between a particular expression of involution and the viability of the organism that exhibits it. Does a given involutive change reflect biological age or is it only a "clock" revealing the time that has elapsed since birth or attainment of sexual maturity? All we know when observing organ weights, reactive astrocytes, or thermal contractility of collagen is that they vary as a function of

Table 3 Cohort size needed to reveal a 10 or 20% departure from assumed life expectancy for each of 12 parameters of biological age[33]

Nature of measurement	Species	Assumed life span (years)	Slope[a]	S.D.	n for given % of life span 10%	20%
Thickness of glomerular basement membrane, 10^3 Å	Rat	3	0.090	0.23	13	5
Neuronal cells, 10^6/g brain	Rat	3	–0.450	1.50	20	7
Chromosomal aberrations, % of abnormal mitoses at anaphase and telophase	Guinea pig	6	0.310	2.00	19	7
Thymus weight, mg	Mouse	2	–0.740	2.20	35	10
Lipofuscin accumulation in the Purkinje cell layer of cerebellum, % tissue volume	Rat	3	0.110	0.48	34	10
Reactive astrocytes in hippocampus, square root of %	Rat	3	0.140	0.85	64	18
Thermic contractility of tail tendon, mm	Rat	3	0.063	0.42	76	20
Physiological capacitance in the stressed organism (gram caloric output)	Mouse	2	–5.300	25.00	86	23
Spleen cell response to T cell mitogens, ratio PHA to Con A tritiated thymidine incorporation, mean count/min	Mouse	2	–0.013	0.10	220	60
Thyroxin degradation rate, mg thyroxin iodine/d	Man	70	–0.055	15.00	220	60
Chromosomal aberrations, % of abnormal mitoses at anaphase and telophase	Hamster	3	0.500	6.40	270	71
Cell doubling potential of skin fibroblasts, number of divisions of cultured cells	Man	70	–0.017	8.00	660	170

[a] *Rate of change per month.*

chronological age. Can we be certain when we alter experimentally the rate at which such a lesion progresses that the viability of the entire organism has been altered accordingly? In nearly all of the published work, such a correlation between whatever is being measured and organismic viability is silently assumed but never documented.[13] To substantiate this assumption when involutive change is measured is a major goal in any further work on measurement of aging.[36] It is also one of the objectives of the biomarker program of the National Institute on Aging.

To document a correlation between a given age-related change and viability, one would need to measure its extent in groups of individuals selected from populations large enough to determine the corresponding mortality rates (with the proviso that environmental pathogenesis is minimal). The age-related increase of glomerular basement membrane thickness may serve as an example. This change is clearly correlated with chronological age, occurs in all mammals including man, and appears to be less variable than many of the quantifiable expressions of involution described in the literature.[33,40] Such a change can be conveniently measured in cohorts aging at demonstrably different rates.[33] If, at a given chronological age, the order of basement membrane thickness is the inverse of the observed rates of aging, measurements would reflect biological age. Experiments of this type are costly and time consuming. They require comparisons between animal populations living in strictly controlled laboratory settings, and whose genetic characteristics are thoroughly understood. Harrison and Archer[13] have attempted this by looking for relationships between collagen changes, renal function, and longevity. Results suggest that aging is timed by more than one mechanism and that strong correlations with chronological age do not necessarily indicate that independent tests will be correlated with longevity or with each other. It is conceivable, however, as Comfort stressed several years ago, that this difficulty can be minimized by measuring a large number of unrelated changes,[7] unrelated in the sense that the different tests of a battery show little or no statistical correlation between themselves, beyond that imposed by their age dependence. Ingram asks whether the individual differences in such measurements reflect individual differences in biological age. The answer, as he points out, must be found through assessment of reliability, construct validity, internal consistency, and predictive validity of the measurements and tests employed.[25]

It should be noted that different inbred strains of the same species show different longevities, but it is far from clear that such differences are due to different rates of aging.[37] Interlaboratory comparisons or comparisons between data collected at different time periods are hampered not only by the interference of uncontrollable environmental variables, but different strains may exhibit different pathologies unrelated to age. It is probably safer to modify longevity by means of caloric restriction or administration of antioxidants than to rely on uncertain genetic differences, when comparisons between short- and long-lived cohorts are intended.

It was pointed out above that genetically conditioned discrepancies between chronological and biological age may require observation of changes different from those underlying artificially induced discrepancies. A set of changes suitable to assess genetically conditioned discrepancies between chronological and biological age[44] may fail to yield dependable readings when such discrepancies are artifacts, i.e., due to certain experimental conditions or preventive treatment. A specific preventive treatment may decelerate neuronal loss, another may be limited to muscular aging, still another may inhibit selectively lipofuscin accumulation. Moreover, measurements of biological age are attempted in organisms in which age is expected to change in response to experimental conditions that may have unknown or uncontrollable side effects. These conditions may affect one parameter of aging selectively, while leaving others unchanged, or influence them in ways which distort or even preclude conclusions regarding age. For instance, if life expectancy is modified by whole-body exposure to ionizing radiation, tumor incidence may respond in ways unrelated to modification of biological age itself.[23] Because empirical data on these contingencies are lacking, projects requiring assessment of biological age in different settings will always require extensive preliminary testing of the methods to be employed.

In conclusion, biological age can be assessed only by quantifying its epiphenomena, to the extent these epiphenomena can be quantified. The rate at which aging progresses varies from organ to organ. This variability between organs is not the same in individuals of the same species. Elucidation of aging at the molecular level will not remove the need for statistical approaches to its quantification, even if aging were traceable to a process common to all cells, extracellular structures, or organs. It would seem, therefore, that error-free ascertainment of an individual's biological age is an unattainable goal at this time. Chronological time is based on inanimate clocks progressing at constant rates, such as the rotation of the earth, chronometers, or radioactive decay, while biological time is based on molecular events, the occurrence of which is only predictable within certain limits. However, the statistical nature of biological aging does not preclude its measurement in cohorts, particularly of inbred experimental animals. In theory, the demonstration of an age-related change that is representative of many other such changes could make its ascertainment in individuals a more realistic goal.

Among the currently known biomarkers that may possibly meet the requirement of being representative of many others, the progressive thickening of capillary basement membranes, which was mentioned earlier in this chapter, deserves particular attention. In the experimental animal, it is probably a biomarker of choice. In man, it is likely to be important as well, despite the fact that it requires "invasive" methodology, although only mildly so. Muscle biopsies are a convenient method to determine the extent of this change in different body areas. The particular interest of capillary basement thickness as a biomarker of aging is suggested by the following.

Thickening of capillary basement is, in contrast to many other biomarkers reported in the literature, a truly universal expression of aging. It has been described in all laboratory animals thus far investigated, is observable in all tissues, and extensively documented in man. It has received relatively little attention among experimental gerontologists, presumably because it has been studied primarily by researchers interested in diabetes. All those studying progressive basement membrane thickening in diabetic patients have pointed out, however, that this change also increases with age in nondiabetic controls. Moreover, it is one of the most regular, if not *the* most regular, among the known morphometric expressions of aging. It should be noted that the data presented here are derived from measurements of the glomerular basement membrane only. Sampling within the same individual from different sites, particularly different skeletal muscles, will in all likelihood allow one to obtain the same result by using a much smaller population sample. Even significant comparisons between individuals may be possible, but here again we are faced with the same question as with other known measurable expressions of aging: does this change reflect viability or does it merely measure chronological age? Once the first is clearly demonstrated, capillary basement thickening may well emerge as a biomarker of choice, certainly in the animal. One should, however, not lose sight of the following: current gerontology, in insisting on empirical evidence for correlation with viability (instead of chronological age), may merely attempt to "force an already open door". Max Planck once wrote: "In science not only pure reason governs but also common sense", and common sense suggests that a diversified (i.e., biologically independent) battery of age-related changes (or an age-related change demonstrable in all organs of all mammalian species so far examined) are indeed biomarkers of aging, in the sense that such a battery will reflect, if properly analyzed, modifications of a normal rate of organismic aging. The concrete experience gathered over time, be it by clinically working physicians or scientists working in the laboratory, will sooner or later confirm or rectify the initial assumption.

If different organs age independently from one another,[13] and if measures designed to decelerate aging interfere with these independent progresses selectively, assessment of biological age will require batteries of tests that are comprehensive, diversified, and flexible, and which will require separate testing before they are applied to a particular clinical or experimental situation.

REFERENCES

1. Ball, J.P. and Squire, J.R., A study of mortality in a burn unit, *Ann. Surg.*, 130, 160, 1949.
2. Brody, H., Structural changes in the aging nervous system, in *The Regulatory Role of the Nervous System in Aging: Interdisciplinary Topics in Gerontology*, Vol. 7, S. Karger, Basel, 1970, 9.
3. Brody, H., An Examination of cerebral cortex and brain stem in aging, in *Neurobiology and Aging*, Terry, R.D. and Gershon, S., Eds., Raven Press, New York, 1976, 177.
4. Brocklehurst, J.C., *Textbook of Geriatric Medicine and Gerontology*, Churchill-Livingstone, Edinburgh, 1978, 341.
5. Comfort, A., *The Biology of Senescence*, Routledge & Kegan Paul, London, 1956, 257.
6. Comfort, A., Mutation, autoimmunity, and aging, *Lancet*, 2, 138, 1963.
7. Comfort, A., Measuring the human aging rate, *Mech. Age. Dev.*, 1, 101, 1972.
8. Curtis, M. and Crowley, C., Chromosome aberrations in liver cells in relation to the somatic mutation theory of aging, *Rad. Res.*, 18/19, 337, 1953.
9. Curtis, M. and Miller, K., Chromosome aberrations in liver cells of guinea pigs, *J. Gerontol.*, 26, 292, 1971.
10. Darmady, E.M., Offer, J., and Woodhouse, M.A., The parameters of the aging kidney, *J. Pathol.*, 109, 195, 1973.
11. Fries, F.F., Aging, natural death, and the compression of morbidity, *N. Engl. J. Med.*, 303, 130, 1980.
12. Goldstein, S., Life span of cultured cells in progeria, *Lancet*, 2, 424, 1969.

13. Harrison, D.E. and Archer, J.R., Physiological assays for biological ageing in mice: relationship of collagen, renal function, and longevity, in *The Measurement of Biological Age*, Ludwig, F.C. and Masoro, E.J., Eds., *Exp. Age. Res.*, (4), 9, 104, 1983.
14. Hayflick, L., The limited *in vitro* lifetime of human diploid cell strains, *Exp. Cell Res.*, 37, 614, 1965.
15. Hayflick, L., The cellular basis of biological age, *Verh. Dtsch. Ges. Pathol.*, 59, 52, 1975.
16. Hayflick, L., The cell biology of human aging, *Sci. Am.*, 242, 58, 1980.
17. Hayflick, L., Prospects for human life extension by genetic manipulation, in *Aging: A Challenge to Science and Society*, Vol. 1, Danon, D., Shock, N.W., and Marois, M., Eds., Oxford University Press, New York, 1981, 346.
18. Hensley, H.C., McWilliams, P.C., and Oakley, G.E., Physiological capacitance: a study in physiological age determination, *J. Gerontol.*, 19, 317, 1964.
19. Hollander, D. and Dadufalza, V.D., Increased intestinal absorption of oleic acid with aging in the rat, *Exp. Gerontol.*, 18, 287, 1983.
20. Hollander, D., Dadufalza, V.D., and Shetten, E.G., Does essential fatty acid absorption change with aging?, *J. Lipid Res.*, 25, 321, 1984.
21. Howell, T.H., Old age, *Geriatrics*, 4, 281, 1949.
22. Howell, T.H., Multiple pathology in nonagenarians, *Geriatrics*, 18, 899, 1963.
23. Howell, T.H. and Piggott, A.P., Morbid anatomy of old age. I and II., *Geriatrics*, 6, 85, 1951.
24. Howell, T.H. and Piggott, A.P., Morbid anatomy of old age. III., *Geriatrics*, 7, 137, 1952.
25. Ingram, D.K., Toward the behavioral assessment of biological aging in the laboratory mouse: concepts, terminology, and objectives, in *The Measurement of Biological Age*, Ludwig, F.C. and Masoro, E.J., Eds., *Exp. Age. Res.*, 9(4), 104, 1983.
26. Landfield, Ph., Rose, G., Sandles, L., Wohlstadler, T.H., and Lynch, G., Patterns of astroglial hypertrophy and neuronal degeneration in the hippocampus of aged, memory-deficient rats, *J. Gerontol.*, 82, 3, 1977.
27. Landfield, Ph., Waymire, J.C., and Lynch, G., Hippocampal aging and adenocorticoids: quantitative correlations, *Science*, 202, 1098, 1978.
28. Lindop, P. and Rotblat, J., Induction of aging by radiation, in *Biological Aspects of Aging*, Shock, N.W., Ed., Columbia University Press, New York, 1962, 216.
29. Linzbach, A.J. and Akuamoa-Boateng, A., Die Altersveranderungen des menschlichen Herzens. I. Das Herzgewicht im Alter, *Klin. Woschenschr.*, 51, 156, 1973.
30. Linzbach, A.J. and Akuamoa-Boateng, A., Die Altersversanderungen des menschlichen Herzens. II. Die Polypathie des Herzens im Alter, *Klin. Woschenschr.*, 51, 164, 1973.
31. Linzbach, A.J., Altern and Krankheit., Abeitung einer neun Alterstheorie auf der Grundlage der Polypathie, *Verh. Dtsch. Ges. Pathol.*, 56, 242, 1975.
32. Ludwig, F.C. and Silverman, L., Measuring biological age in samples of kidney and brain obtained at autopsy from rats, *Verh. Dtsch. Ges. Pathol.*, 59, 242, 1975.
33. Ludwig, F.C. and Smoke, M.E., The measurement of biological age, *Exp. Aging Res.*, 6, 497, 1980.
34. Ludwig, F.C., What to expect from gerontological research? (editorial), *Science*, 209(4461), 1980.
35. Ludwig, F.C., Senescence, pathology facing medicine's ultimate issue, *Arch. Pathol. Lab. Med.*, 105, 445, 1981.
36. Ludwig, F.C. and Masoro, E.J., Introduction, in *The Measurement of Biological Age*, Ludwig, F.C. and Masoro, E.J., Eds., *Exp. Age. Res.*, 9(No. 4), 104, 1983.
37. *Mammalian Models for Research on Aging*, National Academy Press, Washington, D.C., 1981.
38. Meredith, P., Gerbase-Lima, M., and Walford, L., Age-related changes in the PMA: Con A stimulatory ratios of cells from spleens of a long-lived mouse strain, *Exp. Gerontol.*, 10, 247, 1972.
39. Miquel, J., Oro, J., Bensch, K.G., and Johnson, J.E., Lipofuscin: fine-structural and biochemical studies, in *Free Radicals in Biology*, Vol. 3, Academic Press, New York, 1977, 133.
40. Pontes Pacheco, I., Segreto, C., and Iwabuchi, L., The thickness of the glomerular basement membrane in irradiated and unirradiated Wistar rats and C57BL

mice of different age groups, in *The Measurement of Biological Age*, Ludwig, F.C. and Masoro, E.J., Eds., *Exp. Age. Res.*, 9(No. 4), 104, 1983.

41. Soupukova, M. and Holeckova, E., The latent period of explanted organs of newborn, adult and senile rats, *Exp. Cell Res.*, 33, 361, 1964.
42. Strehler, B.L., Mark, D.D., Mildvan, A.S., and Gee, M.V., Rate and magnitude of age pigment accumulation in the human myocardium, *J. Gerontol.*, 14, 430, 1959.
43. Verzar, F., Veranderungen der thermoelastischen Eigenschaften von Sehnenfasern beim Altern, *Experientia*, 11, 230, 1955.
44. Voitenko, V.P. and Tokar, A.V., The assessment of biological age and sex differences of human aging, in *The Measurement of Biological Age*, Ludwig, F.C. and Masoro, E.J., Eds., *Exp. Age. Res.*, 9(4), 104, 1983.
45. Walford, R., *The Immunologic Theory of Aging*, Munksgaard, Copenhagen, 1969.
46. Ludwig, F. et al., unpublished data.

CHAPTER 19

COLLAGEN AS A PARAMETER FOR THE DETERMINATION OF HUMAN PHYSIOLOGICAL AGE

VINCENT M. MONNIER AND DAVID R. SELL

TABLE OF CONTENTS

I. INTRODUCTION

The concept of studying changes occurring in collagen during aging dates back to observations by Bjorksten,[4,5] who noted an analogy between the polymerization curve of gelatin in solution with that of mortality in the human population. This led him to formulate the "cross-linking theory of aging", whereby he envisaged the aging process as a progressive cross-linking of cellular and extracellular molecules mediated by oxidants, metals, "tanning" agents, etc.

The first experimental evidence in favor of this concept was by Verzar,[55] who demonstrated that the resistance to thermal denaturation of rat tail tendons increased with advancing age. The relationship between these parameters appeared to be so high that a number of scientists began to investigate the cause of collagen aging in mammals with the hope that it would provide a clue to the fundamental process responsible for limiting life span. Another incentive for studying the cause of collagen aging was that age-related changes were much more apparent in the extracellular matrix of collagen-rich tissues, such as arteries and lungs, than in cells,[29] suggesting that the life-limiting process might result from a global failure involving these tissues rather than the dying out of specific cells.

Before attempting to evaluate the potential usefulness of collagen changes for determination of human physiological age, we first discuss the concept of fundamental vs. segmental aging process. We ask the question of whether age-related changes in collagen-rich tissues belong

0-8493-0129-7/94/$0.00+$.50

primarily to the former or latter process and what factors affect their rate. The usefulness of these changes for the assessment of human physiological age is examined at the molecular level, whereby special emphasis is placed on fluorophores and cross-links mediated by the Maillard or nonenzymatic glycosylation reaction.

II. FUNDAMENTAL VS. SEGMENTAL AGING PROCESSES

An arbitrary distinction between fundamental and segmental aging process is necessary for the evaluation of the potential usefulness of collagen changes for the assessment of human physiological age. The notion that the two processes should be separated is extrapolated from the article on progeroid syndromes by George Martin.[33] Below, we utilize the word "segmental" to indicate an aging process which occurs in a "segment", i.e. a specific tissue, of the body. Major characteristics of these two entities are summarized in Table 1. If the rate change of a biological parameter correlates highly with age, i.e., the data points scatter minimally around the regression line, this phenomenon suggests the presence of a biological clock (Figure 1). If demonstration can be made that the clock ticks at a rate that is inversely proportional to species longevity, this would strongly suggest that the clock is the expression of the fundamental aging process, i.e., a process responsible for determining the maximal life span of the species. Thus, one expects that those conditions that impact on general aging processes will be mainly able to modify the speed of the biological clock. However, because the biological clock is dependent on the expression of species-specific genes, it is unlikely that external intervention, such as food restriction, would modify dramatically the rate change of the parameter under consideration. In contrast, the rate of a segmental aging process is specific to a particular tissue and is expected to depend strongly on environmental factors and to vary greatly among individuals of the same species. A typical example of a segmental aging process is atherosclerosis, which is found in 100% of autopsied elderly subjects in Western populations. Its extent, however, varies from minimal and localized to diffuse and severe among subjects of the same age.

In contrast to the fundamental aging process, the rate of evolution of a segmental aging process is expected to be more strongly dependent on external factors such as nutrition, smoke, and radiation exposure. Accordingly, it will respond to external interventions such as dietary food restriction and drug treatment, but only to the extent allowed by the individual genetic makeup. The latter argument is again best illustrated by atherosclerosis as an example of a segmental aging process. Both familial and nutritionally induced forms of atherosclerosis are amenable to external intervention. Dietary restriction and exercise, which have moderate, although significant effects on longevity in rodents, are expected to have a dramatic impact on the progression of "secondary" atherosclerosis. In contrast, familial atherosclerosis will progress in spite of nutritional intervention and exercise because the defect in receptor-mediated removal of low density lipoproteins is genetic in nature.

In anticipation of the conclusion of this chapter, the preceding discussion points out that a marker for the fundamental aging process will not necessarily help predict the rate of progression of a segmental aging process, which itself might terminate prematurely the life of an individual. From this argument it already can be concluded that biomarkers of segmental and fundamental aging processes should not be combined together to provide a single parameter of biological age. Because longevity of an individual will depend on the rate at which individual segmental aging processes evolve, it is clear that several time points involving several tissues will be needed for accurate predictions of longevity. Below we evaluate various physical and chemical properties of collagen as measures of segmental and fundamental aging processes.

Table 1 Distinction between fundamental and segmental aging processes[a]

Fundamental aging process	Segmental aging process
Universal; generalized progressive; irreversible; incurable; and nonpreventable	Potentially individual; localized; progressive; and preventable
Quantitative parameter correlates highly with age	Quantitative parameter correlates weakly with age
Process rate is species specific and higher in short- than long-lived species	Process rate varies greatly among individuals
Process rate overall little affected by environmental factors because it is strongly dependent on species-specific genes	Process rate generally more strongly affected by environment and food intake; can be overridden by individual genetic factors
"Antisenescence" genes less efficient in short- than long-lived species	Specific genetic defect present or poor expression of "antisenescent" genes in tissues undergoing accelerated aging
Examples: stiffening of collagen-rich tissue (arteries, lungs, joints), thickening of basement membranes, accumulation of fluorophores, chromophores and cross-links in extracellular lens, matrix and decreased mitogenic response of T cells	Examples: hypertension, neoplasms (e.g., colon, bladder), atherosclerosis, lung, autoimmune diseases, type II diabetes, Alzheimer's disease, and osteoarthritis

[a] *This distinction is purely conceptual and its characteristics remain, for the most part, to be tested experimentally.*

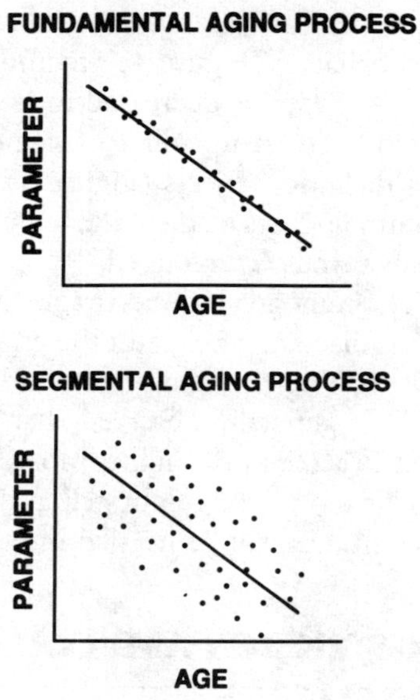

Figure 1 Expected quantitative relationship with age of a segmental vs. fundamental aging process.

III. AGE-RELATED CHANGES IN COLLAGEN-RICH TISSUES

Evidence for the fact that collagen changes in aging may serve for the determination of human physiological age stems from a large number of investigations at organ, tissue, and submicroscopical level. The ubiquitousness and longevity of collagen suggests that aging may also affect the overall function of collagen-rich tissues. This concept was championed by the late Robert Kohn,[29] who pointed out repeatedly that age-related changes in the mammalian organism were more dramatically expressed in the extracellular matrix than in cells. With age, tendons become progressively more resistant to heat denaturation and less soluble and digestible by collagenase.[24,49,55] The elastic modulus of the lung[41] and the elasticity of arteries and skin decrease linearly.[43] The myocardium becomes stiffer and joints lose their flexibility.[8] These changes are thought to contribute to the age-related loss of vital capacity, increased blood pressure, arthropathic changes, and increased susceptibility to infections in aging, the latter being in part attributed to decreased permeability of old collagen to inflammatory cells.

One striking observation is that many of these parameters correlate highly with age, as seen for example in the decreased elasticity modulus of the lungs (Figure 2) and the aorta (Figure 3). This suggests that the age-related stiffening reflects primarily a fundamental rather than a segmental aging process. The increased scattering of the values in the aortic elasticity experiment suggests that a superimposed segmental aging process such as atherosclerosis might affect the degree of stiffness. Yet there is little doubt that the stiffening process in aging arteries occurs independently from the extent of atherosclerosis.[40]

IV. DIABETES AND COLLAGEN AGING

Many age-related phenomena have been noted to occur at an earlier age in diabetes.[31] These include, for example, cardiovascular diseases such as hypertension, myocardial infarction, strokes, and amputation,[10] cataracts, limitation of joint mobility, infections in skin and lungs and loss of vital capacity.[44,45] At the tissue level, capillary basement membranes thicken at a higher rate[28] and fluorescent molecules in lens and collagen (Figure 4) accumulate at a higher rate than in age-matched controls.[7,37] Solubility of collagen is decreased in skin, trachea, and dura mater from diabetic subjects.[49] The age-related decrease in collagenase and cyanogen bromide digestibility of tendons and dura mater from diabetic subjects (Figure 5) is accelerated.[24,30]

Similar studies in rodents confirm findings made in the human. Solubility and thermal denaturation time of tail tendons from diabetic rats is prolonged,[22,60] and increased amounts of fluorescent molecules and high molecular weight cyanogen bromide fragments are present in skin from diabetic rats.[9] All these changes suggest that diabetes accelerates the cross-linking rate of collagen.

The generalized impact of diabetes on the aging rate of tissues suggests that diabetes acts on the fundamental aging process. It is generally observed that the aging rate in these tissues is increased by a factor of 2. Taking into account the higher mortality rate of the diabetic population, it is possible that assaying for specific cross-links might help predict the risk of shortened life span in diabetes. However, prospective studies will be needed in order to address this question.

V. FOOD RESTRICTION AND COLLAGEN AGING

In analogy to diabetes, which accelerates age-related processes throughout the organism, food restriction in rodents delays the onset and progression of a large number of age-related changes. Food restriction in rodents helps maintain their immunologic functions at younger levels relative to their ages.[21] It also improves complex maze and motor performance in rats and mice.[23,26]

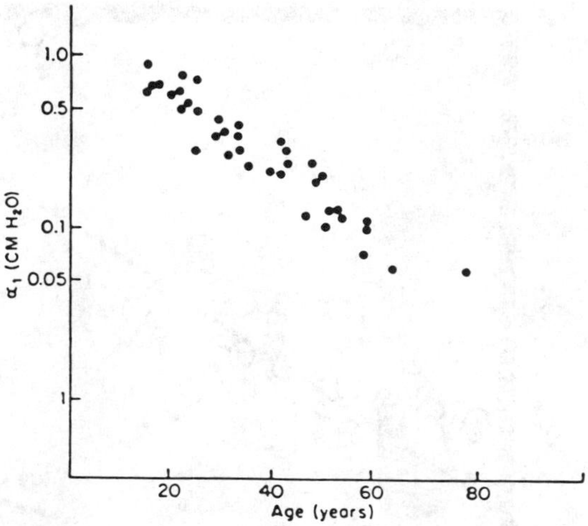

Figure 2 Lung elasticity modulus (α_1) as a function of age in human beings. (From Neiwoehner, D.E. et al., *J. Appl. Physiol.*, 39, 943, 1975. With permission.)

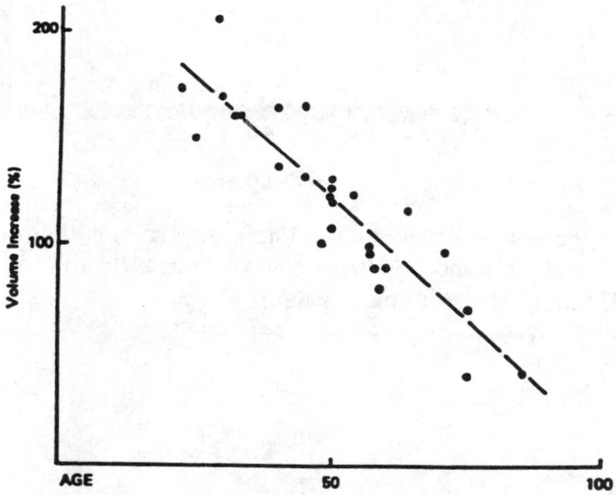

Figure 3 Volume increase of human thoracic aorta under standard pressure as a function of age. (Redrawn from Bader, H., *Circ. Res.*, 20, 354, 1967. By permission of the American Heart Association, Inc.)

Furthermore, there is evidence that food restriction reduces the blood pressure of spontaneously hypertensive rats and the progression of nephrosis.[32,58]

Everitt[13] examined the effects of food restriction on aging rate of collagen as measured by thermal stability in 7 *M* urea. At comparable age, the time needed for tail tendons to break was significantly higher in ***ad libitum*** fed vs. food-restricted animals, suggesting increased cross-linking in the former group. In the same context, Everitt et al.[12] investigated the effect of hypophysectomy and thyroidectomy and found that both decrease the aging rate of collagen. However, in these experiments as well as in many other reports in which specific interventions were used to attempt to decrease the aging rate, it was observed that experimental animals ate less, thus making it difficult to attribute the delayed aging rate to a specific effect of the intervention.

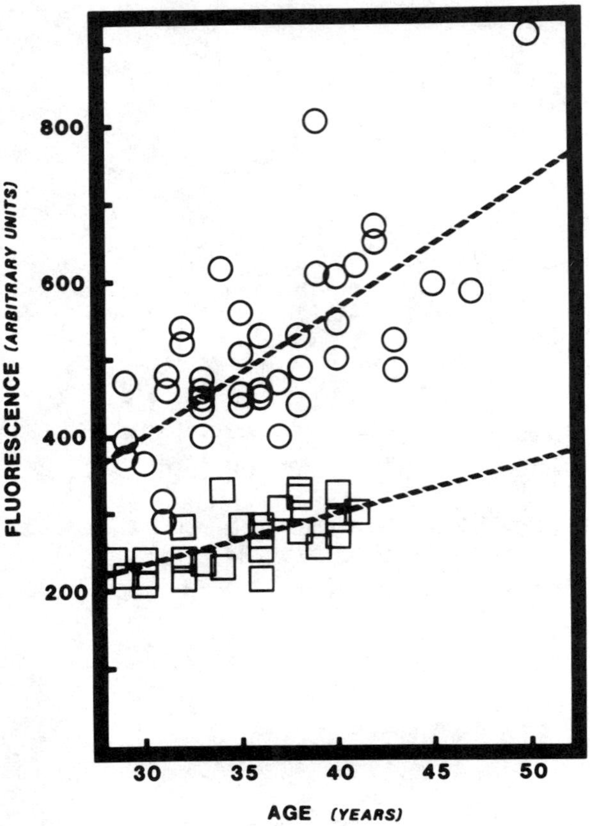

Figure 4 Age-related increase in collagen-linked fluorescence at 440 nm (excitation at 370 nm) in skin from diabetic (○) and nondiabetic subjects (□). (From Monnier, V.M. et al., *J. Clin. Invest.*, 78, 832, 1986. With permission.)

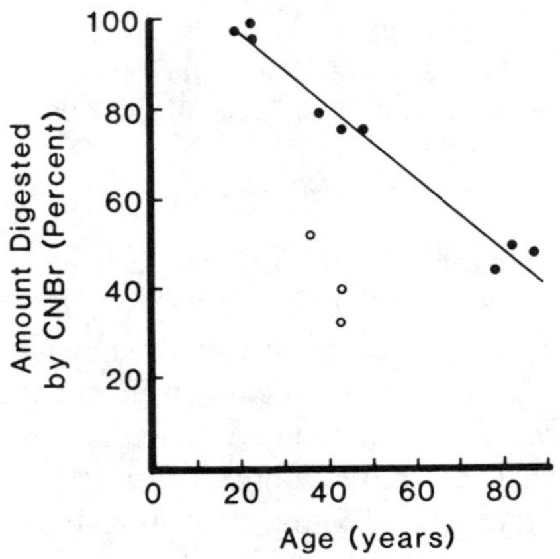

Figure 5 Amount of insoluble dura mater collagen from nondiabetic and diabetic subjects solubilized by cyanogen bromide, plotted as a function of age. Nondiabetic = ●; diabetic = ○. (From Kohn, R.R., *Connect. Tissue Res.*, 121, 169, 1983. With permission.)

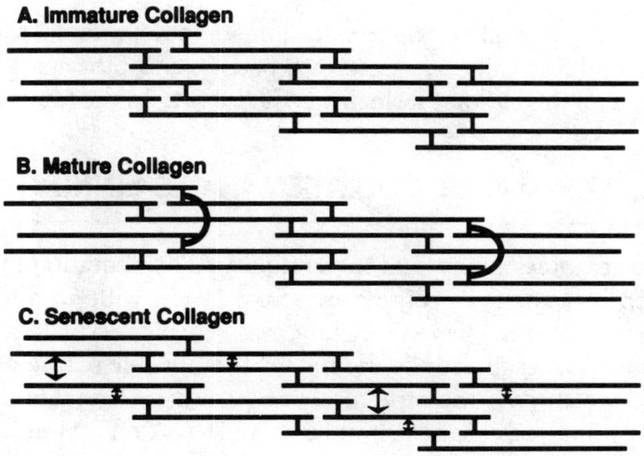

Figure 6 Types of cross-links of fibrillar collagen as a function of age. (From Bailey, A.J., *Eye*, 1, 175, 1987. With permission.)

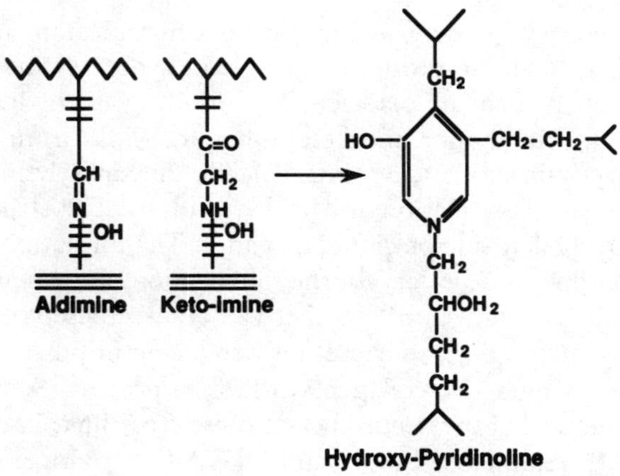

Figure 7 Proposed mechanism for the formation of the fluorescent cross-link pyridinoline. (From Bailey, A.J., *Eye*, 1, 175, 1987. With permission.)

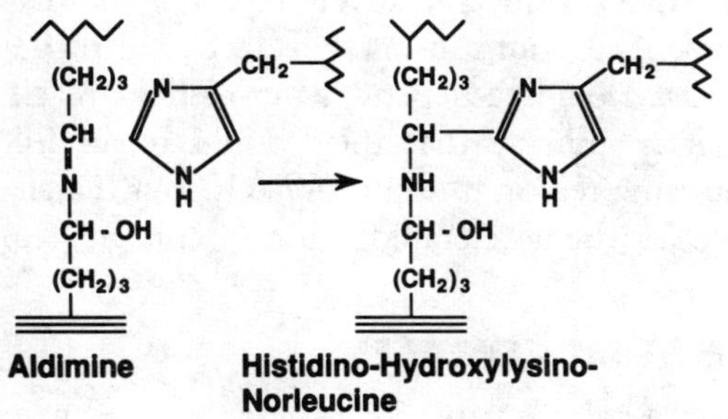

Figure 8 Formation of the trivalent cross-link HHL from the lysyl oxidase-dependent aldimine cross-link. (From Bailey, A.J., *Eye*, 1, 175, 1987. With permission.)

Although one could argue that *ad libitum* feeding might represent a pathological condition, the observation that food restriction acts on several parameters of the aging process suggests that it also modifies the rate of the biological clock, i.e., it also acts on the fundamental aging process.

VI. MECHANISMS OF COLLAGEN CROSS-LINKING IN AGING

The decreased solubility, digestibility, and susceptibility to denaturation by heat of old collagen suggest that collagen is becoming progressively cross-linked with advancing age. Accelerated cross-linking by diabetes and *ad libitum* feeding, respectively, point to a mechanism strongly dependent on glycemia, either directly or indirectly. The possible nature of this mechanism will become apparent as we discuss the structure, mechanism of formation, and occurrence of currently known cross-links of collagen. Emphasis is placed on cross-links from tissues rich in type I collagen. Each of these cross-links will be examined for its potential use as a parameter for estimation of human physiological age.

Basically, three types of cross-links occur in collagen, depending on whether the individual is in the growth, maturation, or senescent phase of his life (Figure 6).

A. CROSS-LINKS OF IMMATURE COLLAGEN

Soon after its synthesis, collagen undergoes postsynthetic modification and cross-linking. Under the action of lysyl oxidase, ε-amino groups of lysine and hydroxylysine residues in telopeptide regions of the tropocollagen chain are oxidized. The resulting aldehydes condense with lysyl or hydroxylysl residues to form aldimine and ketoimine cross-links from which the amino acids lysinonorleucine, hydroxylysinonorleucine (HLNL), and dihydroxylysinonorleucine (DHLNL) are released upon borohydride reduction and acid hydrolysis. The structure of the unreduced cross-link is depicted on the left side of Figures 7 and 8. The formation of these divalent inter- and intramolecular cross-links is necessary for the stabilization of the newly synthesized collagen fibrils in the proper "quarter-staggered" geometry. Because these cross-links are involved in further reactions during maturation, they are not detectable in postpubertal tissues[47] unless a pathological process involving active collagen synthesis is present.

A systematic investigation of the occurrence of these cross-links in diabetic tissues has been performed. Reiser et al.[48] quantitated HLNL and DHLNL in younger diabetic skin and found that the DHLNL/HLNL ratio was associated with degree of hand contracture, skin thickening, and the presence of retinopathy. Thus, it may well be that chronic hyperglycemia might affect lysyl oxidase-dependent pathways of physiological collagen cross-linking.

Another cross-link formed during maturation of collagen is the tetrafunctional borohydride reducible cross-link histidinohydroxymerodesmosine (HHMD). *In vivo* labeling with radioactive lysine showed that HHMD formed relatively rapidly.[46] It was absent from rat bone, but present in skin and tendon. Its amount in rat skin decreased throughout life span.[47]

In summary, because lysyl oxidase-dependent cross-links reach maturity relatively rapidly after collagen synthesis, it is unlikely that they would be useful for estimation of human physiological age. For the same reason it is also unlikely, but remains to be demonstrated, that they would be responsible for the accelerated aging of collagen in diabetes.

B. CROSS-LINKS OF MATURE COLLAGEN

As noted above, the borohydride reducible cross-links undergo further reactions, the products of which depend on the tissue in which they occur. In bone, cartilage, dentin, tendon and ligament, an aldimine and a ketoimine cross-link will condense together under dissociation of the aldimine bond to form the trivalent fluorescent cross-link hydroxylysinopyridinoline[2,18]

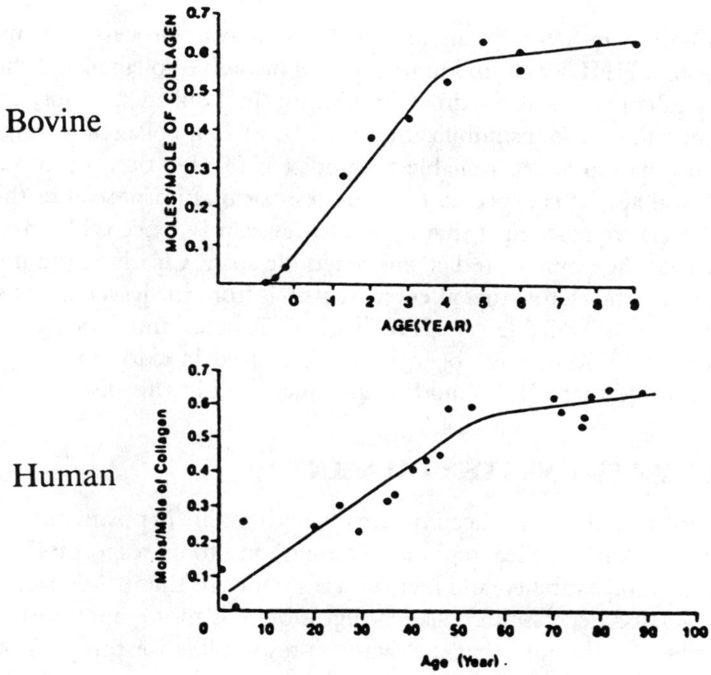

Figure 9 Age-related formation of HHL in bovine (top) and human skin (bottom). (From Yamauchi, M. et al., *Biochem. Biophys. Res. Commun.*, 152, 898, 1988. With permission.)

(Figure 7) as well as its analogue lysinopyridinoline.[14,42] Pyridinoline can be easily assayed by high performance liquid chromatography. It was detected in human cartilage and tendon, but was practically absent from skin, cornea, and rat tail tendon.[38] It was found to increase during puberty in both tissues and reached a plateau at about 20 years of age, after which it decreased in cartilage and remained unchanged in tendon. Lysinopyridinoline was detected in significant amounts only in bone and dentin.[14]

The lack of change in pyridinoline level after puberty and its absence from skin makes it unlikely that it could be used for determination of physiological age. Although pyridinoline may not serve to determine human physiological age, it may, however, serve as a marker for diseases with increased collagen turnover rate, such as osteoarthritis and Paget's disease, in which high levels were detected in the urine.[6]

To our knowledge, no systematic study of pyridinoline level in diabetes has been performed. One study reported no significant increase in the pyridinoline to hydroxylysine ratio in skin from three individuals with unknown type of diabetes.[54] In view of the fact that other authors failed to detect pyridinoline in skin, one wonders if the compound assayed in this study was truly pyridinoline.

In summary, the assay of pyridinoline in skin or urine is not expected to provide information on the rate of the fundamental aging process. It may, however, provide information on segmental aging processes such as osteoarthritis.

The maturation of borohydride-reducible cross-links in skin leads to the formation of a cross-link whose structure was elucidated.[34] Instead of reacting with a ketoimine cross-link, the aldimine precursor of HLNL can react with the imidazole ring of a histidine residue to form the trivalent interhelix cross-link histidinohydroxylysinonorleucine (HHL) (Figure 8). HHL was assayed in aging bovine and human skin.[59] As can be seen in Figure 9 (top and bottom), its amount increases linearly with age to reach plateau level at midlife. Because of lack of progression throughout life and because it is found only in selected tissues such as skin, it represents primarily a maturation rather than an ubiquitous senescent process. Of interest is that the highest proportion of HHL was found in fractions of insoluble collagen and that concentrations in middle-aged adults reaches approximately 0.5 mol/mol collagen. Thus, this cross-link may play an important role in the insolubilization process of skin collagen during aging.

Too little information is yet available to predict if HHL would be of value for assessing human physiological age. It is expected to be useless for that purpose after the age of 50 years because plateau levels are reached at that time. However, it is conceivable that increased rate of synthesis prior to that age might predict shortened life span. Clearly, more information will be needed to understand the factors that affect its synthesis from the lysyl oxidase-dependent cross-links. No information is available on HHL level in diabetes and food restriction. However, because DHLNL and HLNL have been found increased in skin from subjects with type I diabetes,[48] it is possible that HHL could be also increased in this disease.

C. SENESCENT CROSS-LINKS OF COLLAGEN

Senescent cross-links are those that accumulate throughout life in postmature collagen. They are postulated to cross-link interhelical regions (Figure 6) and to be responsible for the age-related decrease in solubility, digestibility, and increased resistance to thermal denaturation of collagen. Because the age-related decrease in collagen digestibility is more rapid in short- vs. long-lived mammalian species, it is thought that the factor(s) responsible for this phenomenon is a direct reflection of the fundamental aging process.[25] In essence, three cross-linking mechanisms are possible, depending on the factors postulated to play a role in the aging process: (1) cross-links resulting from free radical products; (2) cross-links mediated by reducing sugars during Maillard reaction; and (3) cross-links resulting from other reactions.

Free radicals have long been postulated to be responsible for collagen cross-linking and the basic aging process itself. Chio and Tappel[11] showed that malondialdehyde, which arises from lipid oxidation, can condense with free amino groups in proteins to form fluorescent cross-links and adducts that have similar excitation-emission properties with those isolated from aging tissues. Two models have been proposed for the fluorogens. One model is based on conjugated Schiff bases with *N,N*¹-disubstituted-1-amino-3-iminopropene structure.[11] The other model is based on the more recent discovery of 1,4-dihydropyridine-3,5-dicarbaldehydes, which also form from the reaction of malondialdehyde with amino acids.[27,39] Despite the availability of these model compounds, however, no report to date has documented their presence in senescent collagen, thus raising doubts as to whether free radicals generated during lipid oxidation play an important role in the fundamental aging process.

A second mechanism by which collagen might become cross-linked in aging is based on the Maillard or nonenzymatic Browning reaction. This proposition stems from the observation that proteins incubated with reducing sugars, such as glucose, become progressively yellow, fluorescent and cross-linked with time.[35] Similarities observed between the fluorescence properties of old human collagen and collagen incubated *in vitro* with glucose suggested that the Browning reaction might play a fundamental role in aging. As a first step toward testing this hypothesis, and in the absence of available specific probes for the advanced Maillard reaction, collagen-linked fluorescence at 440 nm with excitation at 370 nm was measured in skin collagen from subjects with type I (insulin-dependent) diabetes and in age-matched controls (Figure 4).[37] The fluorescence was increased in 98% of diabetic subjects compared to age-matched controls and its regression line as a function of age was 2.4 times steeper in diabetic than in controlled subjects. Furthermore, the intercept of both lines corresponded precisely to the mean age of diabetes onset (11.6 years), suggesting that acceleration of the Browning rate of collagen was tightly linked to the diabetic condition. The data points that form the two lines in Figure 4 illustrate well the concept of fundamental vs.

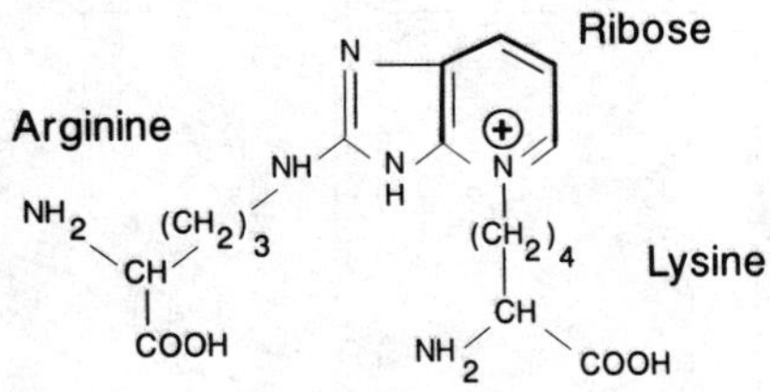

Figure 10 Structure of pentosidine, a protein cross-link involving the ε-amino group of lysine and the guanido group of arginine cross-linked by a reducing pentose.

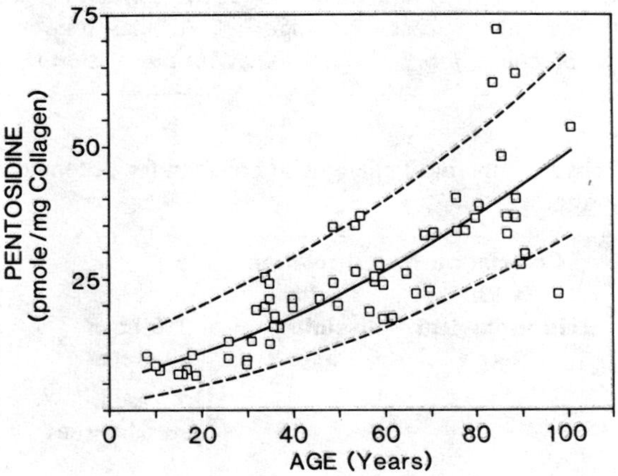

Figure 11 Age-related change in pentosidine in human insoluble skin collagen. (From Sell, D.R. and Monnier, V. M., *J. Clin. Invest.*, 85, 380, 1990. With permission.)

segmental aging process. Very little scattering is observed for the controls, suggesting that fluorescence at 440 nm (excitation at 370 nm) is a reflection of the fundamental aging process. In presence of diabetes, however, the segmental component is predominant and the diabetic data points reflect the sum of genetic and exogenous factors that affect the Browning aging rate of collagen.

The relationship between collagen-linked fluorescence and severity of diabetic complication was evaluated using uni- and multivariate analysis.[37] The amount of fluorescence correlated significantly with age, severity of retinopathy, arterial and joint stiffness, and blood pressure. Multivariate analysis showed that it was most strongly associated with age and presence of retinopathy. Thus, although the association between these parameters could be purely coincidental, the increased amount of fluorescence compared to controls suggests the presence of accelerated collagen aging and higher risk for segmental aging processes that could prematurely terminate the life of the diabetic individual.

Progress in the authors' laboratory led to the isolation of a major fluorophore from aging human skin and dura mater collagen with excitation-emission maxima at 335 and 385 nm, respectively.[51] Structure elucidation revealed the presence of an imidazo [4,5b] pyridinium molecule formed from the guanido group of an arginine residue and the ε-amino group of a lysine residue (Figure 10). The cross-linking moiety is a pentose, which is likely to originate from advanced glycation through fragmentation of glycated proteins, or from glycation by pentoses.[52] The fluorescent cross-link, called pentosidine, was detected in a large variety of human tissues, including plasma proteins and cells in culture. Its level was quantitated in human skin obtained

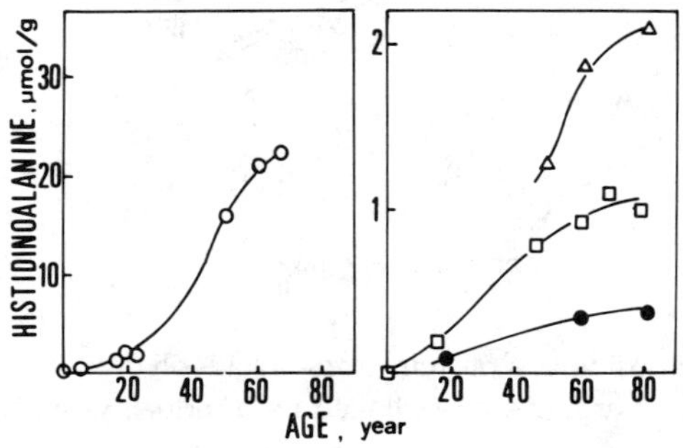

Figure 12 Histidinoalanine content as a function of age. The content is expressed as micromoles per gram of dry weight. ○, Costal cartilage; □, Achilles tendon; Δ, aorta; ●, skin. (From Fujimoto, D., *Biochem. Int.*, 5, 743, 1982. With permission.)

Table 2 Summary of physical-chemical changes in collagen for potential determination of physiological age

Parameter	**Correlation with chronological age**	**Correlation with physiological age**[a]	**Effect of diabetes**	**Effect of food restriction**	**Ref.**
Solubility	Fair	Fair	Decreased in several tissues	Improved	22, 49
Digestibility with					
Collagenase	Excellent	Yes	Decreased	Unknown	24
Cyanogen bromide	Excellent	Yes	Decreased	Unknown	9, 30
Heat denaturation time	Excellent in tail	Yes	Prolonged tendons	Decreased	12, 13, 54, 55
Lysyl oxidase-dependent cross-links	None	None	Increased or unchanged[b]	Unknown	46–48
Pyridinolines	Not beyond puberty	None	Increased[b]	Unknown	18, 31, 53
HHL	Until midlife	Until midlife	Unknown	Unknown	34, 58
370/440 Fluorescence	Expected Expected	Yes	Increased	Unknown	9, 36, 37
Pentosidine	Excellent	Yes	Increased or unchanged	Unknown	50–52
Histidinoalanine	Present in aorta and cartilage	Unknown	Unknown	Unknown	19, 20

[a] *Not tested in prospective studies. Statements above are estimates.*
[b] *Based on preliminary studies.*

at autopsy.[51] Figure 11 shows the age-related increase in pentosidine level in this tissue. Initially linear, it progresses exponentially in late life, suggesting progressive decrease in collagen turnover or a worsening of glucose tolerance in aging. The possibility that not only glucose but also pentoses are involved in postsynthetic modification of proteins in aging is unexpected but potentially very important because ribose is 130 times more reactive than glucose. As it is present in all cells, it might be the predominant aging factor of long-lived cells.

Pentosidine was found to be increased in diabetes and especially uremia, with and without diabetes.[53] The reason for this increase in uremia is currently unknown, but may relate to increased cellular breakdown, as for example, during hemodialysis. Pentosidine levels in skin correlates with the above described 370/440 nm fluorescence, the nature of which might be identical with aldimine cross-link "M" found in skin, bone, and tendon.[3] Thus, the latter fluorophore may also be an advanced Maillard reaction product.

A third type of cross-links whose biosynthesis is not dependent on preformed lysyl oxidase mediated cross-links, free radicals, or sugars is the histidinoalanine cross-link discovered by Fujimoto et al.[19] Histidinoalanine is probably formed by the interaction of a histidine residue in one peptide chain with a serine or cysteine residue in another peptide chain or intramolecularly (Figure 12). The fact that it is found in elevated amounts in calcified human aortas suggests that its formation is catalyzed by alkaline conditions.[19] In human aorta it increases approximately eightfold from 20 to 80 years. In contrast, no significant changes are noted in the levels of pyridinoline, desmosine, and isodesmosine in the same tissue. Histidinoalanine was also detected in large amounts in costal cartilage, with levels being 10 to 20 times higher than in aorta, Achilles tendon, or skin. In the latter tissue, there was only a minor increase.

It is currently unclear what proteins are being cross-linked by histidinoalanine. Solubilization experiments by Fujimoto et al.[19] suggest that a portion of histidinoalanine is very closely associated with elastin and collagen-rich fractions in aortas. The high percentage of acidic amino acids in these fractions suggests the presence of cross-links between these proteins and the so-called acidic structural proteins.

Because of its association with age, histidinoalanine qualifies as a senescent cross-link. In order to establish whether it is an expression of the fundamental aging process or only of a segmental aging process, it will be necessary to demonstrate that histidinoalanine formation is faster in short- vs. long-lived animal species. Also, data in diabetic and food-restricted states will be useful. From a practical viewpoint, however, the absence of an age-related increase in histidinoalanine in skin makes it unlikely that it could serve for the assessment of human physiological age.

VII. CONCLUSION

A number of postsynthetic modifications are known to form during development, maturation, and senescence of human collagen. They are summarized in Table 2. Among them, only changes in solubility, collagenase or cyanogen bromide digestibility, fluorescence at 440 nm upon excitation at 370 nm, HHL, and pentosidine are detectable in the aging human skin and could thus potentially serve as parameters of human physiological age. Evidently, a number of prospective clinical morbidity and mortality studies will be necessary to evaluate each of these modifications in their ability to predict variations in the aging rate of the organism and longevity. Whereas the assay of such parameters in, for example, skin biopsies may provide useful information for initial assessment of the "aging status" of an individual, several months or years may be needed to observe normalization of elevated levels of a collagen cross-link. Thus, additional tests will be necessary to assess short-term effects of specific interventions on the aging process.

As already pointed out in the Introduction, a parameter of the aging process, no matter how good it may be for the assessment of the basic aging rate, is unlikely to be useful as a single measure of life expectancy. Furthermore, the utilization of a general mathematical expression of the aging process that includes a potpourri of various parameters to determine the biological age of an individual is hazardous until enough data are available to establish its validity.

REFERENCES

1. Bader, H., Dependence of wall stress in the human thoracic aorta on age and pressure, *Circ. Res.*, 20, 354, 1967.
2. Bailey, A.J., Structure, function and aging of the collagens of the eye, *Eye*, 1, 175, 1987.
3. Barnard, K., Light, N.D., Sims, T.J., and Bailey, A.J., Chemistry of the collagen cross-links. Origins and partial characterization of a putative mature crosslink of collagen, *Biochem J.*, 244, 303, 1987.
4. Bjorksten, J. and Champion, W.J., Mechanical influence upon tanning, *J. Am. Chem. Soc.*, 64, 868, 1942.
5. Bjorksten, J., A common molecular basis for the aging syndrome, *J. Am. Geriatr. Soc.*, 6, 740, 1958.
6. Black, D., Duncan, A., and Robins, S.P., Quantitative analysis of the pyridinium crosslinks of collagen in urine using ion-paired reversed-phase high performance liquid chromatography, *Anal. Biochem.*, 169, 197, 1988.
7. Bleeker, J.C., vanBest, J.A., Vrij, L., van der Velde, E.A., and Oosterhuis, J.A., Autofluorescence of the lens in diabetic and healthy subjects by fluorometry, *Invest. Opthalmol. Vis. Sci.*, 27, 791, 1986.
8. Borg, T.K., Ranson, W.F., Moslehy, F.A., and Caulfield, J.B., Structural basis of ventricular stiffness, *Lab. Invest.*, 44, 49, 1981.
9. Brownlee, M., Vlassara, H., Kooney, A., Ulrich, P., and Cerami, A., Aminoguanidine prevents diabetes-induced arterial wall protein cross-linking, *Science*, 232, 1629, 1986.
10. The Carter Center, Closing the gap: the problem of diabetes mellitus in the United States, *Diabetes Care*, 8, 391, 1985.
11. Chio, K.S. and Tappel, A.L., Synthesis and characterization of the fluorescent products derived from malonaldehyde and amino acids, *Biochemistry*, 8, 2821, 1969.
12. Everitt, A.V., Seedsman, N.J., and Jones, F., The effects of hypophysectomy and continuous food restriction, begun at ages 70 and 400 days, on collagen aging, proteinuria, incidence of pathology and longevity in the male rat, *Mech. Age. Dev.*, 12, 161, 1980.
13. Everitt, A.V., Food intake, growth and the ageing of collagen in rat tail tendon, *Gerontology*, 17, 98, 1971.
14. Eyre, D.R., Koob, T.J., and Van Ness, K.P., Quantitation of hydroxypyridinium crosslinks in collagen by high performance liquid chromatography, *Anal. Biochem.* 137, 380, 1983.
15. Fernandes, G.E., Yunis, J., and Good R.A., Influence of diet on survival of mice. *Proc. Natl. Acad. Sci. U.S.A.*, 73, 1279, 1976.
16. Fernandes, G.E., Yunis, J., and Good R.A., Influence of protein restriction on immune functions in NZB mice, *J. Immunol.*, 116, 782, 1976.
17. Fernandes, G.E., Yunis, J., and Good, R.A., Suppression of adenocarcinoma in the immunological consequences of caloric restriction, *Nature*, 263, 504, 1976.
18. Fujimoto, D., Moriguchi, T., and Ishida, T., The structure of pyridinoline, a collagen crosslink, *Biochem. Biophys. Res. Comm.*, 84, 52, 1978.
19. Fujimoto, D., Hirama, M., and Iwashita, T., Histidinoalanine, a new crosslinking amino acid, in calcified tissue collagen, *Biochem. Biophys. Res. Commun.*, 104, 1102, 1982.
20. Fujimoto, D., Aging of human connective tissue: increase in the content of a crosslinking amino acid, histidinoalanine, *Biochem. Int.*, 5, 743, 1982.
21. Gerbase-DeLima, M., Meredith, P., and Walford, R.L., Age-related changes, including synergy and suppression, in the mixed lymphocyte reaction in long-lived mice, *Fed. Proc.*, 34, 159, 1975.
22. Golum, L.M., Greenwald, R.A., and Ramamurthy, N.S., The effect of experimental diabetes on the molecular characteristics of soluble rat tail tendon collagen, *Biochem. Biophys. Acta*, 534, 78, 1978.
23. Goodrick, C.L., Effects of lifelong restricted feeding on complex maze performance on rats, *Age*, 7, 1, 1984.
24. Hamlin, C.R., Kohn, R.R., and Luschin, J.H., Apparent accelerated aging of human collagen in diabetes mellitus, *Diabetes*, 24, 902, 1975.
25. Hamlin, C.R., Luschin, J.H., and Kohn R.R., Aging of collagen: comparative rates in four mammalian species, *Exp. Gerontol.*, 15, 393, 1980.

26. Ingram, D.K., Weindruch, R., Spangler, E.L., Freeman, J.R., and Walford, R.L., Dietary restriction benefits learning and motor performance of aged mice, *J. Gerontol.,* 42, 78, 1987.
27. Kikugawa, K. and Bebba, M., Involvement of lipid oxidation products in the formation of fluorescent and cross-linked proteins, *Chem. Phys. Lipids,* 44, 277, 1987.
28. Kilo, C., Volger, N., and Williamson, J.R., Muscle capillary basement membrane changes related to aging and to diabetes mellitus, *Diabetes,* 21, 881, 1972.
29. Kohn, R., Evidence against cellular aging theories, in *Testing the Theories of Aging,* Adelman, R.C. and Roth, G.S., Eds., CRC Press, Boca Raton, FL, 1982, 221.
30. Kohn, R.R., Effects of age and diabetes mellitus on cyanogen bromide digestion of human dura mater collagen, *Connect. Tissue Res.,* 11, 169, 1983.
31. Kohn, R.R. and Schneider, S.L., Glycosylation of human collagen, *Diabetes,* 31(Suppl. 3), 47, 1982.
32. Maeda, H., Gleiser, C.A., Masoro, E.J., Murata, I., McMahan C.A., and Yu, B.P., Nutritional influences on aging of Fischer 344 rats. II. Pathology, *J. Gerontol.,* 40, 671, 1985.
33. Martin, G., Genetic syndromes in man with potential relevance to the pathobiology of aging, in *Birth Defects: Original Article Series,* Vol. 14, Bergsma, D. and Harrison, D.E., Eds., Alan R. Liss, New York, 1978, 5.
34. Mechanic, G.F., Katz, E.P., Henmi, M., Noyes, C., and Yamauchi M., Locus of a histidine-based, stable trifunctional, helix to helix collagen crosslink: stereospecific collagen structure of type I skin fibrils, *Biochemistry,* 26, 3500, 1987.
35. Monnier, V.M. and Cerami, A., Nonenzymatic browning in vivo: possible process for aging of long-lived proteins, *Science,* 211, 491, 1981.
36. Monnier, V.M., Kohn, R.R., and Cerami, A., Accelerated age-related browning of human collagen in diabetes mellitus, *Proc. Natl. Acad. U.S.A.,* 81, 583, 1984.
37. Monnier, V.M., Vishwanath, V., Elmets, C.A., Frank, K.E., and Yamashita, T., Age-related normalization of the browning rate of collagen in diabetic subjects without retinopathy, *J. Clin. Invest.,* 78, 832, 1986.
38. Moriguchi, T. and Fujimoto, D., Age-related changes in the content of the collagen crosslink pyridinoline, *J. Biochem.,* 84, 933, 1978.
39. Nair, V., Offerman, R.J., and Turner, G.A., Novel fluorescent 1,4-dihydropyridines, *J. Am. Chem. Soc.,* 108, 8283, 1986.
40. Nakashima, T. and Tanikawa, J., A study of human aortic distensibility with relation to atherosclerosis and aging, *Angiology,* 22, 477, 1971.
41. Niewoehner D.E., Kleinerman, J., and Liotta, L., Elastic behavior of postmortem human lungs: effects of aging and mild emphysema, *J. Appl. Physiol.,* 39, 943, 1975.
42. Ogawa, T., Ono, T., Tsuda, M., and Kawanishi, Y., A novel fluorophor in insoluble collagen: a crosslinking moiety in collagen molecule, *Biochem. Biophys. Res. Commun.,* 107, 1252, 1982.
43. Pillsbury, H.C., Hung, W., Kyle, M.C., and Freis, E.D., Arterial pulse waves velocity and systolic time intervals in diabetic children, *Am. Heart. J.,* 87, 783, 1974.
44. Primhak, R.A., Whincup, G., Tsanakas, J.N., and Milner, R.D.G., Reduced vital capacity in insulin-dependent diabetes, *Diabetes,* 36, 324, 1987.
45. Rayfield, E.J., Ault, M.J., Keusch, G.T., Brother, M.J., Nechemias, C., and Smith, H., Infection and diabetes, the case of glucose control, *Am. J. Med.,* 72, 439, 1982.
46. Reiser, K.M. and Last, J.A., Biosynthesis of collagen crosslinks: in vivo labelling of neonatal skin, tendon and bone in rats, *Connect. Tissue Res.,* 14, 293, 1986.
47. Reiser, K.M., Hennessy, S.M., and Last, J.A., Analysis of age-associated changes in collagen crosslinking in skin and lung in monkeys and rats, *Biochem. Biophys. Acta,* 926, 339, 1987.
48. Reiser, K., Buckingham, J., Larson, M., Ruper, R., and Uitto, J., Nonenzymatic glycosylation of lysine and hydroxylysine is related to glycohemoglobin levels, changes in collagen crosslinks, and diabetic complications, *Diabetes,* 37(Suppl. 1), 179, 1988.

49. Schneider, S.L. and Kohn, R.R., Effects of age and diabetes mellitus on the solubility of collagen from human skin, tracheal cartilage and dura mater, *Exp. Gerontol.*, 17, 185, 1982.
50. Sell, D.R. and Monnier, V.M., Isolation, purification and partial characterization of fluorophores from aging human extracellular matrix, *Connect. Tissue Res.*, 19, 77, 1989.
51. Sell, D.R. and Monnier, V.M., Structure elucidation of a senescence crosslink from human extracellular matrix. Implication of pentoses in the aging process, *J. Biol. Chem.*, 264, 21597, 1989.
52. Sell, D.R., Nagaraj, R.H., Grandhee, S.K., Odetti, P., Lapolla, A., Fogarty, J., and Monnier, V.M., Pentosidine: a molecular marker for the cumulative damage to proteins in diabetes, aging and uremia, *Diabetes/Metab. Rev.*, 7, 239, 1991.
53. Sell, D.R. and Monnier, V.M., Endstage renal disease and diabetes catalyze the formation of a pentose-derived crosslink from aging collagen, *J. Clin. Invest.*, 85, 380, 1990.
54. Tilson, M.D., Further studies of a putative crosslinking amino acid (3-deoxypyridnoline) in skin from patients with abdominal aneurysm, *Surgery*, 98, 888, 1985.
55. Verzar, F., Veranderungen der thermoelastichen Kontraktion der Sehnenfasern im Alter, *Helv. Physiol. Pharmacol. Acta*, 13, C64, 1955.
56. Verzar, F., Aging of the collagen fiber, *Int. Rev. Connect. Tissue Res.*, 2, 245, 1964.
57. Walford, R.L., Harris, S.B. and Weindruch, R., Dietary restriction and aging: historical phases, mechanisms and current directions, *J. Nutr.*, 117, 1650, 1987.
58. Wright, G.L., McMurty, J.P., and Wexler, B.C., Food restriction reduces the blood pressure of spontaneously hypertensive rats, *Life Sci.*, 28, 1253, 1981.
59. Yamauchi, M., Woodley, D.T. and Mechanic, G.L., Aging and crosslinking of skin collagen, *Biochem. Biophys. Res. Commun.*, 152, 898, 1988.
60. Yue, D.K., McLennan, S., and Turtle, J.R., The thermal stability of collagen in diabetic rats: correlation with severity of diabetes and nonenzymatic glycosylation, *Diabetologia*, 24, 282, 1983.
61. Richard, S., Sell, D.R., Katz, M.S., Masoro, E.J., Monnier, V.M., Food restriction in F344 rats delays tail tendon crosslinking and formation of advanced glycosylation endproducts, *Gerontologist*, 30, 321A, 1990.

CHAPTER 20

SKIN CHANGES AS A REFLECTION OF BIOLOGIC AGE

ARTHUR K. BALIN

TABLE OF CONTENTS

I. INTRODUCTION

Studies measuring alterations in the skin in the same individuals on a longitudinal basis have been few. There have been several attempts, however, to determine a group of parameters that would indicate the rate of human aging. The Atomic Bomb Casualty Commission (ABCC) in Hiroshima and Nagasaki was one of the initial attempts to define the physiologic age of an individual. Hollingsworth and colleagues[37,38] studied the 17 parameters indicated in Table 1 and found that the two items correlating best with chronologic age are the hair-graying score and skin elasticity. Few biologic parameters change so dramatically with aging. Nevertheless, in a conference on nonlethal biological markers of physiological aging conducted by the National Institute on Aging, there was neither reference to nor discussion of cutaneous manifestations of aging.[78] It is hoped

0-8493-0129-7/94/$0.00+$.50

Table 1 Correlation between age and physiologic tests for aging

Test Item	Correlation with age
Hair graying score	+0.717
Skin elasticity	+0.604
Audiometry at 4000 cyc/s	+0.596
Vibrometer	+0.537
Systolic blood pressure	+0.519
Light extinction test	+0.488
Audiometry at 200 cyc/s	+0.445
Diastolic blood pressure	+0.409
Heart size	+0.294
Serum cholesterol	+0.234
Tidal volume	—
Thorax size	–0.124
One-second expiratory volume	–0.126
Total serum albumin	–0.267
Hand grip strength	–0.323
Total vital capacity	–0.402
Visual acuity	–0.423

Note: Approximately 400 individuals were examined for each test.

Data from Hollinsworth, J.W., Hashizuma, A., and Jablon, S., Yale J. Biol. Med., *33, 11, 1965.*

that this review of physiologic alterations of the skin with aging will facilitate the development and application of several cutaneous biomarkers of aging.

In the longitudinal study of aging conducted at the Gerontology Research Center of the National Institute on Aging there are virtually no objective measurements of alterations in the skin being measured.[82] These are serious oversights because our best visual clues to the estimation of an individual's biologic age come from direct assessment of the skin. A number of age-related cutaneous changes have been documented in cross-sectional studies and exist in the literature in places diverse in time and location. Unfortunately, some conclusions about age-related skin changes are common wisdom but are based on studies of inadequate numbers of subjects.

One of the aims of this chapter is to summarize the best of the studies documenting skin changes with age in order to demonstrate the amount of data supporting each of the "conclusions" that have been reached and to facilitate the choice of appropriate cutaneous parameters to include in a battery of tests designed to estimate biologic age. Validation of the predictive value of tests employed to measure biologic age will take many years. The best predictive indices likely will be obtained by determining the rate of change in an individual in any specific parameter as a function of the percent life span completed at the time of the measurement, with the measurements obtained prospectively and the percent life span completed determined retrospectively after the subject's death. The initial validation will take years and because it is not known which measurements will prove to be the most useful it would seem prudent to serially measure as many subjects and parameters as possible.

Table 2 Prevalence rate for significant skin conditions among individuals from 1 to 74 years of age in the U.S.[44]

	Rate per 1000 people								
Age	**5**	**10**	**15**	**20**	**30**	**40**	**50**	**60**	**70**
All significant skin conditions	180	260	480	490	450	480	530	560	660
Diseases of sebaceous glands	8	71	240	210	96	42	21	33	38
Dermatophyte	4	16	32	54	88	125	154	146	125
Tumors	20	20	32	37	38	42	85	133	183
Seborrheic dermatitis	8	10	16	32	38	42	31	29	25

Physical appearance of the skin is one of the most obvious visual clues to the age of an individual. Substantial scientific data shows that there is a progressive alteration in the physiological function of the skin with age. These changes lead to a progressive reduction in the individual's ability to adapt to environmental change and predisposes the individual to skin diseases that frequently accompany the aging process. That skin "ages" hardly comes as a surprise, but comprehension of the alterations provides a framework for understanding the pathological changes that occur with aging and represents a starting point for discovering the molecular mechanisms responsible.

In a Health and Nutritional Examination survey conducted in the U.S. from 1971 to 1974, 20,749 individuals selected by the U.S. Census Bureau as representative of noninstitutionalized individuals 1 to 74 years of age were examined by a dermatologist, and all conditions judged serious enough to be seen by a physician at least once were considered significant.[44] The presence of skin pathology and significant conditions was shown to increase with age (Table 2). Of individuals over 70, 66% have a dermatosis serious enough to require treatment by a physician.

Surveys in different countries show the incidence of many skin conditions varies considerably with race, complexion, climate, and occupation.

Tables 3 to 5 summarize the prevalence of skin changes in selected populations of elderly individuals. These differ from Table 2 in including those not considered in the above survey of skin changes serious enough to require treatment by a physician. Tindall and Smith[90] found that loss of skin elasticity occurred in 94% of persons over the age of 64, while seborrheic keratoses occurred in 80%, comedones in 81%, xerosis in 77% and cherry angiomata in 75% of the individuals studied. Although not included in the list of medical problems requiring professional medical attention, these are almost universal and represent the most common changes found in aging skin. The absolute frequency of the lesions varies with race (Table 4) and population studied (Table 5),[95] but the same general trends are seen.

Young[94] noted abnormal pathologic skin conditions in 96% of elderly patients (average age 80 years) in two chronic-care facilities in New York. Droller[20] reported 521 dermatologic conditions in 476 elderly persons living at home. Lentigos or "liver spots" occur in 90% of those over 80.[36] Vascular dysplasias, in the form of focal capillary proliferation, such as cherry angiomata, de Morgan spots, angiokeratomas, and telangiectasias are almost universal in persons over 70 years. Benign epidermal growths such as seborrheic keratoses, as well as dry skin and wrinkled skin due to loss of elastic and of subcutaneous tissue are especially common accompaniments of the aging process.

Isaki[41] studied the incidence of gray hair in a Japanese population and found a correlation with the age of the individual (Table 6). A survey in a large Australian population (Table 7) confirms the correlation of graying with age.[46]

Table 3 Frequency of skin abnormalities in individuals over 64 years of age

Rank	Percent
Lax skin	94
Seborrheic keratoses	88
Comedones	81
Dermatophytosis	79
Xerosis	77
Cherry angioma	75
Nevi	63
Skin tags	56
Lentigo	51
Varicosities	48
Seborrheic dermatitis	31
Schamberg's disease	31
Spider angiomas	29
Actinic keratoses	28
Rosacea	12
Neurogenic excoriations	12

Note *163 individuals 64 years or greater were examined. The population was composed of 52 white males, 52 white females, 28 black males, and 31 black females..*

Data from Tindall, J.P. and Smith, J.G., JAMA, *186, 1039, 1963.*

Table 4 Distribution of some common lesions by race in individuals over 64 years of age

	Seborrheic keratoses (10 or more)	Nevi (5 or more)	Cherry angiomas (5 or more)	Varicosities
White females ($N = 52$)	38%	23%	77%	58%
White males ($N = 52$)	54%	37%	77%	56%
Black females ($N = 31$)	61%	27%	45%	39%
Black males ($N = 28$)	61%	46%	11%	29%

Note: *163 individuals 64 years or greater were examined. The population was composed of 52 white males, 52 white females, 28 black males and 31 black females.*

Data from Tindall, J.P. and Smith, J.G., JAMA, *186, 1039, 1963.*

II. PHYSICAL ALTERATIONS OF SKIN WITH AGING

There are notable differences in the structure and composition of the skin from region to region on the body. These differences include thickness, number of cells in a layer, development of the granular layer and stratum lucidum, compaction of the stratum corneum, and the presence or

Table 5 Frequency of skin lesions in 222 residents of The Orthodox Jewish Home for the Aged

Diagnosis	Males N	Males %	Females N	Females %
Senile angioma	70	71.4	109	87.9
Comedones	44	44.8	35	28.1
Nevus	41	41.8	66	53.2
Lentigo	35	35.8	67	54.0
Seborrheic keratosis	29	29.3	47	37.9
Tinea pedis	22	22.4	42	33.8
Tinea cruris	13	13.2	0	0
Seborrheic dermatitis	11	11.2	7	5.6
Shamberg's disease	10	10.2	8	6.4
Fordyce disease	9	9.1	15	12.1
Hallux valgus	1	1	22	17.7
Intertrigo	1	1	18	14.5

Note: *222 residents of The Orthodox Jewish Home for the Aged were examined. The group was comprised of 98 males and 124 females and had the following age distribution: 60 to 70 years, 12; 71 to 80 years, 98; 81 to 90 years, 84; 91 years and older, 23.*

Data from Zakon, S., Goldberg, A., and Forman, I., Ill. Med. J., *101, 37, 1952.*

Table 6 Occurrence of gray hairs with age in a Japanese population

Age	Sex	N	Head (%)	Eyebrow (%)	Beard (%)	Axilla (%)	Pubic area (%)
31–41	Female	56	5	0	—	0	0
	Male	97	33	0	7	0	0
41–50	Female	57	65	0	—	0	0
	Male	84	75	5	56	0	18
51–60	Female	59	95	3	—	2	27
	Male	67	95	25	93	13	49
61–70	Female	42	100	17	—	2	81
	Male	63	100	45	100	11	94
71+	Female	36	100	28	—	3	100
	Male	24	100	63	100	42	100

Data from Isaki, Keio Igaku, *28, 59, 1951.*

absence of the cutaneous appendages (apocrine glands, eccrine glands, sebaceous glands, cutaneous vasculature, terminal or vellus hair follicles, cutaneous nerves, etc.). Marked differences appear in biopsy specimens taken only 1 or 2 cm apart;[66,68] for this reason morphologic studies should be performed on skin obtained from identical sites in individuals from various age groups. Systematic study of the morphologic changes of aging skin has been performed on only a few locations of the body, and the number of individuals examined has been small;[34] thus the

Table 7 Incidence of gray hair in an Australian population

	25–34		35–44		45–54		55+	
Age	**Male**	**Female**	**Male**	**Female**	**Male**	**Female**	**Male**	**Female**
Number	2574	698	2156	625	1493	553	429	189
Any graying (%)	22	23	61	66	89	88	94	96
Complete graying (%)	0.23	0.14	2.2	1.6	13	10	30	29

Data from Keogh, E.V. and Walsh, R.J., Nature, *207, 877, 1965.*

Table 8 Distribution of epidermal melanocytes with age (av. no./mm² ± S.D.)

	0–15 years	**(*N*)**	**16–70 years**	**(*N*)**	**70 years**	**(*N*)**
Thigh	1600 ± 200	(4)	1000 ± 390	(34)	560 ± 150	(4)
Ear	2580 ± 80	(10)	1400 ± 260	(12)	1530	(1)
Forehead			2010 ± 20[a]	(8)	1145 ± 85[a]	(4)
Arm			1600 ± 170	(20)	630 ± 400	(4)

[a] *S.E. (standard error, not standard deviation).*

Data from References 24 and 87.

information available to date should be considered fragmentary. In addition, because of extensive damage to skin induced by sunlight, aging changes in skin should be studied as much as possible in individuals lacking a history of excessive sun exposure.

III. EPIDERMAL HISTOLOGY AND AGE

The epidermis of older individuals exhibits a marked variation in thickness (often in the same histologic section) and a disparity in the size, shape, and staining quality of the basal cell nuclei under light microscopy. There is also a loss of the orderly alignment of cells along the basement membrane and a disruption of the gradual upward uniform differentiation present in the epidermis of younger individuals. There is a variable deposition of glycogen in the older epidermis, occasional keratinocyte nuclear atypia, and a flattening of the dermal-epidermal junction.[1,34,66,67] Electron microscopic studies show that the basal cells of the flattened epidermis of old individuals lack villi.[54,67]

Melanocyte density has been reported to decline approximately 10% per decade.[84,85] Table 8 illustrates the average number of melanocytes per square millimeter in several age groups.[24,87] It should be noted, however, that the number of subjects in the over-70 group is quite small in this study.

IV. EPIDERMAL THICKNESS AND AGE

It is commonly accepted that the epidermis atrophies with age, though data on this point conflict. Histologic studies of the thickness of the epidermis between the rete pegs show about a 20% decrease in the thickness of the epidermis over the human life span. For example, Evans et al.[22] reported that the average thickness of the epidermis from the antecubital fossa of seven people 19 to 30 years old was 33.8 μm and from seven people 80 to 94 years was 27.3 μm.

Table 9 Epidermal thickness and age in males (μm)

Age	Trunk	(N)	Extremities	(N)	Face	(N)
10–19			42	(2)		
20–29	41	(6)	40	(2)	39	(2)
30–39	46	(5)			50	(5)
40–49	43	(4)	55	(4)	55	(4)
50–59	45	(14)	58	(8)	60	(6)
60–69	42	(4)	62	(12)	59	(3)
70–79	39	(2)	95	(2)	65	(1)
80+					60	(5)

Note: N = *number of individuals. The average thickness of epidermis from male and female individuals of all ages combined was: face 49.8 ± 2.19 μm,* N *= 30; trunk 42.8 ± 12.4 μm,* N *= 36; and extremities 60.1 ± 18.7 μm,* N *= 45.*

Data from Whitton, J. and Everall, J.D., Br. J. Dermatol., *89, 467, 1973.*

Table 10 The area of the D-E junction in human abdominal skin

Age	0–20	21–40	41–60	61–80	80–100
No.	13	15	17	14	1
Area/mm² body surface ± S.D.	2.75 ± 0.48	2.67 ± 0.68	2.15 ± 0.62	1.90 ± 0.41	1.16

Data from Katzberg, A., Anat. Rec., *131, 717, 1958.*

Artifacts may distort histologic measurements of epidermal thickness. For example, an excised sample will shrink, making the tissue appear thicker than *in vivo.* As described below, skin from older individuals loses its elasticity and after excision or stretching, contracts less than skin from younger individuals.

To avoid such artifacts, Whitton and Everall[93] have measured epidermal thickness by separating the epidermis from the dermis with sodium bromide and then weighing the dried epidermis. The weight of a fixed area of epidermis was determined with a template technique initially devised by Southwood.[88] The measurements are calibrated by restretching the excised specimen to an original template diameter. Although the number of individuals studied was not great, no dramatic difference in the overall thickness of the epidermis was found with age (Table 9). The authors felt the data from the trunk were the most reliable, as it varies least in thickness from site to site.

Histologic studies of the length of the undulating dermal-epidermal (D-E) junction allow for calculation of the area of D-E contact. Table 10 summarizes the average area of the D-E junction of abdominal skin specimens from individuals of various ages.[45] The mean area declines from 2.67 ± 0.68 mm at 21 to 40 years to 1.90 ± 0.41 mm at 61 to 80 years. However, this figure is calculated using the square of the linear measurement of the length of the D-E junction on a histological section of skin. If the undulations in younger skin are more prominent due to greater contraction of the biopsy after excision, the observed difference indicated in Table 10 would be magnified because it is squared and may not accurately reflect the *in vivo* state.

Lavker et al.[54,55] performed electron microscopic studies of upper inner arm and dorsal forearm skin from individuals 20 to 25 and 68 to 84 years old and found no differences in nonsun-exposed skin between the two groups with respect to the fine structural features of the basal, spinous, granular, or horny layers. Basal cells from light-exposed regions of elderly

Table 11 Effect of age on mitotic index of epidermis

Age	0–20	21–40	41–60	61–80
No.	8	21	13	12
Average age	7.7	33.0	49.0	70.0
Mitosis per 100,000 cells	24.5 ± 18	36.8 ± 22	49.7 ± 22	48.9 ± 21
Mitotic index	0.245	0.368	0.497	0.489

Data from Thuringer, J.M. and Katzberg, A.A., J. Invest. Dermatol., *54, 19, 1959.*

subjects showed greater variability in size, shape, and electron density than did similar regions from young donors; otherwise the fine epidermal structure was similar.[54] Electron microscopic studies of the D-E junction in young individuals showed numerous villous cytoplasmic projections of basal cells into the dermis. Old skin lacks these projections, thus exhibiting a flat D-E interface.[54,55] Hull and Warfel[40] studied the epidermal surface of the basal lamina of 26 individuals with scanning electron microscopy. Abdominal skin from 26 individuals ranging from 16 to 92 years was obtained at autopsy and the epidermis was separated from the dermis using 2 N sodium bromide. Although no objective measurements were taken, it was noted that skin from individuals in the 7th to 10th decades showed progressive loss of dermal valleys, flattening and widening of dermal papillae, and loss of corrugation of the basal lamina that was seen in younger individuals.

V. MEASUREMENTS OF EPIDERMAL CELL TURNOVER

Conflicting information exists concerning change in the mitotic rate of the epidermis with age. Clearly, both epidermal and full-thickness wounds heal faster in younger individuals. Thuringer and Katzberg[89] determined the mitotic index of human abdominal skin freshly excised in the morning at surgical operations. Counting mitoses in 100,000 epidermal cells for each person studied, they found the mitotic index to increase with age from 0.245 at an average age of 8 to 0.489 at an average age of 70 (Table 11). This difference is significant at $p < 0.05$, but there are no significant differences between the other age values.

Kligman[52] examined the labeling index of the epidermis 45 min after intradermal injection of ^3H-thymidine in adult and aged men. He found that there were about one half as many labeled basal cell nuclei in the aged population after the 45-min labeling period (Table 12).

The turnover of the human epidermis can be estimated by staining the stratum corneum with a fluorescent marker such as tetrachlorsalicylanilide and measuring the time required for the dye to vanish. Assuming the fluorescent dye does not disturb the steady state, this technique will reflect the replacement rate of the stratum corneum and indirectly the turnover of the epidermis. Using this technique, Baker and Blair[5] found the stratum corneum replacement time of the volar surface of the mid-forearm to be 20.4 ± 3.1 d in five women with an average age of 87.6 ± 4 years and 26.3 ± 5.1 d in six men of 73 ± 10 years. The mean transit time in 9 young men (age not specified) was 13.3 d and in four women between 21 and 40

Table 12 Labeling index of epidermal basal layer in men

Age range	Mean age	*(N)*	Back	Leg
18–25	19	(9)	4.84 ± 0.42	5.44 ± 0.51
69–86	77	(10)	2.73 ± 0.87	2.99 ± 0.95

Data from Kligman, A.M., J. Invest. Dermatol., *73, 39, 1979.*

Table 13 Epidermal renewal as a function of age

Age	(N)	Corneocyte size (mm²) (±S.D.)	Transit time (d) (±S.D.)	Cell layers (±S.D.)	Replacement rate (layers/d, ±S.D.)	Replacement rate (cells/ mm²/d, ±S.D.)
20–25	(10)	938 ± 39	18.6 ± 3.1	16.2 ± 1.0	0.89 ± 0.11	952 ± 154
40–45	(10)	988 ± 94	17.8 ± 2.0	16.0 ± 1.6	0.90 ± 0.11	939 ± 227
60–65	(10)	1143 ± 162	27.7 ± 7.2	16.3 ± 1.5	0.62 ± 0.12	560 ± 177

Data from Grove, G., in Aging and the Skin, *Balin, A. and Kligman, A., Eds., Raven Press, NY, 1989, 193.*

years the forearm transit time was 13.5 ± 2 d.[5-7] Roberts and Marks[77] confirmed that it took longer for the fluorescent dye dansyl chloride to disappear from the stratum corneum of older men than younger men, but not enough individuals were examined to develop reliable statistics with respect to age.

Grove[30] found age-associated diminution in the turnover rate of the epidermis. He measured the time it took for a marker dye to disappear from the stratum corneum and did not find a linear decline with age. The replacement rate of the epidermis was similar in people ranging from 20 to 45 years, but declined in the 60 to 64 year group (Table 13).

The number of corneocytes that can be scrubbed off the skin per square centimeter in a 4-d period is also an indirect measure of epidermal renewal which has been shown to decline with age. The average number decreases from 746,000 (average age 22, $N = 30$) to 351,000 (average age 67, $N = 30$).[59]

VI. DERMAL CHANGES ASSOCIATED WITH AGING

In fetal dermis the collagen fibers are fine and fibrillar. These fibers thicken until about the 20th year. Light microscopic studies reveal that the collagen bundles of nonsun-exposed buttock skin are thinner and less dense throughout the dermis in aged individuals. The interstitial tissue between the collagen bundles stains strongly for hyaluronic acid.[12] The dermal papillae, as mentioned above, flatten with age, and the number of superficial capillary vessels decreases; cutaneous nerves are not noticeably affected. In very old skin degeneration of elastic tissue becomes apparent by tintorial alterations in staining.[54,66,67]

Elastic fibers run from the reticular into the papillary dermis and split to form fibers running parallel to the epidermis, forming an arcade below the D-E junction. From this arcade run fine elastic fibers perpendicular to the basement membrane and even finer fibers in a brush-like pattern going directly to the basal lamina of the D-E junction.[64] The finest fibers are called oxytalan fibers, and the arcade fibers elaunin fibers. The oxytalan fibers consist of bundles of 10 to 12 nm elastic microfibrils, while the elaunin fibers are bundles of microfibrils that are partially infiltrated with elastin.[12] Both Braverman and Montagna[67] have shown that in the sun-protected areas of aged individuals the terminal elastic fibers and arcades become progressively thickened and some terminal fibers disappear.

Braverman found that only a small portion of the elastic fibers were abnormal in the 30 to 50 year age group. The most common abnormality in this age group was the beginning of cystic spaces within the bundles of elastic microfibrils. In people between 50 and 79 years the cystic spaces became larger and produced lacunae that result in the separation of the elastic microfibrils from each other. Some of the lacunae contain granular material. Ruthenium red dye, which stains mucopolysaccharides, is able to penetrate the interstices of elastic fibers in older individuals, indicating that the elastic fiber becomes porous with age-related degeneration.[12] Most of the elastic fibers were abnormal in individuals over 70 years.

Table 14 Histologic evaluation of marked elastosis (grade 3,4) in facial malar skin

Individuals with grade 3, 4 elastosis (%)				
Age	**Black**	***(N)***	**White**	***(N)***
16–20	—	—	10	(18)
21–30	5	(33)	30	(26)
31–40	30	(40)	75	(31)
41–50	35	(58)	90	(39)
51–60	55	(27)	100	(22)
61–70	45	(16)	100	(17)
71–80	75	(14)	100	(10)

Note: *Elastic tissue changes are graded as follows: 0, no change; 1^+, simple increase without thickening; 2^+, greater hyperplasia plus thickening and curling; 3^+, marked hyperplasia, thickening, curling, and frequent branching; 4^+, almost complete replacement of the dermis by a dense tangle of thickened, disorderly fibers accompanied by disorganization into murky, amorphous masses.*

Data from Kligman, A.M., in Sunlight and Man, *Fitzpatrick, T., Ed., University of Tokyo Press, Tokyo, 1974, 157.*

These abnormalities included haphazardly arranged, short, elastic microfibrils associated with amorphous, electron-dense, granular material. The short fibers may be an artifact of sectioning tightly coiled fibers. There was no evidence that alterations in collagen contributed to the abnormal elastic fibers. There was no inflammatory infiltrate among the degenerated elastic fibers of aged skin.[12]

Light microscopy of sun-damaged skin shows marked proliferations of fibers that stain with elastic stains throughout the papillary dermis and superficial reticular dermis. These elastotic fibers are thickened and form large granular and amorphous-appearing bodies. By electron microscopy Lavker[54,55] has demonstrated increased amounts of elastic fibers in the papillary dermis of actinically damaged skin of aged individuals. Electron microscopy of the elastotic staining granules and the amorphous deposits seen by light microscopy in actinically damaged skin shows them to be composed of masses of 8 to 11 nm microfibrils.[54,55] This confirms that the elastotic staining material in actinically damaged skin is due to degenerating elastic fibers, rather than collagen. Additionally, the desmosine concentration of the elastotic material has been shown by radioimmunoassay to be increased fourfold compared to normal skin, further supporting that the elastotically degenerated material derives from elastic tissue.[48]

Sun-damaged skin contains dense conglomerates of tightly packed colinear collagen fibrils. These fibrils are located primarily parallel to the surface of the skin, immediately below the basal lamina, resulting in a grenz zone believed to represent a reparative process.[54] Table 14 illustrates the magnitude of marked elastotic change in facial skin of whites and blacks; 75% of whites show marked elastotic degeneration by age 40.[50,51]

Table 15 Total number of cells in dermis of human abdominal skin in 34,810 μm²

Age	Japanese female	(N)	Japanese male	(N)	Caucasian male	(N)
1	106.6 ± 5.0[a]	(8)	109.1 ± 7.1	(7)	90.9 ± 4.8	(11)
1–10	73.0	(10)	85.8 ± 5.1	(7)	83.5 ± 4.0	(10)
11–20	66.4 ± 4.5	(7)	72.4 ± 3.3	(15)	76.7 ± 2.4	(10)
21–30	61.1 ± 2.4	(1)	64.2 ± 2.7	(17)	69.2 ± 2.4	(11)
31–40	62.9 ± 2.6	(16)	63.1 ± 2.6	(23)	58.7 ± 4.4	(12)
41–50	66.7 ± 3.1	(14)	64.3 ± 2.4	(20)	50.9 ± 4.5	(11)
51–60	61.0 ± 2.2	(12)	58.2 ± 1.7	(35)	54.2 ± 4.0	(10)
61–70	55.7 ± 2.2	(16)	55.5 ± 1.6	(29)	45.5 ± 1.8	(24)
71–80	50.1 ± 2.3	(13)	42.2 ± 1.2	(16)	50.7 ± 1.9	(25)
81+	39.3 ± 1.4	(6)	45.3 ± 1.4	(3)	46.2 ± 1.6	(20)

[a] *Standard deviation.*

Data from Andrew, W., Behnke, R., and Sato, T., Gerontologica, *10, 1, 1964.*

VII. CHANGES IN THE DERMAL CELL POPULATION WITH AGE

The number of cells in the dermis declines with age. Andrew and associates conducted an extensive study of the number of nuclei in abdominal skin surgically excised from Caucasians and Japanese. The data are summarized in Table 15 and demonstrate a decline of at least 50% in the number of cells in the dermis.[2] Approximately 50% of the cells in each category were fibroblasts. This observation is important for *in vitro* studies of aging, because initial 3-mm punch biopsies from donors of different ages will contain different numbers of fibroblasts. Accordingly, fibroblasts from older individuals will have to undergo more population doublings or have a larger proportion of the fibroblasts in the biopsy grow out of the biopsy to achieve confluence in the first tissue culture flask (designated passage 0). Some of the apparent age-related decline in *in vitro* population doublings from older individuals may be due to the fact that the experiments are started with fewer cells from older individuals. These cells will have had to undergo more population doublings before the experiments start. Unambiguous data comparing the *in vitro* life span of cells from individuals of various ages could be obtained by establishing the cultures with a known quantity of fibroblasts isolated from the primary biopsy. Also, the age-related proliferation decrement may prove to be underestimated by the current technique and could be of more prognostic utility if the total cumulative life span of all the fibroblasts within the biopsy were determined instead of simply the proliferative life span of the first crop or outgrowth to fill the initial (primary) flask.

VIII. THICKNESS OF THE DERMIS WITH AGE

Skin thickness can be determined by a radiographic method which allows *in vivo* measurement. This obviates the problem of potential differences in contraction of the specimen due to age, an objection to micrometer measurements of excised dermis. Excised specimens, however, can be restretched to an original template diameter, as described by Southwood[88] and as discussed above. Black[10] has applied this radiographic technique and has confirmed that skin thickness decreases with age. His results show that the average skin thickness declines from 1.3 mm in

Table 16 Radiographic measurement of skin thickness with age (radial aspect forearm)

	Average age	N	Average skin thickness (mm) (S.E.)
Female	35.1	53	1.1 ± 0.005
Male	32	51	1.3 ± 0.02
Female	77.2	22	0.9 ± 0.03
Male	78.6	14	0.9 ± 0.041

Data from Black, M., Br. J. Dermatol., *81, 661, 1969.*

adult males (1.1 mm in females) to 0.9 mm in aged individuals of either sex (Table 16). Both epidermis and dermis are measured, but as we see from Table 9, the epidermal contribution is uniform and <5%.

IX. ALTERATIONS IN DERMAL COLLAGEN WITH AGE

An extensive literature has developed documenting alterations in collagen during the aging process. Most of these studies have been performed on collagen from tendon, dura mater or other sites, but not human skin. Recently, advanced nonenzymatic glycosylation products have been found to accumulate with age and to cross-link with collagen.

X. SKIN ELASTICITY AND AGE

Marked changes in skin elasticity occur with age. Skin elasticity was defined by Hollingsworth as the time required for a standard "pinch" to flatten.[37,38] Table 17 quantifies the marked decrease in elasticity that occurs with aging. Few biologic parameters change so dramatically with aging. Skin elasticity seems to be one of the best biologic parameters correlating with chronological age, and there are several techniques for its determination that provide quantitative, reproducible data.

Table 17 Skin elasticity and age

	Time (s) ± S.D.			
Age	**Female**	***(N)***	**Male**	***(N)***
10–19	0	(4)	0	(3)
20–29	0	(34)	0	(23)
30–39	0.2 ± 0.5	(90)	0.02 ± 0.1	(45)
40–49	1.9 ± 2.4	(43)	1.2 ± 1.0	(19)
50–59	11.8 ± 15.7	(59)	3.9 ± 5.3	(40)
60–69	21.6 ± 23.8	(26)	19.9 ± 20.8	(30)
70+	57.3 ± 31.6	(12)	43.1 ± 28.4	(9)

Note: Skin elasticity is defined as the time required for a standard pinch to flatten.

Data from Hollingsworth, J.W., Hashizuma, A., and Jablon, S., Yale J. Biol. Med., *33, 11, 1965.*

Obviously, those tests that can be performed repeatedly and noninvasively are of greater utility for the measurement of changes that may correlate with physiological age.

Lee[57] measured the elasticity of 10 × 35 mm strips of antecubital and forehead skin excised from autopsied individuals of various ages. She placed ink marks 20 mm apart and measured the distance between the marks after a 10-g weight had been allowed to stretch the skin (to equilibrium) and again after the weight had been removed and the skin allowed to recover. She found that with increasing age the skin stretches less and then recovers a smaller fraction of the length. This study gives an estimate of the differences in contraction to be expected when excisional (or punch) biopsies are obtained from individuals of different ages (Table 18).

Kirk and Chieffi[49] used a Schade elastometer to determine the degree of indentation following the application of a 50-g weight on the skin surface and the recovery that occurred after removal of the weight. The measurements were made over the medial surface of the tibia 10 cm above the medial malleolus in patients with no evidence of edema. Recovery from this procedure was inversely related to the age of the donor (Table 19). Although it is difficult to determine precisely the relative contribution of all of the parameters involved in influencing the results of this test, this simple procedure may prove a useful aid in constructing a physiological aging index.

Grahame and Holt[27] have developed a suction technique to measure the elastic modulus of human skin *in vivo* and have been able to quantitate skin distensibility in dynes per square centimeter. Their studies show that dorsal forearm skin is more distensible in older individuals (Table 20). Skin already stretched *in vivo* will be lax and thus more distensible with this suction technique. When excised it will neither contract nor stretch much more if a weight is applied, as seen in Table 18.

XI. ALLERGIC CONTACT SENSITIZATION AND AGE

Several teams of investigators have compared the ability of adult and aged individuals to develop contact sensitivity. Waldorf et al.[92] attempted to induce contact sensitivity to 2,4-dinitrochlorobenzene (DNCB) by application of a 5-d occlusive patch test containing 2 mg of DNCB. They found that only 69% of individuals over the age of 70 would react compared to 96% of individuals under 70 (Table 21). Of the 104 subjects, 60 showed a positive reaction to tuberculin; 16 of these could not be sensitized to the DNCB.[92]

It should be mentioned, however, that several studies have not been able to demonstrate a difference in the ability to sensitize adult and aged individuals. Catalona et al.[16] could show no age-related change in the ability to sensitize to DNCB and found that 96% of 143 healthy volunteers between 20 and 80 could be so sensitized. Smith and Kiem[83] found no difference in the ability of young (18 to 42 years) and old (66 to 97 years) individuals to be sensitized to a single application of 0.00125 mol of DNCB or 0.00125 mol of paranitrodimethylaniline (NDMA). This amount of antigen was sufficient, however, to sensitize only 60% of the DNCB-challenged individuals and 44 to 50% of the NDMA-challenged individuals. Epstein and Jessar[21] studied 119 people aged 60 to 97 and found no decreased susceptibility to sensitization with DNCB or NDMA.

Langerhans cells are involved in the initial processing and presentation of antigens to the immune system. Gilchrest et al.[26] have examined the number of epidermal Langerhans cells in four young and seven old individuals. They counted the number of Langerhans cells in a single 1 μm section of a 3-mm punch biopsy from each of the donors and found that young adults (22 to 26 years) had 10.0 ± 0.8 ($N = 4$) Langerhans cells per 3 mm wide section and aged adults (62 to 86, mean age 69) had 5.8 ± 1.1 ($N = 7$) Langerhans cells (Table 22).

Table 18 Stretch and recovery of 20-mm strip of antecubital skin after application of a 10-g weight

Age	*N*	Forearm skin length during suspension (mm ± S.D.)	Forearm skin length after recovery (mm ± S.D.)
73–84	2	23.6 ± 2.0	21 ± 0.6
62–65	2	26.1 ± 1.3	22 ± 0
47–54	4	27.4 ± 1.3	21.7 ± 0.5
40–45	7	29.0 ± 1.3	21.4 ± 0.4
30–35	4	29.9 ± 3.4	21.1 ± 0.2
23–29	4	32.8 ± 2.6	21.4 ± 0.4
13–15	3	32.5 ± 0.2	20.8 ± 0.2
4–10	5	32.4 ± 2.4	21 ± 0.5
4 months–1 year	4	26.5 ± 1.2	21.4 ± 0.8

Data from Lee, M., Anat. Rec., *129, 473, 1957.*

Table 19 Standard elasticity in males over the medial surface of tibia

Age	*N*	Indentation, 2-min (mm ± S.D.)	Immediate rebound as % 2-min indentation (mm ± S.D.)	Rebound, 3-min, as % 2-min indentation (mm ± S.D.)
100–104	1	1.60	40	81
95–99	1	2.70	26	59
90–94	2	1.98	31	68
85–89	8	2.15 ± 1.02	25 ± 10	65 ± 10
80–84	17	1.96 ± 0.85	35 ± 11	76 ± 8
75–79	20	2.25 ± 0.80	37 ± 16	71 ± 13
70–74	32	2.18 ± 0.90	34 ± 12	73 ± 9
65–69	33	2.42 ± 0.82	42 ± 11	78 ± 12
60–64	43	2.25 ± 1.10	39 ± 11	75 ± 13
55–59	11	1.91 ± 0.65	41 ± 19	74 ± 15
50–54	15	1.88 ± 0.77	38 ± 12	74 ± 15
45–49	16	1.95 ± 0.78	48 ± 12	74 ± 10
40–44	13	2.31 ± 0.84	47 ± 4.0	79 ± 12
35–39	19	2.54 ± 1.07	55 ± 17	77 ± 14
30–34	9	2.52 ± 0.65	53 ± 14	84 ± 9
25–29	15	2.31 ± 1.02	55 ± 11	83 ± 11
20–24	14	2.56 ± 0.79	68 ± 17	85.4 ± 14
18–19	9	3.32 ± 0.86	77 ± 11	99 ± 5

Data from Kirk, J. and Chieffi, M., J. Gerontol., *17, 373, 1962.*

Table 20 *In vivo* elastic modulus of dorsal forearm skin from humans with age (dyn/cm^2 × 10^8 ± S.E.)

Age	Male	*N*	Female	*N*
20–44	1.8 ± 0.17	12	2.6 ± 0.17	11
45–69	2.2 ± 0.15	10	3.4 ± 0.29	12
70	3.2 ± 0.51	5	5.7 ± 0.71	9

Data from Grahame, R. and Holt, P., Gerontologist, *15, 121, 1969.*

Mackay and co-workers[76] examined the age-related ability to respond with a delayed hypersensitivity skin response to five common antigens: *Candida,* trichophyton, tuberculin, mumps, and streptokinase/streptodornase. Their results are shown in Table 23. No person under 25 years had fewer than two positive reactions while 57% of those over 60 years had fewer than two positive reactions. They found a significantly greater mortality in the people over 80 years who had fewer than two positive reactions (80% of 35 people vs. 35% of 17 people $p < 0.005$) than in those with two or more positive reactions during the 2 years following their measurement. The mean age of survivors was 85.1 years at the time of testing but 85.9 for nonsurvivors. Pneumonia, stroke, and cardiac failure were the most common causes of death in these individuals.[76] Augener et al.[4] showed that the number of circulating T lymphocytes declines more than 50% with age, while the number of B lymphocytes remains steady (Table 24). T lymphocytes were identified by their ability to form spontaneous sheep red blood cell rosettes and B lymphocytes were identified by positive surface immumoglobulin. These findings have been confirmed by other investigators.[15] The decline in T lymphocytes is a possible explanation for the decreased recall-delayed hypersensitivity responses discussed above. Many recent studies have confirmed the decline in T-cell mediated immunity with age. Murasko et al.,[69] for example, have shown that mitogen-induced proliferative responses of lymphocytes in the elderly are significantly lower than in young individuals. They have also found a significant association between lack of response to all three of the mitogens (phytohemagglutinin, concanavalin A, pokeweed mitogen) they tested and mortality.

Table 21 Ability to sensitize to DNCB as a function of age

	Age	No.	DNCB, no. reactive	DNCB, % reactive
Control	35–69	26	25	96
Study	59–69	17	16	94
	70–79	62	43	69
	80–89	35	24	68
	90–99	2	1	50

Note: 60 of 104 subjects showed a positive tuberculin test. The frequency of the positive did not vary significantly with age. A total of 16 individuals who reacted to tuberculin could not be sensitized to DNCB.

Data from Staricco, R.J. and Pinkus, J., J. Invest. Dermatol., *28, 33, 1957.*

Table 22 Epidermal Langerhans cells in young and older adults

Av. age	(N)	Mean ± SEM	Range
69	(7)	5.8 ± 1.1	2–10
23	(4)	10 ± 0.8	8–12

Note: The number of Langerhans cells in a 1-μm section of a 3-mm biopsy from the buttock was determined.

Data from Gilchrest, B.A., Murphy, G., and Soter, N.A., J. Invest. Dermatol., *79, 85, 1982.*

Table 23 Delayed hypersensitivity response to common test antigens

	Number of people	
Total no. of positive	**Young, 25 years (N = 20)**	**Old, 60 years (N = 68)**
5	4	0
4	8	4
3	6	8
2	2	17
1	0	15
0	0	24

Data from Roberts-Thomson, I.C., Whittingham, S., Youngchaiyud, U., and Mackay, I.R., Lancet, *2, 368, 1974.*

XII. AGE-RELATED CHANGES IN SUCTION BLISTER FORMATION

Kiistala[47] has reported an age-related change in the ability to form suction blisters. Dermal-epidermal separation can be achieved by the application of a suction cup device to the skin with negative pressure over time. Suction-induced blisters split at the D-E junction, with the periodic acid Schiff- (PAS) positive basement membrane adhering to the dermal blister base. Electron microscopy shows that the basal lamina also remains at the dermal base of the blister.

Blistering time is defined as the interval between the onset of suction and the appearance of the earliest minute vesicles. There is a progressive decline in the time it takes to form a suction blister as an individual ages. For the experimental data presented in Table 25, 200 mm of negative pressure was maintained with a vacuum pump and applied using a diaphragm with five holes, each 6 mm in diameter. The procedure was done at room temperature (22° to 25°C), but the temperature at the blister site was not controlled or monitored. Maximum resistance to blister formation occurs in the younger age groups and declines progressively with age (116 ± 27 min, age 20 to 29; 36 ± 12 min, age 90 to 99; see Table 25).

Although the mechanisms responsible are not fully established, an inverse relationship exists between the amount of suction pressure applied and the time to blister formation.[60,72] Skin temperature is an important determinant of blistering time; blistering occurs more rapidly at higher skin temperatures. Data obtained by Peachey show that skin blisters are raised twice as fast in both adult and aged individuals at 40°C compared to 34°C (Table 26).[72,73] Neither local vasodilatation (achieved by histamine iontophoresis) nor local vasoconstriction (achieved by

Table 24 Circulating lymphocyte population and age

Age	*(N)*	Total lymphocytes/ mm³ ± S.D.	Total B lymphocytes/ mm³ ± S.D.	Total T lymphocytes/ mm³ ± S.D.
3–12	(12)	2490 ± 850	399 ± 130	1890 ± 600
19–25	(10)	1770 ± 230	350 ± 70	1260 ± 210
32–50	(11)	1560 ± 500	330 ± 100	980 ± 340
67–83	(11)	1250 ± 570	270 ± 140	780 ± 400

Data from Augener, W., Cohnen, G., Reuter, A., and Brittinger, G., Lancet, *1, 1164, 1974.*

Table 25 Epidermal suction blister formation time as a function of age

Age	No.	Antecubital blistering time (mean ± S.D. min)
90–99	11	36 ± 12
80–89	31	45 ± 21
70–79	45	56 ± 20
60–69	51	70 ± 23
50–59	40	85 ± 28
40–49	34	89 ± 23
30–39	49	99 ± 25
20–29	88	116 ± 27
15–19	38	117 ± 35

Note: Performed with 200 mm suction pressure at room temperature (22° to 25°C).

Data from Kiistala, U., Ann. Clin. Res., *4, 10, 1972.*

Table 26 Minutes to blister at 300 mmHg

Age	No.	40°C	*(N)*	37°C	*(N)*	34°C	*(N)*
72.5 ± 5	12	14.1 ± 5.8	(48)	17.8 ± 7.3	(48)	26.1 ± 11	(48)
25 ± 3	12	31.5 ± 8.7	(48)	42.7 ± 11.5	(48)	59.0 ± 15	(48)

Note: Suction cup applied to forearm.

Data from Peachey, R., Br. J. Dermatol., *84, 447, 1971.*

adrenalin iontophoresis) affected the mean blistering time in four 22-year old men when 355 mmHg of suction was applied at 37°C.[73] Presumably the decrease in blistering time in the elderly is a physiological manifestation of the anatomically observed flattening of the rete pegs, which reflects the interdigitation of the epidermis and dermis. Shearing of the skin of aged individuals commonly occurs with minor trauma and represents a pathologic manifestation of these factors.

XIII. PERMEABILITY

The protective barrier function of the skin is primarily due to its low permeability. The stratum corneum presents the major diffusion barrier of the skin.[81] Its permeability has been examined in young and old adults. Despite the histologically evident flattening of the epidermal rete ridges in aged epidermis, the thickness of the stratum corneum and the number of cell layers in the stratum corneum remains the same in young and old individuals. Intact sheets of stratum corneum have been obtained by a cantharidin blister technique,[53] stained with alkaline methylene blue and counted[17]. There are about 15 cell layers (range 14 to 17) in the stratum corneum from the mid-back of young and old individuals.[17,18] These findings have been confirmed by assessing the thickness of the stratum corneum with an electronic thickness gauge, after 10 min and after 24 h of immersion in water. The results indicate that there is no difference in the thickness of the stratum corneum from young and old adults (Table 27).

Potts et al.[75] measured the propagation and attenuation of shear waves generated by frequencies from 8 to 1016 Hz in the skin of the back of the hand in 16 men aged 24 to 63 years. These parameters largely reflect the water content of the stratum corneum and their results suggest that aged stratum corneum has a lower water content than the stratum corneum of younger men.

The functional ability of the stratum corneum to retard water loss appears unimpaired with aging. Christophers and Kligman[18] obtained stratum corneum from the mid-back of young and old individuals and determined the rate of evaporation of water from a chamber through the stratum corneum (Table 28). The water permeance was similar in young and old individuals. It was determined that water is transferred in the vapor phase because the diffusion rate was the same whether the stratum corneum was in physical contact with water or with water vapor.[81]

Although aged stratum corneum is not more permeable to water, it is to some chemical substances. The permeability of the stratum corneum to sodium fluorescein was determined by measuring the diffusion of the fluorescein from one chamber, across a stratum corneum sheet (from the mid-back, as described above), into a second chamber. The transfer across the stratum corneum from aged men was much greater than that from younger men (Table 29). In addition, extreme individual variation was present through the stratum corneum of aged individuals. The large standard deviation present in the aged values of Table 29 resulted from a permeability of 22.1 μg/h/cm^2 in one individual. If this result is omitted the mean is 4.9 ± 3.0. A similar increase in the permeability of the stratum corneum from aged individuals to tetrachlorsalicylanilide was also found.[18]

Grove et al.[28] have created intraepidermal blisters in young and old adults by applying a 50% solution of NH_4OH to the skin. This technique was developed by Frosch and Kligman,[25] and it has been shown that prolonged exposure (10 min greater than the minimal blistering time) to this agent will produce total destruction of the epidermis; marked vascular damage with hemorrhage; and a deep inflammatory infiltrate in the dermis.[25] The minimal exposure time required to induce a blister is an indicator of the barrier property of the stratum corneum (see

Table 27 Thickness of the stratum corneum (μm) after water immersion

Age ± S.D.	(N)	10 min ± S.D.	24 h ± S.D.
76.8 ± 3.8	(15)	9.2 ± 1.4	18.9 ± 3.1
24.2 ± 2.4	(13)	10.8 ± 1.4	22.2 ± 2.2

Note: Stratum corneum obtained by cantharidin blister technique from the midback.

Data from Christophers, E. and Kligman, A.M., in Advances in the Biology of the Skin, *Vol. 6, Montagna, W., Ed., Pergamon Press, New York, 1965, 163.*

Table 28 Water permeance of stratum corneum

Age ± S.D.	(N)	mg/h/cm²
74 ± 4	(12)	0.74 ± 0.33
24 ± 2	(11)	0.82 ± 0.18

Note: *Stratum corneum obtained by cantharidin blister technique from the midback. The stratum corneum was sealed over water in diffusion chambers, kept at 37°C in a desiccator, and weighed daily for 6 d.*

Data from Christophers, E. and Kligman, A.M., in Advances in the Biology of the Skin, *Vol. 6, Montagna, W., Ed., Pergamon Press, New York, 1965, 163.*

below). The initial blistering response, as measured by Grove et al.,[28] was the time for tiny follicular vesicles to develop. The average time for an initial blistering response to develop on the volar forearm decreased from 11.6 ± 4.3 min in 12 individuals aged 18 to 30 to 6.6 ± 3.0 min in 12 individuals aged 65 to 78. This decreased initial blistering time is thought to reflect either increased diffusion through appendageal shunts or loss of stratum corneum integrity.

XIV. PERCUTANEOUS ABSORPTION

Percutaneous absorption involves several steps: absorption to the stratum corneum; diffusion through the stratum corneum, epidermis and papillary dermis; and removal by the microcirculation. Penetration through the stratum corneum, the rate-limiting step under most circumstances, was discussed above. The physical variations in skin morphology contribute to regional differences in percutaneous penetration of some substances, such as ^{14}C cortisol.[23] Despite the increased permeability of aged stratum corneum to some chemical agents (but not to water), *in vivo* percutaneous absorption has been shown to be markedly reduced when absorption through mid-back skin of aged men is compared with that of young men. *In vivo* absorption of ^{14}C testosterone was determined on the mid-back skin of young and old individuals by the residual analysis method of Malkinson.[61] Absorption is three times greater in 24-year-old men than in 75-year-old men (Table 30).

This reduced absorption is due, as least in part, to a diminished clearance of the substance by the microcirculation in the aged individuals. Physiologic $^{22}NaCl$ was injected into the upper dermal layer of the mid-back skin of young and aged individuals. A continuous recording of the radioactivity was determined with a γ-ray probe, and the halftime for disappearance of the $^{22}NaCl$ was determined. Clearance was significantly slower in older individuals (Table 31).[18] This result

Table 29 Permeability of stratum corneum to fluorescein

Age ± S.D.	(N)	μg/h/cm² ± S.D.
71.2 ± 3.3	(9)	6.97 ± 6.39
25 ± 2.4	(7)	0.95 ± 0.47

Note: *Stratum corneum obtained from midback by cantharidin blister technique.*

Data from Christophers, E. and Kligman, A.M., in Advances in the Biology of the Skin, *Vol. 6, Montagna, W., Ed., Pergamon Press, New York, 1965, 163.*

Table 30 Percutaneous absorption of testosterone

Age ± S.D.	(N)	Absorbed in 24 h (%)
75 ± 4	(10)	12.6 ± 7.1
24 ± 3	(10)	34.9 ± 12.7

Note: In vivo *determination of residual* ^{14}C *testosterone on back skin by method of Malkinson (1958).*

Data from Christophers, E. and Kligman, A.M., in Advances in the Biology of the Skin, *Vol. 6, Montagna, W., Ed., Pergamon Press, New York, 1965, 163.*

Table 31 Clearance of intradermally injected $^{22}NaCl$ from midback skin

Age ± S.D.	(N)	Clearance half-time (min)
76 ± 7	(11)	13.3 ± 2.8
23 ± 1	(10)	8.8 ± 2.0

Note: In vivo *determination of disappearance of* $^{22}NaCl$ *monitored continuously by atomic γ-ray probe.*

Data from Christophers, E. and Kligman, A.M., in Advances in the Biology of the Skin, *Vol. 6, Montagna, W., Ed., Pergamon Press, New York, 1965, 163.*

was confirmed by duplicate intradermal injections of fluorescein in six young and six old individuals, and monitoring the time to disappearance of the fluorescein under a Wood's light (UVA 365 nm). The average time to disappearance of the fluorescein was 96 min in the young and 133 min in the aged. Heite[33] also found that removal of fluorescein dye was slower in the aged.

DeSalve and Thompson[19] have also measured $^{22}NaCl$ clearance with aging, but with fewer subjects per age group, different body locations, and somewhat contradictory results. They noted a decrease in NaCl clearance with age in forearm skin, an increase with age in hand skin, a decrease in facial skin from 20 to 60 years, and then an increase from 60 to 90 years. Individual measurements were not presented, and statistical significance could not be ascertained from their report.

The McClure-Aldrich test measures the time required for a wheal raised by an intradermal injection of 0.2 cm^3 of isotonic saline to flatten. McClure and Aldrich[63] found that it took 66 ± 9 min for a volar forearm wheal to flatten in 12 control children and adults. Ascher[3] determined the wheal resorption time from the volar forearm in aged individuals who were physically healthy but institutionalized for chronic mental disorders. As the age of the individual increased, so did the time required for the wheal to resorb (Table 32). Kligman[52] has repeated this test with 0.5 cm^3 of intradermal isotonic saline, on both the lower back and the volar forearm of young (21 to 30) and old (70 to 83) individuals. He found that the wheals took twice as long to resolve in the aged population (Table 33).

Rougier et al.[79] found that there was an inverse correlation between epidermal cell proliferation and corneocyte size. They determined that there was no difference in radioactive benzoic acid absorption between 20- to 30-year-old men and 44- to 55-year-old men, but a fourfold decrease in the percutaneous absorption of benzoic acid in 65- to 80-year-old men (Table 34). Because the transepidermal water loss was similar in all age groups, this finding may reflect alterations in the dermal vascular supply leading to a decreased clearance of substances absorbed.

Table 32 Wheal resorption time with age

Age ± S.D.	(N)	Wheal resorption time (min) ± S.D.
72 ± 1.3	(4)	128 ± 34
68 ± 1.4	(11)	122 ± 25
63 ± 1.1	(7)	95 ± 18
38 ± 9	(6)	67 ± 14

Note: Duplicate intradermal wheals were injected into the volar forearm with 0.2 cm³ of physiologic saline. Resorption of the wheal was defined as the time the wheal could no longer be seen or palpated. These patients were physically healthy but were institutionalized for chronic mental disorders. N = *number of individuals.*

Data from Ascher, B., Exp. Med. Surg., *18, 17, 1960.*

Table 33 Wheal resorption time (min)

	Lower back		Volar forearm	
Age	(N)	(min ± S.D.)	(N)	(min ± S.D.)
21–30	(21)	40 ± 9	(22)	47 ± 11
70–83	(26)	83 ± 19	(24)	86 ± 18

Note: Wheal resorption measured after intradermal injection of 0.5 ml isotonic saline.

Data from Kligman, A.M., J. Invest. Dermatol., *73, 39, 1979.*

Table 34 **Skin permeability and corneocyte size as a function of age**

Male	(N)	TEWL ± S.D.	Benzoic acid penetration (± S.D. in 4 d)	Corneocyte surface (mm² area ± S.D.)
20–30	(8)	4.24 ± 0.35	9.15 ± 1.01	980 ± 34
45–55	(8)	5.07 ± 0.23	10.02 ± 1.02	994 ± 56
65–80	(7)	4.73 ± 0.45	2.53 ± 0.82	1141 ± 63

Data from Rougier, A., Lotte, C., Corcuff, P., and Maibach, H.I., J. Soc. Cosmet. Chem., *39, 15, 1988.*

Grove et al.[28] noted that it took at least twice as long for full-tense blisters to develop after 50% NH_4OH application in aged adults compared to young adults. These were the same people described above in the section on stratum corneum permeability. Although the aged individuals had a much shorter initial follicular blistering response, it took twice as long to fill a tense blister as the younger cohort (volar forearm: $N = 12$, age 13 to 30, 11.8 ± 7.1 min to blister formations vs. $N = 12$, age 65 to 78, 24.6 ± 12.3 min). This age-associated increase in blister time appears to reflect the impairment in the microvasculature's ability to supply fluid. This impairment manifests itself clinically as a decreased cutaneous inflammatory response (redness, warmth, swelling) to noxious agents.

XV. MICROVASCULATURE CHANGES IN AGED SKIN

Alkaline phosphatase stained histological sections highlight the cutaneous vasculature. Deletion and derangement of small blood vessels is found in aged skin, with sun-damaged skin with extensive elastosis being the most severely affected.[52]

Braverman et al.[13,14] have examined the dermal microvasculature of aged individuals by electron microscopy. In actinically damaged extensor forearm skin the walls of the microcirculatory vessels were thickened. The postcapillary venules were more severely involved than the terminal arterioles and capillaries. The thickening was produced by a perivascular layer of basement membrane-like material mixed with collagen fibers. A veil cell was usually seen in the space between the vessel and the newly deposited material. The thickness of the walls of the affected vessels was increased by 0.5 to 2 um. The vascular wall thickening was not seen in individuals under the age of 40, whose extensor forearm skin appeared normal.

Biopsies from the buttocks of several 80- to 93-year-old individuals revealed vessels with abnormally thin walls. The changes were confined primarily to the postcapillary venules, with the venous and arterial capillaries affected to a lesser degree. The deposition of basement membrane material in the wall of the vessel was normal in some areas of the vessel and reduced to a single basal lamina between the endothelial cell and the surrounding dermal collagen in other areas. The basement membrane material normally present in lamellae of the vascular wall was decreased. The walls of the thin vessels measured 0.5 to 1.0 μm (normal 2 to 3 μm). The veil cells surrounding the thin vessels of older individuals were absent or fewer in number.[13,14]

XVI. NAIL GROWTH AND AGE

Nail growth has been shown to decline with age.[8,9,32,35,70] Data from two large cross-sectional studies are presented in Table 35. In these studies growth of thumbnails was recorded over a 6- to 8-week interval. Overall the mean growth rate declined from approximately 0.75 mm/week at ages 20 to 29 to 0.5 mm/week at ages 80 to 89 (Table 36).[32,70] It should be noted that these tables were derived from graphs of mean data presented in the original publications, and the standard deviation within the age groups was not published. Scattergrams of individual data points from these publications reveal extensive individual variation within the age groups.

Hillman[35] studied 12 males and 17 females from ages 30 to 39 and found a mean ± S.D. nail growth rate of 0.80 ± 0.07 mm/week and 0.72 ± 0.11 mm/week. These standard deviations are not applicable to the data presented in Tables 35 and 36 but do give an idea of the range of individual variation within a particular age group.

Studies of nail growth rate have revealed no differences between the right and left hands.[32,58] Fingernails grow faster than toenails; the third fingernail grows the fastest, about 9% faster than the thumbnail.[32] Nail growth is retarded during severe illness, starvation, and lactation[8,9] and is increased in nailbiters, with pregnancy, and warm weather.[71] It is decreased in a paralyzed limb; and ischemia slows nail growth, most commonly on the feet.[9]

Bean[9] has performed a longitudinal study by marking his left thumbnail every month for 31 years and recording the interval required for the mark to move to the distal free margin of his nail. He has noted a slow but irregular decline in the rate of growth: 0.87 mm/week at age 32; 0.82 mm/week at age 42; 0.73 mm/week at age 52; and 0.70 mm/week at age 61. He has noted a marked decrease in nail growth with illness but no variation with geographic locations, physical activity, or season.

Transonychial water loss decreases with increasing age and appears independent of nail thickness.[43]

Table 35 Thumbnail growth (mm/week) in various age groups of Japanese and Caucasian males and females

	OMG[a]			
Age	**Female**	***(N)***	**Male**	***(N)***
5–10				
10–19	0.74	(8)	0.89	(8)
20–29	0.78	(16)	0.94	(8)
30–39	0.72	(10)	0.74	(11)
40–49	0.70	(17)	0.84	(6)
50–59	0.66	(12)	0.68	(1)
60–69	0.70	(12)	0.67	(2)
70–79	0.59	(45)	0.56	(12)
80–89	0.57	(55)	0.53	(20)
90–99	0.54	(10)	0.45	(3)

	Hamilton[b]							
	Caucasian				**Japanese**			
Age	**Female**	***(N)***	**Male**	***(N)***	**Female**	***(N)***	**Male**	***(N)***
5–10					0.72	(24)	0.75	(23)
10–19					0.72	(71)	0.76	(77)
20–29	0.74	(20)	0.75	(126)	0.70	(56)	0.73	(52)
30–39	0.69	(10)	0.71	(12)	0.67	(29)	0.71	(24)
40–49	0.64	(17)	0.63	(17)	0.63	(27)	0.67	(22)
50–59	0.62	(20)	0.60	(14)	0.62	(23)	0.65	(25)
60–69	0.62	(22)	0.49	(42)	0.56	(20)	0.64	(19)
70–79	0.55	(30)	0.53	(34)	0.54	(15)	0.55	(14)
80–89	0.54	(49)	0.49	(35)	0.57	(15)	0.54	(15)
90–99	0.50	(13)						

[a] *OMG: data from Orentreich and Sharp.*[70]
[b] *Hamilton: data from Hamilton, Terada and Mestler.*[32]

Note: The rate of growth of the thumbnail was measured over a 6 to 8-week interval. The left thumbnail was used for most measurements. N = *number of subjects.*

XVII. WOUND HEALING AND AGE

Although dermatologic surgeons may sometimes prefer aged patients, who, in contrast to younger subjects, have more lax skin, less tendency to form hypertrophic scars or keloids, and lower cosmetic expectations, investigators studying age-related alterations in physiologic function have observed a decreased rate of healing and a decreased final wound strength in older mammals. Hard experimental data in humans are limited but do support the contention that wound healing is slower in the elderly population.

Healing of skin blisters raised by applications of NH_4OH has been compared in two groups of 12 younger (18 to 25) and 12 older (65 to 75) adults; restoration of skin-line markings was used as an indication of complete healing. The younger subjects healed in 3.6 ± 0.7 weeks, the older in 5.4 ± 1.2 weeks.[29]

Table 36 Thumbnail growth vs. age

Age	*(N)*	Growth/week (mm)
90–99	(26)	0.51
80–89	(190)	0.54
70–79	(150)	0.56
60–69	(117)	0.61
50–59	(95)	0.63
40–49	(106)	0.66
30–39	(96)	0.70
20–29	(278)	0.74
10–19	(164)	0.75
5–10	(47)	0.73

Note: Weighed average of all data presented by subject class in Table 33. N = *number of subjects.*

Orentreich and Selmanowitz[71] have reported their observations in a series of 12,000 dermabrasions, a procedure in which a rapidly rotating wire brush was used to remove the epidermis and the upper third of the dermis on the full face. Healing and epithelialization occurred sooner in younger patients: in 10 d for 25 year olds; 15 d for 50 year olds; and 21 d for 75 year olds.

Grove examined the stratum corneum transit time and the time to repair epidermal defects in 12 individuals ranging in age from 65 to 70 years. He found that those individuals who were judged younger than their stated age had a faster stratum corneum transit time and repaired epidermal defects quicker than those who were judged to look their stated age or to look older than their stated age (Table 37).

The incidence of wound dehiscence has been used as a functional criterion for wound healing of full-thickness surgical wounds. In several retrospective studies it has been shown that this increases with age.[31,65] For example, in a cooperative study at 19 Veterans Administration hospitals, the incidence of wound dehiscence after surgery for duodenal ulcer increased from 1% in patients 30 to 39 to 5% in those over 70 (Table 38).[65]

The tensile strength of healing wounds, as defined by the force required to disrupt wounds, was examined in a few patients 5 d after an experimental surgical incision was created. Less force was required to disrupt wounds in four individuals over 70 than in seven persons under 70.[80] The tensile strength of healing wounds in old rats is also decreased.[86] However, many experimental studies supposedly performed to study wound healing as a function of age, were actually planned to compare juvenile with adult animals rather than adult with aged animals.[39,56]

Regeneration of connective tissue has been studied in a few subjects using a technique in which a cellulose sponge is implanted subcutaneously. After 7 d of implantation, the sponge is removed and analyzed for hydroxyproline content. Less hydroxyproline is recovered from sponges removed from older individuals compared to younger subjects.[90] Despite the clinical importance of wound healing problems, the influence of age on wound healing has been inadequately explored scientifically.

Table 37 The relation between epidermal renewal time and appearing younger or older than actual age

Stratum corneum transit time (d)	Time to repair epidermal defects (d)	Estimated age
20	22	<65
25	25	<65
25	39	<65
28	28	<65
30	29	<65
41	35	65–70
43	38	65–70
43	38	65–70
45	41	65–70
47	41	65–70
50	44	>70
60	58	>70

Note: *Stratum corneum transit time was measured by the danoyl chloride dye disappearance method. The time to repair epidermal defects was measured by restoration of skin surface markings. All subjects were between ages 65–70 years. Estimated age was determined by a visual assessment.*

Data from Grove, G., in Aging and the Skin, *Balin, A. and Kligman, A., Eds., Raven Press, NY, 1989, 193.*

Table 38 Incidence of wound dehiscence with age

Age	Patients	Disrupted wound	(%)
80–99	18	1	4.4
70–79	274	13	4.7
60–69	495	22	4.4
50–59	523	13	2.5
40–49	991	13	1.3
30–39	589	5	0.9
20–29	98	0	0
Total	2988	67	2.3

Data from Mendoza, C.B., Postlethwaite, R.W., and Johanson, W.D., Arch. Surg., *101, 396, 1970.*

XVIII. SYNTHESIS OF VITAMIN D

MacLaughlin and Holick[62] measured the relation between aging and the ability of human skin to synthesize vitamin D_3. As shown in Table 39, there is a twofold decrease in the concentration of 7-dehydrocholesterol of epidermis from adult to old age. The data in this table are representative of that obtained with skin from 28 individuals from the age 8 to 92. The ability of aging skin to convert previtamin D_3 to provitamin D_3 under the influence of UV light was also examined. As shown in Table 40, postirradiation levels of previtamin D_3 in 82-year-old skin was 40% that of 8-year-old skin. These results are important, because vitamin D deficiency can contribute to osteomalacia and osteoporosis, conditions commonly seen in the elderly. Because skin is the major site for the synthesis of vitamin D precursors, it has long been held that vitamin D deficiency in the elderly is due to decreased sun exposure. This work shows that elderly skin is actually less responsive to the effect of UV irradiation in converting provitamin D_3 to previtamin D_3.[62]

XIX. SEBACEOUS GLANDS

Sebaceous wax ester secretion in men and women was shown to decline after age 15 to 35. Jacobsen et al.[42] measured the sebaceous wax ester secretion in 109 men and 167 women, aged 15 to 97. The cutaneous sebum reservoir on the forehead was first depleted by overnight lipid absorption onto a layer of bentonite clay. Fresh clay embedded with 2-cm cloth disks was then used to absorb lipid for 3 h. Ether was used to extract the absorbed lipid from the disk, and wax ester content analyzed by thin layer chromatography. The wax ester secretion rate was found to be highest in the 15- to 35-year-old group, and declined afterward. The data suggested that sebum secretion declines about 23%/decade in men and 32%/decade in women.

Table 39 Effect of aging on concentration of 7-dehydrocholesterol (7-DHC) in the epidermis in six individuals

Age	7-DHC conc. (μg/g)	7-DHC conc. (ng/cm²)
88	6.98	838
77	2.41	338
58	8.81	1409
47	9.00	1350
29	11.53	1614
21	11.65	1747

Note: Caucasian skin samples were obtained from patients undergoing operations such as reduction mammoplasty and limb amputation. Epidermal concentrations of 7-DHC were determined and expressed per area and per weight of sample.

Data from MacLaughlin, J. and Holick, M.F., J. Clin. Invest., *76, 1536, 1985.*

Table 40 Previtamin D_3 content after exposure to UV radiation and the percentage of previtamin D_3 formed in the epidermis and dermis relative to an 8-year-old subject

Age	Previtamin D_3 (ng/cm^2)	Previtamin D_3 formation relative to an 8-year-old subject (%)
82	183	40
77	168	37
18	368	80
8	442	100

Note: Skin samples were irradiated with 295 ± 5 nm and concentration of previtamin D_3 measured.

Data from MacLaughlin, J. and Holick, M.F., J. Clin. Invest., *76, 1536, 1985.*

The size of the sebaceous glands, in contrast, increases with age. Plewig and Kligman[74] compared the sebaceous gland size of three different age groups by planimetry. They obtained cheek biopsies from 16 aged subjects (mean 65 ± 5 years), five adults (mean 50 ± 3 years), and 15 young adults (mean 28 ± 8 years). On all biopsies, they measured the average mean cross-sectional area of all sebaceous glands, the size of the individual largest sebaceous glands, and the proportion of total surface occupied by sebaceous glands. As shown in Table 41, there was a gradual increase of all three parameters from young adults to old adults. It was also noted that the population of demodex mites within the follicular canals increased with age.

XX. SUMMARY AND CONCLUSIONS

The cutaneous changes associated with the aging process are widespread and extensive. They affect the epidermis, dermis, appendageal structures, subcutaneous tissue, and the integrated physiologic functioning of the skin. Longitudinal studies correlating changes in specific cutaneous parameters with biologic age do not exist. However, recently data have become available to support the common contention that the overall visual assessment of an individual represents one of the best ways to estimate a person's biological age. The Baltimore Longitudinal Study has been underway at the Gerontology Research Center of the National Institute on Aging since 1958 and has involved the serial measurement of 24 tests of physiologic age in over 1000 males.

Table 41 Variation of sebaceous gland size with age

Age ± S.D.	*(N)*	Largest gland (mm^2) ± S.D.	Av. mean size of sebaceous glands (mm^2) ± S.D.	Mean % surface area ± S.D.
69 ± 5	(21)	0.5060 ± 23	0.4003 ± 0.21	45.7 ± 24.2
50 ± 3	(5)	0.3563 ± 14	0.2532 ± 0.13	44.3 ± 19.6
28 ± 8	(15)	0.3614 ± 15	0.2258 ± 0.08	37.6 ± 17.2

Note: Sizes of sebaceous glands were measured in skin biopsies obtained from the cheek in 41 subjects

Data from Plewig, G. and Kligman, A.M., J. Invest. Dermatol., *70, 314, 1978.*

Borkan and Norris[11] compared the men who were judged to look the oldest for their stated age with those who appeared the youngest for their stated age. These groups were compared with respect to several biologic measurements. On 19 of 24 tests, the subgroup who looked oldest for their stated age were biologically older as well. Further, the subjects who died since the start of the study were biologically older in 19 of the 24 variables.

Except for this visual estimate and the proliferative life span of fibroblasts obtained from skin biopsy, no cutaneous parameters are included for the assessment of biologic age in the Baltimore Longitudinal Study. In addition, in a recent National Institutes of Health conference for the development of biomarkers to measure human age, more than 28 tests were discussed; none involved any cutaneous parameter.[78] It is hoped that cutaneous measurements will be included in future longitudinal studies designed to measure biological age.

In general, most of the measurements presented here demonstrate progressive differences throughout the life span. These trends are seen when groups of young and old are compared. Within each age group a range of variability exists in the measured value and it has been impossible to determine an individual's physiological age based on any single measurement. The past approach to measurement of biologic age and the determination of the rate of human aging should be modified slightly for future studies. The value obtained when any single measurement is performed is likely to be less useful than the rate of change in that measurement in the same individual over time. In order to establish the rate of aging, measurements selected for study must be easily performed in order to be frequently repeated in the same individual. Many of the cutaneous parameters discussed above meet this criteria.

REFERENCES

1. Andrew, W., Aging of the skin and related structures, in *Structural Aspects of Aging*, Bourne, G.H., Ed., Hafner Publishing, New York, 1961.
2. Andrew, W., Behnke, R., and Sato, T., Changes with advancing age in the cell population of human dermis, *Gerontologica*, 10, 1, 1964.
3. Ascher, B., Intradermal salt solution text in elderly patients, *Exp. Med. Surg.*, 18, 17, 1960.
4. Augener, W., Cohnen, G., Reuter, A., and Brittinger, G., Decrease of T lymphocytes during aging, *Lancet*, 1, 1164, 1974.
5. Baker, H. and Blair, C., Cell replacement in the human stratum corneum in old age, *Br. J. Dermatol.*, 80, 367, 1968.
6. Baker, H. and Kligman, A.M., Technique for estimating turnover time of human stratum corneum, *Arch. Dermatol.*, 95, 408, 1967.
7. Baker, H. and Kligman, A.M., A simple in vivo method for studying the permeability of the human stratum corneum, *J. Invest. Dermatol.*, 48, 273, 1967.
8. Bean, W., A note on fingernail growth, *J. Invest. Dermatol.*, 20, 27, 1953.
9. Bean, W., Nail growth: 30 years of observation, *Arch. Intern. Med.*, 134, 497, 1974.
10. Black, M., A modified radiographic method for measuring skin thickness, *Br. J. Dermatol.*, 81, 661, 1969.
11. Borkan, G.A. and Norris, A.H., Assessment of biological age using a profile of physical parameters, *J. Gerontol.*, 35, 177, 1980.
12. Braverman, I.M. and Fonferko, E., Studies in cutaneous aging. I. The elastic fiber network, *J. Invest. Dermatol.*, 78, 434, 1982.
13. Braverman, I.M. and Fonferko, E., Studies in cutaneous aging. II. The microvasculature, *J. Invest. Dermatol.*, 78, 444, 1982.
14. Braverman, I.M., Sibley, J., and Keh-Yen, A., A study of the veil cells around normal, diabetic and aged cutaneous microvessels, *J. Invest. Dermatol.*, 86, 57, 1986.
15. Carosella, E., Mochanko, K., and Braun, M., Rosette-forming T cells in human peripheral blood at different ages, *Cell. Immunol.*, 12, 323, 1974.
16. Catalona, W., Taylor, P., and Chretien, P., Quantitative dinitrochlorobenzine contact sensitization in a normal population, *Clin. Exp. Immunol.*, 12, 325, 1972.

17. Christophers, E. and Kligman, A.M., Visualization of the cell layers of the stratum corneum, *J. Invest. Dermatol.,* 42, 407, 1964.
18. Christophers, E. and Kligman, A.M., Percutaneous absorption in aged skin, in *Advances in the Biology of the Skin,* Vol. 6, Montagna, W., Ed., Pergamon Press, New York, 1965, 163.
19. De Salve, S.J. and Thompson, G., $Na^{23}Cl$ skin clearance in humans and its relation to skin age, *J. Invest. Dermatol.,* 45, 315, 1965.
20. Droller, H., Dermatologic findings in a random sample of old persons, *Geriatrics,* 10, 421, 1955.
21. Epstein, W.L. and Jessar, R.A., Contact type delayed hypersensitivity in patients with rheumatoid arthritis, *Arthritis Rheumatism,* 2, 178, 1959.
22. Evans, R., Cowdry, E., and Nielson, P., Aging of human skin. I. Influence of dermal shrinkage on appearance of the epidermis in young and old fixed tissues, *Anat. Rec.,* 86, 545, 1959.
23. Feldmann, R.J. and Maibach, H., Regional variation in percutaneous penetration of ^{14}C cortisol in man, *J. Invest. Dermatol.,* 48, 181, 1967.
24. Fitzpatrick, T., Szabo, G., and Mitchell, R., Age changes in the human melanocyte system, in *Advances in the Biology of Skin,* Vol. 6, Montagna, W., Ed., Pergamon Press, New York, 1965, 35.
25. Frosch, P. and Kligman, A.M., Rapid blister formation in human skin with ammonium hydroxide, *Br. J. Dermatol.,* 96, 461, 1977.
26. Gilchrest, B.A., Murphy, G., and Soter, N.A., Effect of chronologic aging and ultraviolet irradiation on Langerhans cells in human epidermis, *J. Invest. Dermatol.,* 79, 85, 1982.
27. Grahame, R. and Holt, P., The influence of aging on the in vivo elasticity of human skin, *Gerontologist,* 15, 121, 1969.
28. Grove, G., Duncan, S., and Kligman, A.M., Effect of aging on the blistering of human skin with ammonium hydroxide, *Br. J. Derm,* 107, 393, 1982.
29. Grove, G., Age related differences in healing of superficial skin wounds in humans, *Arch. Dermatol. Res.,* 272, 381, 1982.
30. Grove, G., Age-associated changes in human epidermal cell renewal and repair, in *Aging and the Skin,* Balin, A. and Kligman, A., Eds., Raven Press, New York, 1989, 193.
31. Halasz, N.A., Dehiscence of laparotomy wounds, *Am. J. Surg.,* 116, 210, 1968.
32. Hamilton, J.B., Terada, H., and Mestler, G.E., Studies of growth throughout the lifespan in Japanese: growth and size of nails and their relationship to age, sex, heredity, and other factors, *J. Gerontol.,* 10, 400, 1955.
33. Heite, H.J., Der Funktionzusand der kleinem Gefaesse im Lichte gleichzeitig gemessener Quaddelund fluorescein Resorptionsgesch-windigkeit, *Arch. Klin. Exp. Dermatol.,* 206, 216, 1957.
34. Hill, W. and Montgomery, H., Regional changes and changes caused by age in the normal skin. A histologic study, *J. Invest. Dermatol.,* 3, 231, 1940.
35. Hillman, R., Fingernail growth in the human subject: rates and variation in 300 individuals, *Hum. Biol.,* 27, 274, 1955.
36. Hodgson, G., Senile lentigo, *Arch. Dermatol.,* 87, 197, 1963.
37. Hollingsworth, J.W., Hashizuma, A., and Jablon, S., Correlations between tests of aging in Hiroshima subjects — an attempt to define "physiologic age", *Yale J. Biol. Med.,* 33, 11, 1965.
38. Hollingsworth, J.W., Ishii, G., and Conrad, R., Skin aging and hair graying in Hiroshima, *Geriatrics,* 16, 27, 1961.
39. Holm-Pederson, P. and Zederfeldt, B., Strength development of skin incisions in young and old rats, *Scand. J. Plast. Reconst. Surg.,* 5, 7, 1971.
40. Hull, M.T. and Warfel, K.A., Age-related changes in the cutaneous basal lamina: scanning electron microscopic study, *J Invest. Dermatol.,* 81, 378, 1983.
41. Isaki, M., Studies on senile changes in the skin. I. Statistical observations, *Keio Igaku,* 28, 59, 1951.
42. Jacobsen, E., Billings, J., Frantz, R., Kinney, C., Stewart, M., Downing, D., Age-related changes in sebaceous wax ester secretion rates in men and women, *J. Invest. Dermatol.,* 85, 483, 1985.
43. Jemec, G.B.E., Agner, T. and Serup, J., Transonychial water loss: relation to sex, age and nail-plate thickness, *Br. J. Dermatol.,* 121, 443, 1989.
44. Johnson, M.L.D. and Roberts, J., Prevalence of Dermatological Disease Among Persons 1-74 Years of Age, U.S. Advance

Data No. 4, U.S. Department of Health, Education and Welfare, Washington, D.C., 1977.
45. Katzberg, A., The area of the dermal-epidermal junction in human skin, *Anat. Rec.*, 131, 717, 1958.
46. Keogh, E.V. and Walsh, R.J., Rate of greying of human hair, *Nature,* 207, 877, 1965.
47. Kiistala, U., Dermal-epidermal separation. I. The influence of age, sex and body region on suction blister formation in human skin, *Ann. Clin. Res.,* 4, 10, 1972.
48. King, G.S., Mohan, V.S., and Starche, B.S., Radioimmunoassay for desmosine, *Connect. Tissue Res.,* 7, 263, 1980.
49. Kirk, J. and Chieffi, M., Variations with age in elasticity of skin and subcutaneous tissue in human individuals, *J. Gerontol.,* 17, 373, 1962.
50. Kligman, A.M., Early destructive effect of sunlight on human skin, *JAMA,* 210, 2377, 1969.
51. Kligman, A.M., Solar elastosis in relation to pigmentation, in *Sunlight and Man,* Fitzpatrick, T., Ed., University of Tokyo Press, Tokyo, 1974, 157.
52. Kligman, A.M., Perspectives and problems in cutaneous gerontology, *J. Invest. Dermatol.,* 73, 39, 1979.
53. Kligman, A.M. and Christophers, E., Preparation of isolated sheets of human stratum corneum, *Arch. Dermatol.,* 88, 702, 1963.
54. Lavker, R., Structural alterations in exposed and unexposed aged skin, *J. Invest. Dermatol.,* 73, 59, 1979.
55. Lavker, R., Zheng, P., and Dong, G., Aged skin: a study by light, transmission electron, and scanning electron microscopy, *J. Invest. Dermatol.,* 88, 44s, 1987.
56. Leaming, D.B., The influence of age on wound healing, *J. Surg. Rest.,* 3, 43, 1963.
57. Lee, M., Physical and structural age changes in human skin, *Anat. Rec.,* 129, 473, 1957.
58. Legros-Clark, W.E., and Buxton, L., Studies in nail growth, *Br. J. Dermatol.,* 50, 221, 1938.
59. Leyden, J., McGinley, K., Grove, G. and Kligman, A.M., Age-related differences in the rate of desquamation of skin surface cells, in *Advances in Experimental Medicine and Biology,* Roberts, J. and Cristofalo, V., Eds., 1978, 297.
60. Lowe, L.B. and Van der Leun, J.C., Suction blisters and dermal-epidermal adherence, *J. Invest. Dermatol.,* 50, 308, 1968.
61. Malkinson, F.D., Studies on the percutaneous absorption of C^{14} labelled steroids by use of the gas flow cell, *J. Invest. Dermatol.,* 31, 19, 1958.
62. MacLaughlin, J. and Holick, M.F., Aging decreases the capacity of human skin to produce vitamin D_3, *J. Clin. Invest.,* 76, 1536, 1985.
63. McClure, W. and Aldrich, C., Time required for disappearance of intradermally injected salt solution, *JAMA,* 81, 293, 1923.
64. Meema, H.E., Sheppard, R., and Rapoport, A., Roentgenographic visualization and measurement of skin thickness and its diagnostic application of acromegaly, *Radiology,* 82, 411, 1964.
65. Mendoza, C.B., Postlethwaite, R.W., and Johnson, W.D., Incidence of wound disruption following operation, *Arch. Surg.,* 101, 396, 1970.
66. Montagna, W., Morphology of the aging skin: the cutaneous appendages, in *Advances in the Biology of the Skin,* Vol. 6, Montagna, W., Ed., Pergamon Press, New York, 1965, 1.
67. Montagna, W. and Carlisle, K., Structural changes in aging human skin, *J. Invest. Dermatol.,* 73, 47,
68. Montagna, W. and Parakkal, P., *The Structure and Function of Skin,* 3rd ed., Academic Press, New York, 1974.
69. Murasko, D.M., Weiner, P., and Kaye, D., Decline in mitogen induced proliferation of lymphocytes with increasing age, *Clin. Exp. Immunol.,* 70, 440, 1987.
70. Orentreich, N. and Sharp, N., Keratin replacement as an aging parameter, *J. Soc. Cosmet. Chem.,* 18, 537, 1967.
71. Orentreich, N. and Selmanowitz, V.J., Levels of biological functions with aging, *Trans. N.Y. Acad. Sci., Ser. II,* 31, 992, 1969.
72. Peachey, R., Some factors affecting the speed of suction blister formation in normal subjects, *Br. J. Dermatol.,* 84, 435, 1971.
73. Peachey, R., Skin temperature and blood flow in relation to the speed of suction blister formation, *Br. J. Dermatol.,* 84, 447, 1971.
74. Plewig, G. and Kligman, A.M., Proliferative activity of the sebaceous glands of the aged, *J. Invest. Dermatol.,* 70, 314, 1978.

75. Potts, R.O., Buras, E.M., and Chrisman, D.A., Changes with age in the moisture content of human skin, *J. Invest. Dermatol.*, 82, 97, 1984.
76. Roberts-Thomson, I., Whittingham, S., Youngchaiyud, U., and Mackay, I.R., Aging, immune response and mortality, *Lancet,* 2, 368, 1974.
77. Roberts, D. and Marks, R., The determination of regional and age variations in the rate of desquamation: a comparison of four techniques, *J. Invest. Dermatol.*, 74, 13, 1980.
78. Reff, M. and Schneider, E., Biological Markers of Physiologic Aging, NIH Publ. No. 82-2221, National Institutes of Health, Bethesda, MD, 1982.
79. Rougier, A., Lotte, C., Corcuff, P., and Maibach, H.I., Relationship between skin permeability and corneocyte size according to anatomic site, age, and sex in man, *J. Soc. Cosmet. Chem.*, 39, 15, 1988.
80. Sandblom, P., Peterson, P., Muren, A., Determination of the tensile strength of the healing wound as a clinical test, Acta Chir. Scand., 105, 252, 1953.
81. Scheuplein, R.J. and Blank, I.H., Permeability of the skin, *Physiol. Rev.*, 51, 702, 1971.
82. Shock, N., Greulich, R.C., Andres, R., Arenberg, D., Costa, P., Lakatta, E., and Tobin, J., Normal Human Aging: The Baltimore Longitudinal Study of Aging, NIH Publ. 84-2450, U.S. Department of Health and Human Services, and Washington, D.C., 1984.
83. Smith, J.G. and Kiem, I., Allergic contact sensitivity in the aged, *J. Gerontol.*, 16, 118, 1961.
84. Snell, R.S. and Bischitz, P.G., The melanocytes and melanin in human abdominal wall skin: a survey made at different ages in both sexes and during pregnancy, *J. Anat.*, 97, 361, 1963.
85. Staricco, R.J. and Pinkus, J., Quantitative and qualitative data on the pigment cells of adult human epidermis, *J. Invest. Dermatol.*, 28, 33, 1957.
86. Sussman, M., Aging of connective tissue: physical properties of healing wounds in young and old rats, *Am. J. Physiol.*, 224, 1167, 1973.
87. Szabo, G., The regional anatomy of the human integument with special reference to the distribution of hair follicles, sweat glands and melanocytes, *Philos. Trans. R. Soc.*, 252, 447, 1967.
88. Southwood, W., The thickness of the skin, *Plastic Reconstruct. Surg.*, 15, 423,.
89. Thuringer, J.M. and Katzberger, A.A., The effect of age on mitosis in the human epidermis, *J. Invest. Dermatol.*, 54, 19, 1959.
90. Tindall, J.P. and Smith, J.G., Skin lesions of the aged and their association with internal changes, *JAMA,* 186, 1039, 1963.
91. Viljanto, J., A sponge implantation method for testing connective tissues regeneration in surgical patients, *Acta Chir. Scand.*, 135, 297, 1969.
92. Waldorf, D., Willkens, R., and Decker, J., Impaired delayed hypersensitivity in an aging population, *JAMA,* 203, 111, 1968.
93. Whitton, J. and Everall, J.D., The thickness of the epidermis, *Br. J. Dermatol.*, 89, 467, 1973.
94. Young, A.M., Dermatogeriatric problems in the chronic disease hospital, *N.Y. State J. Med.*, 65, 1748, 1965.
95. Zakon, S., Goldberg, A., and Forman I., Geriatric dermatoses: a survey of the skin of the aged, *Ill. Med. J.*, 101, 37, 1952.

CHAPTER 21

HAIR CHANGES WITH AGING AS A PARAMETER TO UTILIZE IN THE ESTIMATION OF HUMAN BIOLOGICAL AGE

David S. Orentreich and Norman Orentreich

TABLE OF CONTENTS

I. INTRODUCTION

The human hair follicle is a complex, diverse cutaneous adnexa. The type of hair produced by a given follicle, vellus or terminal, short or long, pigmented or nonpigmented, is determined by embryologic development and the genetic characteristics of the particular body region, e.g., scalp, beard, axilla, eyebrow, etc. Each variety of hair is unique in its duration of cyclic activity and response to hormonal influences.

The changes in hair associated with aging are related to an interplay of endocrinologic, chronologic, and physiologic factors. There is a variable genetic predisposition of hair follicles to respond to androgens. For example, dihydrotestosterone prolongs the anagen phase of beard hair follicles; shortens the anagen phase of the balding scalp follicles in male pattern alopecia, called more precisely androgenetic alopecia[49] or androchronogenetic alopecia (ACGA);[52] and has no effect on the nonbalding scalp, axillary, and pubic hair follicles. Testosterone prolongs the anagen phase of axillary, pubic, and some body hair follicles.

0-8493-0129-7/94/$0.00+$.50

The hair growth cycle is divided into three stages: catagen, telogen, and anagen. During the transitional catagen stage the lower portion of the growing (anagen) hair follicle involutes, and hair production ceases. The follicle then enters the quiescent telogen stage when little or no metabolic activity is evident. Hairs are shed, brushed out, or otherwise lost during the end of the telogen phase because the hair shaft is loosely anchored in the dormant follicle. After an interval of time characteristic of the hair type, the telogen follicle undergoes a period of dramatic cytoarchitectural remodeling. It enters the anagen stage of active growth and differentiation. The new hair produced pushes out any residual unshed hair remaining in the follicle. The duration of anagen is variable, depending on hair type, genetic expression, age, and endocrine factors, e.g., beard and scalp hair can grow for 2 to 6 years or longer, whereas eyebrow hair grows for only 1 to 2 months. We have observed that maximal scalp hair length diminishes with age in postpubertal women who let their scalp hair grow without cutting. The marked decrease in the duration of anagen, not the minimal decline in the rate of growth, is the major cause of diminished maximum scalp hair length with age. In the uncommon angora variant a cyclic growth and rest cycle does not occur in the scalp hair follicles, so hair is produced uninterruptedly throughout life.

In the aging adult, the quality of hair undergoes a change which results in an increase in the number of vellus hairs on the scalp, a decrease in facial hair in men, and an increasing thickness of hair on the face of women. The eyebrows become thicker and longer.[70] Both the duration of the growth phase and the size of hair follicles change with age. For example, from the third decade on there is a progressive transition of vellus hairs into terminal hairs on the tragus and antitragus of male ears. The opposite transition, from terminal to vellus hair growth, occurs in both sexes in age-associated ACGA of the scalp.[6] The number of hair follicles on the scalp decreases about one-third, resulting in a distinctively patterned hair loss. Androchronogenetic baldness is not only an expression of age but also of genotype and androgen activity. In general, the sequence of terminal hair loss with advancing age on the trunk, limbs, pubes, and axillae reverses that of its appearance, but axillary and pubic hair are lost earlier and more completely in females than in males.[66]

With aging, the total undersculpture of the epidermis and the number, arrangement, and types of hair follicles become altered. With advancing age, a statistically significant increase in the number of single and bunched hair follicles takes place at the expense of grouped follicles. Groups of three hair follicles do not appear in the skin until after the age of 20 and groups of four or more do not appear until after the age of 50. With increasing age, new follicles seem to sprout from existing follicles, the processes varying in individual regions of the body and in men and women.[48]

The follicle itself undergoes a relentless change in ACGA: the coarse, terminal (young adult) hair is replaced by a fine, less pigmented vellus hair. Some but not all of these vellus hairs may then be lost. Hair follicles are usually clustered in groups of four or five. The vellus hair formation that occurs with aging occurs first within the groups, then affects entire groups, and lastly entire areas.

II. ALOPECIA

In The Netherlands, 1000 healthy women and 1000 healthy men aged 10 to 65 and older were examined in a cross-sectional study for the extent and distribution of their hair.[9] With puberty an increased growth of body hairs was noted especially in men. With the climacteric (age 45) a loss of body hair was observed which was more marked in women. By contrast, the female climacteric period showed an increased growth of beard and moustache and the development of calvities frontalis (ACGA). Baldness continued to increase steadily with age involving 75% of both men and women.

In all races the incidence and the degree of baldness increase with age. In a study, baldness was found positively correlated in relation to age in 312 males and 214 females who were either students or staff members at Yale, Missouri, and New York State Universities, or inmates or staff members at Riker's Island Prison, New York, Fairfield State Hospital in Newton, CT, Jewish Sanitorium in Brooklyn, and in 77 normal Chinese males in New York.[25]

In the Caucasian male ACGA appeared in the latter half of the second decade of life and reached a peak in the seventh decade, when it included over 80%. It then leveled off through the ninth decade. In Caucasian females ACGA was less common, 30%, and peaked in the fifth decade of life. In Chinese males, baldness was less common than in Caucasian males but had a similar increased incidence with advancing age.

The severity of ACGA according to the age of the patient was studied in 302 subjects living in or near Genoa, Italy. The scores revealed a linear regression with age. In 81 additional subjects, all over 70 years of age, the disease did not seem to have developed any further.[12]

On Honshu Island in Japan, 21 monozygotic twins were compared to 6 dizygotic twins and 16 pairs of siblings. All were healthy and ranged in age from 41 to 90. The onset and pattern of alopecia senilis was found to be subject mainly to hereditary control.[47]

In eunuchs castrated prepubertally hair stays luxuriant into old age. If they are genetically predisposed to baldness, eunuchs who receive exogenous androgens from the second decade on lose their hair slowly over a period of years as do normal young men.[23]

If a eunuch reaches the sixth decade of life and then receives androgen therapy, he loses his hair within a few months. In "male pattern" alopecia (ACGA) genetic, endocrine, and aging factors are interdependent. The aging factor was clearly evident in a study of identical male twins.[23] One twin, castrated before puberty, retained his original full complement of scalp hair at age 40. The uncastrated twin had gradually gone bald over a 20-year period. At age 40, the castrated twin received injections of testosterone. Within a 6-month period he became as bald as his twin brother had become in 20 years. Decades of exposure to androgens were not required to reach this degree of baldness, indicating that time-dependent selective changes in gene expression can be operative but not expressed in the absence of hormonal influence. On the basis of this observation, it would appear possible to inhibit or perhaps reverse balding by the effective use of antiandrogens to block activation of genetic expression. In fact, there is no unequivocal evidence that the "bald" hair follicles are permanently repressed. In one case, treatment with a variety of antiandrogenic modalities partially restored hair growth in a 50-year-old, bald, male-to-female transsexual.[52]

A study of androgen stimulation of beard hair illustrates the wide variation of hair follicle response and the influence of genetics and aging on endocrine expression. The repeated injections subcutaneously at intervals of 5 to 6 weeks for 1 year of a long-acting testosterone ester (testosterone cyclopentylproprionate) into a single site in the lateral chin beard area of five postmenopausal women 50 to 65 years of age produced in two women a vigorous growth of terminal hair at the injection site in 4 months; two had sparse hair growth in 1 year; and one showed no growth.[37] Prior to the testosterone injections, all the women had typically very short, non-pigmented, thin vellus facial hair which was barely noticeable on close visual inspection; however, the action of a potent androgenic steroid hormone effected a transformation to terminal hair. Six of seven postmenopausal women 49 to 67 years of age with alopecic skin in the pubic area developed localized hair growth at the injection site of testosterone cyclopentylproprionate. Maguire[38] injected 10 mg at 4- to 6-week intervals for 2 to 5 months before hair first appeared.

III. THE HISTOLOGY OF ANDROCHRONOGENETIC ALOPECIA AND THE AGED SCALP

The hair in the aged scalp is very small compared to the sebaceous gland to which it is attached.[40] In addition, strands of arrectores pilorum muscles, once attached to the follicles before they became involuted, are found free in the dermis.[40] In the follicles of guard hairs of aged individuals, the bulge, to which is attached the arrector pili muscle, is caruncular; in young skin the bulge is usually smooth. The entire lower third of the follicles from very old individuals becomes wrinkled, like a partially collapsed sac; in young individuals the bulb assumes this condition only at the beginning of catagen, otherwise it is turgid.[40]

A histologic study of hairless skin obtained from the heads of six males aged 52 to 72 showed a variable reduction of hair follicles; thicker, united, and fused elastic fibers; and thickening of the walls and tunica intima of arterioles. The latter two findings probably do not play an etiologic role in the development of baldness but are a result of actinic damage incurred after the processes of ACGA and aging denude the scalp and expose it to sunlight. An electron microscopic study was undertaken in Japan with anagen hairs removed from 11 normal subjects of both sexes, ranging in age from 10 to 56 years.[67] In the peribulbar region of the hair follicle, the perivascular basal lamina was found to consist of double or triple thin layers. On the other hand, in the hair dermal papilla of the same specimen, the basal lamina was characterized by a concentric multilamellar arrangement. With regard to the effect of age on the extent of the thickening, this study showed that the number of the basal lamina increases with age. These findings suggest a possible relationship between the degree of stratification and the number of hair cycles.

IV. SCALP

The thickness of normal hairy human scalp was studied in 22 male and 22 female cadavers 16 to 85 years of age and in 19 living male subjects 16 to 59 years of age, of whom eight had a normal scalp, seven had early ACGA, and four had advanced ACGA.[27] The epidermis was similar in men and women; it increased in thickness up to age 40 in women and age 50 in men and decreased thereafter. The dermis of the hair-bearing scalp was thicker in women than men and reached its maximum around 35 years in women and 55 in men. It then decreased in men to age 80 and in women to age 70, when a renewed rise was noted in women over 70.

The hypodermis (subcutaneous fat) made up 50% of the thickness of the scalp. It was thicker in women than men. In men it reached a plateau in their 30s and did not change significantly with age. In women it reached its peak in their early 30s, decreased until 70, and rose again up to 85.[27]

The galea was thicker in men. In both sexes it increased until age 55, then decreased to age 80.[27]

In early ACGA no significant changes in the scalp layers were observed. In advanced ACGA a definite decrease in the thickness of the epidermis, dermis, and hypodermis was observed. No change was noted in the galea. There is about a 40% decrease in total thickness with advanced ACGA.[27] This change is of clinical importance in performing hair transplants because it is partially responsible for "cobblestoning".[53]

V. RATE AND DURATION OF GROWTH AND REGENERATION TIME AFTER PLUCKING

Although the rate of scalp hair growth declines with age, the rate of body hair growth appears to be greatest between 50 and 70 years of age in both men and women.[58]

The prolonged regeneration time after plucking reflects the hair follicle's diminished reserve capacity with aging. Although alopecia and graying of hair do not normally occur during aging in mice, a prolonged regeneration time after plucking does. The replacement of plucked hair was slowed in a subpopulation of C57Bl/6J male mice aged 24 months or older; such delays are often associated with degenerative diseases of senescence.[18]

A study of the long-term effect of repeated pluckings on the function of the mouse vibrissal follicles[28] has shown results analogous to the human situation. Single mouse vibrissae were plucked repeatedly at the same time of the cycle (10 to 15 d after eruption) for ten successive cycles from eight individual follicles. After three pluckings the first gray whisker appeared; after six pluckings all were gray. Two follicles stopped producing whiskers after seven pluckings and another two after eight. Henceforth, only 50% of the follicles continued producing whiskers until the end of the experiment. All the follicles that ceased to produce whiskers had a keratogenous cyst occupying most of the follicle in direct contact with the dermal papilla. In all cases the isolated dermal papilla was condensed and rounded in shape. Both loss of pigment and cyst formation could be due to the mechanical damage in the follicle caused by repeated plucking.

Women who repeatedly pluck the hair of the glabella area and the eyebrows report the occasional regeneration of gray hairs and the eventual cessation of regrowth after years of routine pluckings.

The rate of growth of hairs and the regeneration of 90% of hairs after plucking was studied in 54 residents of New York State institutions of mental disease.[45] The range of age was 9 to 84 years (24 males and 28 females). Hair growth was normal in institutionalized subjects in good physical health. Though the rate of hair growth on the scalp, thigh, and eyebrow did not change with age, the chin and especially the axillary hair growth rates decreased with age. Age did not affect the rate of regeneration after plucking of scalp or eyebrow hairs. However, the chin, axilla, and thigh required a longer interval with increasing age.

In Rosario, Argentina measurements on 104 normal individuals (53 males and 51 females) aged 10 to 74 years showed a 20% decrease in the growth rate of their central axillary hairs.[57]

Phenotypically, some hairs are vellus (fine, short, and nonpigmented), while others are terminal (coarse, longer, and pigmented). The duration of anagen and the size of the hair follicle determine whether a hair is vellus or terminal. Aging has a dramatic effect on these two parameters in some hair types. For example, as noted before, after the third decade of life, there is a progressive transition of the vellus hairs in the ears of males into terminal hairs, usually on the tragus and antitragus.[42] In West Bengal, India, 168 families were studied for hypertrichosis of the ear rims, baldness, and chest hairiness. All were positively correlated with increasing age.[63] The opposite transition, from terminal to vellus hair growth, occurs in age-associated common baldness of the scalp,[6] also called androgenetic or ACGA alopecia, in both men and women.[52] Both transitions are examples of selective patterns of sequential gene modification by steroid hormones. The miniaturization of terminal hair follicles in common baldness is not associated with a decrease in their number except in very advanced age. Individuals predisposed to ACGA will not express the trait in absence of androgens, but genetic and aging influences are still operative.

VI. MASS

Trotter,[74] using a shaving technique, measured the weekly growth of the hairs of the axilla, arms, and legs and noted that the daily growth rate of leg hair increased with advancing age between 14 and 45 years. On the other hand, axillary and pubic hair showed the opposite trend.

Age-associated loss of axillary and pubic hair reflects diminished endocrine function and the effects of aging. In a quantitative measurement of axillary hair[24] subjects who lived in New York State institutions for mental health were selected. They consisted of 260 males and 188 females between 15 and 92 years of age. A total of 70 eunuchs and 10 oophorectomized women were also studied.

The total weight of axillary hair was measured by shaving the axilla, defatting the hair in ether, and then dehydrating the hair in a desiccator. The weight produced per day was determined by repeating the same procedures 42 d later.

In eunuchs the axillary hair was markedly diminished, especially if the castration occurred before puberty. The axillary hair was more plentiful in men castrated as adults, but was still considerably below that of normal men of the same age.

In normal males the mass of axillary hair reaches a peak in the third decade and linearly decreases 90% until the ninth decade. In normal females the weight is maximal in the fourth decade and decreases with aging more rapidly than in men. Axillary hair loss begins with the menopause and the adrenopause and is almost complete by the sixth decade. Maximal female axillary hair mass is only two thirds that of males. However, in the second decade female axillary hair mass is greater than that of the male.

The daily growth rate of hair on the pubis, axilla, scalp, and thigh was measured using a shave technique.[58] The growth rate in subjects 50 to 69 years old was higher than in subjects either 40 to 49 or 70 to 79; the daily rate of hair growth was higher in men than in women. The daily growth rate showed a regional variation with the rate decreasing progressively for the following areas: pubis, axilla, scalp, thigh. The diameter decreased in the same order. Another study employed a shave and weigh technique to show that daily growth rates of hair were greater in summer than in winter.[11]

A normal male weighed the mass of his beard growth from age 66 to age 81. There was a 30% diminution in annual weight over this 15-year period. Several illnesses and surgical procedures produced significant decreases in beard growth mass.[62]

VII. DENSITY AND DIAMETER

A. AXILLARY AND PUBIC HAIR

Careful mensuration of pubic hair with age showed a decline in hair density (population per area) and rate of growth in men and women.[2] Hair shaft diameter did not change. It was further observed that during pregnancy and postpartum the parameters of the pubic hair trichogram were not affected. This observation is of interest because scalp hair is frequently affected by these conditions.[36,51]

Pubic hair pattern in aging males showed a decrease in the horizontal and sagittal directions and an increase in a disperse distribution; no significant changes were found in females. A horizontal pattern of pubic hair in men tended to be associated with sparse chest hair. Only 20% of the younger group had conspicuous chest hair compared with 71% of the older group.[16]

The hair density in the axilla decreases over 50% with age. Unlike the pubic area but like the scalp hair, there was a significant decrease in the postpartum period.[57]

In women, androgens from the adrenal cortex (reticular zone) are primarily responsible for axillary and pubic hair growth. Because the plasma concentrations of the major adrenal androgens, dehydroepiandrosterone (DHEA) and its sulfate (DHEA-S), decline dramatically after the third decade of life,[54] loss of axillary and pubic hair with age is invariably observed in women especially after the menopause. Moreover, in women with Addison's disease pubic and axillary hair is lost. However, hair in these areas can be regrown in aged individuals by local or systemic administration of androgens, e.g., 1 to 2% testosterone propionate tincture or lotion.[50] In the male, testicular androgens are present in so much greater quantity than adrenal androgens that axillary and pubic hair growth are maintained, even in Addison's disease. Because testosterone remains high in men even into the sixth decade of life their pubic, axillary, and beard hair density and rate of growth decline only moderately. This decline may represent cellular aging or diminished androgen receptors in the pilosebaceous end organ with age. As free testosterone declines with age, due to an increase in androgen binding globulin starting in the fifth decade of life, it contributes to the diminution (miniaturization) of androgen-stimulated hairs.[61,77]

B. SCALP HAIR

Sixty-two specimens of scalp from the vertex of the skull were obtained postmortem (within 4 to 5 h of death) from subjects of both sexes ranging from fetal life to 90 years of age.[21] All types of hair follicles were counted, terminal and vellus, in all stages of the hair growth cycle. The adult scalp of individuals 20 to 30 years has 615 hair follicles per square centimeter while the mean hair follicle density in the newborn is 1135/cm^2. There is a gradual reduction in the density of hair follicles with advancing age. Szabo[73] determined the regional frequency distribution of hair follicles (number of hair follicles of all types per square centimeter) and its change with development and aging. He concluded that there is a correlation between the differential rate of growth of the body surface and the regional frequency distribution of skin appendages. There is no large-scale destruction of hair follicles during postnatal development, but rather a dilution of the original dense population of hairs during the growth of the body surface. During postnatal development, which extends up to 24 years of age, the total surface of the scalp increases about threefold[10] so the dense hair follicles of the newborn gradually become spaced farther apart. With advancing age there is an inexorable loss of hair follicles. This is evident in some subjects as early as 30 years of age; others may not show any changes until 40 years, but hair follicles are noticeably fewer in the scalp of men 50 years of age and older.

Heredity, sex, and age influence the cross-sectional diameter (thickness) of scalp hair. The maximum cross-sectional area (8000 m^2) at age 20 is slightly larger for Japanese males than females.[29] By age 80 the cross-sectional area is reduced 50%. The regression is almost linear when large numbers of males (1059) and females (2062) are averaged. Females maintain a slightly larger cross-sectional area of scalp hair than males after age 30.

In a study of 81 healthy Japanese male subjects in Tokyo whose ages ranged from 2 to 91 years, the diameter of the scalp hair showed a peak at 15 years of age. A gradual decrease of one third occurred with advancing age.[46]

In Sheffield, England, 58 Caucasian women aged 13 to 72 with diffuse hair loss and 73 normal Caucasian women had their mean anagen hair diameters determined. Both groups evinced a decline with age, but the data were significant only in the women with diffuse alopecia.[31]

In New York, 20 specimens from the vertex scalp were obtained at autopsy and examined histologically after cutting the sections horizontal to the skin surface. Specimens were obtained for every decade of life from prematurity to age 88. These data confirmed that the maximum diameter is reached by the second decade and diminished only slightly with age.[3]

In Argentina, 17 males and 22 females (aged 16 to 48) had surface trichograms of 100 hairs performed on five areas of the scalp (right and left parietal, frontal, crown, and occipital). The density (population per square centimeter) decreased with age in all regions. The thickness (diameter) of hair and the percent of hairs in anagen decreased with age over the entire scalp in both sexes.[5]

VIII. GRAYING

Graying hair is at once a normal part and usually an important marker of the aging process, but it can also begin in early adulthood in genetically predisposed individuals. Premature graying is a dominant familial trait. Graying usually starts at the temples and moves toward the scalp's vertex. The hairy areas away from the head may, uncommonly, participate in the graying phenomenon. In Caucasians, white hairs first appear in the region of the temples at the age of 34.2 +9.6 years; by the age of 50, half the population has at least 50% gray hairs.[17]

The pigmentation in a hair produced by a given follicle can be interrupted intermittently before permanent graying is established.[13] Their observations imply that melanocytes are not completely lost in follicles as a result of the aging process, but rather that their function is first impaired.

Rapid graying or whitening of the hair after severe emotional stresses, as judged by the overall appearance of the scalp, has been so often recorded by reliable observers that its occurrence must be accepted. However, the belief that this is due to destruction of pigment in individual hairs has no foundation. The phenomenon is adequately explained by a preferential shed of pigmented hairs from a mixed population as a result of either telogen effluvium or alopecia areata of rapid onset.[17]

The loss of pigment from the hair shafts is associated with a progressive loss of tyrosinase activity in the melanocytes of the hair bulbs. In a histologic study of 49 gray-haired subjects with 11 young controls depigmentation was associated with a great reduction or total absence of melanocytes in the hair bulb. No Langerhans cells were found, as in the depigmentation of vitiligo.[26]

There are various differences in the fine structure of hair between older and younger people: the cuticle of hair in older people is thinner, the number of osmiophilic inclusions is reduced, and some of the cuticular cells have become fully keratinized. The fibrils of the cortex keratin show no changes, but the matrix between the fibrils is loosened and, especially in white hair, interspersed with vacuoles of 0.15 to 0.3 μm in size, which are optically empty. Furthermore, in contrast to the black hair of the same person, white hair shows only occasionally intact melanin granules, but large quantities of pigment detritus. Melanocytes in older people probably produce only a few imperfect granules of melanin, which disintegrate in the hair shaft. The blanching of the hair in age is not due to a corpuscular color. It is a color impression arising from the actual color of the hair keratin and from the reflection of light on the boundary surfaces and the islets of the interfibrillar matrix.[55]

Pernicious anemia (PA) is associated with an increased incidence of premature graying of the hair. In Scotland, 121 PA patients (39 males and 82 females) and 200 normal subjects (96 males and 104 females) aged 20 to over 80 years were studied. Graying occurred earlier in subjects with PA up to the age of 60; no difference between PA patients and normal subjects was observed after this age. This study did not show a statistical difference for sex and graying.[14]

Gray hair may present as an associated finding of other disease states, e.g., Vogt-Koyanagi-Harada syndrome, vitiligo, or alopecia areata. Loss of sympathetic innervation by sympathectomy has been reported to retard the development of gray hair in the lumbar[56] and cervical[35] regions.

Some strains of C57BL/10 H-2 congenic mice were found to exhibit graying with age, whereas others did not. Two patterns of graying were observed: diffuse graying beginning at 4 to 6 months of age and patterned graying beginning at 4 to 6 weeks. Strains exhibiting either graying pattern expressed high levels of infectious ecotropic and mink cell focus-inducing murine leukemia viruses (MuLV) in tests of thymus and spleen and in cultures from skin or tail biopsies, whereas nongraying strains expressed little virus until late in life. Electron microscopy demonstrated large accumulations of MuLV in gray but not in black areas of skin from a mouse with patterned graying. Infectious MuLV was produced spontaneously by embryos of graying but not of nongraying mice; pups of nongraying strains fostered on graying mothers turned gray after 3 months. These results suggest that graying with age results from melanocyte dysfunction which occurs subsequent to pre- or early postnatal infection with MuLV.[43]

In a study of 1008 German men aged 20 to 65, 50% showed that 10% of their scalp hair turned gray by age 40. By 65 years of age, almost all showed graying of scalp hair with an average of 70% of the hairs involved.[19]

Hair grayness in 480 adult Mexicans was recorded in 1948. By 1969, 21 years later, 101 persons of the original sample had died. Those between 35 to 69 years of age in 1948 who had died from natural causes in the intervening years were significantly grayer than average for their respective sex and 5-year age group.[34]

In one clinical report, a 13-year-old girl suffering from prolidase deficiency was shown to have premature gray hairs.[1] Other symptoms included chronic, recurrent ulcers on the legs and feet, diffuse telangiectasia, shallow, scar-like atrophic lesions on the face and arms, and unusually thin abdominal skin. Enzyme studies of the patient's fibroblasts grown in culture revealed the absence of prolidase. Genetic mutations of this nature yield important clues to understanding the biochemistry and physiology of melanocyte activity and the effects of aging.

Longitudinal studies of American children 6 to 18 years of age[71] and Czechoslovakian children 4 to 9 years of age[4] confirmed that children's hair became darker with age. Sex differences must also be considered because among adults there are more females than males with dark hair.[33]

In the Japanese twin study referred to above (alopecia section), the onset and number of gray hairs on the head was subject mainly to hereditary control.[47]

Hair color changes during early childhood were studied in American Caucasian twins 3 months to 6 years of age (169 female pairs, 161 male pairs, and 60 opposite sex pairs).[39] The trend for both sexes was clearly toward higher percentages of darker hair with increasing age. However, a sex difference was apparent: males tended to be more represented in the light category and females in the medium or dark. By 6 years of age, there were more than twice as many light-haired males as females.

A greater incidence of more darkly pigmented hair occurs among adults than among children in Caucasian populations.[75] Similar findings have resulted from cross-sectional studies of the hair color of French Canadians[76] and a mixture of ethnic groups.[8]

Hair samples from 274 Faroe Islanders (mean age 16.7 years) and 246 Orkney Islanders (mean age 13.5 years) were classified and divided into eight color categories by matching them to standard samples on the "Haarfarbentafel nach Fischer-Saller".[72] Sex differences in the proportions in each category in both the Faroese (144 males, 130 females) and Orcadians (120 males, 126 females) were not significant. However, a highly significant difference was found in the proportions in the eight categories between the total Faroese and Orcadian samples. The Faroese subjects, despite their higher mean age, had a higher proportion of light-haired individuals. Hair of a "smoky-gray" tone, clearly unrelated to graying with age and not represented on the Fischer-Saller scale, was reported and found to be a feature predominantly of Orcadian males.

IX. ELEMENTAL ANALYSIS

Elemental analysis of hair is a useful adjunct in forensic medicine and possibly nutritional studies, but its application in aging research has not been rigorously controlled. Metals are incorporated into the hair shaft at the follicular stage of hair growth, or they may be absorbed to the hair surface upon exposure to extraneous contaminants. Hair is often subjected to years of environmental exposure, which includes solar irradiation, atmospheric elements, hydrocarbons, soaps, shampoos (some containing metal salts), sweat, skin surface lipids, and numerous dyes and pomades. Perhaps more important are influences such as sex, geographic location, nutritional status, and certain metabolic diseases, all of which contribute to the highly variable nature of hair composition. Many studies have attempted to relate elemental composition to age, but most have failed to account for these numerous variables. For example, hair zinc levels are markedly influenced by dietary zinc supplementation;[22] therefore, any attempt to relate hair zinc to age would have to control for the influence of diet.

Activation analyses of 26 German subjects for trace elements in hair showed that sodium, chlorine, antimony, chromium, gold, and cobalt were higher in males; zinc, mercury, calcium, and manganese were higher in females; and iron and selenium showed no sex difference. Manganese, calcium, sodium, chlorine, and cobalt first increased by the third decade of life and then decreased after the fifth decade. Selenium, mercury, gold, zinc, iron, and chromium decreased by the third decade of life and then remained unchanged after the fifth decade.[32]

Hair samples analyzed from 211 American males and females (95% Caucasian and 5% Negro) aged 1 to 80 years showed that for males zinc and copper levels increased until age 12 then slowly decreased until age 80. The average zinc content in the hair of females and males of comparable age was very similar. Apparently, though, the copper content in the hair of females follows a different pattern in relation to age from that in the hair of males. The seemingly slight increase, with age, of copper content in the hair of females was not, however, statistically significant.[59]

Lead level in human hair did not show a sex or age difference in 250 New Zealand subjects (133 males and 117 females) aged 1 to 87 years.[64] Previous studies showed a decrease[68,78] and an increase[68] with age.

Antique hair (1871 to 1923) contained a significantly greater amount of lead than did contemporary (1971) hair.[78] These results indicate that the lead content of human hair has markedly decreased in the last 50 years in spite of a general increase in atmospheric lead concentrations. No significant differences due to sex or hair color were found. The significantly lower lead content observed in adult (persons older than 16 years) hair compared with that of children (persons younger than 16 years) is consistent with other reports[68] and probably reflects a generally higher metabolic level in children and the fact that absorption decreases with age.

Hair samples analyzed for cadmium and lead from 95 white American males (2 to 88 years) and from 83 females (14 to 84 years) showed that (1) cadmium had a peak level at age 12 for males and age 50 for females, and (2) lead showed no change with age for males and had a peak level at age 30 for females.[60]

In 11 male and 16 female Americans, analysis of hair for zinc, copper, magnesium, and iron showed higher zinc levels in female subjects.[15] For both males and females, only zinc levels in scalp hair decreased after 40 years of age. This substantiates the findings of Petering et al.,[59] who found that hair zinc declined from age 12 to age 80 for males and females. Forty-nine normal white individuals (26 males and 23 females), ranging in age from 15 months to 63 years in Washington, D.C., had hair sample determinations for zinc content.[20] Up to 20 years of age a statistically significant positive linear correlation was noted; from 20 to 63 years of age there was no significant correlation for age. The reader is referred to D. L. Moyer's critique, "Is Hair Analysis Useful: An Evaluation of Health and Disease by Hair Analysis".[44]

Although hair analysis has value, albeit limited, in screening for heavy metal exposure, its correlation with specific deficiency or disease states remains unproven. In the opinion of most experts the chemical condition of the hair and the state of health of the body are so unreliably related that hair analysis provides little useful information.[30] Nonetheless, many commercial laboratories that claim hair analysis can provide valuable clues to deficiency states and diseases offer this service, along with detailed recommendations for therapy, to health stores, beauticians, nutrition consultants, and physicians. A recent report suggests that commercial use of hair analysis is unscientific, economically wasteful, and of little clinical utility.[7]

X. CUTICULAR SCALE AND RHEOLOGY

The size of cuticular scales from scalp hairs is significantly smaller in older than younger individuals.[79] These measurements were performed by scanning electron microscopy (SEM) on 178 healthy volunteers at the University of Hull, Hull, England. The 108 younger people had a mean age of 22.7, range 18 to 26 years, and the 60 in the older group had a mean age of 43.9, range 37 to 55 years. The mean scale number, determined as the mean of six readings, was a reciprocal function of the linear size of the exposed cuticular scales.

In a subsequent SEM study of normal human subjects, scale edge number depended on site, sex, and age and correlated with hair growth rate.[65]

The rheology of male scalp hair studied in 81 healthy Japanese, 2 to 91 years of age, showed a breaking strength that peaked at age 20 and diminished by more than half with advanced age; these findings are in support of a 1934 study by Sasaki.[46]

XI. SUMMARY

Hair follicles and hair are unique biological materials for research in developmental biology, metabolism, nutrition, biorhythms, dermal-epidermal interaction, endocrinology, and aging. For aging, each hair type responds differently, most diminishing but some, as yet inexplicably, increasing in growth function with age. Many of the changes can be related to the altered endocrine function, but some seem to be related to chronologic and physiologic aging, such as the inexorable gradual decrease in scalp hair diameter.

In studying organ functions, it is the reserve capacity that changes most with age. For the hair follicle, reserve capacity can be evaluated by measuring the regeneration time after plucking anagen hair. Regeneration time may be particularly useful for measuring physiologic age. Because of the difficulties in avoiding nutritional variations and environmental contamination, the conflicting results of the elemental analyses of hair have been of little use. On the other hand, a change as obvious as graying has proven to be a measurable parameter useful in studies of aging and also related to longevity.

REFERENCES

1. Arata, J., Umemura, S., Yamamoto, Y., Hagiyama, M., and Nohara, N., Prolidase deficiency: its dermatological manifestations and some additional biochemical studies, *Arch. Dermatol.*, 115, 62, 1979.
2. Astore, I.P.L., Pecoraro, V., and Pecoraro, E.G., The normal trichogram of pubic hair, *Br. J. Dermatol.*, 101, 441, 1979.
3. Atkinson, S.C., Cormia, F.E., and Unrau, S.A., The diameter and growth phase of hair in relation to age, *Br. J. Dermatol.*, 71, 309, 1959.
4. Babickova, D., and Halkova, M., The colour of hair and eyes in a group of children observed from 4 to 9 years of age in a long term study, *Cs. Pediatr.*, 25, 551, 1970.
5. Barman, J.M., Astore, I., and Pecoraro, V., The normal trichogram of the adult, *J. Invest. Dermatol.*, 44, 233, 1965.
6. Barman, J.M., Pecoraro, V., and Astore, I., Biological basis of the inception and evolution of baldness, *J. Gerontol.*, 24, 163, 1969.
7. Barrett, S., Commercial hair analysis: science or scam?, *JAMA*, 254, 1041, 1985.
8. Bean, R.B., Hair and eye color in old Virginians, *Am. J. Phys. Anthropol.*, 20, 171, 1935.
9. Beek, C.H., A study on extension and distribution of the human body-hair, *Dermatologica*, 101, 317, 1951.
10. Boyd, E., *The Growth of the Surface Area of the Human Body.* University of Minnesota Press, Minneapolis, 1935.
11. Casey, J.H., Burger, H.G., Kent, J.R., Kellie, A.E., Moxham, A., Nabarro, J., and Nabarro, J.D.N., Treatment of hirsutism by adrenal and ovarian suppression, *J. Clin. Endocrinol. Metabol.*, 26, 1370, 1966.
12. Cervia, M. and Rebora, A., Age-related severity of male-pattern alopecia, *Dermatologica*, 166, 81, 1983.
13. Comaish, S., White scalp hairs turning black—an unusual reversal of the aging process, *Br. J. Dermatol.*, 86, 513, 1972.

14. Dawson, A. and Ogston, D., The effect of age on the diagnostic value of greying of the hair in Addisonian pernicious anaemia, *Gerontol. Clin.*, 14, 317, 1972.
15. Deeming, S.B. and Weber, C.W., Hair analysis of trace minerals in human subjects as influenced by age, sex, and contraceptive drugs, *Am. J. Clin. Nutr.*, 31, 1175, 1978.
16. Dupertuis, C.W., Atkinson, W.B., and Elftman, H., Sex differences in pubic hair distribution, *Hum. Biol.*, 15, 136, 1945.
17. Ebling, F.J., The physiology of hair growth, in *Cosmetic Science*, Vol. 2, Breuer, M.M., Ed., Academic Press, London, 1980, 181.
18. Finch, C.E., Retardation of hair regrowth, a phenomenon of senescence in C57B1/6J male mice, *J. Gerontol.*, 28, 13, 1973.
19. von Flugel, B., Des Ergrauen der Haare als Kriterium des biologischen Alters, *Z. Alternsforsch.*, 23, 397, 1971.
20. Gentile, P., Trentalange, M.J., and Coleman, M., The relationship of hair zinc concentrations to height, weight, age, and sex in the normal population, *Pediatr. Res.*, 15, 123, 1981.
21. Giacometti, L., The anatomy of the human scalp, in *Advances in the Biology of the Skin,* Vol. 6, *Aging,* Montagna, W., Ed., Pergamon Press, New York, 1965, 97.
22. Greger, J.L. and Geissler, A.H., Effect of zinc supplementation on taste acuity of the aged, *Am. J. Clin. Nutr.*, 31, 633, 1978.
23. Hamilton, J.B., Male hormone stimulation is prerequisite and an incitant in common baldness, *Am. J. Anat.*, 71, 451, 1942.
24. Hamilton, J.B., Quantitative measurement of a secondary sex character, axillary hair, *Ann. N.Y. Acad. Sci.*, 53, 585, 1951.
25. Hamilton, J.B., Patterned loss of hair in man: types and incidence, *Ann. N.Y. Acad. Sci.*, 53, 708, 1951.
26. Herzberg, J. and Gusek, W., The greying of hair: histochemical and electronmicroscopical investigations, *Arch. Clin. Exp. Dermatol.*, 236, 368, 1970.
27. Hori, H., Moretti, G., Rebora, A., and Crovato, F., The thickness of human scalp: normal and bald, *J. Invest. Dermatol.*, 58, 396, 1972.
28. Ibrahim, L. and Wright, E.A., The long term effect of repeated pluckings on the function of the mouse vibrissal follicles, *Br. J. Dermatol.*, 99, 371, 1978.
29. Ikoma, E. and Tsumoto, S., A study of the thickness of human parietal hair in reference to genetics, *Wakayama Med. Rep.*, 15, 65, 1971.
30. *Internal Medicine Alert,* Commercial Hair Analysis—Unscientific and Misleading, Vol. 7(19), 1985, 74.
31. Jackson, D., Church, R.E., and Ebling, F.J., Hair diameter in female baldness, *Br. J. Dermatol.*, 87, 361, 1972.
32. Kasperek, K., Feinendegen, L.E., and Siller, V., Aktivierungsanalyse von Spurenelementkonzentrationen im menschlichen Kopfhaar; Einfluß von Geschlecht, Alter und Umwelt, *Nucl. Med. Stuttgart*, 9, 123, 1971.
33. Keogh, E.V. and Read, G., The distribution of skin, hair and eye colours in an Australian population, *Austr. J. Exp. Biol.*, 41, 405, 1963.
34. Lasker, G.W. and Kaplan, B., Graying of the hair and mortality, *Social Biol.*, 21, 290, 1974.
35. Lerner, A.B., Gray hair and sympathectomy: report of a case, *Arch. Dermatol.*, 93, 235, 1966.
36. Lynfield, Y.L., Effect of pregnancy on the human hair cycle, *J. Invest. Dermatol.*, 35, 323, 1960.
37. Maguire, H.C., Facial hair growth over site of testosterone injection in women, *Lancet*, 1, 864, 1964.
38. Maguire, H.C., Terminal hair growth confined to the site of locally administered testosterone in the adult women, *J. Invest. Dermatol.*, 35, 323, 1965.
39. Matheny, A.P., Jr. and Dolan, A.B., Sex and genetic differences in hair color changes during early childhood, *Am. J. Phys. Anthropol.*, 42, 53, 1975.
40. Montagna, W., Morphology of aging skin: the cutaneous appendages, in *Advances in the Biology of the Skin,* Vol. 6, *Aging,* Montagna, W., Ed., Pergamon Press, New York, 1965, 1.
41. Montagna, W., Histology and cytochemistry of human skin. XXXIV. The eyebrows, *Arch. Dermatol.*, 101, 257, 1970.
42. Montagna, W. and Giacometti, L., Histology and cytochemistry of human skin. XXXII. The external ear, *Arch. Dermatol.*, 99, 757, 1969.
43. Morse, H.C., III, Yetter, R.A., Stimpfling, J.H., Pitts, O.M., Fredrickson, T.N., and

Hartley, J.W., Greying with age in mice: relation to expression of murine leukemia viruses, *Cell,* 41, 439, 1985.
44. Moyer, D.L., Is hair analysis useful: an evaluation of health and disease by hair analysis, *J. Appl. Nutr.*, 29, 55, 1977.
45. Myers, R.J. and Hamilton, J.B., Regeneration and rate of growth of hairs in man, *Ann. N.Y. Acad. Sci.*, 53, 562, 1951.
46. Naruse, N. and Fujita, T., Changes in the physical properties of human hair with age, *J. Am. Geriatr. Soc.*, 19, 308, 1971.
47. Nishimura, H. and Shimizu, S., Studies on various aging phenomena in Japanese twins and siblings, *Acta Genet. Med. Gemell.*, 12, 22, 1963.
48. Oberste-Lehn, H., Effects of aging on the papillary body of the hair follicles and on the eccrine sweat glands, in *Advances in the Biology of the Skin,* Vol. 6, *Aging*, Montagna, W., Ed., Pergamon Press, New York, 1965, 17.
49. Orentreich, N., Pathogenesis of alopecia, *J. Soc. Cosmet. Chem.*, II, 479, 1960.
50. Orentreich, N., Preventive and therapeutic measures for aging skin. *Proc. Sci. Sect. Toilet Goods Association.*, 41, 37, 1964.
51. Orentreich, N., Hair problems, *J. Am. Med. Women's Assoc.*, 21, 481, 1966.
52. Orentreich, N. and Rizer, R.L., Medical treatment of androgenetic alopecia, in *Hair, Trace Elements and Human Illness, Part IV, Hirsutism and Alopecia*, Brown, A.C. and Crounse, R.A., Eds., Praeger Press, New York, 1980, 294.
53. Orentreich, N., The problems of hair transplantation, in *Hair Research*, Orfanos, C.E., Stuttgen, G., and Montagna, G., Eds., Springer-Verlag, Berlin, 1981, 650.
54. Orentreich, N., Brind, J.L., Rizer, R.L., and Vogelman, J.H., Age changes and sex differences in serum dehydroepiandrosterone sulfate concentrations throughout adulthood, *J. Clin. Endocrinol. Metabol.*, 59, 551, 1984.
55. Orfanos, C., Ruska, H., and Mahrle, G., White hair in older people. IV. Fine structure of human hair, *Arch. Klin. Exp. Dermatol.*, 236, 395, 1970.
56. Ortonne, J.P., Thivolet, J., and Guillet, R., Greying of hair with age and sympathectomy, *Arch. Dermatol.*, 118, 876, 1982.
57. Pecoraro, V., Astore, I., and Barman, J.M., Growth rate and hair density of the human axilla. A. Comparative study of normal males and females and pregnant and post-partum females, *J. Invest. Dermatol.*, 56, 362, 1971.
58. Pelfini, C., Cerimele, D., and Pisanu, G., Aging of the skin and hair growth in man, in *Advances in the Biology of the Skin,* Vol. 9, *Hair Growth*, Montagna, W. and Dobson, R.L., Eds., Pergamon Press, New York, 1969, 153.
59. Petering, H.G., Yeager, D.W., and Witherup, S.O., Trace metal content of hair. I. Zinc and copper content of human hair in relation to age and sex, *Arch. Environ. Health*, 23, 202, 1971.
60. Petering, H.G., Yeager, D.W., and Witherup, S.O., Trace metal content of hair. II. Cadmium and lead of human hair in relation to age and sex, *Arch. Environ. Health*, 27, 327, 1973.
61. Pirke, K.M. and Doerr, P., Age related changes and interrelations between plasma testosterone, estradiol, and androgen binding globulin in normal adult males, *Acta Endocrinol.*, 74, 792, 1973.
62. von Radig, K., Uber das Wachstum der Barthaare und dessen Beeinflußung durch Krankheiten, *Dermatol. Monatsschr.*, 160, 335.
63. Rao, D.C., A contribution of the genetics of hypertrichosis of the ear rims, *Hum. Hered.*, 20, 486, 1970.
64. Reeves, R.D., Jolley, K.W., and Buckley, P.D., Lead in human hair: relation to age, sex and environmental factors, *Bull. Environ. Contam. Toxicol.*, 14, 579, 1975.
65. Riggott, J.M. and Wyatt, E.H., A mathematical approach to the study of hair using the scanning electron microscope, *J. Cutaneous. Pathol.*, 8, 473, 1981.
66. Rook, A., Endocrine influences on hair growth, *Br. Med. J.*, 1, 609, 1965.
67. Sato, S., Nishijima, A., Hiraga, K., and Hidano, A., Changes in basal lamina of blood vessels within hair dermal papilla: a possible relation to the hair cycle, in *Biology and Diseases of the Hair*, Kabori, T. and Montagna, W., Eds., University of Tokyo Press, Tokyo, 1975, 87.
68. Schroeder, H.A. and Nason, A.P., Trace metals in human hair, *J. Invest. Dermatol.*, 53, 71, 1969.
69. Shabel'nik, D.Y., *Mikrolem. Med.*, 1, 184, 1968.

70. Soloman, L.M. and Virtue, C., The biology of cutaneous aging. *Int. J. Dermatol.*, 14, 172, 1975.
71. Steggerda, M., Change in hair color with age, *J. Hered.*, 32, 402, 1941.
72. Suter, D., Hair colour in the Faroe and Orkney Islands, *Ann. Hum. Biol.*, 1, 89, 1979.
73. Szabo, G., The regional frequency and distribution of hair follicles in human skin, in *The Biology of Hair Growth*, Montagna, W. and Ellis, R.A., Eds., Academic Press, New York, 1958, 33.
74. Trotter, N., The life cycles of hair in selected regions of the body, *Am. J. Phys. Anthropol.*, 7, 427, 1924.
75. Trotter, N., The form, size, and color of head hair in American nell'eta senile, *Minerva Med.*, 60, 3651, 1930.
76. Trotter, N. and Dawson, H.L., The hair of French Canadians, *Am. J. Phys. Anthropol.*, 18, 443, 1934.
77. Vmeulen, A., Rubens, R., and Verdonck, L., Testosterone secretion and metabolism in male senescence, *J. Clin. Endocrinol. Metabol.*, 34, 730, 1972.
78. Weiss, D., Whitten, B., and Leddy, D., Lead content of human hair (1871-1971), *Science*, 178, 69, 1972.
79. Wyatt, E.H., and Riggott, J.M., Scanning electron microscopy of hair. Observations on surface morphology with respect to site, sex and age in man, *Br. J. Dermatol.*, 96, 627, 1977.
80. Zaun, H., Altersveranderungen des Haarkleides, *Fette, Seifen, Anstrichm.*, 72, 807, 1970.

BIOCHEMICAL MEASUREMENTS

CHAPTER 22

DEHYDROEPIANDROSTERONE: MARKER OR MODIFIER OF AGING?

NORMAN ORENTREICH, JAY A. ZIMMERMAN, AND JONATHAN R. MATIAS

Dehydroepiandrosterone (DHEA, 3β-hydroxy-5-androsten-17-one) and its sulfate (DS) are abundantly produced adrenal steroids that have been recognized for more than 50 years. These steroids have attracted considerable attention because of their apparent ability to modify a variety of physiological, pharmacological, and metabolic functions, including but not limited to chemical carcinogenesis,[25,27] tumor growth,[4,7] age-related memory loss,[19,28] obesity,[5,15] diabetes mellitus,[30] immunological function,[24,31] and, possibly, human immunodeficiency virus (HIV) infection.[9] Of great interest is whether these ubiquitous steroids act in senescence to modify the rate of aging, or to indicate chronological or clinical age. Studies in the authors' laboratories and elsewhere indicate that this molecule may serve both roles.

The principal source of DHEA is the zona reticularis of the adrenal glands. Secretion of DHEA and glucocorticoids is often parallel, but there is a dissociation between the circulating levels of these two hormones in patients who have had surgery, compared to others who were hospitalized for medical problems. This observation, along with the finding that in senescent human subjects there is a loss of diurnal periodicity for cortisol, but not DS, suggests that in some circumstances secretion of glucocorticoids and DHEA is regulated by separate trophic agents,[10,22] the one regulating DHEA called cortical androgen-stimulating hormone (CASH).[21]

In humans, DHEA secreted by the adrenal glands is rapidly conjugated in the liver, or may be conjugated prior to secretion in the adrenal glands themselves to form DS.[1] The more water-soluble DS is the predominant form found in the human circulation, where it probably serves as a transport function. Large amounts of DHEA are stored in adipose tissue.

Despite the recent report of a possible receptor or binding protein for DHEA in rodent liver,[11] it is not clear that this steroid, which acts on a wide variety of tissues, interacts in the normal steroid-receptor fashion with target tissues. Rather, it is likely that DS functions as a prohormone, undergoing intracellular bioconversion to a variety of active hormones.[8,13] In the corpus luteum, placenta and brain DHEA is converted into 17β-estradiol, estrone, and even some testosterone. Thus, administration of DS to prepubescent females leads to the stimulation of pudendal and uterine growth.[12] In males DHEA is converted to androstenedione, and then to testosterone and dihydrotestosterone in androgen target tissues. As a consequence, DS administration to immature males produces prostatic and genital enlargement. Although DHEA and DS are commonly termed "adrenal androgens", this is probably a misnomer in view of the need for bioconversion to active androgens and estrogens. It might even be better to call this steroid a "presexogen".

Many of the varied physiological and pharmacological effects of DHEA probably stem from the steroid interconversions discussed above, leading to active and well-known steroids (e.g., estrone, testosterone, etc.). Nevertheless, DHEA and some of its analogues which are not

0-8493-0129-7/94/$0.00+$.50

capable of being metabolized to estrogens or androgens, retain specific biological activities.[29] Some of these analogues, as well as DHEA itself, modulate target cell metabolism through their ability to directly inhibit glucose-6-phosphate dehydrogenase (G6PD). Among the actions linked to DHEA-related G6PD reduction is reduced susceptibility to chemical carcinogenesis,[17,18,23] and reduced growth rate for already-established tumors.[16] These actions have been associated with reduced G6PD levels, rather than with the genotrophic actions of DHEA-derived steroid hormones.

Senescence in virtually all mammalian species is accompanied by a wide variety of disorders, including increased tumorigenesis, diabetes mellitus, reduced immune function, and others. Many of these age-related alterations in function resemble, to some extent, the inverse of the actions of DHEA. It is then of interest to know whether serum DS levels decline with age, and whether such a decline can be related causally to the changes accompanying aging. In order to explore such a possible relationship the authors have measured circulating DS levels longitudinally and cross-sectionally in a large number of human beings spanning ages 10 to 75 years (Figure 1).[20] In both males and females, serum DS rises beginning with adrenarche,[6] peaking in the mid-20s at >3500 ng/ml in males and 2500 ng/ml in females. Thereafter, serum DS levels decline steadily in both sexes at a rate of approximately 10%/decade (in males) between ages 30 and 70. The decline is more rapid in males, so that by age 75 a sexual dichotomy no longer exists in the survivors.

In normal human serum DS levels are modified by a variety of physiological, behavioral, and metabolic factors, including, for example, hypertension, gout, psoriasis, meditation, obesity, stress, and smoking.[26] We believe that DS levels are a marker of aging in the sense that on a population-wide basis, a reproducible age-related decline occurs in the plasma concentration of this steroid. However, while DS levels also decline on an individual basis, disease and probably other as yet undefined factors can add an overlay to the age-related decline, reducing the power of the test to discern true age. Although reduced circulating levels of DS have been associated with increased risk of breast cancer in women, and with a history of heart disease in men,[2] there have been no studies correlating either DS levels or changes in DS over time with subsequent survival.

In addition to being a marker of age, the age-related decline in DS seen in human beings and the great apes may be a cause of biological aging. Should this be true, then experimentally increasing circulating DS levels should be associated with relief from some of the symptoms of senescence. Accordingly, we have fed male C57Bl/6J mice from weaning with a diet supplemented with 0.4% DHEA in order to determine whether such treatment would produce an alteration in the rate of aging of the animals. The diet was well tolerated because neither food consumption nor body weight was altered by the presence of DHEA in the food. Lifelong consumption of 0.4% DHEA-supplemented food altered neither median nor maximum life span (Figure 2).

The C57Bl/6J mouse is considered to be a low-tumor strain, and does not develop diabetes as it ages. The failure of lifelong feeding with DHEA to extend life span may reflect the ability of DHEA to influence only a portion of the total disability spectrum of senescence, a portion which is not important in the senescence of this particular biological model. Nevertheless, DHEA feeding at this level clearly did not alter the intrinsic rate of aging, and cannot be considered to be a modifier of the rate of aging in mice. This does not preclude a role for DHEA in modifying the progress of certain diseases that are associated with aging, such as cancer, diabetes, etc.

It is important to note that DS is found in substantial quantities only in the circulation of the primates. This probably reflects the inability of subprimate species to carry out the sulfation reaction leading from DHEA to the water- (and blood-) soluble DS. DHEA fed to rodents is likely to raise adipose stores, and is known to elevate the serum concentration of DHEA by up to fourfold, while not altering DS.[13]

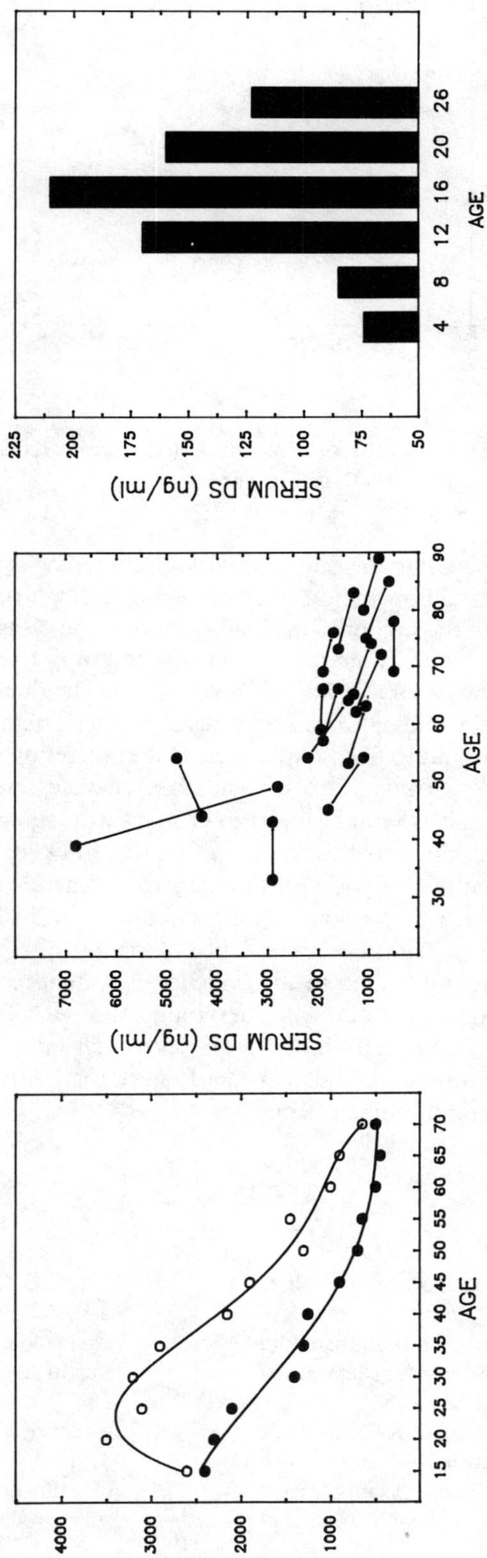

Figure 1 Age-related changes in serum dehydroepiandrosterone sulfate in primates. (Left) Cross-sectional data from 981 human males (open circles) and 481 females (closed circles). (Center) Longitudinal measures in 15 individuals. (Right) Cross-sectional measures in 83 pigtailed macaques.

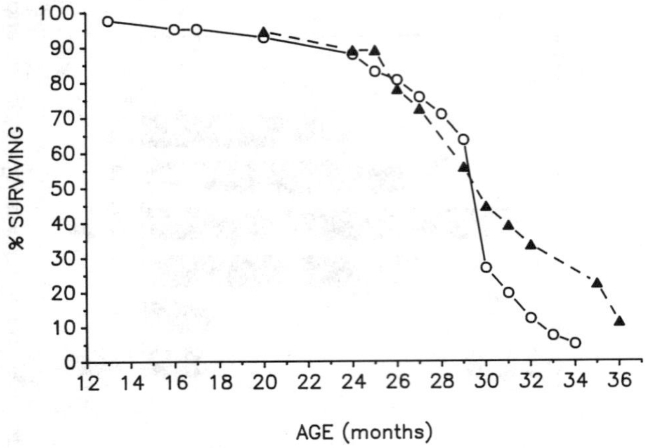

Figure 2 Survival curves for C57B1/6J male mice fed normal diets (triangles) or normal diets supplemented with 0.4% DHEA (circles).

The determination that some measure is a biological marker of senescence is fraught with hazards. Does "marker" mean an indicator of chronological age or a predictor of death and disability brought about by those conditions that we have come to associate with advanced age? At this stage, it is not possible to assign plasma DS concentration to either category because it is not clear why the concentration of this steroid falls with age. The dramatic and reproducible age-related decline in serum DS could reflect altered rates of synthesis stemming from reduced adrenal capability, altered release resulting from diminished CASH secretion, or increased conversion to other steroids. Alternatively, regulation of the sulfatase enzyme responsible for regulating the partition between DHEA and DS might undergo changes with aging. Of these possibilities, the age-related reduction in the kinetics of conversion of DHEA to DS has been documented,[3] as has the enhanced aromatization of DHEA in postmenopausal women.[14] Nevertheless, low DS levels in individuals, as judged either by previous measures in that individual or by age-adjusted norms, should be viewed with some alarm because of the association of reduced DS with a variety of serious diseases. On the other hand, no strong evidence exists that restoring normal (or elevated) circulating levels of DS will prevent or delay the development of such illnesses. Based on our animal studies, we cannot demonstrate that elevating DS levels will influence the underlying rate of biological aging, but we cannot rule out beneficial effects of DHEA on some of the diseases associated with clinical aging in human beings.

REFERENCES

1. Adams, J.B. and McDonald, D., Enzymatic synthesis of steroid sulfates. XVI. Specificity and regulation of human adrenal hydroxysteroid sulfotransferase, *Steroids,* 41(5), 375, 1983.
2. Barrett-Conner, E., Khaw, K.-T., and Yen, S.S.C., A prospective study of dehydroepiandrosterone sulfate, mortality and cardiovascular disease, *N. Engl. J. Med.,* 315, 1519, 1986.
3. Bird, C.E., Tremblay, J., Masters, V., and Clark, A.F., Delta 5-androstenediol: kinetics of metabolism and binding to plasma proteins in normal post-menopausal women, *Acta Endocrinol.,* 99, 309, 1982.
4. Boccuzzi, B., Brignardello, E., DiMonaco, M., Forte, C., Leonardi, L., and Pizzini, A., Influence of dehydroepiandrosterone and 5-en-androstene-3b, 17b-diol on the growth of MCF-7 human breast cancer

cells induced by 17b-estradiol, *Anticancer Res.,* 12, 799, 1992.
5. Cleary, M.P., The antiobesity effect of dehydroepiandrosterone in rats, *Proc. Soc. Exp. Biol. Med.,* 196, 8, 1991.
6. Cutler, G.B., Glenn, M., Bush, M., Hodgen, G.D., Graham, C.E., and Loriaux, D.L., Adrenarche: a survey of rodents, domestic animals and primates, *Endocrinology,* 103, 2112, 1978.
7. Hamilton, S.R., Gordon, G.B., Floyd, J., and Golightly, S., Evaluation of the dietary dehydroepiandrosterone for chemoprotection against tumorigenesis in premalignant colonic epithelium of male F344 rats, *Cancer Res.,* 51, 476, 1991.
8. Haning, R.V., Jr., Flood, C.A., Hackett, R.J., Loughlin, J.S., McClure, N. and Longcope, C., Metabolic clearance rate of dehydroepiandrosterone sulfate, its metabolism to testosterone, and its intra-follicular metabolism to dehydroepiandrosterone, androstenedione, testosterone, and dihydrotestosterone *in vivo*, *J. Clin. Endocrinol. Metab.,* 72, 1088, 1991.
9. Henderson, E., Yang, J.Y., and Schwartz, A., Dehydroepiandrosterone (DHEA) and synthetic DHEA analogs are modest inhibitors of HIV-1 IIIB replication, *AIDS Res. Hum. Retroviruses,* 8, 625, 1992.
10. Hung, T.T. and LeMaire, W.H., The effects of corticotropin, opioid peptides and crude pituitary extract on the production of dehydroepiandrosterone and corticosterone by mature rat adrenal cells in tissue culture, *J. Steroid Biochem.,* 29, 721, 1988.
11. Kalimi, M. and Regelson, W., Physiochemical characterization of [3H]DHEA binding in rat liver, *Biochem. Biophys. Res. Commun.,* 158, 22, 1988.
12. Knudsen, T.T. and Mahesh, V.B., Initiation of precocious sexual maturation in the immature rat treated with dehydroepiandrosterone, *Endocrinology,* 97, 458, 1972.
13. Leiter, E.H., Beamer, W.G., Coleman, D.L., and Longcope, C., Androgenic and estrogenic metabolites in serum of mice fed dehydroepiandrosterone: relationship to antihyperglycemic effects, *Metabolism,* 36(9), 863, 1987.
14. Longcope, D., Bourget, C., and Flood, C., The production and aromatization of dehydroepiandrosterone in post-menopausal women, *Maturitas,* 4, 325, 1982.
15. Macewen, E.G. and Kurzman, I.D., Obesity in the dog: role of the adrenal steroid dehydroepiandrosterone (DHEA), *J. Nutr.,* 121(Suppl.), S51, 1991.
16. Matias, J.R., DeFeo, C.P., Malloy, V., and Orentreich, N., Inhibition of prostate cancer in rats by the administration of dehydroepiandrosterone, *Ann. N.Y. Acad. Sci.,* 494, 316, 1987.
17. Moore, M.A., Thamavit, W., Hiasa, Y., and Ito, N., Early lesions induced by DHPN in Syrian golden hamsters, Influence of concomitant *Opisthorchis* infestation, dehydroepiandrosterone or butylated hydroxyanisole administration, *Carcinogenesis,* 9, 1185, 1988.
18. Moore, M.A., Weber, E., Thornton, M., and Bannasch, P., Sex-dependent, tissue-specific opposing effects of dehydroepiandrosterone on initiation and modulation stages of liver and lung carcinogenesis induced by dihydroxy-di-*n*-propylnitrosamine in F344 rats, *Carcinogenesis,* 9, 1507, 1988.
19. Nasman, B., Olsson, T., Backstrom, T. et al., Serum dehydroepiandrosterone sulfate in Alzheimer's disease and in multi-infarct dementia, *Biol. Psych.,* 30, 684, 1991.
20. Orentreich, N., Brind, J.L., Rizer, R.L., and Vogelman, J.H., Age changes and sex differences in serum dehydroepiandrosterone sulfate concentrations throughout adulthood, *J. Clin. Endocrinol. Metab.,* 59, 551, 1984.
21. Parker, L.N., Lifrak, E.T., and Odell, W.D., A 60,000 molecular weight human pituitary glycopeptide stimulates adrenal androgen secretion, *Endocrinology,* 113(6), 2092, 1983.
22. Parker, L.N. and Odell, W.D., Control of adrenal androgen secretion, *Endocr. Rev.,* 1(4), 392, 1980.
23. Paskho, L.L., Hard, G.C., Rovito, R.J., Williams, J.R., Sobel, E.L., and Schwartz, A.G., Inhibition of 7,12-dimethylbenz(a) anthracene-induced skin papillomas and carcinomas by dehydroepiandrosterone and 3-B-methylandrost-5-en-17-one in mice, *Cancer Res.,* 45, 164, 1985.

24. Rasmussen, K.R., Arrowood, M.J., and Healey, M.D., Effectiveness of dehydroepiandrosterone in reduction of cryptosporidial activity in immunosuppressed rats, *Antimicrob. Agents Chemother.*, 36, 220, 1992.
25. Ratko, T.A., Detrisac, C.J., Mehta, R.G., Kelloff, G.J. and Moon, R.C., Inhibition of rat mammary gland chemical carcinogenesis by dietary dehydroepiandrosterone or a fluorinated analogue of dehydroepiandrosterone, *Cancer Res.*, 51, 481, 1991.
26. Salvini, S., Stampfer, M.J., Barbieri, R.L., and Hennekens, C.H., Effects of age, smoking and vitamins on plasma DHEA levels: a cross-sectional study in men, *J. Clin. Endocrinol. Metab.*, 74, 139, 1992.
27. Sambasiva Rao, M., Subburao, V., Yeldandi, A.V., and Reddy, J.K., Hepa-tocarcinogenicity of dehydroepian-drosterone in the rat, *Cancer Res.*, 52, 2977, 1992.
28. Schneider, L.S., Hinsey, M., and Lyness, S., Plasma dehydroepiandrosterone sulfate in Alzheimer's disease, *Biol. Psych.*, 31, 205, 1992.
29. Schwartz, A.G., Lewbart, M.L., and Pashko, L.L., Novel dehydroepiandrosterone analogues with enhanced biological activity and reduced side effects in mice and rats, *Cancer Res.*, 48, 4817, 1988.
30. Small, M., Gray, C.E., Beastall, G.H., and MacCuish, A.C., Adrenal androgens in insulin-dependent diabetes mellitus, *Diabetes Res.*, 11, 93, 1989.
31. Suzuki, T., Suzuki, N., Daynes, R.A., and Engleman, E.G., Dehydroepiandrosterone enhances IL2 production and cytotoxic effector function of human T cells, *Clin. Immunol. Immunopathol.*, 61, 202, 1991.

CHAPTER 23

THE ASSAY OF ENDOGENOUS OXIDATIVE DNA DAMAGE AS RELATED TO AGING

Bruce N. Ames

TABLE OF CONTENTS

ABSTRACT

Progress in identifying the important endogenous processes damaging DNA and developing methods to assay this damage in individuals is presented. This approach may aid studies on nutritional modulation of the aging process.

The endogenous background level of oxidant-induced DNA damage *in vivo* has been assayed by measuring 8-hydroxydeoxyguanosine (oh^{8}dG), thymine glycol and thymidine glycol in urine, and oh^{8}dG in DNA. oh^{8}dG is one of about 20 adducts found on oxidizing DNA, e.g., by radiation. The level of oxidative DNA damage as measured by oh^{8}dG in normal rat liver is shown to be extensive, especially in mtDNA (1/130,000 bases in nuclear DNA and 1/8000 bases in mitochondrial DNA). Three hitherto unrecognized antioxidants in man are also discussed.

I. ENDOGENOUS SOURCES OF DNA DAMAGE, AGING, AND CANCER

The marked increase in life span that has occurred in 60 million years of primate evolution has been accompanied by a marked decrease in age-specific cancer rates. Cumulative cancer risk increases with approximately the fourth power of age (Figure 1), both in short-lived species such as rats and mice (about 30% have cancer by the end of their 2- to 3-year life span) and in long-lived species such as humans (about 30% have cancer by the end of their 85-year life span). Thus, cancer is fundamentally

0-8493-0129-7/94/$0.00+$.50

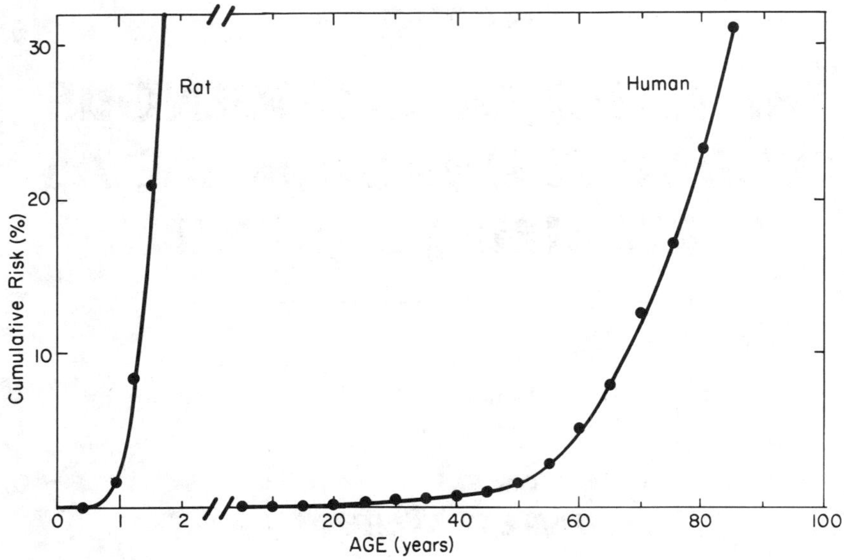

Figure 1 Cumulative net risk of death from cancer for rats and humans. (From Ames, B.N. et al., in *Molecular Biology of Aging: Gene Stability and Gene Expression,* Sohal, R.S. et al., Eds., Raven Press, New York, 1985, 137. With permission.)

a degenerative disease of old age, though it can be increased (e.g., cigarette smoking in humans) or decreased (e.g., calorie restriction in rodents) by exogenous factors.

One important factor in longevity appears to be basal metabolic rate (BMR),[15] which is much lower in man than in rodents and could markedly affect the level of endogenous mutagens produced by normal metabolism. We assume that DNA damage is likely to be critical for both cancer and aging. One view of the somatic damage theory of aging is that the amount of maintenance and repair of somatic tissues is always less than that required for indefinite survival. Thus, some DNA damage in somatic cells induced by endogenous mutagens will accumulate with time.

Four important endogenous processes leading to significant DNA damage are likely to be oxidation,[2,15,39] methylation, deamination, and depurination.[33] In support of this are the existence of specific DNA repair glycosylases for oxidative, methylated, and deaminated adducts, and a repair system for apurinic sites produced by spontaneous depurination.[29] The measurement of DNA adducts by new methods shows that oxidation is a major type of DNA damage (see below).

II. THE MEASUREMENT OF OXIDATIVE DNA DAMAGE

Oxidants are produced as by-products of normal metabolism and of lipid peroxidation (Figures 2 and 3). Oxidative damage of cellular DNA has been detected by chemical, physical, enzymatic, and immunochemical methods. The methods have been sensitive enough to detect DNA damage induced by severe stresses such as kilorad doses of radiation, but have not been useful generally for examining the background levels of damage products formed from normal aerobic metabolism. Our laboratory has overcome this problem by using an approach based on the pathways shown in Figure 4. Nonspecific DNA repair enzymes excise DNA adducts to release deoxynucleotides, or specific DNA repair glycosylases release free bases. Deoxynucleotides are enzymatically hydrolyzed to the deoxynucleosides which are not usually further metabolized, and both these and the free bases may be recovered in the urine. Two products of oxidative damage to DNA are thymine glycol and 5-hydroxymethyluracil. Ames and co-workers[25] have described a specific DNA repair enzyme, a DNA

$$O_2 \xrightarrow{e^-} O_2^{\dot{-}} \xrightarrow{e^-} H_2O_2 \xrightarrow{e^-} \cdot OH \xrightarrow{e^-} H_2O$$

$$O_2 \xrightarrow[\text{LIGHT}]{\text{DYE}} {}^1O_2$$

Figure 2 The formation of superoxide, hydrogen peroxide, and hydroxyl radicals by successive additions of electrons to oxygen. Cytochrome oxidase adds four electrons fairly efficiently during energy generation in mitochondria, but some of these toxic intermediates leak out. Singlet oxygen is generated from oxygen by the absorption of energy from a dye activated by light. (From Ames, B.N. and Gold, L.S., *Mutat. Res.,* 250, 3, 1991. With permission.)

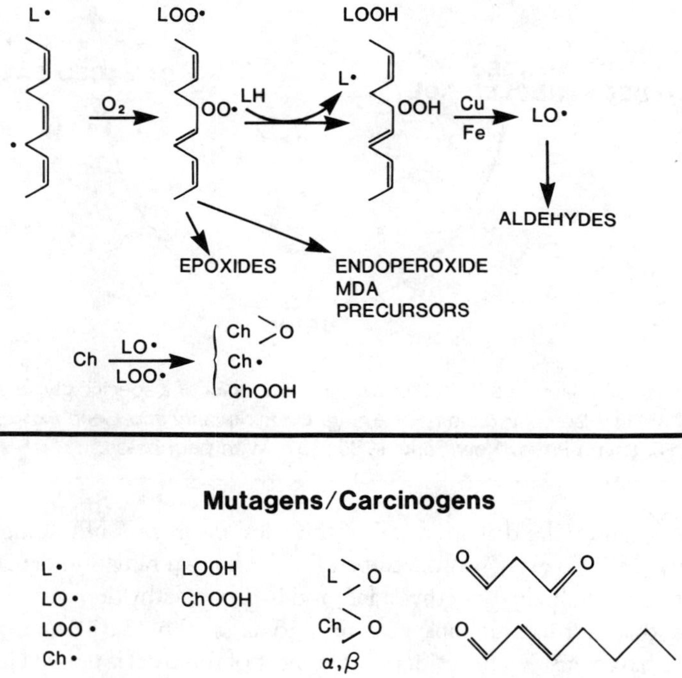

Figure 3 Lipid peroxidation. L = lipid radical; L· = alkoxy lipid radical; LOO· = hydroperoxy lipid radical; LOOH = lipid hydroperoxide; Ch = cholesterol; Ch>O = cholesterol epoxide; L>O = lipid epoxide; MDA = malondialdehyde. (From Ames, B.N., in *Methods for Detecting DNA Damaging Agents in Humans: Applications in Cancer Epidemiology and Prevention,* IARC Sci. Publ. No. 89, Bartsch, H. et al., Eds., International Agency for Research on Cancer, Lyon, 1988, 407. With permission.)

glycosylase from mouse cells, which repairs 5-hydroxymethyluracil and differs from the specific DNA glycosylase repair enzyme for thymine glycol in mouse cells. The existence of these specific repair enzymes points to the importance of this type of DNA damage *in vivo.*

Our method suffers from being an indirect measurement of what was in the DNA and being potentially subject to artifacts. Nevertheless, it has two very powerful advantages. It can be made extremely sensitive, in part because DNA lesions from all the cells in the body are concentrated in a relatively small volume of urine, and it is noninvasive.

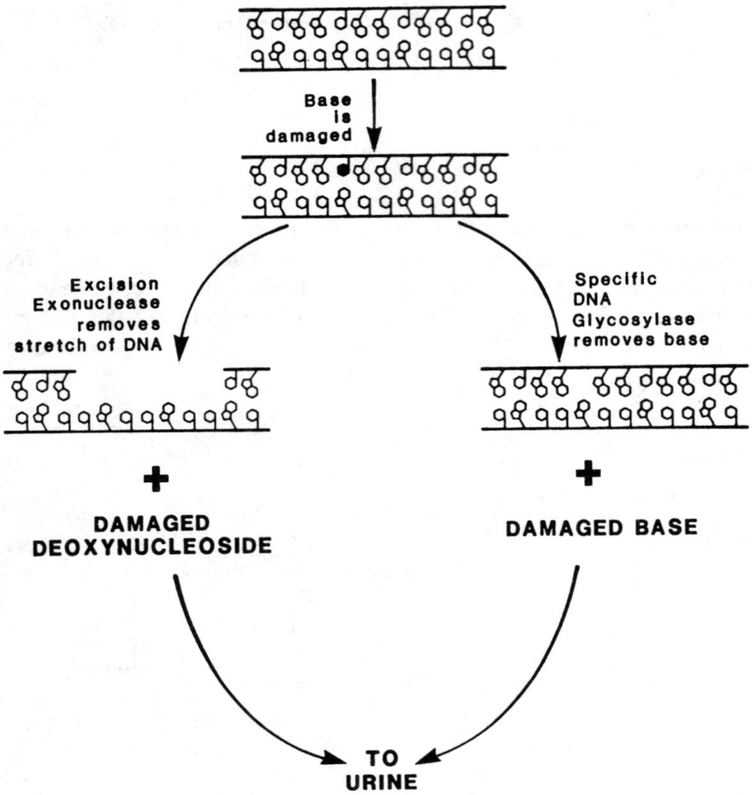

Figure 4 Repair of a damaged DNA base by excision repair or a specific glycosylase. (From Ames, B.N. et al., in *Molecular Biology of Aging: Gene Stability and Gene Expression,* Sohal, R.S. et al., Eds., Raven Press, New York, 1985, 137. With permission.)

In order to quantify the daily removal of these lesions from DNA, a high performance liquid chromatography (HPLC) assay was developed for the known radiation damage products thymine glycol, thymidine glycol, hydroxymethyluracil, and hydroxymethyldeoxyuridine in urine.[11,34,43] Our results indicate that normal humans excrete a total of about 100 nmol/d of the first three compounds. We have considerable evidence that most of this total is derived from repair of oxidized DNA, rather than from alternative sources, e.g., diet or bacterial flora.[6,11,34] This total may therefore represent an average of about 10^3 oxidized thymine residues per day for each of the body's 6×10^{13} cells. Because these products are only 3 of about 20 products of oxidative damage of DNA,[9,40] the total number of all types of oxidative hits of DNA per cell per day in man may be $>10^4$.

III. OXIDANT-INDUCED DNA DAMAGE AS RELATED TO METABOLIC RATE

Although considerable speculation about the relationships among oxidants, cancer, and aging abounds, the experimental evidence is still weak. The impressive inverse interspecies correlation between the specific metabolic rate and the rate of aging, i.e., species with high metabolic rates also have a high age-specific cancer incidence (Figure 1), is circumstantial evidence implicating oxidants in aging. The faster rate of aging and the faster accumulation of carcinogenic events for mammals with higher specific metabolic rates may be explained by assuming that these species have higher rates of production of oxidants per cell, leading to faster accumulation of somatic damage, carcinogenic events, and aging. We now have data on four species that provide additional circumstantial evidence for this theory and are consistent with the possibility that DNA is a critical target in aging. Rats, which have a higher specific metabolic rate and a shorter life span than humans, excrete about 15 times more thymine glycol and thymidine glycol per kilogram of body weight than do humans (Figure 5).[1,11] Mice have an even higher metabolic rate and a shorter life span, and they have higher levels of thymine glycol and thymidine glycol than rats. Data obtained with monkeys are consistent with this relationship.[1]

We have now tested urines for thymine glycol and thymidine glycol from normal human volunteers aged 22 to 84 years.[34] The preliminary evidence is that their urinary outputs are age independent, which suggests that the rate of oxidative DNA damage in man does not change substantially with age. This is consistent with age-independent somatic damage theories of aging.[31]

IV. URINARY 8-HYDROXYDEOXYGUANOSINE

Our urinary thymine glycol assay is difficult and takes about 3 weeks. We thus developed a simpler urinary assay for 8-hydroxydeoxyguanosine (oh^8dG), which has been measured in DNA by electrochemical detection at about 1000 times the sensitivity of UV detection.[16,26,28] This assay[14,35] can be done quickly and thus is a much more rapid and simpler assay of urine for oxidized DNA. The level in human urine is of the same order as thymidine glycol (dTg) and is much lower than the level in rodents. We also have evidence for the presence of 8-hydroxyguanosine, a measure of oxidative damage to RNA.[35] We have used this assay to measure oh^8dG in the urine of humans with chronic granulomatous disease.[14] These people lack the respiratory burst from phagocytic cells, yet they still produce oh^8dG in their urine. This is evidence that the presence of oxidized DNA bases in urine cannot be accounted for by normal cell turnover.

V. 8-HYDROXYDEOXYGUANOSINE IN DNA

Because our work on urinary excretion of oxidized bases did not distinguish between damage to nuclear and mitochondrial DNA we have examined the level of oh^8dG, one of about 20 known radiation damage products, in both mitochondrial and nuclear DNA of normal rat liver.[32] It is present at a level of 1/130,000 bases in nuclear DNA and 1/8000 bases in mitochondrial DNA. Our preliminary evidence suggests that the level of oh^8dG increases with age. The extremely high level in mitochondrial DNA may be caused by the immense oxygen metabolism, relatively inefficient DNA repair, and the absence of histones in mitochondria. Thus, mitochondria may be accumulating mutations with age which could compromise energy supplies to the cell. Mitochondria are likely to be a major source of the oxidants damaging nuclear DNA.

VI. DEFENSES AGAINST OXIDANTS

Many defense mechanisms within the organism have evolved to limit the levels of reactive O_2 species and the damage they induce. Among the defenses are superoxide dismutase (SOD), catalase, and GSH peroxidase as well as the antioxidants β-carotene, tocopherols, and vitamin C. We have discussed several previously unappreciated antioxidants that have appeared in evolution. Uric acid is a powerful antioxidant that appeared in primate evolution concomitant with the development of a long life span and large, metabolically active brain.[7] Uric acid is the main antioxidant in saliva and is 300 μM in human blood. It is present in much lower amounts in animals before the primates. Uric acid levels increased in primate evolution at about the same time as we lost the ability to synthesize ascorbic acid, so that these events may be related.

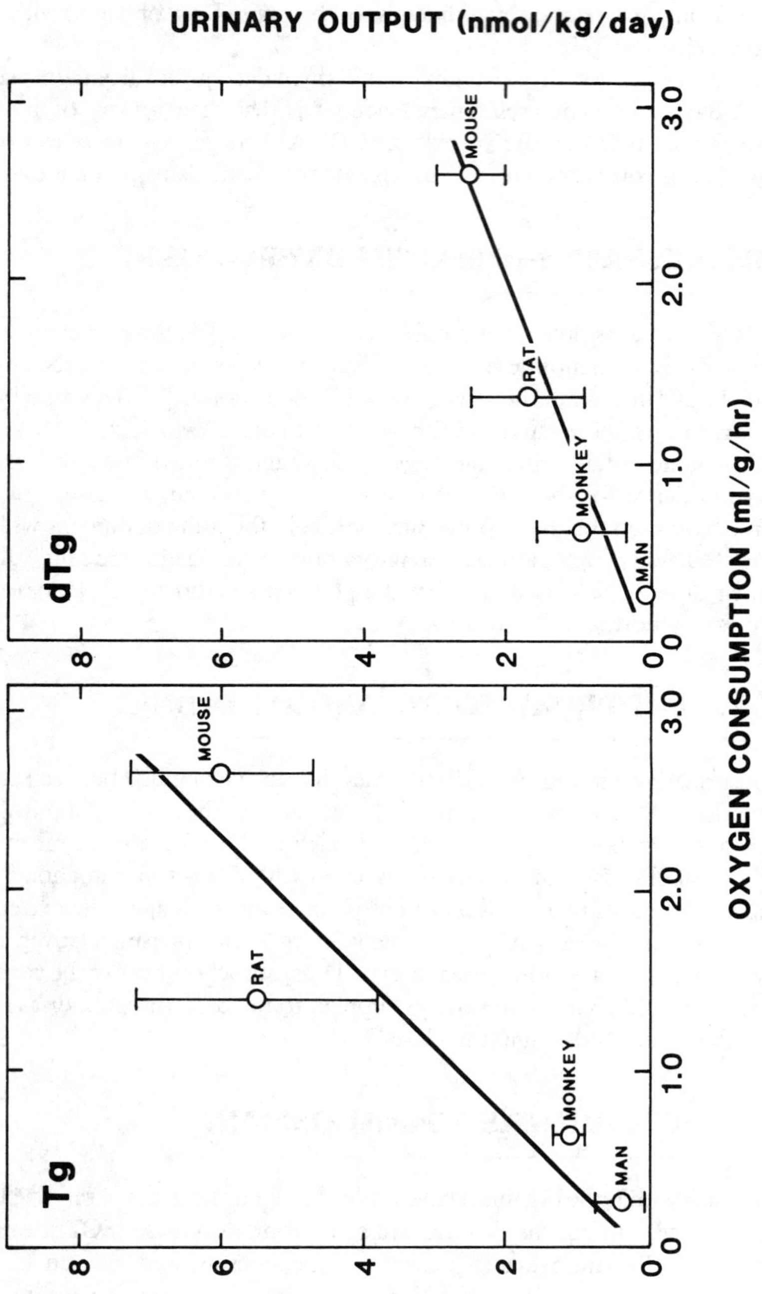

Figure 5 Average urinary output of thymine glycol (Tg) and thymidine glycol (dTg) for four different species, expressed as a function of the specific metabolic rate.

Heme is degraded to biliverdin, and in mammals biliverdin is converted to bilirubin, both of which are shown to be powerful antioxidants.[36-38] The bilirubin in human blood is bound at a specific site on albumin at a concentration of 20 μM.[36-38] This is a much higher level than in rat blood. Conjugated bilirubin also appears to be the most important antioxidant in bile, and with the copper ions present in bile forms a powerful redox system for oxidizing xenobiotics and destroying hydroperoxides.[36]

Carnosine, which is present in high concentrations in human muscle and brain, has been shown to have antioxidant properties and to chelate copper and iron ions so as to inhibit oxidative reactions. We have postulated that it is a physiologically significant antioxidant.[27]

Because of the finite time between generation of oxidants and their destruction by a defense mechanism, low levels can exist for sufficient time to produce damage to cellular macromolecules.[12] For nuclear DNA, however, the mammalian cell has three more levels of defense. First, nuclear DNA is compartmentalized away from mitochondria and peroxisomes where most oxidants are probably generated. Second, most nonreplicating nuclear DNA is surrounded by histones and polyamines which may protect against oxidants. Finally, most of the types of DNA damage produced can be repaired by efficient enzyme systems. The net result of this multilevel defense is that nuclear DNA is very well, but not completely, protected from oxidants.

VII. ENDOGENOUS DNA DAMAGE COULD CAUSE AGING BY VARIOUS MECHANISMS

Several models relate endogenous DNA damage, cancer, and aging. One possibility is that mutagens react with nuclear DNA to produce somatic mutations, both point mutations and clastogenic events such as deletions. The sources of mutagenic oxidants could include: long-lived oxidants generated outside the nucleus in the mitochondria and cytoplasm and capable of crossing the nuclear membrane, lipid-soluble oxidants generated in the nuclear membrane itself, and oxidants generated within the nucleus. Somatic mutation could disrupt the cell by altering gene products or by altering their regulation.

Another model for mutagenic damage is that the high rate of oxidative damage to mitochondria causes an accumulation of mutations with age in mitochondrial DNA that results in energy deficiencies in old cells. This would, in turn, lead to deficiencies in repair enzymes or to cell death.

In addition to mutation, DNA damage can prevent DNA replication and lead to cell death. This can cause neighboring cells to proliferate, a promotional stimulus for carcinogenesis in cells that do not normally undergo DNA replication. In addition, oxidative cell damage activates the protooncogenes c-*fos* and c-*myc*, thus acting as a promotional carcinogen.[13]

Oxidation could also cause loss of 5-methylcytosine, an epigenetic change. 5-Methylcytosine is important in turning off genes in differentiation so that its loss by DNA damage could cause dedifferentiation and contribute to cancer and aging.[24,42] By analogy with 5-hydroxymethyluracil, 5-hydroxymethylcytosine could be formed by oxidative damage.[10] This could lead to lack of methylation after DNA replication as the DNA maintenance methylase is not likely to recognize 5-hydroxymethylcytosine as 5-methylcytosine. Similarly, 8-hydroxyguanine is likely to interfere with maintenance methylation at neighboring or base-paired cytosines and cause loss of 5-methylcytosine.

More recent studies extend these findings.[3,8a,17-23,30,41]

ACKNOWLEDGMENTS

This work was supported by National Cancer Institute Outstanding Investigator Grant CA39910 and by National Institute of Environmental Health Sciences Center Grant ES01896. This paper was adapted in part from Reference 4.

REFERENCES

1. Adelman, R., Saul, R.L., and Ames, B.N., Oxidative damage to DNA: relation to species metabolic rate and life span, *Proc. Natl. Acad. Sci. U.S.A.*, 85, 2706, 1988.
2. Ames, B.N., Dietary carcinogens and anticarcinogens. Oxygen radicals and degenerative diseases, *Science*, 221, 1256, 1983.
3. Ames, B.N. and Shigenaga, M.K., Oxidants are a major contributor to aging, *Ann. N.Y. Acad. Sci.*, 663, 85, 1992.
4. Ames, B.N., Endogenous DNA damage as related to cancer and aging, *Mutat. Res.*, 214, 41, 1989.
5. Ames, B.N., Measuring oxidative damage in humans: relation to cancer and ageing, in *Methods for Detecting DNA Damaging Agents in Humans: Applications in Cancer Epidemiology and Prevention*, IARC Sci. Publ. No. 89, Bartsch, H., Hemminki K., and O'Neill, I.K., Eds., International Agency for Research on Cancer, Lyon, 1988, 407.
6. Ames, B.N. and Saul, R.L., Cancer, aging, and oxidative DNA damage, in *Theories of Carcinogenesis*, Iversen, O.H., Ed., Hemisphere, Washington, D.C., 1988, 203.
7. Ames, B.N., Cathcart, R., Schwiers, E., and Hochstein, P., Uric acid provides an antioxidant defense in humans against oxidant- and radical-caused aging and cancer: a hypothesis, *Proc. Natl. Acad. Sci. U.S.A.*, 78, 6858, 1981.
8. Ames, B.N., Saul, R.L., Schwiers, E., Adelman, R., and Cathcart, R., Oxidative DNA damage as related to cancer and aging: the assay of thymine glycol, thymidine glycol, and hydroxymethyluracil in human and rat urine, in *Molecular Biology of Aging: Gene Stability and Gene Expression*, Sohal, R.S., Birnbaum, L.S., and Cutler, R.G., Eds., Raven Press, New York, 1985, 137.

8a. Ames, B.N., Shigenaga, M.K., and Hagen, T.M., Oxidants, antioxidants, and the degenerative diseases of aging, *Proc. Natl. Acad. Sci. U.S.A.*, 90, 7915, 1993.

9. Cadet, J. and Berger, M., Radiation-induced decomposition of the purine bases within DNA and related model compounds, *Int. J. Radiat. Biol.*, 47, 127, 1985.
10. Cannon, S.V., Cummings, A., and Teebor, G.W., 5-Hydroxymethylcytosine DNA glycosylase activity in mammalian tissue, *Biochem. Biophys. Res. Commun.*, 151, 1173, 1988.
11. Cathcart, R., Schwiers, E., Saul, R.L., and Ames, B.N., Thymine glycol and thymidine glycol in human and rat urine: a possible assay for oxidative DNA damage, *Proc. Natl. Acad. Sci. U.S.A.*, 81, 5633, 1984.
12. Chance, B., Sies, H., and Boveris, A., Hydroperoxide metabolism in mammalian organs, *Phys. Rev.*, 59, 527, 1979.
13. Crawford, D. and Cerutti, P., Expression of oxidant stress-related genes in tumor promotion of mouse epidermal cells JB6, in *Anticarcinogenesis and Radiation Protection*, Nygaard, O., Simic, M., and Cerutti, P., Eds., Plenum Press, New York, 1988, 183.
14. Cundy, K., Kohen, R., and Ames, B.N., Determination of 8-hydroxydeoxyguanosine in human urine: a possible assay for *in vivo* oxidative DNA damage, in *Oxygen Radicals in Biology and Medicine*, Simic, M.G., Taylor, K.A., Ward J.F., and von Sonntag, C., Plenum Press, New York, 1988, 479.
15. Cutler, R.G., Antioxidants, aging, and longevity, in *Free Radicals in Biology*, Vol. 6, Pryor, W.A., Ed., Academic Press, New York, 1984, 371.
16. Floyd, R.A., Watson, J.J., Wong, P.K., Altmiller, D.H., and Rickard, R.C., Hydroxyl free radical adduct of deoxyguanosine: sensitive detection and mechanisms of formation, *Free Rad. Res. Commun.*, 1, 163, 1986.
17. Fraga, C.G., Shigenaga, M.K., Park, J.-W., Degan, P., and Ames, B.N., Oxidative damage to DNA during aging: 8-hydroxy-2'-deoxyguanosine in rat organ DNA and urine, *Proc. Natl. Acad. Sci. U.S.A.*, 87, 4533, 1990.
18. Fraga, C.G., Motchnik, P.A., Shigenaga, M.K., Helbock, H.J., Jacob, R., and Ames, B.N., Ascorbic acid protects against endogenous oxidative DNA damage in human sperm, *Proc. Natl. Acad. Sci. U.S.A.*, 88, 11003, 1991.
19. Frei, B., Stocker, R., and Ames, B.N., Antioxidant defenses and lipid peroxidation in human blood plasma, *Proc. Natl. Acad. Sci. U.S.A.*, 85, 9748, 1988.
20. Frei, B., England, L., and Ames, B.N., Ascorbate is an outstanding antioxidant in human blood plasma, *Proc. Natl. Acad. Sci. U.S.A.*, 86, 6377, 1989.

21. Frei, B., Kim, M.C., and Ames, B.N., Ubiquinol-10 is an effective lipid-soluble antioxidant at physiological concentrations, *Proc. Natl. Acad. Sci. U.S.A.*, 87, 4879, 1990.
22. Frei, B., Forte, T.M., Ames, B.N., and Cross, C.E., Gas phase oxidants of cigarette smoke induce lipid peroxidation and changes in lipoprotein properties in human blood plasma: protective effects of ascorbic acid, *Biochem. J.*, 277, 133, 1991.
23. Frei, B., Stocker, R., and Ames, B.N., Small molecule antioxidant defenses in human extracellular fluids, in *Molecular Biology of Free Radical Scavenging Systems*, Scandalios, J., Ed., Cold Spring Harbor Laboratory Press, Cold Spring Harbor, NY, 1992, 23.
24. Holliday, R., The inheritance of epigenetic defects, *Science*, 238, 163, 1987.
25. Hollstein, M.C., Brooks, P., Linn, S., and Ames, B.N., Hydroxymethyluracil DNA glycosylase in mammalian cells, *Proc. Natl. Acad. Sci. U.S.A.*, 81, 4003, 1984.
26. Kasai, H., Crain, P.F., Kuchino, Y., Nishimura, S., Ootsuyama, A., and Tanooka, H., Formation of 8-hydroxyguanine moiety in cellular DNA by agents producing oxygen radicals and evidence for its repair, *Carcinogenesis*, 7, 1849, 1986.
27. Kohen, R., Yamamoto, Y., Cundy, K., and Ames, B.N., Antioxidant activity of carnosine, homocarnosine, and anserine present in muscle and brain, *Proc. Natl. Acad. Sci. U.S.A.*, 85, 3175, 1988.
28. Kuchino, Y., Mori, F., Kasai, H., Inoue, H., Iwai, S., Miura, K., Ohtsuka, E., and Nishimura, S., Misreading of DNA templates containing 8-hydroxydeoxyguanosine at the modified base and at adjacent residues, *Nature*, 327, 77, 1987.
29. Lindahl, T., DNA repair enzymes, *Annu. Rev. Biochem.*, 51, 61, 1982.
30. Park, E.-M., Shigenaga, M.K., Degan, P., Korn, T.S., Kitzler, J.W., Wehr, C.M., Kolachana, P., and Ames, B.N., The assay of oxidative DNA lesions: isolation of 8-oxoguanine and its nucleoside derivatives from biological fluids with a monoclonal antibody column, *Proc. Natl. Acad. Sci. U.S.A.*, 89, 3375, 1992.
31. Peto, R., Parish, S.E., and Gray, R.G., There is no such thing as ageing, and cancer is not related to it, in *Age-Related Factors in Carcinogenesis*, IARC Sci. Publ. No. 58, Likhachev, A., Anismov V., and Montesano, R., Eds., International Agency for Research on Cancer, Lyon, 1985, 43.
32. Richter, C., Park, J.-W., and Ames, B.N., Normal oxidative damage to mitochondrial and nuclear DNA is extensive, *Proc. Natl. Acad. Sci., U.S.A.*, 85, 6465, 1988.
33. Saul, R.L. and Ames, B.N., Background levels of DNA damage in the population, in *Mechanisms of DNA Damage and Repair: Implications for Carcinogenesis and Risk Assessment*, Simic, M.G., Grossman L., and Upton, A.C., Eds., Plenum Press, New York, 1986, 529.
34. Saul, R.L., Gee, P., and Ames, B.N., Free radicals, DNA damage, and aging, in *Modern Biological Theories of Aging*, Warner, H.R., Butler, R.N., Sprott R.L., and Schneider, E.L., Eds., Raven Press, New York, 1987, 113.
35. Shigenaga, M.K., Gimeno, C.J., and Ames, B.N., Urinary 8-hydroxy-2'-deoxyguanosine as a biological marker of *in vivo* oxidative DNA damage, *Proc. Natl. Acad. Sci. U.S.A.*, 86, 9697, 1989.
36. Stocker, R. and Ames, B.N., Potential role of conjugated bilirubin and copper in the metabolism of lipid peroxides in bile, *Proc. Natl. Acad. Sci. U.S.A.*, 84, 8130, 1987.
37. Stocker, R., Glazer, A.N., and Ames, B.N., Antioxidant activity of albumin-bound bilirubin, *Proc. Natl. Acad. Sci. U.S.A.*, 84, 5918, 1987.
38. Stocker, R., Yamamoto, Y., McDonagh, A.F., Glazer, A.N., and Ames, B.N., Bilirubin is an antioxidant of possible physiological importance, *Science*, 235, 1043, 1987.
39. Totter, J.R., Spontaneous cancer and its possible relationship to oxygen metabolism, *Proc. Natl. Acad. Sci. U.S.A.*, 77, 1763, 1980.
40. von Sonntag, C., *The Chemical Basis of Radiation Biology*, Taylor & Francis, London, 1987.
41. Wagner, J.R., Hu, C.-C., and Ames, B.N., Endogenous oxidative damage of deoxycytidine in DNA, *Proc. Natl. Acad. Sci. U.S.A.*, 89, 3380, 1992.
42. Wilson, V.L., Smith, R.A., Ma, S., and Cutler, R.G., Genomic 5-methyldeoxycytidine decreases with age, *J. Biol. Chem.*, 21, 9948, 1987.
43. Ames, B.N. and Saul, R.L., unpublished observations.

NONHUMAN MODEL STUDIES

CHAPTER 24
MODELING BIOLOGICAL AGING IN A NONHUMAN PRIMATE

Robert A. Short, Darrell D. Williams, and Douglas M. Bowden

TABLE OF CONTENTS

I. RATIONALE AND THEORY

Interventions with the potential to extend the maximum human life span must be tested experimentally. Those that have proven promising in short-lived species should be tested in nonhuman primates before progressing to human testing. The nonhuman primate affords the opportunity to assess the effectiveness of interventions in retarding senescence and to discover possible undesirable side effects in long-lived species phylogenetically close to humans.

The conventional approach to assessing the influence of an intervention on life span in short-lived mammals, such as rodents, has been to construct a survival curve from measures of longevity for a group of subjects exposed to an intervention and to compare it with the survival curve of a suitable control group.[13] The use of this technique in a study of Old World primates would require a study lasting a minimum of 15 years. In macaques, the most commonly studied genus of nonhuman primate, it would require a study lasting approximately 35 years.[3] The measurement of longevity as an outcome variable using long-lived primates as subjects is clearly not practical.

An alternative to longevity as an outcome variable is the rate of aging.[2] The rate of aging is the inverse of the life span. It presumably reflects the vulnerability of an individual to death from normal aging processes. More to the point, a measurement of the aging rate should be possible within a period of time considerably shorter than that required to construct a survival curve.

The use of nonhuman primate subjects helps to bridge the gap, theoretically and empirically, between human studies and studies of insects and inbred rodents. It gives us the opportunity to exert experimental control over many of the important variables that could confound a measurement of the aging rate. For example, the diet of human subjects is difficult to control experimentally for long periods of time, and diet exerts an influence on numerous biological variables[19] that can easily be

0-8493-0129-7/94/$0.00+$.50

mistaken for an influence of aging. Additionally, because the life span of a nonhuman primate is one third that of a human, measurements requiring 15 years in a human life can be accomplished in 5 years in a nonhuman primate.

Aging has been defined as all biochemical, structural, and functional changes that normally take place in the postpubertal period of a life span.[3] While a direct measure of the genetic and environmental mechanisms that determine the rate of these changes is not available, effects on the phenotypic characteristics of the organism can be measured. A major challenge of gerontologic research is to measure that phenotypic change.[11] Although such variables are inherently susceptible to influences from the environment and genetic factors that are unrelated to the aging process, and although any such variable taken singly is likely to be a noisy index of the underlying mechanism that governs the aging rate, by combining a variety of age-sensitive variables that are relatively insensitive to direct environmental manipulations, it should be possible to measure aging rate as a phenotypic outcome variable.

The purpose of this chapter is to outline and discuss the authors' approach to constructing a valid and reliable index of the aging rate. It entails a series of steps utilizing standard statistical and psychometric concepts which can be easily adapted to different numbers and kinds of variables.[17]

II. IDENTIFYING AGING MARKERS

A plethora of cross-sectional studies provide mean values for animals of different age groups on a plethora of characteristics that can change with age.[10] From this body of data one can obtain an estimate of the biological age of an individual in comparison to other members of its cohort.[6] However, these cross-sectional data do not provide a reliable estimate of the rate of biological aging.[6,15]

Research in our laboratory has been directed toward measuring the rate of aging by gathering innocuous measurements on a broad set of variables in a longitudinal study of a nonhuman primate, the pigtailed macaque (*Macaca nemestrina*). Some 250 characteristics were screened in cross-sectional study for ones that might be expected to change with age in longitudinal study.[1] Another set of 40 characteristics were evaluated that had been identified as showing age effects in cross-sectional studies of rodents and humans.[12] Of these candidate variables, 72 proved sufficiently feasible, innocuous, and inexpensive to be studied in a cross-sectional experiment in which the effects of age, sex, and diet were tested on each variable.[19] Twenty variables were found to covary with age and were provisionally included in a variable set for continued longitudinal study. Many variables that did not show age covariance cross-sectionally continued to be studied, however, because as several authors[15,20] have noted, estimates of change, based on cross-sectional data, do not always match those based on longitudinal data. Indeed, some variables in this study failed to show an effect of age in the cross-sectional phase of the study, only to be found in longitudinal study to change with age. Conversely, many variables that showed age effects in cross-sectional study did not show change in longitudinal study.

III. LONGITUDINAL ANALYSIS

The measurement of an individual's rate of aging depends on the ability to measure change in a representative sample of many diverse attributes,[5] which may be changing at different rates.[14] The more measurements taken on a particular variable, the more confidence that can be placed on the estimate of the individual's change score. For analysis, we required enough data points on each variable to detect statistically a change if a change had taken place. Variables were measured at 6-month or shorter intervals for 3 to 5 years. In humans, this would correspond to obtaining a measure every 12 to 18 months for 10 to 15 years. In a preliminary analysis[4] variables were included if at

Table 1 Variables showing within-subject change by a *t*-test on linear regression coefficients

Rate of change variable	Abbreviation
Fingernail growth rate	FNG*
Serum sodium	NA*
Serum chloride	CL*
Immuglobulin A	IGA*
Serum total protein	TP*
Serum creatinine	CRE*
Blood urea nitrogen	BUN
Lymphocytes in WBC (%)	LYM*
Neutrophils in WBC (%)	NEU
Mean corpuscular hemoglobin	MCH*
Mean corpuscular volume	MCV
Mean corpuscular hemoglobin conc.	MCHC

Note: *Variables that were retained as biomarkers of the aging rate and were included in the BIA are indicated by an asterisk (*). WBC stands for white blood cell count.*

least 6 data points, collected over a period of at least 2.5 years, were available (for immunoglobulin A a minimum of 5 points over a minimum of 1.8 years was accepted). Data meeting these criteria were available on 28 variables from 24 females varying in age from about 4 years to about 31 years, i.e., from puberty to very old age.

For a variable to be considered a manifestation of central aging process, it should show evidence of change with the passage of time. The mathematical function that best describes the change in an attribute over the entire life span is undoubtedly not linear, but change can be approximated by a linear function if the time span is not great. Because the measurements in this study were taken over a relatively short period of time, rate-of-change was estimated by a straight line. For each animal and each variable, the line of best fit was computed by linear regression using the animal's age at which measurements were taken as the independent variable. The slope of the line was taken as the measure of the rate-of-change of that variable.

The mean of slope measures for each variable across animals was tested by a Student *t*-test to determine whether it differed statistically from zero. Those variables with means different from zero were retained for further analysis. Of the 28 variables tested, 12 showed significant longitudinal change (Table 1). Within the time spans that the animals were studied, the linear component of the change was sufficiently strong that the slope coefficient appeared to be a reasonable measure of the rate-of-change.

Three of the 12 variables were omitted from further analysis because of dependencies.[16] MCV and MCHC were excluded because they were derived from the same hemoglobin measure as MCH. NEU was excluded because it was highly correlated with LYM.

IV. FORMING THE BIOLOGICAL INDEX OF AGING

If there is a common, underlying mechanism that governs a global rate of aging, the measured rates of change of the characteristics should covary. Animals showing a rapid aging rate on any given variable should show high rates of change on other variables, and animals with low rates of change on a variable should show low rates of change on other variables. If the indicators covary we have some confidence that they measure a central aging process.

To show, in a correlational analysis, that the indicators covary, the common influence of variables outside the variable set must be removed. Because measures in this study were taken from one gender and from animals in the same environment, the major between-subject factor that needed to be controlled statistically was age. Animals of different ages may show different rates of change on a given variable. This possible source of covariance was removed by cross-sectional multiple regression; the line of best fit for each set of slopes was computed, using the average age of the subjects when the measurements were taken as the independent variable. The residuals, i.e., the age-corrected change scores, were retained for further analysis. The age-corrected score represented the difference between the individual's change score and the score predicted for animals of that chronological age as estimated by the line of best fit.

A histogram was then formed for each set of residuals and outliers that could unduly influence subsequent correlations, and other oddities of distribution, such as skewness, were eliminated by recoding scores into three to five groups of approximately equal size. These recoded residual scores were then standardized for each variable by setting the mean equal to zero and the variance equal to one. The recoded, standardized residual variables represented the portion of the rate of change scores that were independent of the animal's chronological age.

A correlation matrix was formed from the standardized rate of change scores, and the first principal component extracted. It was found that eight variables (indicated by asterisks in Table 1) had nonzero loadings. Based on the signs of these components loadings, the signs of the coefficients in the correlation matrix were reflected such that all eight variables were positively correlated with the first principal component. These eight variables were interpreted as age-sensitive variables that merited inclusion in a global index of aging, and thus were considered biological markers of the aging rate. The standardized scores were averaged to produce the biological index of aging (BIA). The sign of each biomarker used in the summation depended on the sign of its correlation with the principal component.

Internal consistency reliability was computed from the sign adjusted matrix of correlations for the eight biomarkers and found to be about 0.7. Internal consistency reliability assesses the extent of agreement among a number of independently measured variables and quantifies how well they measure a common phenomenon. Using the rate of change data for the BIA was critical for obtaining an internal consistency reliability of this magnitude. Using the mean value as the basic data yielded a reliability of only 0.6.

V. CONSTRUCTING A MODEL OF BIOLOGICAL AGING

It is instructive to express the relationships among variables thought to be relevant to the aging process into a concise mathematical/statistical model. The BIA provides a basis from which to develop such a model, as it has high reliability and high face validity.

The measurement model for the BIA (Figure 1) illustrates graphically the pattern of correlations among the biomarkers. In this and subsequent figures, variable names enclosed in rectangles represent measured variables, variable names enclosed in ovals represent latent, or unmeasured, variables, and arrows represent directed relations between variables.[17] The postulated latent variable, labeled "Rate of Biological Aging" in Figure 1, is enclosed by an oval. The eight biomarkers are each enclosed in a rectangle. Because the "Rate of Biological Aging" is hypothesized to be manifest through the eight age-corrected biomarkers, single-headed arrows are drawn emanating from the oval and pointing to each rectangle. Directed relations between "Chronological Age" and each biomarker are also illustrated by arrows. The variables at the arrowheads are presumed to be, in part, determined by the variable from which the arrow comes; thus, each score on each biomarker is

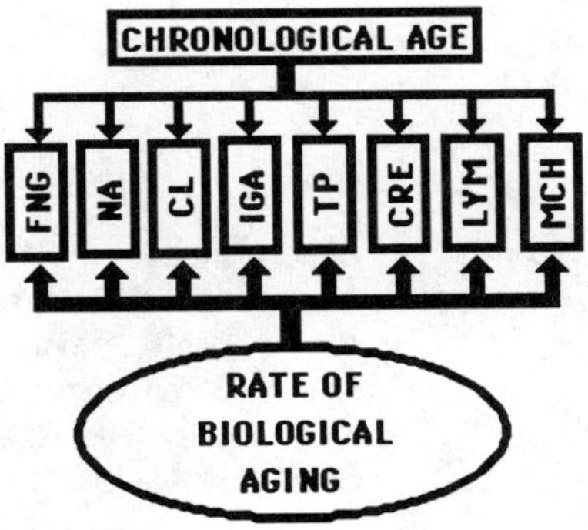

Figure 1 Measurement model for the rate of biological aging. (See Table 1 for abbreviations.)

represented by having two major determinants: the individual's chronological age and the individual's rate of aging.

The model in Figure 1 meets an important validity criterion in terms of internal consistency reliability. Another form of validity that one might assess concerns correlations between the variable of interest and variables outside of the measurement model. This type of validity is sometimes referred to as concurrent validity.[9] There are a number of variables that could help establish concurrent validity of the BIA. Here we examine the relationship of the BIA to two sets of measures presumed to relate in different ways to biological aging, namely sexual behavior and antioxidant activity. Sexual behavior is represented as a latent variable composed of several measured variables. We illustrate how this measurement, based on cross-sectional data, can be integrated into the model of the biological aging rate. Antioxidant activity is also a latent variable represented by several measured variables. Its inclusion illustrates how the model can accommodate variables postulated to influence the rate of biological aging.

VI. MEASUREMENT MODEL OF SEXUAL BEHAVIOR

Studies of several primate species indicate that reproductive function declines with age.[3] The frequency and regularity of ovarian cycles decrease, changes are noted in morphological sex characteristics, blood estradiol concentrations decrease, blood luteinizing hormone and follicle-stimulating hormone concentrations increase, and sexual behavior declines.[18] One might predict that animals that are aging rapidly, as evidenced by high BIA scores, would exhibit low sexual behavior for their age, and animals that are aging slowly, as evidenced by low BIA scores, would exhibit high sexual behavior for their age.

The sexual behavior of 22 of the 24 females for which we had measures of the BIA was observed in a mating situation with unfamiliar males of various ages on three occasions during the early follicular phase of two ovarian cycles.[18] Two types of sexual behavior were found on cross-sectional study to vary as a function of age: the presenting behavior of the female and the number of times the female was mounted by the male. General activity in the test situation was also found to be lower in old than in young females. The intercorrelations among these three behavioral measures were sufficiently large to suggest that the behaviors were measuring the same underlying phenomenon. Each variable was therefore standardized and linearly combined by summation. The internal consistency reliability of the measures was 0.7. Part of the variance in the measure could be accounted for by chronological age. The question of interest, however, was whether the part left over, i.e., the residuals left after regressing the scores on chronological age, were related to the rate of biological aging. The correlation between the age-corrected sexual behavior and the BIA was –0.5, which was significant (p <0.05), and thus served as a concurrent validation of the BIA.

The relations described above are summarized and integrated into the model in Figure 2. Note that two arrows impinge on the latent variable "SEX". One is from "Chronological Age", which

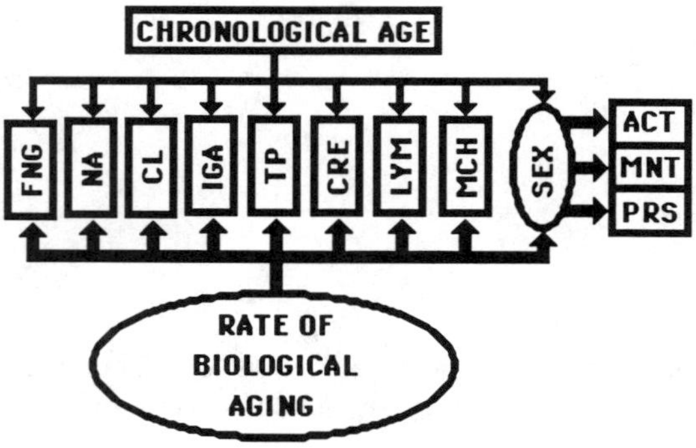

Figure 2 Measurement model for sexual behavior, SEX, integrated into the model. MNT: female mounted by male; PRS: female presented to male; ACT: activity level. (See Table 1 for other abbreviations.)

represents the idea that the "SEX" measure is influenced by the chronological age of the subjects. The second is from the "Rate of Biological Aging" and specifies the hypothesis that sexual behavior is influenced by that variable. The model illustrates that conceptually the sexual behavior variable can be considered equivalent to any one of the other eight biomarkers, i.e., as an additional marker of the BIA.

VII. MEASUREMENT MODEL OF ANTIOXIDANT ACTIVITY

Some investigators[7] have suggested that antioxidant compounds circulating in the bloodstream may play a protective role in the body by neutralizing damaging oxidizing agents. One might postulate that if true, a higher level of antioxidant activity should be found in individuals that are aging slowly, and lower levels of antioxidant activity should be found in individuals that are aging more rapidly.

To test this hypothesis we obtained serum to measure the antioxidants vitamin C, vitamin E, and carotenoids on two occasions from 19 of the 24 animals on which we had BIA measures. The mean value from the two determinations on each of the three variables was used to form a correlation matrix. The correlations among these measures yielded an internal consistency reliability of 0.7. When the standardized scores for these variables were summed, the correlation with the BIA was found to be –0.3. While this correlation was not statistically significant, the sign was in the predicted direction and the magnitude suggestive that as predicted, high levels of these putative protective compounds were associated with low scores on the BIA and low levels were associated with high scores on the BIA.

Protection mechanisms, such as antioxidant activity, are not equivalent conceptually to the biomarkers, and were therefore entered into the model differently (Figure 3). Theory suggests that compounds that protect tissues from aging directly affect the rate of aging; thus an arrow is drawn from the "Aging Rate Modulator" variable toward the "Rate of Biological Aging" variable.

From these considerations, it is evident that not all variables important to the aging process should necessarily be expected to covary with chronological age in longitudinal or cross-sectional study. Measures of antioxidant activity, for example, may influence the rate of aging without undergoing significant change themselves. Indeed, in preliminary study, we found no significant effect of age on the three antioxidants studied.

An important feature of the BIA, and the model of biological aging, is its generality. As suggested in Figure 4, the number and nature of the biomarkers that can be used to estimate the rate of biological aging are not limited to those presented. Any number of variables that meet the criteria for categorization as biomarkers of aging rate can be accommodated. The more heterogeneous the biomarkers, the greater the face validity of the BIA.[5] Likewise, variables can easily be incorporated, either as latent variables or as measured variables, into the model as contributing to the "Aging Rate Modulator" variable.

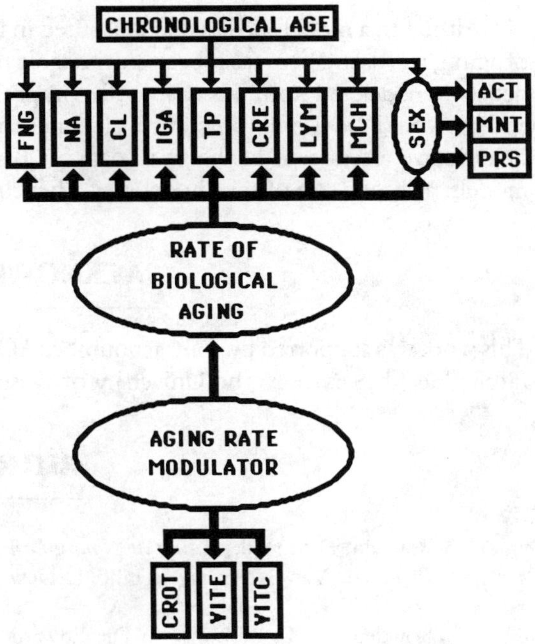

Figure 3 Measurement model for antioxidant activity integrated into the model. VITC: vitamin C; VITE: vitamin E; CROT: carotenoids. (See Table 1 and Figure 2 for other abbreviations.)

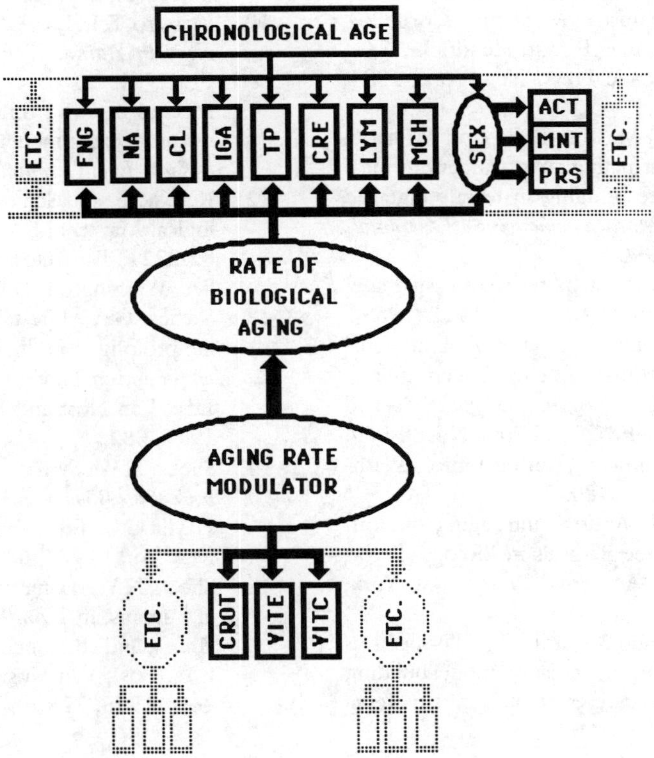

Figure 4 Generalized model for biological aging. (See Table 1 and previous figures for abbreviations.)

Although a model such as that illustrated in Figure 4 is an obvious simplification of our concept of aging, it is useful because it helps put testable hypotheses in perspective. Although some technical details were deleted from this chapter for simplicity, the complete model could easily be completed and it would be isomorphic with algebraic model equations. The model would then allow quantitative assessment of the fit to data.[8,17] Because a model is usually tested against alternative models, a second use of this model is as a benchmark against which other models may be viewed.

ACKNOWLEDGMENTS

This work was supported by contract number AG42101 and grant number RR00166 from the U.S. Public Health Service to the University of Washington.

REFERENCES

1. Bowden, D.M., Ed., *Aging in Nonhuman Primates,* Van Nostrand Reinhold, New York, 1979.
2. Bowden, D.M., Response to Dr. Edward Masoro, *Exp. Gerontol.,* 23, 395, 1988.
3. Bowden, D.M. and Williams, D.D., Aging, in *Research on Nonhuman Primates,* Vol. 2 of Advances in Veterinary Science and Comparative Medicine, Cornelius, E.E., Simpson C.F., and Hendricks, A.G., Eds., Academic Press, New York, 1984, 305.
4. Bowden, D.M., Short. R., and Williams, D.D., Constructing an instrument to measure the rate of aging in female pigtailed macaques (*Macaca nemestrina*), *J. Gerontol.,* 45, B59, 1990.
5. Comfort, A., Test-battery to measure ageing-rate in man, *Lancet,* 2, 1411, 1969.
6. Costa, P.T. and McCrae, R.R., Functional age: a conceptual and empirical critique, in *Epidemiology of Aging,* Hayes, S.B. and Feinleib, M., Eds., NIH Publ. No. 80-969, U.S. Government Printing Office, Washington, D.C., 1980, 23.
7. Cutler, R.G., Antioxidants, aging and longevity, in Free Radicals in Biology, Pryor, W.A., Ed., Academic Press, New York, 1984, 371.
8. Horn, J.L. and McArdle, J.J., Perspectives on mathematical/statistical model building (MASMOB) in research on aging, in *Aging in the 1980's: Psychological Issues,* Poon, L.W., Ed., American Psychological Association, Washington, D.C., 1980, 503.
9. Ingram, D.K., Toward the behavioral assessment of biological aging in the laboratory mouse: concepts, terminology, and objectives, *Exp. Age. Res.,* 9, 225, 1983.
10. Massaro, E.J., Ed., *CRC Handbook of Physiology in Aging,* CRC Press, Boca Raton, FL, 1981.
11. McClearn, G.E., Strategies for biomarker research: experimental and methodological design, *Exp. Gerontol.,* 23, 245, 1988.
12. Reff, M.E. and Schneider, E.L., Eds., Biological Markers of Aging, NIH Publ. No. 82-2221, U.S. Government Printing Office, Washington, D.C., 1982.
13. Sacher, G.A., Life table modification and life prolongation, in *Handbook of the Biology of Aging,* Finch, C.E. and Hayflick, L., Eds., Van Nostrand Reinhold, New York, 1977, 582.
14. Shock, N.W., Systems integration, in *Handbook of the Biology of Aging,* Finch, C.E. and Hayflick, L., Eds., Van Nostrand Reinhold, New York, 1977, 639.
15. Shock, N.W., Longitudinal studies of aging in humans, in *Handbook of The Biology Of Aging,* 2nd ed., Finch, C.E. and Schneider, E.L., Eds., Van Nostrand Reinhold, New York, 1985, 721.

16. Short, R. and Horn, J.L., Some notes on factor analysis of behavioral data, *Behaviour,* 90, 203, 1984.
17. Short, R., Horn, J.L. and McArdle, J.J., Mathematical-statistical model building in analysis of developmental data, in *Continuities and Discontinuities in Development,* Emde, R.N. and Harmon, R.J., Eds., Plenum Press, New York, 1984, 371.
18. Short, R., England, N., Bridson, W.E., and Bowden, D.M., Ovarian cyclicity, hormones, and behavior as markers of aging in female pigtailed macaques (*Macaca nemestrina*), *J. Gerontol.,* 44, B131, 1989.
19. Short, R., Williams, D.D. and Bowden, D.M., Cross-sectional evaluation of potential biological markers of aging in pigtailed macaques, effects of age, sex, and diet, *J. Gerontol.,* 42, 644, 1987.
20. Williams, D.D., Short, R. and Bowden, D.M., Fingernail growth rate as a biomarker of aging in the pigtailed macaque (*Macaca nemestrina*), *Exp. Gerontol.,* 25, 423, 1990.

CHAPTER 25

WHAT ANIMAL EXPERIMENTS CAN TELL US ABOUT HUMAN BIOLOGICAL AGE

GERHARD HOFECKER, MONIKA SKALICKY, AND HANS NIEDERMÜLLER

TABLE OF CONTENTS

I. INTRODUCTION

For the physiologist as well as for other scientists working in experimental medical research, structural and functional homology in evolution and, in particular, within the class of mammals, is an evident phenomenon. Homology is seen in a variety of biochemical and physiological principles of function such as protein synthesis, action potentials or regulatory mechanisms of the circulatory system. Regardless of the differences in life span, aging seems to be so universal a phenomenon that seen within the frame of life span, a number of age changes at the molecular, cellular, organ, or system level show striking similarities in pattern. This may be essential for research into human aging because strictly controlled animal experiments can reveal those basic principles of aging which are obscured in man by a variety of uncontrollable factors. The intention of this chapter is to show that animal models of biological age reveal a number of regularities of multicellular aging which may also be relevant to human aging.

0-8493-0129-7/94/$0.00+$.50

II. BIOLOGICAL AGE AND VITALITY

According to Hruza's[21] definition, aging is "increase in vulnerability and decrease in vitality finally leading to death". This decrease in vitality proceeds in such a characteristic manner that we are able to estimate intuitively an individual's chronological age. This age, estimated from the remaining vitality, is termed "biological age". If we try to objectivate biological age, we try to do three things:

1. We estimate vitality according to an operational definition.
2. We establish the respective average vitality for different age groups in a defined population. This relation provides the regularity of normal aging in this population.
3. We estimate the vitality of an individual or the average vitality of a subgroup of this population and look up in the "normal aging curve" what chronological age would correspond to this vitality.

Consequently, as a metric of the multicellular aging process, biological age is usually expressed as the chronological age one would assign to an individual according to his biological state (or vitality) by making reference to a "normal aging population".

III. ESTIMATION OF BIOLOGICAL AGE

In experimental gerontology, estimations of biological age are aimed mainly at two goals: to describe the patterns and dynamics of normal aging and to use these patterns as a standard against which influences on the aging process can be measured. The study of potential influences on multicellular aging reveals the major problem of measuring biological age: the complex process to be measured does not presently allow for the development of simple, well-defined models. Obviously, the normal aging of the organism does not simply emerge from changes in a particular type of molecule, cell, organ, or functional system, but is probably a systemic process shaped by numerous interactions in a biological hierarchy.[36] If we use a comparatively simple, well-defined test model such as collagen aging or the clonal aging of mitotically active cells, we will see the effects of intervention on the molecules or cells, but we will not be able to predict what consequences this will have on the aging of the organism as a whole. However, it is this complex pattern of effects that will determine the success of intervention.

On the other hand, a model at a high level in the biological hierarchy (e.g., a behavioral model) will not solve the problem for two reasons: (1) uncontrollable normal variations in the internal status of the organism (e.g., in motivation) are frequently much more pronounced than the gradual change with age and may either obscure or simulate an effect of intervention; (2) an improvement in the function of a complex system also may be obtained without any interference with the aging process, e.g., by training of adaptive mechanisms.

A more promising solution to the problem of objectivation of influences on multicellular aging can be obtained by multivariate models of biological age, which make use of a larger number of significantly age-related parameters obtained from various levels of the biological hierarchy.[11,12,17,28,29,32] Multivariate estimations of biological age are based on the following considerations:

1. Multicellular aging seems to follow a regular pattern of changes, which may be obscured by age-independent functional variations in particular systems. To minimize the influence of these variations, estimations of biological age should make use of a greater number of parameters covering as many systems as possible.
2. Aging proceeds gradually from maturity to death. Shorter fluctuations may appear, but they are due to environmental changes, biological rhythms, or pathological processes.

Therefore, parameters for the assessment of biological age should be followed during the whole period of senescence to make sure that the measured process in fact is aging.

3. The aging changes of the organism are apparently the result of at least two types of processes: primary aging at the molecular or subcellular level, which should be very similar in all systems of the body, and system-specific secondary events, which may worsen or ameliorate the deleterious effects of primary aging.

Human studies of biological age are hampered by methodological problems which are difficult to overcome: the long duration of the necessary longitudinal studies, the need for a large population of clinically healthy persons who abide by the study for a considerable length of time, and the different genetic background, life history, living conditions, and lifestyle, which reduce the accuracy and sensitivity of estimations of biological age.

In contrast, laboratory animals, e.g., the rat, allow for longitudinal or cohort studies over a few years, are genetically far more homogenous, and can be kept in large numbers under standardized conditions. We think that such models can reveal basic regularities of mammalian aging which are very likely to apply also to human aging patterns.

IV. STUDIES OF BIOLOGICAL AGE IN RATS

In order to obtain and test a multivariate model of the biological age of the rat, we performed a long-term cohort study with an initial number of 1100 male Sprague-Dawley rats. The animals were assigned to five groups, one of which (A) served as a normal aging control. The other groups were used to test the following influences, all of which started after the attainment of maturity (6 months): dietary restriction (2 fast days per week, group B), regular exercise (treadmill running, 30 m, 25 m/min, 5 days per week, group C), fast days plus exercise (group D), and, as a test of the revitalizing effects described in 1889 by the French physiologist Brown-Séquard, the parenteral administration of heterologous fetal testis material* to the animals of group T.[19,32]

A total of 23 age parameters were measured at the ages of 10, 17, 25, and 30 months. The test battery comprised age parameters of various body systems and levels of organization (Table 1). The parameters were selected from an initial number of 42 variables according to the following criteria:

1. They should show a unidirectional change of at least 10% of the initial value between 10 and 30 months.
2. Variables which did not further improve the multiple correlation were eliminated by the computer program.
3. Variables with an unclear behavior during senescence (such as succinate dehydrogenase) were eliminated.
4. Parameters which could not be measured in all age groups had to be eliminated. This was necessary, for instance, with the ECG parameters since in the 25- and 30-month-old rats up to 90% of the ECGs were irregular and could not be quantified.

A. NORMAL AGING

All parameters showed a more or less pronounced nonlinear change with age (Figure 1), which could be described by exponential or logarithmic functions.[32] The parameter values as a function of chronological age were submitted to three kinds of multivariate statistics in order to assess the normal aging patterns: multiple regression analysis, factor analysis, and discriminant analysis.

* Lyophilized fetal sheep testis, Siccacell®, Cybila, Heidelberg, Germany.

Table 1 List of variables used in the multivariate analyses

V2	Running capacity[a]
V4	Hexosamine, coreum
V6	Magnesium, heart
V7	Copper, heart
V8	Zinc, heart
V10	Magnesium, kidney
V13	Calcium, heart
V15	Iron, kidney
V18	Tendon y_0 ("cross-links")[b]
V19	Tendon k_1 ("stability")[b]
V20	Tendon k_2 ("permeability")[b]
V26	Aorta b ("elastic fibers")[c]
V27	Aorta c ("collagen fiber spiral")[c]
V28	Aorta d ("collagen stability")[c]
V29	Aorta K_3t (maximum load, transverse extension)[c]
V30	Aorta K_3l (maximum load, longitudinal extension)[c]
V31	Triglycerides, plasma
V32	Cholesterol, plasma
V38	Lipofuscin, heart
V39	Lipofuscin, brain
V40	Spontaneous motor activity[d]
V41	Reactive locomotion (2)[e]
V42	Reactive activity (1+2)[e]

[a] *Treadmill endurance (in meters), 20 m/min, 15° ascent.*
[b] *Parameters from chemical contraction-relaxation of tail tendon fibers.*[16]
[c] *Parameters from stress-strain hysteresis loops.*[27]
[d] *Animex Activity Meter®, 45 μA.*[15]
[e] *Cinematographic method, activity grades: 0 (rest or sleep), 1 (partial movements), 2 (locomotion).*[15]

1. Multiple Regression Analysis

By this method, a metric of biological age is calculated by a linear combination of the parameter values in each individual. According to its correlation with the chronological age, each parameter is given a certain weight (see equation in Figure 2a). Because we found a nonlinear fashion of the parameters' change with age, we calculated two regression models (Figure 2): one model based on the assumption of a linear relationship between the chronological and biological ages (Figure 2a), the other model on an exponential relationship (Figure 2b).

According to our definition of biological age, its estimate should match exactly the chronological age in a normal aging population. Therefore, the predicted function is represented by the 45° lines in Figure 1. No dramatic difference is found between the models, which both meet the prediction very well. However, there is a continuous bend in the linear model which requires a correction, whereas the exponential model is practically the predicted one; the deflection at the age of 30 months is obviously due to the well-known cohort effect, i.e., the oldest group comprised those animals that had the best vitality of all.

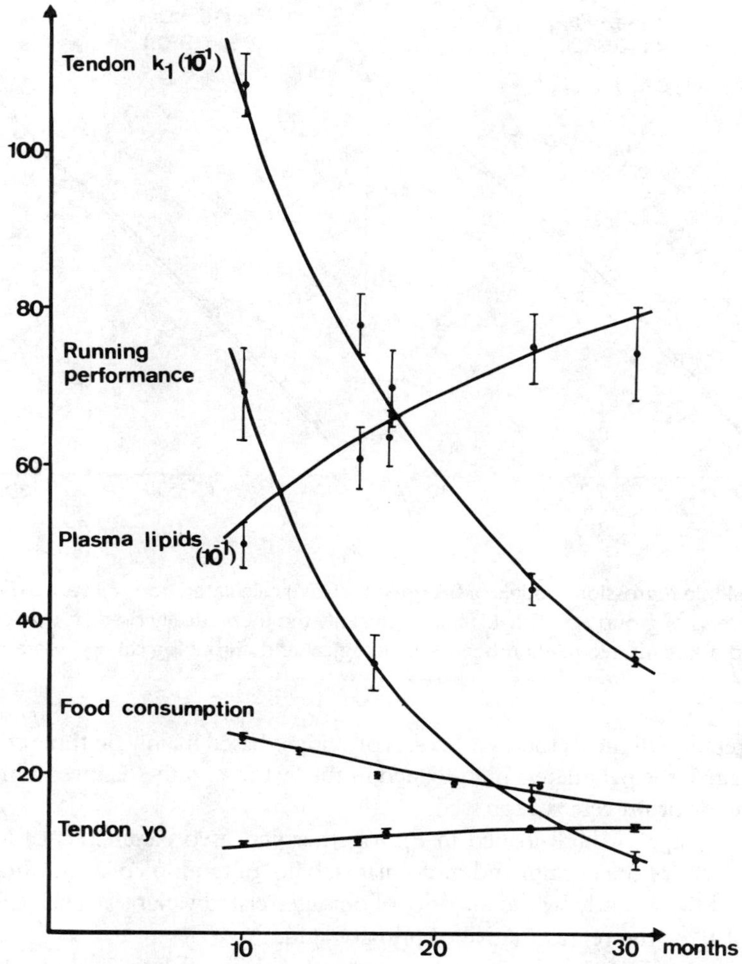

Figure 1 Changes in various parameter values during senescence of the rat. (Mean ± SEM.)

2. Factor Analysis

A problem that is still to be solved in the assessment of biological age is constituted by the fact that the parameters are selected without sufficient knowledge of their actual significance to multicellular aging. We have tried to deal with this problem by factor analysis. The objective of this multivariate procedure is to disclose the latent structures and relations within a complex phenomenon. Applied to models of biological age, it may elucidate the regularities that underlie the mutual variation of the parameters in the course of aging. By means of factor analysis, a large number of age-dependent parameters is replaced by a set of a few complex variables (factors), representing those underlying processes that cause the parameters to change in combination. One may expect that aging processes will dominate these patterns.

Table 2 presents the factor pattern of the variables given in Table 1 (principal factor analysis plus VARIMAX rotation[34]). The natural logarithm of chronological age (ln age) was also added as a vector representing the dynamics of stochastic processes, which we hypothesize to be the cause of primary aging. Six factors could be extracted from the multiple correlation matrix. Each factor or process is represented by the variables in which it is significantly expressed. The extent to which a parameter is influenced by the process (correlation with the factor) is given by the "factor loadings" together with the variables.[17]

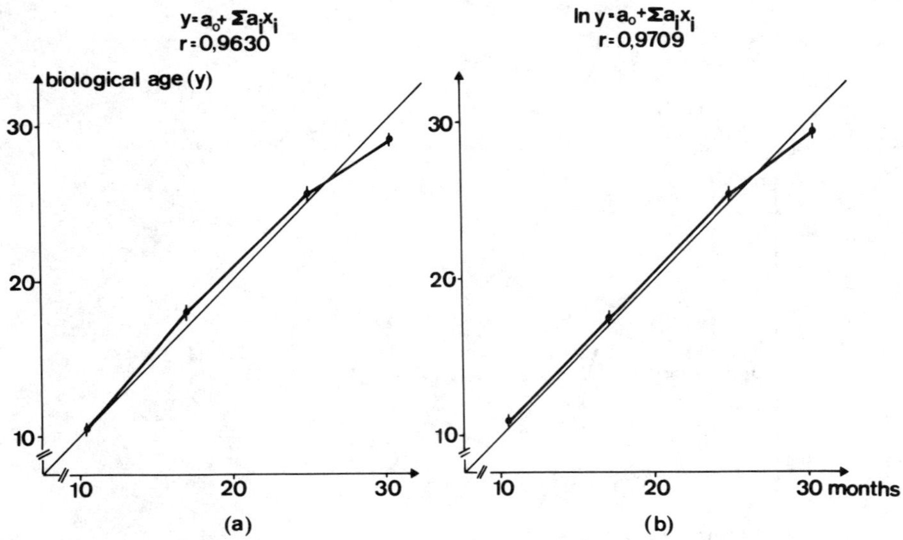

Figure 2 Multiple regression models of BA (mean ± SEM) calculated from 23 variables measured in 71 animals of group A.[32] The 45° line represents the theoretically predicted values. Both a linear and a logarithmic relation between biological and chronological age were tested.

The interpretation of the factors as processes of aging is based mainly on three criteria: the factor loading of "ln age", the parameters high-loaded in the factor, and the relative number of variables by which the factor or process is expressed.

The vector "ln age" is high-loaded in F_1, together with two parameters of molecular aging (hexosamine content of the corium and molecular stability of tendon collagen). Furthermore, this factor is expressed significantly by the majority of our age-related variables. This seems to justify an interpretation of F_1 as the representative of primary aging.

The vector "ln age" is also significantly correlated with the factors F_2 to F_5, but with clearly lower loadings than in F_1. Therefore, we may tentatively apostrophize these factors as representative of secondary processes of aging. This answer of the organism to the deleterious effects of primary aging is obviously dependent on specific features of the individual body systems. Because this answer is certainly of a complex nature (deleterious as well as compensatory reactions), it seems conceivable that there can be no simple linear relation (linearly independent factors). The idea of system-specific secondary aging being expressed by the factors F_2 to F_5 implies that parameters specific to a system must dominate each factor. This consideration underlies the following attempts at an interpretation.

Factor 2, which is high-loaded with three aortic parameters and the reactive motor activity, might be a "circulatory factor". Factor 3, loaded initially with variables of the heart and the locomotor activity, can be apostrophized as a "cardiac factor". Factor 4 is mainly loaded with connective tissue variables measured in the tendon and aorta and may reflect the secondary aging of this system. Factor 5 is high-loaded with parameters of tissues made up of postmitotic cells, namely the brain and myocardium. We propose calling it a "postmitotic factor". These factor interpretations are preliminary and hypothetical and must be proven by the introduction of additional parameters characteristic of the respective system.

3. Discriminant Analysis

From the nonlinearity and the differences in the type of the age change of the parameters used, a methodological problem emerges which can be demonstrated by means of discriminant analysis. This multivariate analysis can show which variables of an age test program are most effective in

Table 2 Factor loadings arranged according to the correlation of the parameters with the respective factor

Factor 1	**(68)**	**Factor 2**	**(9.5)**	**Factor 3**	**(8.0)**	**Factor 4**	**(5.9)**	**Factor 5**	**(5.4)**	**Factor 6**	**(4.5)**
Hexosamine	0.80	Aorta d	0.67	Zn heart	0.71	Tendon k_2	0.97	Lipofuscin heart	0.70	Triglycerides	0.70
ln age	–0.75	Aorta b	–0.64	Cu heart	0.67	Tendon y_0	–0.61	Lipofuscin brain	0.65	Cholesterol	0.42
Tendon k_1	0.66	Reactive activity	0.60	Mg heart	0.58	Aorta c	0.41	Ca heart	0.38	Aorta K_3l	0.32
Aorta K_3t	–0.65	Aorta K_3l	–0.51	Reactive locomotion	0.41	Running	0.37	Mg heart	–0.33	Ca heart	0.29
Spontaneous activity	0.64	Mg kidney	0.39	**ln age**	–0.35	Tendon k_1	0.33	**ln age**	0.31	Aorta c	–0.26
Aorta c	0.60	Running	0.37	Hexosamine	0.31	Aorta K_3l	–0.28	Cholesterol	0.30	Mg heart	–0.23
Ca heart	–0.53	**ln age**	–0.34	Lipofuscin brain	–0.29	**ln age**	–0.28	Tendon k_1	–0.28		
Running	0.52	Aorta c	0.29	Reactive activity	0.29	Hexosamine	–0.24				
Cu heart	0.49	Mg heart	0.26	Tendon k_1	0.27						
Aorta K_3l	–0.46	Tendon k_1	0.26	Aorta c	0.26						
Cholesterol	–0.44	Aorta K_3l	–0.25								
Fe kidney	–0.43										
Reactive locomotion	0.41										
Mg heart	0.40										
Mg kidney	0.39										
Lipofuscin brain	–0.27										
Lipofuscin heart	–0.24										

Note: *Variables not significantly correlated at the 5% level have been rejected. The figures given with the factor number indicate the share of combined variance explained by the respective factors*

Table 3 Standardized discriminant function coefficients of the comparison of adjacent age groups

10 and 17 months		17 and 25 months		25 and 30 months	
Lipofuscin heart	1.419	Aorta $K_3$1	1.933	Reactive activity	1.672
Aorta d	1.244	Aorta K_3t	1.887	Triglycerides	1.085
Hexosamine	1.243	Aorta b	1.218	Cu heart	1.077
Mg kidney	1.098	Tendon k_1	0.850	Spontaneous activity	1.074
Ca heart	1.024	Zn heart	0.797	Tendon k_1	0.593
Fe kidney	0.885	Lipofuscin brain	0.729	Aorta d	0.588
Cu heart	0.849	Lipofuscin heart	0.630	Ca heart	0.587
Mg heart	0.727	Cholesterol	0.614	Aorta b	0.582
Tendon k_1	0.722	Mg kidney	0.588		
Zn heart	0.570	Triglycerides	0.576		
Cholesterol	0.525	Running	0.563		
		Spontaneous activity	0.561		

separating various age groups. Discriminant analysis attempts to do this by forming one or more linear combinations of distinctive variables. The coefficients obtained by the analysis reflect the parameter's value in distinguishing between the groups.

The power of aging parameters to discriminate between groups of different biological age varies during senescence. We were able to show this by analysis of the adjacent age groups in our study: the age groups 10 and 17 months, 17 and 25 months, and 25 and 30 months (Table 3). Table 3 shows the standardized coefficients that represent the power of the individual parameters to discriminate between the age groups under consideration. In the early phase of senescence, the most important parameters are the lipofuscin and calcium content of the heart, a collagen parameter of the aorta, the hexosamine content of the skin, and the magnesium content of the kidney. In the second phase, extensibility parameters of the aorta show the highest discriminating power. In the last phase, which ends in senility, two parameters of the motor activity, the plasma triglycerides and the copper content of the heart, are found at the top of the column.

These findings suggest that models of biological age will show an optimal sensitivity when testing influences on the aging process, if the parameters used in the age test battery have been analyzed by these three multivariate methods. They are a first attempt to objectively quantify multicellular aging. In the authors' opinion, this is a presupposition for an understanding of this complex phenomenon and for studies on influencing aging.

B. INFLUENCES ON BIOLOGICAL AGE

The estimates of the biological age of the animals in groups B, C, D, and T were calculated for each individual using the constants of the logarithmic model. The means and standard errors of the estimated biological age are shown in Figure 3. All influences caused slight shifts in the curve of biological age. The differences between the controls and the individual experimental groups proved significant by discrimination analysis, with $p < 0.001$. Food restriction (B) caused a drop in the estimated biological age in the groups of 25 and 30 months of age. In group C (physical training) lower values were found only at an age of 25 months, whereas at 30 months the average biological age exceeds the value of the controls. Fast days plus exercise showed only minimal effects, whereas the most obvious lowering of biological age was found in group T. Beginning at an age of 17 months, the curve of the testis group remained constantly below that of the controls. Because this

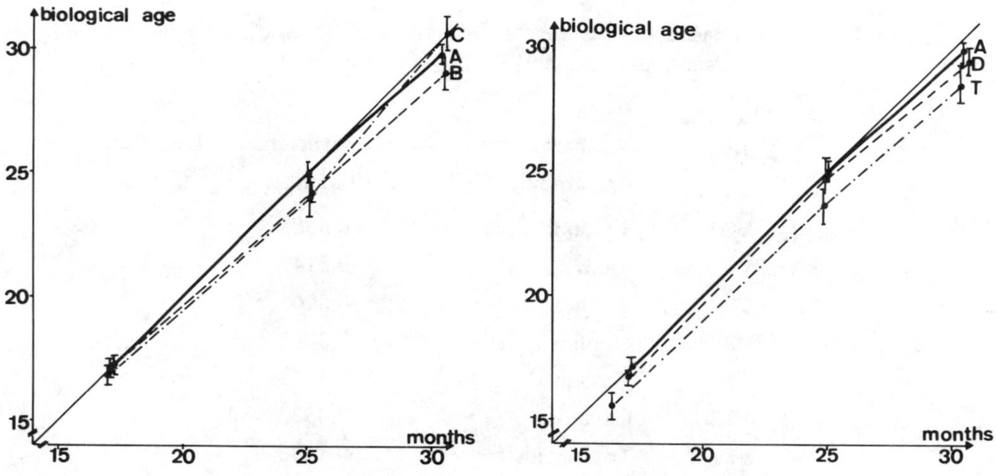

Figure 3 Multiple regression models of biological aging (mean ± SEM) of the experimental groups B (dietary restriction), C (exercise), D (dietary restriction + exercise), and T (lyophilized heterologous fetal testis) as compared to the "normal aging group" A.

effect was the most pronounced, further analysis and a follow-up study were performed, the results of which can be regarded as an example of how to test influences on the aging process by multivariate methods.[20]

In order to find out which of the variables were the most important in bringing about the difference in biological age between the "testis group" and the controls, we submitted the data to a stepwise discriminant analysis. The analysis was calculated with two sets of data, one covering the whole range of age from 17 to 30 months, the other selecting the older animals aged 25 and 30 months (Table 4). The number of significantly discriminating variables and also the values of the coefficients increased with advancing age. With the exception of Ca^{2+}-heart, Mg^{2+}-kidney, and lipofuscin brain, the overwhelming number of distinctive variables shifted to a lower age in group T. We speculate that the results of treatment may indicate that parts of the material were used by an increasing number of functionally deficient cells to substitute for progressive aging losses in certain elements or factors.

However, the phenomenological analysis provides no insight into the real mode of action. In their present state, the models of biological age may be regarded only as hypothesis-finding instruments for testing possible ways of retarding biological aging or its consequences. Wherever an effect on aging is indicated by the multiple regression model, a discriminant analysis may point to those variables that bring about the changes in biological age. This may enable us to formulate hypotheses that can be tested by more specific models of particular aging processes at various levels of the organismic hierarchy. In the present case, the high-level parameters of running performance and motor activity were of special interest and were investigated in a follow-up study,[18] which confirmed the earlier findings. Because one possible explanation of these results and others (e.g., the effects on tendon collagen) pointed to an involvement of androgenes, we also measured the plasma testosterone levels in the two-year-old male rats 4 months after the last application of fetal testis material. Testosterone levels were found to be significantly higher in group T than in the age-matched controls. As testosterone levels decrease with age in the male rat,[25] an effect of the fetal testis material on androgen-producing cells may be postulated.

The question remained as to what effect this treatment may have on the longevity of rats, particularly with regard to the finding that testosterone administration can shorten life.[1] This problem was attacked in a survival study. A cohort of 180 male Sprague-Dawley rats was randomly

Table 4 Standardized discriminant function coefficients of the functions separating groups A and T

Variable no.	Parameter	Coefficient	Direction
	Age groups: 17, 25, and 30 months		
V20	Tendon k_2	–0.5589	–
V2	Running	–0.5142	–
V7	Cu, heart	–0.5101	–
V38	Lipofuscin, heart	0.3755	–
V19	Tendon k_1	0.3554	–
V13	Ca, heart	–0.3323	+
V31	Triglycerides	0.3106	–
V10	Mg, kidney	0.2929	+
V29	Aorta K_3t	–0.2488	–
V41	Spontaneous activity	–0.2210	–
	Age groups: 25 and 30 months		
V41	Reactive locomotion	–0.7293	–
V20	Tendon k_2	–0.6747	–
V19	Tendon k_1	0.6195	–
V39	Lipofuscin, brain	–0.6146	+
V32	Cholesterol	0.4776	–
V2	Running	–0.4562	–
V38	Lipofuscin, heart	0.4406	–
V10	Mg, kidney	0.4309	+
V28	Aorta d	0.3756	0
V30	Aorta K_3l	0.3483	–
V8	Zn, heart	–0.3239	–
V18	Tendon y_0	–0.2958	–
V29	Aorta K_3t	–0.2523	–
V6	Mg, heart	–0.2305	–

Note: The "+" and "–" indicate that in group T the mean values (all age groups) shifted toward "older" or "younger", whereas "0" indicates that the discriminating features of the variable are not expressed by the arithmetic mean.

divided into two groups, one of which (T) was injected subcutaneously four times with lyophilized fetal testis (between 60 and 120 weeks of age), the control animals (C) receiving Ringer's solution at the same points of time. At the age of 50% survival, the survival curves separated, showing a slightly better characteristic for the testis group with a gain in maximum life span of approximately 4 months.[20] The Gompertz curves of age-specific mortality rates (Figure 4) deflected toward lower values after the age of 20 months. The difference between the mortality lines of group C and T was significant (p <0.05) by straight line regression analysis. According to Sacher's hypothesis,[30] this means that in those rats surviving to the age of 20 months the rate of aging must have been reduced by the applied material. Only a subgroup of the cohort may have benefitted from the treatment, i.e., those animals free from a disposition to an early lethal disease.

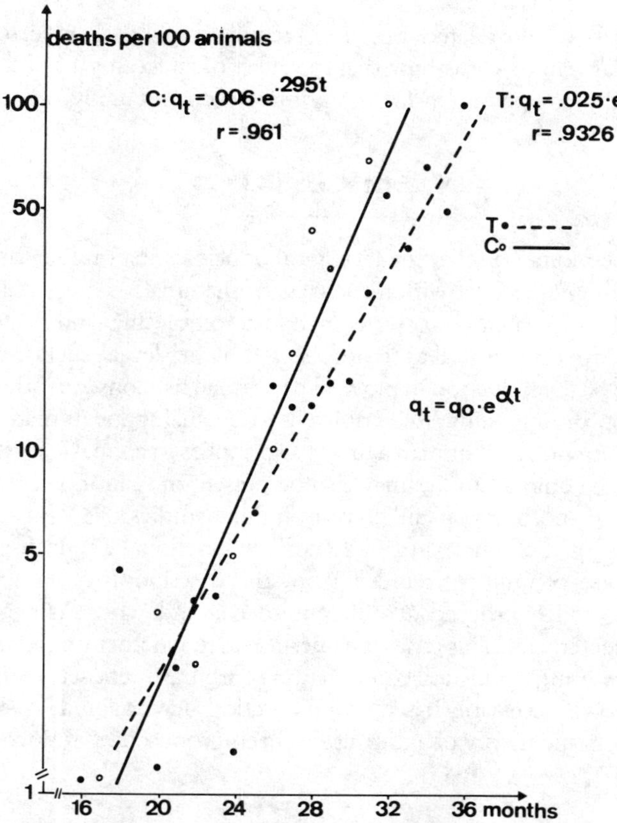

Figure 4 Age-specific mortality rates of groups T (fetal testis) and C (controls).[20]

Nevertheless, we do not believe that these effects may be termed a "rejuvenation" in the sense of a general reversal or even a general retardation of the aging process. This follows from the aging pattern obtained by factor analysis of all the experimental groups (Table 5): If the treatment had a general impact on all the basic processes of aging, one would expect the aging pattern to be about the same in the treated groups as in the controls. However, all experimental conditions caused a more or less pronounced disintegration of the normal factor pattern. This disintegration is most obvious in the "testis group". Instead of six factors, as in "normal aging" (one primary aging, four secondary aging, one without age relation), eight factors were extracted from the values of the "testis

Table 5 Number of factors in the various experimental groups as opposed to the "normal aging controls"

	No. of factors			
Group	**Total**	**Primary aging**	**Secondary aging**	**No age correlation**
Control	6	1	4	1
Dietary restricted	6	1	3	2
Exercise	7	1	4	2
Dietary restricted + exercise	7	1	1	5
Testis	8	1	0	7

group", only one of which was age related. Because "secondary aging" disappeared completely from the factor pattern, we may tentatively assume that the effect of fetal testis may have been mainly due to an improvement of the compensation for the primary events of aging.

V. DISCUSSION

Aging is so universal a phenomenon that the biological principles responsible for its intrinsic nature are very likely to be the same, at least within the class of mammals. This pertains to a number of molecular and cellular changes, such as cross-linking of macromolecules and the limited proliferative capacity of mitotically active cells, as well as to processes at higher levels, such as the progressive loss of immune competence or the reduction in physical performance. Consequently, the basic regularities in system interaction during aging are very likely to be analogous in man and rat. Thus, the criticism applied to measurements of human aging[8,9] also applies to animal (rat) studies. Regularities found in tightly controlled animal studies may also be present in man, however masked they may be by the methodological shortcomings inherent in human studies.

The major criticism of the concept of biological or functional age expressed by Costa and McCrae[8] refers to the use of multiple regression for the description of an apparently unrelated multiplicity of changes, which proceed at different speeds and whose change with age shows different, nonlinear characteristics. This raises the question as to whether we can measure the evident phenomenon of aging by using a statistical combination of arbitrarily chosen age-related parameters. An answer to this question is necessarily based on a theoretical view of aging. We would like to argue on the grounds of a stochastic theory of aging, as has been proposed by Kirkwood,[22] Cutler,[10] and others.

A. REGULARITIES IN MULTICELLULAR AGING

The concept of biological age is based on the assumption that in the course of normal aging each chronological age is characterized by a certain vitality, i.e., a specified functional state of the organism as a whole. This implies that multicellular aging follows a fixed aging pattern, which is found in all individuals of the respective population. The results of factor analysis support this view. The factor pattern in our study explains approximately 60% of the total variation.[17] The pattern and time course of the changes of the parameters are obviously the result of two types of processes:

1. A stochastic process, which represents the random changes that affect the organism simply with the lapse of time. Its dynamic is expressed in most of our parameters, in particular in the molecular.
2. The action of stochastic aging on the mutually dependent body systems, interlinked by the organism's homeostatic mechanisms. These secondary actions apparently include biosenescent as well as antibiosenescent processes at all levels of organization,[10] and thus are responsible for the extent to which the fundamental processes affect the vitality of the organism.

Therefore, we assume that the aging pattern that enables us to estimate an organism's age is the reflection of the bionomic order of the organism affected by the progressive accumulation of stochastic, i.e., deleterious, changes. Because in senescence no new principles of function emerge and no homeostatic principle of function disappears, the basic aging pattern (as shown by the factor pattern in our study) can be seen throughout senescence as long as homeostasis is maintained. Therefore, in healthy individuals of an ideal "normal aging population", the change in age-related parameters seems to be a reliable reflection of the rate of aging. Furthermore, this pattern seems to be the only criterion that allows us to distinguish biological aging from other processes that reduce vitality, for example, disease or uncontrollable environmental factors.

The linearity of aging changes has been postulated in a number of studies,[12,14,31,35] though this concept is hardly compatible with any theoretical concept or the Gompertz law. Brown and Forbes,[5] Comfort,[7] and Lohmann[24] found some evidence that the functional capabilities of the organism change in an exponential rather than in a linear mode. Our own results support this latter view. As has been shown in our multiple regression model, the logarithmic transformation of the chronological age provides the better estimates. Because in many parameters the gradual change with age is small compared to age-independent variations, both the linear and exponential model provide similar results. However, in agreement with convincing evidence from human data,[24] we think that the "dogma of linearity" of functional decline with age is merely a consequence of the high variations of human age parameters that allow for a number of mathematical descriptions, the most attractive being naturally the linear one.

B. CHANGES IN VITALITY WITH AGE

The changes in vitality with age (or biomorphosis) may explain the different shape and type of change of age-related parameters, one of the problems addressed by Costa and McCrae. Vitality has been defined by Beier et al.[4] as "a measure of an organism's capacity to realize all functions essential to life". According to this concept, vitality is a complex variable that comprises all essential functions. The parameters of these functions can, in turn, be used to estimate vitality.

If we look at age-related changes in physiological functions such as the glomerular filtration rate, renal plasma flow, maximum breathing capacity, vital capacity, and maximum O_2 uptake, we find that a phase of rapid increase in functional capacity during development is followed by a progressive functional decline during adulthood.[2] If we infer the change in vitality with age from these parameters, this change can be described by a two-factor model of the interaction of development and error accumulation[3] with the following characteristics (Figure 5). The vitality curve begins at time 0, corresponding to conception or birth. During development, vitality increases to a peak which exceeds by far the level required to cope with the basic demands of the everyday environment. This excess capacity, or biological redundancy, reflects the great adaptability of the young adult organism. In senescence, vitality declines and the adaptability of the organism is reduced. However, this reduction only becomes fully evident if the organism is stressed to the limits of its adaptability. The basic demands of the environment can be met up to an advanced age. It is only when vitality

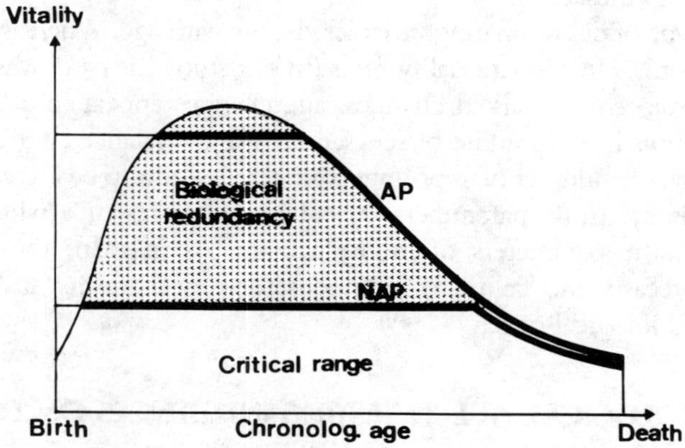

Figure 5 Estimated changes in vitality according to the biophysical model of Beier[3] and the behavior of "adaptive parameters" (AP) and "nonadaptive parameters" NAP. (For details see text.)

falls to the critical level required for normal daily life that slight additional stresses or minor infections lead to a fatal failure or terminal disease.

With regard to this concept of vitality, age parameters can be located between two extremes depicted in Figure 5: adaptive (AP) and non-adaptive (NAP) parameters. Adaptive parameters, such as maximum O_2 uptake or, in our studies, the running capacity of rats, make use of the full biological redundancy and show a continuous decline in senescence. Nonadaptive parameters, which measure only basal functions, will not show dramatic changes until an advanced age on the verge of senility. In our study, this second type of parameter is, for instance, represented by spontaneous motor activity. A special case is given by homeostatic parameters of the *milieu interieur*, e.g., pH, blood volume, osmotic pressure, and electrolyte content, mentioned by Costa and McCrae. The constant levels of these parameters are of vital importance to the survival of the organism and are maintained by homeostatic mechanisms throughout life without significant changes. In normal aging, a permanent change in homeostatic parameters indicates the breakdown of regulation and, consequently, the terminal phase of life. It is clear that this type of parameter will be a predictor of vitality or biological age only if the regulatory capacity is challenged by some kind of perturbation, e.g., pH regulation by an acid load.

C. CHANGES WITH AGE IN THE DISCRIMINATING POWER OF PARAMETERS

Costa and McCrae conclude that the difference in the parameters' rates and curves in age-related decline changes their usefulness in predicting functional age according to the age group under study. This criticism is supported by the discriminant analysis of our data. This means that in order to obtain an optimum sensitivity of models of biological age it is sensible to calculate two or more multiple regression curves for different phases of senescence by selecting different sets of parameters according to the results of discrimination analyses. In studies into influences on the aging process, models of biological age covering the whole period of senescence will tend to underestimate the differences between the groups.

From the results of discriminant analysis, the following conclusions can be drawn with regard to the ability of parameters to discriminate between adjacent age groups:

1. Age parameters of the heart, aorta, and connective tissue are important distinctive features in all phases of senescence and should be included in every model of biological age.
2. Models of biological age based on a short observational period are not optimal for the whole period of senescence.
3. Number and type of discriminating variables change with age. Whereas at the beginning of senescence only a few functional systems (in our study the cardiovascular system and connective tissue) show marked changes, age changes appear in a larger number of functional systems in the middle of senescence. At an advanced age, probably on the verge of senility, the number of important parameters seems to be increasingly restricted. Most interestingly, those parameters prevail which represent a wide range of body functions, i.e., the parameters of motor activity. As in man, the decline in these parameters forecasts the failure of compensatory mechanisms and the impending breakdown of biological order.

D. MODELS OF BIOLOGICAL AGE IN TESTING INFLUENCES ON THE RATE OF AGING

One of the main tasks of models of biological age is to serve as a standard against which potential intervention into aging can be tested. Regardless of the drawbacks mentioned above, multiple regression models can be used as indicators of an effect on aging: a significant shift in the multiple regression curve will only be shown if the overwhelming number of parameters tend to change in the same direction, e.g., to values of a lower biological age. In order to ensure that the measured process is in fact aging and not a change in a restricted domain of the organism, parameters should originate from various systems and levels of organization and be followed over as long a period of senescence as possible.

Discriminant analysis can complement the multiple regression model by showing which of the variables are the most important in discriminating between the groups. This may provide a clue as to the mode of action of the influence. Another criterion is provided by factor analysis which shows the aging pattern, i.e. the interdependence of various systems and levels in the aging process. In the authors' opinion, a shift in biological age to lower values may be termed a true retardation of aging or a "rejuvenation" only if the basic factor pattern is still present in the treated group. The influences implemented in the reported studies meet this demand to various degrees (Table 5). The group with dietary restriction (B) was very similar in pattern to the controls. This indicates that food restriction actually causes a true retardation of the aging process. In the "testis group" (T), factor analysis revealed a marked disintegration of the normal pattern, indicating that the apparent improvement of vitality has not been brought about by a simple retardation of the normal aging process. For this kind of effect, Kment[23] proposed the term "revitalization", defined as a "prolonged maintenance or recovery of a vitality level appropriate to a significantly lower biological age than is in accordance with the chronological age of the organism".

As an additional criterion, survival should be checked in animal experiments as this is certainly the most problematic and time-consuming task in human studies. Harrison[13] has shown that the relation between functional changes with age and age-related mortality is far from being clear. In a study into stress and aging,[26,33] we were able to show that parameters at different levels of organization are of a different value as predictors of survival. Rats submitted to persistent crowding showed accelerated aging in molecular and subcellular parameters such as lipofuscin accumulation in the heart and collagen cross-linking. However, there was a significant improvement in motor activity and maze learning. The survival function of the stressed rats was improved as compared to that of control rats of the same age cohort.

Regardless of the unsolved problem of functional decline and mortality, we feel that an improved vitality in the individuals of a population should also be reflected at the population level, i.e., in improved survival. In our study of the "Brown-Séquard effect", the survival curve of group T separated from that of the controls (C) not before the age of 50% survival, an age at which mortality is mainly due to aging rather than to a disposition toward an early lethal disease. This means that intervention in aging does not necessarily prevent premature deaths from causes other than aging. Consequently, if survival is used as a parameter of the rate of aging, it seems to be necessary to study the influence of the respective treatment or condition at an advanced age, i.e., after the age of 50% survival.

VI. CONCLUSION

From its very beginning, gerontology has taken on the task of developing objective criteria for the measurement of aging and for the assessment of intervention into this process. However, aging is poorly defined and there is no standard procedure for its assessment. It is obvious that aging is a complex phenomenon made up of countless partial processes and events that are interlinked in an unknown manner. Thus, all attempts at measuring aging basically depend on theories about the primary causes and the relationships between the partial processes within this complex phenomenon.

Animal models have contributed significantly to our understanding of mammalian aging and are valuable tools in testing the theoretical bases of aging measurements in man. Our rat studies indicate that multicellular aging is not a completely random process without any regularity, but follows a pattern which is determined by the organism's principles of order and its response to the stochastic events of primary aging. Based on this theoretical concept, multicellular aging can be described by a single complex variable, biological age, which allows us to compare the aging rates of different individuals or different subgroups of a population. However, the assessment of the effect of intervention into aging is a far more difficult task because intervention may affect the normal aging pattern in an unpredictable way. Consequently, if the index of biological age indicates an improvement in vitality, this does not necessarily mean that this change has been brought about by a modification of the rate of aging. Thus, only the combination of the various multivariate methods, i.e., multiple regression analysis, discriminant analysis, and factor analysis, with survival studies will provide clues to what has really happened to the aging organism. Whether the effect of treatment may be termed a rejuvenation, a revitalization, or retardation of aging depends on our theories and definitions of aging.

In conclusion, we state that though aging is a familiar and obvious phenomenon, there is still no generally accepted measurement at hand that allows us to assess its dynamics and the effect of possible intervention. Multivariate models of biological age are at present the only approach based on a plausible theoretical view of aging. Any progress in this field will not depend on a refinement of measuring skills but rather on an improvement of our theoretical understanding of the fundamental processes, their interactions, and the homeostatic response of the aging organism.

REFERENCES

1. Asdell, S.A., Doornenbal, H., Joshi, S.R., and Sperling, G.A., The effects of sex steroid hormones upon longevity in rats, *J. Reprod. Fertil.*, 14: 113, 1967.
2. Bafitis, H. and Sargent, F., Human physiological adaptability through the life sequence, *J. Gerontol.*, 32, 402, 1977.
3. Beier, W., Biomorphose, in *Biophysikalische Grundlagen der Medizin*, Beier, W. and Rosen, R., Eds., Georg Fischer, Stuttgart, 1980, 502.
4. Beier, W., Brehme, K.H., and Wiegel, D., *Biophysikalische Aspekte des Alterns Multizellulärer Systeme*, VEB Thieme, Leipzig, 1973.
5. Brown, K.S. and Forbes, W.F., A mathematical model of aging processes. IV. A multivariate analysis of blood pressure in a Montreal and a Utah population, *J. Gerontol.*, 31, 385, 1976.
6. Brown-Séquard, C.E., Des effects produits chez l'homme par des injections souscutanèes d'un liquide retiré des testicles de cobaye et de chien, *C. R. Soc. Biol.*, 41, 415, 1889.
7. Comfort, A., *The Biology of Senescence*, Churchill Livingstone, Edinburgh, 1979.
8. Costa, P. and McCrae, R.R., Functional age: a conceptual and empirical critique, in *Proc. 2nd Conf. Epidemiology of Aging*, Haynes, S.G. and Feinleib, M., Eds., National Institutes of Health, Bethesda, MD, 1980, 22.
9. Costa, P. and McCrae, R.R., Concepts of functional or biological age: a critical view, in *Principles of Geriatric Medicine*, Andres, R., Bierman, E.L., and Hazzard, W.R., McGraw Hill, New York, 1985, 30.
10. Cutler, R.G., Evolution of longevity in primates, *J. Hum. Evol.*, 5, 169, 1976.
11. Dubina, T.L., Mints A.Ya., and Zhuk, E.V., Biological age and its estimation. III., *Exp. Gerontol.* 19, 133, 1984.
12. Furukawa, T., Inoue, M., Kajiya, F., Inada, H., Takasugi, S., Takeda, H., and Abe, H., Assessment of biological age by multiple regression analysis, *J. Gerontol.* 30, 422, 1975.
13. Harrison, D.E., Experiences in developing assays of physiological age, in *Biomarkers of Aging*, Reff, M.E. and Schneider, E.L., Eds., National Institutes of Health, Bethesda, MD, 1982, 2.
14. Heikkinen, E., Kiiskinen, A., Käythy, B., Rimpelä, M., and Vouri, I., Assessment of biological age: methodological study of two Finnish populations, *Gerontologia*, 20, 33, 1974.
15. Hofecker, G., Kment, A., and Niedermüller, H., Die motorische Aktivität als Altersparameter der Ratte, *Akt. Gerontol.*, 8, 271, 1978.

16. Hofecker, G., Niedermüller, H., Skalicky, M., and Jahn, J., Die chemische Kontraktion von Schwanzsehnenfäden der Ratte als Altersparameter: Mathematische Analyse der Kontraktions-Relaxationskurven, *Akt. Gerontol.*, 9, 269, 1979.
17. Hofecker, G., Skalicky, M., Kment, A., and Niedermüller H., Models of the biological age of the rat. I. A factor model of age parameters, *Mech. Age. Dev.*, 14, 345, 1980.
18. Hofecker, G., Niedermüller, H., and Skalicky, M., Der altersbedingte Leistungsabfall und seine Beeinflussung im Tierexperiment, *Akt. Gerontol.*,11, 188, 1981.
19. Hofecker, G., Skalicky, M., Niedermüller, H., and Kment, A., Long-term effects of heterologous fetal testis material on the biological age of the male rat, in *Drugs and Aging*, Platt, D., Ed., Springer-Verlag Berlin, 1986, 171.
20. Hofecker, G., Niedermüller, H., Skalicky, M., and Kment, A., Revitalization studies in laboratory rats, in *Biological Age and Aging Risk Factors*, Ruiz-Torres, A., Ed., Tecnipublicaciones, Madrid, 1987, 273.
21. Hruza, Z., Aging of cells and molecules, in *Handbuch der Allgemeinen Pathologie, Vol. 6/4: Altern*, Holle, G., Ed., Springer, Berlin, 1972, 83.
22. Kirkwood, T., Ageing and evolution, in *The Theoretical Basis of Ageing Research. Proc. 7th Wiener Symp. Experimental Gerontology, 1990*, Robert, F. and Hofecker, G., Eds., Facultas, Vienna, 1990, 21.
23. Kment, A., Altern und Geriatrica aus der Sicht der experimentellen Gerontologie, *Akt. Gerontol.*, 8, 241, 1978.
24. Lohmann, W., Altersindex und Interpretation der Absterbekurven, *Z. Alternsforsch.*, 32, 461, 1977.
25. Miller, A.E. and Riegle, G.D., Serum testosterone and testicular response to HCG in young and aged male rats, *J. Gerontol.*, 33, 197, 1978.
26. Niedermüller, H., Bubna-Littitz, H., Skalicky, M., and Hofecker, G., Stress and aging of the rat, in *Biological Age and Aging Risk Factors*, Ruiz-Torres, A., Ed., Tecnipublicaciones, Madrid, 1979, 217.
27. Pav, E., Hofecker, G., and Skalicky, M., A mathematical model of mechanical properties of the rat's aorta, *Adv. Physiol. Sci.*, 34, 37, 1981.
28. Pöthig, D., Experimentelle Entwicklung eines klinischen Diagnostikmodells zur Objektivierung des biologischen Alters des Menschen, Dissertation zur Promotion B, Leipzig, 1984.
29. Ries, W., Problems associated with biological age, *Exp. Gerontol.*, 9, 145 , 1974.
30. Sacher, G.A., Life table modification and life prolongation, in *Handbook of the Biology of Aging*, Finch, C.E. and Hayflick, L., Eds., Van Nostrand Reinhold, New York, 1977, 582.
31. Shock, N.W., System integration, in *Handbook of the Biology of Aging*, Finch, C.E. and Hayflick, L., Eds., Van Nostrand Reinhold, New York, 1977, 639.
32. Skalicky, M., Hofecker, G., Kment, A., and Niedermüller, H., Models of the biological age of the rat. II. Multiple regression models in the study on influencing aging, *Mech. Age. Dev.*, 14, 361, 1980.
33. Skalicky, M., Bubna-Littitz, H., and Hofecker, G., The influence of persistent crowding on the age changes of behavioral parameters and survival characteristics of rats, *Mech. Age. Dev.*, 28, 325, 1984.
34. Weber, E., *Einführung in die Faktorenanalyse*, VEB Georg Fischer, Jena, 1974.
35. Webster, I.W. and Logie, A.R., A relationship between functional age and health status in female subjects, *J. Gerontol.*, 31, 546, 1976.
36. Witten, M., A return to time, cells, systems and aging. II. Relational and reliability theoretical approaches to the study of senescence in living systems, *Mech. Age. Dev.*, 27, 323, 1984.

STATISTICAL ANALYSIS

CHAPTER 26

STATISTICAL APPROACH FOR THE ASSESSMENT OF BIOLOGICAL AGE

EITARO NAKAMURA

TABLE OF CONTENTS

I. INTRODUCTION

Since World War II, the average life span of humans has increased dramatically in many industrial nations. As a result of "population aging" and the greater visibility of elderly persons, many developed nations are confronted with the practical and economic problems created by a rapidly expanding geriatric population.[44]

What is obviously needed is a well-planned health administration to care for elderly citizens. To develop a system of primary health care for elderly people and to reinforce the health administration to care for elderly people, we must have enough knowledge about normal aging in elderly people. In addition, we must have a measure for assessing an individual's aging rate or their "biological age". However, a standardized system for measuring biological age has not been developed.[23,27,37]

Although aging is a universal biological phenomenon, its diverse morphological and physiological manifestations make it difficult to propose a single process or theory which adequately describes aging.[17,27,34,39] This complexity has generated many definitions of aging as well as various statistical approaches for the prediction of biological age.

One of the early attempts to assess the biological age of an individual was made by Benjamin[1] in 1947. An index of aging based on data covering life history and clinical examinations was devised,

0-8493-0129-7/94/$0.00+$.50

but Benjamin did not propose an actual method of quantification in predicting one's biological age. Many years later, Birren,[3] Comfort,[9] Shock,[37] and Bourliere[5] expressed the need for developing indices of biological age and suggested possible approaches to the problem.

The most widely used approach for the assessment of biological age has been to combine a large number of age-related physiological variables into a multiple regression equation, taking chronological age as the dependent variable and the value predicted by the multiple regression equation viewed as the biological age of the individual.[2,11,14,15,19,21,28,42,43] Dean[13] summarized the information about measuring "biological age" or "functional age" in humans presented up to the present. This approach gives fairly satisfactory results in estimating various influences on aging, but it has been noted that this method suffers from the following serious problems. One relates to the distortion of individual biological age because of regression to the mean, i.e., the multiple regression equation overestimates individual biological ages for younger persons and underestimates those for older persons.[14,28,43] The other problem is a theoretical contradiction in that a "perfect model ($r = 1.0$)" would merely be predicting the subject's chronological age, not his biological age.[6,10]

In recent years, some gerontologists cast considerable doubt on the existence of a unitary aging factor that controls the rate of aging in different organs and functions.[10,27,39] Most physiological variables do not necessarily change with age in the same way nor at the same rate that produces the large range in the performance of most physiological variables among subjects of the same chronological age.[10,27,39] For example, a 60-year-old subject may have a cardiac output equivalent to the average values for 50 year olds, but a renal function equal to the average value for 70 year olds. At present, there is little evidence for the existence of fixed laws governing and underlying the process of human aging. However, we notice that most biological changes after nearly 30 years old continue an irreversible path of normal decline into the 70s and 80s.[5,39] Changes in physical appearance, e.g., facial changes, are one of the most obvious manifestations of the aging process. This means that in a sense biological aging seems to proceed according to a fixed pattern. If the laws are known, an objective measure of assessing one's biological age could be obtained. Therefore, it is a prerequisite to discern the laws controlling the aging process.

Clark[8] applied a factor analysis to data for 25 physiological and psychological measurements, and revealed that the 25 parameters were grouped into five factors. The first factor, which was loaded significantly with 19 of the 25 parameters and accounted for almost all the variance of age, could be interpreted as a single general aging factor. A similar study has been reported by Hofecker et al.,[20] who applied a factor analysis to data for 23 parameters obtained from rats, and extracted five factors. They interpreted the first factor as representing primary aging, and factors two to five as system-specific secondary aging factors. These studies suggest that biological aging seems to proceed according to a fixed pattern. However, in similar analyses, Jalavisto and Makkonen[24] and Costa and McCrae[10] failed to identify a single general aging factor. There are many problems that remain unsolved, and the existence of fixed laws governing aging processes is not yet confirmed.

This chapter examines the assumptions that biological age changes can be separated into primary and secondary aging processes, and develops a new and more reliable method for the assessment of biological age through the application of principal component analysis, if the laws are known. The idea discussed is based on previously published data.[30,31]

II. MODELS FOR MEASURING BIOLOGICAL AGING

A. DEFINITIONS

As we grow older, there appear to be losses in functional capacity at the cellular level, the tissue level, the organ level, and the system level of organization.[34,37,38] However, there are considerable individual variations in the changes in physiological functions with age. In other words, individuals

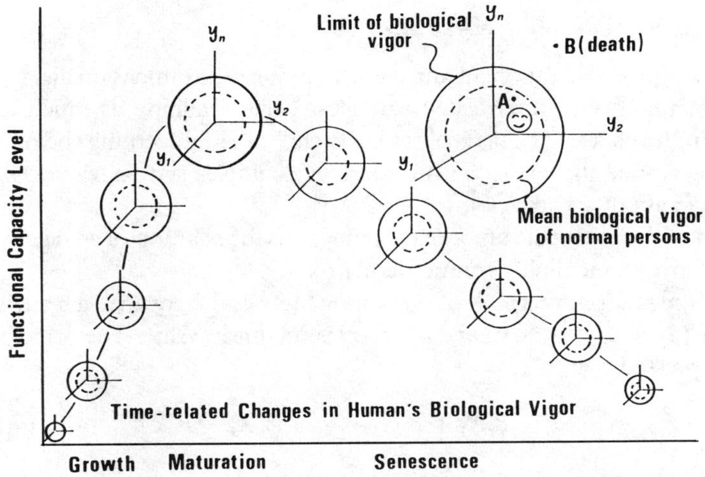

Figure 1 A model for measuring individual's biological aging. The individual state of biological vigor is estimated as a point in *N*-space represented by *N*-physiological variables (y_1, y_2, ..., y_n).

at the same chronological age are not necessarily at the same age in terms of physiological functions; i.e., they may manifest a quite different functional organic integrity for survival, i.e., so-called biological age.

In this chapter, biological aging is defined as a process or group processes that result in the progressive decrement of viability of the organism with advancing age, following the definitions of Comfort,[9] Hofecker et al.,[20] and Ingram:[22] whether a person is younger or older biologically suggests the quality of functioning organ systems and reflects the probability of death. Biological age, therefore, can be viewed as an objective measure for the assessment of one's biological vigor, which inevitably declines with advancing age.

B. MODEL FOR MEASURING BIOLOGICAL AGING

A biological age has been proposed as a general marker of aging based on the assumption that there is a unitary aging process that controls the rate of aging in a number of different functions. Based on the above-mentioned definition of biological aging and the assumption of the existence of a unitary aging process, the individual state of biological vigor was estimated as a conceptual sum of a large number of physiological variables closely related to the maintenance of life.

Figure 1 shows a hypothetical diagram for the changes in human biological vigor with advancing age. Although aging is a process that occurs over the entire life span,[34,36] this chapter is concerned with the biological changes that occur after sexual maturation. In Figure 1, the individual state of biological vigor is estimated as a point in *N*-space represented by *N*-physiological variables (y_1, y_2, ..., y_n). The outside circle is a closed curved surface representing the limit of one's biological vigor, and the inner dotted circle is a curved surface representing the mean biological vigor of normal persons. If a point in *N*-space falls in the inside (e.g., A) of the dotted circle, physiological conditions are assessed as being in good condition and we are considered to be younger biologically. If a point in *N*-space falls in the outside (e.g., B) of the closed curved surface by means of the internal and external causes, our body can no longer maintain the effectiveness of homeostatic control, a state which can lead to death. This is the hypothesis for measuring one's biological aging.

However, problems are posed by the question as to how we estimate an individual's location in *N*-space or an individual's biological vigor. In this study, the first principal component obtained from principal component analysis was used to estimate a point in *N*-space. We will describe its validity in more detail later.

C. PRINCIPAL COMPONENT ANALYSIS

The main idea of a principal component analysis is to reduce the dimensionality of a data set, which consists of a large number of interrelated variables, while retaining as much as possible of the variation present in the data set.[18] This analysis is a useful tool in discerning the underlying structure of interrelationship among the test scores measured in a complex system or process, especially when not much is known about an area of investigation.[22]

Computation of the principal components reduces to the solution of an eigenvalue-eigenvector problem for a positive-semidefinite symmetric matrix.

Suppose that the random vector X of n-components has the covariance matrix V, and X is also a deviation vector ($x_1 - m$, $x_2 - m$, ..., $x_n - m$), where m is the mean value. The principal component of the vector Z is expressed by:

$$Z = B_1X_1 + B_2X_2 + \cdots + B_nX_n = B'X \qquad (1)$$

where B is a weight vector.

The basic task is accomplished by solving for a set of n-homogeneous equations which results from partial differentiation of the function to be maximized, subject to a restriction that is introduced by use of Lagrange multipliers (λ).

The resulting equation in matrix notation is expressed as

$$(V - \lambda I)\, B = 0 \qquad (2)$$

where I is an identity matrix, and 0 is a null vector.

In order to solve Equation 2, with $B = 1$, we must have $V - \lambda I$ singular

$$|V - \lambda I| = 0 \qquad (3)$$

Equation 3 is the so-called characteristic equation, and has n-eigenvalues; let these be $\lambda_1 > \lambda_2 > \lambda_3 > \ldots > \lambda_4$. The weight vector B of the first principal component is obtained as an eigenvector corresponding to the largest eigenvalue λ_1.[18]

III. METHODS

A. SUBJECTS

From 6000 Japanese middle-aged and elderly men who underwent a 2-d health examination at the Kyoto Red Cross Hospital between 1979 and 1982, 462 healthy men were arbitrarily selected in such a way that the number of subjects exceeded 100 men in most of the decades studied except that of the 7th decade. The subjects ranged in age from 30 to 80 years, with a mean age of 50.8 years. In addition, the data for 62 hypertensive and 65 diabetic men was used to compare their biological ages with those of healthy subjects. The subject's occupations and residence and the criteria for clinical normality have been reported in detail previously.[30]

B. TEST ITEMS AND TEST PROCEDURES

The 2-day health examination consisted of more than 60 test items, including anthropometric measurements, cardiovascular and respiratory functions, and physical and chemical properties of blood and urine. Excluding results of tests expressed by binary variables, and considering the connection of the results of tests with the aging process, the following 30 variables were chosen for further analysis.

Results of urine examination: (1) urine specific gravity (urine SG), (2) urine pH. Results of blood examination: (3) hemoglobin concentration (Hb, g/dl), (4) hematocrit (Ht, %), (5) red blood cell count (RBC, $10^4/mm^3$), (6) white blood cell count (WBC, $/mm^3$). Results of biochemical examination of serum: (7) total protein (g/dl), (8) albumin (g/dl), (9) ratio of albumin to globulin (A/G ratio), (10) total cholesterol (mg/dl), (11) triglyceride (mg/dl), (12) urea nitrogen (mg/dl), (13) creatinine (mg/dl), (14) uric acid (mg/dl), (15) total bilirubin (mg/dl), (16) zinc sulfate test (ZTT, unit), (17) glutamate oxaloacetate transaminase (GOT, K-unit), (18) glutamic pyruvic transaminase (GPT, K-unit), (19) alkaline phosphatase (ALP, KA-unit). Results of oral glucose tolerance test: (20) OGTT (mg/dl), (21) OGTT (1 h), (22) OGTT (2 h). Results of vision test: (23) visual acuity for right eye (Vision (R), index measured by Landolt C chart), (24) visual acuity for left eye (Vision (L). Results of cardiorespiratory function test: (25) pulse rate at rest (beats per minute), (26) respiratory rate (numbers per minute), (27) forced vital capacity (FVC, ml), (28) percentage of forced vital capacity to predicted vital capacity (%FVC, ml), (29) systolic blood pressure (SBP, mmHg), and (30) diastolic blood pressure (DBP, mmHg).

Of the above-mentioned tests, urine SG was measured by the Fishburg method. Urine pH was measured by the litmus paper method. Blood analyses were undertaken by a TOA Automatic Blood Analyzer (Model CC-710, Towa Special Electric Company Ltd., Kobe, Japan). Biochemical measurements on heparinized blood were made by a Hitachi Automatic Analyzer (Model 726, Tokyo). Oral glucose tolerance tests (50 g glucose load) were conducted according to the procedure prescribed by the Japanese Society of Diabetes.[33] Visual acuity was measured by the Landolt Ring Test. Respiratory functions were measured by an electric spirometer (Model LAM-10, Fukuda Electric Company Ltd., Osaka) three times while standing, and the best record was adopted. Blood pressure was measured manually after 10 min rest in the supine position.

IV. RESULTS

A. FACTOR ANALYSIS OF AGE PARAMETERS

Table 1 shows the mean and standard deviation of the 30 physiological variables by 5-year chronological age groups from 30 to 80 years. The differences of means among age groups were tested by one-way analysis of variance for each variable. In most variables except for urine pH, triglyceride, bilirubin, GPT, and ALP, the differences of means among age groups were statistically significant at the 5% level. With the advance of the age, mean Hb, Ht, RBC, albumin, A/G ratio, vision, FVC, and %FVC decreased gradually, while those of total cholesterol, urea nitrogen, creatinine, OGTT (1 and 2 h) and DBP showed gradual increases. For some variables, the means were relatively constant among age groups younger than 60 years old, but showed a sharp decrease (WBC, uric acid) or increase (ZTT, OGT, pulse rate, SBP) after the age of 60.

To discern the underlying structure of intercorrelations among the 30 physiological variables, a principal component analysis was applied to the correlation matrix of the 30 physiological variables and chronological age. This multivariate statistical method is a highly useful technique for summarizing the unique patterns of covariance among a large set of variables, i.e., to identify principal components of intercorrelations. In this analysis, chronological age was included with the 30 physiological variables due to discerning whether principal components could be formulated as a function of chronological age. Twelve principal components with corresponding eigenvalues (the variance of component) >1.0 were obtained, following the recommendations of Guttman[16] (Table 2). Over two thirds of total variance (71%) was accounted for by these 12 principal components. The first principal component was loaded with 20 significantly correlated variables, and explained 13.5% of the total variance of all variables. In particular, chronological age showed an extremely high

Table 1 Means and standard deviations of the physiological variables by age group

Test item	Age group 30 Mean	30 S.D.	35 Mean	35 S.D.	40 Mean	40 S.D.	45 Mean	45 S.D.	50 Mean	50 S.D.	55 Mean	55 S.D.	60 Mean	60 S.D.	65 Mean	65 S.D.	70 Mean	70 S.D.	75 Mean	75 S.D.	F ratio
1. Urine SG	1.024	0.006	1.026	0.010	1.025	0.006	1.024	0.006	1.023	0.007	1.024	0.007	1.021	0.006	1.023	0.007	1.024	0.007	1.020	0.004	[a]2.742
2. Urine pH	6.0	0.5	5.9	0.5	5.7	0.4	6.0	0.4	6.0	0.7	6.0	0.4	6.0	0.6	6.1	0.6	6.0	0.6	5.9	0.8	1.714
3. Hb	15.70	0.94	15.66	1.03	15.48	1.03	15.58	1.11	15.15	1.02	15.30	0.88	14.89	1.07	14.96	1.40	14.99	1.33	14.78	1.03	[b]8.995
4. Ht	46.6	2.4	46.5	3.0	45.9	2.9	46.3	3.1	45.1	2.9	45.5	2.7	45.0	3.1	45.3	4.1	44.9	3.5	44.6	2.7	[b]4.749
5. RBC	490	32	491	40	476	37	478	36	471	34	465	33	464	41	467	49	472	49	443	33	[b]8.613
6. WBC	5829	1561	6082	1429	6191	1383	6498	1712	6370	1772	6316	1505	5648	1195	5576	1274	5456	1399	5364	1223	[b]5.342
7. Total protein	7.30	0.30	7.16	0.38	7.17	0.36	7.06	0.34	7.07	0.36	7.03	0.28	7.29	0.32	7.34	0.46	7.39	0.40	7.25	0.60	[b]8.909
8. Albumin	4.50	0.18	4.40	0.41	4.43	0.18	4.34	0.19	4.29	0.22	4.31	0.21	4.29	0.27	4.33	0.20	4.22	0.26	4.12	0.19	[b]9.206
9. A/G ratio	1.63	0.17	1.66	0.17	1.66	0.24	1.60	0.14	1.56	0.15	1.61	0.22	1.45	0.15	1.45	0.18	1.44	0.46	1.36	0.24	[b]21.861
10. Total cholesterol	187.1	34.4	190.7	32.9	193.3	35.6	202.0	36.2	197.9	33.4	214.6	39.6	204.7	34.3	213.2	29.2	209.3	28.2	200.8	28.6	[b]4.708
11. Triglyceride	104.3	45.2	108.6	46.1	113.9	60.2	110.7	47.2	108.0	36.9	106.0	42.2	101.3	32.4	100.6	39.6	100.3	22.4	85.3	18.9	1.609

15. Total bilirubin	0.81	0.32	0.85	0.30	0.80	0.36	0.82	0.29	0.79	0.31	0.80	0.29	0.76	0.29	0.77	0.28	0.83	0.27	0.69	0.17	0.831
16. ZTT	5.8	2.7	5.6	2.2	5.8	2.4	5.7	2.3	5.9	2.5	6.0	2.4	7.0	2.7	7.2	2.7	7.9	3.0	7.4	3.4	[b]7.773
17. GOT	20.1	8.3	19.6	4.9	21.3	8.0	21.4	7.2	20.6	7.1	20.7	6.3	22.3	10.3	21.8	4.3	24.9	7.3	23.7	8.4	[a]3.008
18. GPT	17.8	10.3	18.4	10.0	18.7	8.9	20.2	10.6	18.7	8.3	16.8	8.2	18.5	10.5	16.3	5.9	17.8	7.5	16.6	8.6	0.751
19. ALP	6.4	1.6	6.2	1.5	6.3	1.8	5.9	1.9	6.9	2.3	6.1	1.4	6.5	1.9	6.2	1.7	6.5	2.2	7.0	2.2	1.434
20. OGTT	86.8	6.7	86.7	7.4	89.2	9.3	87.6	7.9	89.0	14.7	89.3	18.3	88.7	9.5	88.7	8.4	95.9	10.8	92.1	6.7	[a]2.822
21. OGTT (1 h)	108.1	25.4	106.0	27.8	121.5	34.5	121.0	32.6	123.5	45.2	123.3	46.8	125.3	32.5	138.7	30.3	153.6	38.0	132.6	21.2	[b]9.333
22. OGTT (2 h)	71.3	14.7	76.2	16.7	81.6	23.7	82.1	24.1	83.3	25.6	87.4	37.6	86.3	24.4	96.3	24.0	109.1	29.6	96.9	20.2	[b]10.179
23. Vision (R)	0.57	0.54	0.86	0.56	0.83	0.60	0.90	0.50	0.70	0.53	0.63	0.39	0.50	0.38	0.52	0.38	0.31	0.24	0.39	0.27	[b]11.523
24. Vision (L)	0.54	0.54	0.95	0.59	0.85	0.57	0.93	0.49	0.75	0.48	0.64	0.41	0.52	0.43	0.48	0.37	0.32	0.25	0.40	0.26	[b]13.410
25. Pulse rate	66.5	6.5	64.4	5.9	65.0	6.6	65.3	6.8	66.7	8.2	67.0	7.4	66.2	7.7	72.0	6.8	70.7	9.0	72.8	6.3	[b]7.725
26. Respiratory rate	17.6	2.3	17.4	2.0	17.1	2.3	17.2	2.3	17.6	2.4	17.5	2.6	17.6	2.8	18.3	2.1	18.0	2.1	19.1	2.1	[a]2.550
27. FVC	3985	470	3899	495	3709	524	3479	483	3324	400	3195	589	2996	524	2887	448	2625	306	2691	350	[b]75.329
28. %FVC	98.0	10.3	98.7	10.8	97.4	12.2	94.7	11.8	92.9	10.1	92.0	16.2	98.8	14.6	90.9	11.4	82.5	8.2	91.6	11.5	[b]9.756
29. SBP	111.4	12.5	1.8.8	10.9	111.0	14.9	110.7	12.6	109.9	12.4	119.4	14.3	125.0	15.3	137.3	14.7	136.5	22.2	150.1	17.6	[b]56.195
30. DBP	69.5	7.9	71.1	9.5	71.2	11.9	73.6	14.4	74.1	10.4	78.4	9.6	80.4	9.4	85.6	8.0	81.8	13.0	82.9	13.0	[b]21.095
No. of Subjects	35	71	57	57	65	49	60	38	16	14											

[a] $p<0.05$.
[b] $p<0.01$.

Data from Nakamura, E., Mech. Age Dev., *46, 1, 1988. With permission.*

Table 2 Principal components for age and 30 physiological variables

Variable (*j*)	F_1	F_2	F_3	F_4	F_5	F_6	F_7	F_8	F_9	F_{10}	F_{11}	F_{12}	h_j^2
1. Age	0.79	–0.15	0.01	–0.15	–0.16	0.18	0.01	–0.03	0.08	–0.03	–0.05	–0.05	0.75
2. Urine SG	–0.15	0.01	0.37	–0.02	0.21	–0.20	0.09	0.46	0.20	0.09	0.04	0.11	0.54
3. Urine pH	0.07	0.05	–0.18	0.02	–0.22	–0.76	0.00	–0.56	0.08	0.08	–0.11	0.00	0.46
4. Hb	–0.27	0.78	–0.16	–0.26	–0.08	–0.16	0.12	–0.02	0.22	0.03	0.11	–0.10	0.89
5. Ht	–0.23	0.74	–0.21	–0.32	–0.15	0.02	0.13	–0.01	0.23	–0.00	0.14	–0.10	0.88
6. RBC	–0.27	0.73	–0.19	–0.24	–0.07	0.02	0.18	0.02	0.19	–0.01	0.04	–0.08	0.78
7. WBC	–0.12	0.16	–0.18	–0.03	–0.27	–0.09	–0.01	0.12	–0.16	0.37	0.09	0.59	0.70
8. Total protein	0.29	0.31	–0.41	0.07	0.40	0.18	0.30	0.21	–0.30	0.07	–0.26	–0.05	0.87
9. Albumin	–0.36	0.33	0.03	–0.16	0.28	0.10	0.24	0.12	–0.45	–0.35	–0.35	0.16	0.84
10. A/G ratio	–0.56	0.01	0.43	–0.23	–0.18	–0.09	–0.04	–0.08	–0.16	–0.38	0.01	0.15	0.78
11. Total cholesterol	0.16	0.30	0.17	–0.32	–0.12	0.34	–0.18	0.04	–0.32	0.17	–0.15	–0.12	0.58
12. Triglyceride	–0.01	0.53	0.04	0.05	–0.02	0.06	–0.37	0.12	–0.29	0.26	0.07	0.01	0.61
13. Urea nitrogen	0.18	–0.14	0.32	–0.08	0.03	0.18	–0.09	0.43	0.38	0.04	–0.27	0.07	0.62
14. Serum creatinine	0.08	0.01	0.26	–0.21	0.11	0.43	–0.17	0.11	0.09	–0.27	0.22	–0.32	0.59
15. Uric acid	–0.10	0.16	0.12	–0.08	0.06	0.11	–0.51	0.23	0.06	0.31	0.11	0.08	0.51
16. Total bilirubin	0.01	0.24	0.10	–0.04	0.15	–0.19	–0.00	0.06	0.38	–0.01	–0.35	0.04	0.41
17. ZTT	0.37	–0.14	–0.52	0.19	0.21	–0.01	0.04	0.16	0.16	0.24	–0.04	–0.26	0.71
18. GOT	0.36	0.40	–0.10	0.41	0.14	–0.21	–0.41	–0.02	–0.01	–0.26	0.03	–0.03	0.80
19. GPT	0.19	0.58	–0.04	0.37	0.08	–0.17	–0.40	0.02	–0.10	–0.27	0.08	–0.06	0.82
20. ALP	0.07	0.16	–0.32	0.21	0.02	–0.18	–0.02	0.21	0.27	–0.29	–0.10	0.28	0.50
21. OGTT	0.35	0.35	0.46	0.24	0.06	–0.25	0.28	–0.08	–0.05	0.13	0.01	–0.10	0.70
22. OGTT (1 h)	0.44	0.34	0.50	0.12	–0.05	–0.18	0.19	–0.10	0.02	0.13	0.04	–0.01	0.68
23. OGTT (2 h)	0.49	0.31	0.47	0.07	0.06	–0.18	0.23	–0.04	–0.08	0.14	–0.01	–0.06	0.69
24. Vision (R)	–0.37	0.13	0.12	0.63	–0.31	0.44	0.17	0.04	0.06	0.02	–0.07	–0.02	0.91
25. Vision (L)	–0.38	0.21	0.09	0.62	–0.32	0.42	0.14	0.06	0.05	0.01	–0.03	0.00	0.91
26. Pulse rate	0.38	0.01	–0.09	0.01	0.15	0.06	0.22	0.00	–0.15	–0.04	0.43	0.16	0.47
27. Respiratory rate	0.22	–0.12	–0.04	0.05	0.04	0.07	0.29	0.33	0.01	–0.20	0.52	0.08	0.60
28. FVC	–0.67	0.04	0.08	0.13	0.60	0.07	–0.01	–0.23	0.11	0.10	0.11	0.07	0.94
29. %FVC	–0.48	–0.05	0.10	0.11	0.69	0.18	–0.01	–0.31	0.14	0.14	0.10	0.09	0.86
30. SBP	0.69	0.12	0.01	–0.10	0.06	0.34	–0.01	–0.21	0.16	–0.10	–0.03	0.30	0.80
31. DBP	0.58	0.25	0.07	–0.05	0.10	0.34	–0.06	–0.24	0.18	–0.07	–0.02	0.35	0.77
Variance	4.20	3.51	2.06	1.83	1.72	1.44	1.41	1.37	1.29	1.16	1.06	1.01	22.06

Note: "h_j^2" *is called the communality, which can be expressed by the sum of the squared factor loading of the extracted factors. This value presents the fraction of the variable's variance.*

From Nakamura, E., Mech. Age. Dev., *46, 1, 1988. With permission.*

factor loading (correlation) of 0.79 with this component. Principal components 2 through 12 showed a considerably lower loading for chronological age, and were high-loaded only with a few variables related to a single system or organ. These results suggested that there was a fixed pattern which showed a hierarchical factor structure in the variation of these variables.

Based on the results of principal component analysis, we deduced that biological age changes may be separated into primary and secondary aging processes. However, it was difficult to ascertain this assumption directly from only the results of this analysis because a principal component analysis is originally devised to reduce the dimensionality of a data set which consists of a large number of interrelated variables. To ascertain this assumption, a hierarchical factor analysis,[35] which makes explicit the hierarchical ordering of factors above the first-order domain, was applied to the same correlation matrix. Three variables (WBC, creatinine, and ALP) were excluded from this analysis. In the hierarchical factor analysis, it was necessary to group all variables into subsets in advance. However, because these three variables were independent of other variables, they were not suited for this analysis. The principle of hierarchical factor analysis was developed by Schmid and Leiman.[35] This model presents a procedure for transforming an oblique factor analysis solution containing a hierarchy of higher-order factors into an orthogonal solution which preserves simple structure and also provides orthogonal reference axes. The mathematical theorem of this analysis has been described in more detail elsewhere.[31]

Table 3 shows the final hierarchical factor solution. In this hierarchical factor solution, three group factors functioning at different levels of complexity composed of the 16 common factors were extracted. Of these group factors, the first and third group factors can be referred to the aging process. The first group factor, the so-called factor 1, loaded with most of the physiological variables, was interpreted as a primary aging factor which presented the primary process of human aging. The second group factors, the so-called factors 2 to 5, were the next most complex factors, but it was difficult to explain these factors because they were not loaded with the variables representing the same organs or systems. The third group factor, the so-called factors 6 to 16, loaded only with a few variables related to a single physiological system or organ, and was thus interpreted as representing a system-specific aging factor. These factors could be named on the basis of the nature of the variables loading the factor. For example, factor 6 was relatively highly loaded with three variables of Hb, Ht, and RBC. Thus, factor 6 was interpreted as a "hematologic factor". Factors 7 to 12 were interpreted in the same manner as follows: factor 7 was a "visual factor"; factor 8, a "pulmonary function factor"; factor 9, a "liver function factor"; factor 10, a "clinical hypertensive factor"; factor 11, a "glucose tolerance factor"; factor 12, a "protein metabolic factor"; factor 13, a "circulatory factor"; factor 14, an "unknown factor"; factor 15, a "lipid metabolic factor"; and factor 16, a "renal function factor". Factor 14 was relatively highly loaded only with three variables of urine SG, blood urea nitrogen (BUN), and bilirubin. However, it was difficult to name this factor because urine SG and BUN were used for the diagnosis of renal function, while bilirubin was used for the diagnosis of liver function. Thus, factor 14 was interpreted as the unknown factor. These results will be made useful in explaining the factor extracted by principal factor analysis.

Table 4 shows a summary of interpretation of the factors extracted by principal component analysis, and their degrees of contribution to total variance of all variables. The interpretation of factors that form system-specific aging factors were determined considering the results of hierarchical factor solution. The degrees of contribution of a general aging factor, system-specific aging factors, and uniqueness (individual variance inherent in every variable) to the total variance of all variables were 13.5, 57.5, and 29.0%, respectively. In human studies, a general aging factor has a relatively small percentage of the parameters' variance. This means that as for the assessment of the human's aging process, we have to consider the existence of system-specific aging factors as well as a single general aging factor. As for the explanation of factors extracted as system-specific aging factors, they could be named as follows: factor 2 as a "hematologic factor"; factor 3, a "glucose tolerance factor"; factor 4, a "visual factor"; factor 5, a "pulmonary function factor"; factor 6, an "unknown factor"; factor 7, a "liver function factor"; factor 8, a "renal function factor"; factor 9, a "serum lipid metabolic factor"; factor 10, a "protein metabolic factor"; factor 11, a "respiratory function factor"; and factor 12, a "hypertensive factor".

These results afford proof of Strehler's[40] hypothesis that "multicellular aging is the expression of a hierarchy of events proceeding from elementary interactions of molecules at the cellular and subcellular level to the very complex interactions of the whole organism" (p. 18). Therefore, biological age changes can be viewed as a time-dependent complex integration of primary and

Table 3 Hierarchical factor solution for 27 physiological variables

Variable	F1	F2	F3	F4	F5	F6	F7	F8	F9	F10	F11	F12	F13	F14	F15	F16	*h*
1. IIb	0.13	0.41				0.73											0.76
2. IIt	0.15	0.49				0.72											0.833
3. RBC	0.14	0.40				0.67											0.650
4. Albumin	0.14	0.21				0.43											0.271
5. Vision (R)	0.36	0.55					0.66										0.899
6. Vision (L)	0.33	0.53					0.67										0.857
7. FVC	0.53		0.40					0.68									0.963
8. %FVC	0.38		0.31					0.75									0.832
9. GOT	0.32		0.33						0.77								0.850
10. GPT	0.20	–0.22	0.30						0.73								0.757
11. SBP	0.56	0.11	0.41							0.55							0.817
12. DBP	0.50		0.38							0.55							0.728
13. Glucose	0.27		0.23								0.69						0.631
14. OGTT (1 h)	0.35		0.26								0.62						0.597
15. OGTT (2 h)	0.39		0.26								0.63						0.638
16. A/G ratio	0.38		0.28									0.64					0.689
17. ZTT	0.22	0.13	0.16		–0.16							0.62					0.544
18. Protein	0.23	–0.11	0.25			–0.23						0.64					0.631
19. HR	0.32			0.17									0.37	–0.22			0.362
20. Respiratory rate	0.50			0.47									0.33	0.22			0.663
21. Urine SG	0.11			0.28									–0.13	0.40			0.316
22. BUN	0.48			0.47									0.21	0.31			0.648
23. Bilirubin	0.16			0.19									–0.18	0.37			0.279
24. Cholesterol	0.17				0.39										0.51		0.482
25. Triglyceride		–0.14			0.42				0.12						0.49		0.480
26. Uric acid					0.46											0.28	0.320
27. Creatine	0.11				0.39											0.30	0.281
Variance	2.78	1.42	1.24	0.60	0.89	1.83	0.93	1.08	1.20	0.66	1.31	1.26	0.41	0.48	0.56	0.19	16.84

Note: Factor loading of 0.11 needed to reach significance at 0.05 level. Variables not significantly correlated (5% level) have been rejected.

Data from Nakamjura, E., Mech. Age. Dev., *60, 153, 1991. With permission.*

Table 4 Interpretation of the factors extracted and their degrees of contribution to total variance

	System-specific aging factor	
	F2: Hematologic factor	
	F3: Gulcose tolerance factor	
	F4: Visual factor	
	F5: Pulmonary function factor	
	F6: —	
A general aging factor (F1)	F7: Liver function factor	Uniqueness
	F8: Runal function factor	
	F9: Serum lipid metabolic factor	
	F10: Protein metabolic factor	
	F11: Respiratory function factor	
	F12: Hypertensive factor	
←13.5%→	←57.5%→	←29.0%→
←	Total Variance	→

secondary aging processes. From the facts described above, the score of first principal component can be used as a unitary index related to the aging process of various physiological functions.

B. A TEST BATTERY

From the above-mentioned perspective, the variables that were included in a test battery to measure biological aging should be selected from variables which correlated well with the first principal component. However, as pointed out by Comfort[9] and Bourliere,[5] the variables must be sufficiently diverse to give a balanced picture of the overall changes in physiological functions with advancing age. Thus, a test battery for measuring biological aging was determined considering (1) the variables that correlated well with a general aging factor extracted, (2) the physiological meaning of each test, e.g., select one variable among those related to functions of the same organ or the same physiological system, and (3) the loss of the informative value being caused by redundant correlation among several of the variables of the test battery.[32]

Finally, the following 11 variables were selected from the test battery to estimate biological age: Hb, albumin, A/G ratio, total cholesterol, urea nitrogen, GOT, OGTT (1 h), vision (L), pulse rate, FVC, and SBP.

Figure 2 shows the relative changes in means of the selected 11 physiological tests among age groups (30 to 34, 35 to 39, ..., 70 to 74 and 75+), putting the mean in the youngest age group (30 to 34 years old) as 100%. The majority of means for the physiological tests began to change only at ages 40 and older, and sharp changes were observed thereafter. However, the rates of change with age varied greatly for different tests. Therefore, it was necessary to establish a unitary index based on a combination of a number of age-related physiological variables for assessing an individual's biological age.

C. ASSESSMENT OF BIOLOGICAL AGE BY PRINCIPAL COMPONENT ANALYSIS

To establish a unitary index related to the aging process of the selected physiological variables, a principal component analysis was applied to the correlation matrix, which was calculated from the selected 11 physiological variables. Four principal components with corresponding eigenvalues >1.0 were obtained (Table 5). Of these four components, the first principal component accounts for 20.6% of the total variance in the battery of the 11 physiological variables. In this study, the first

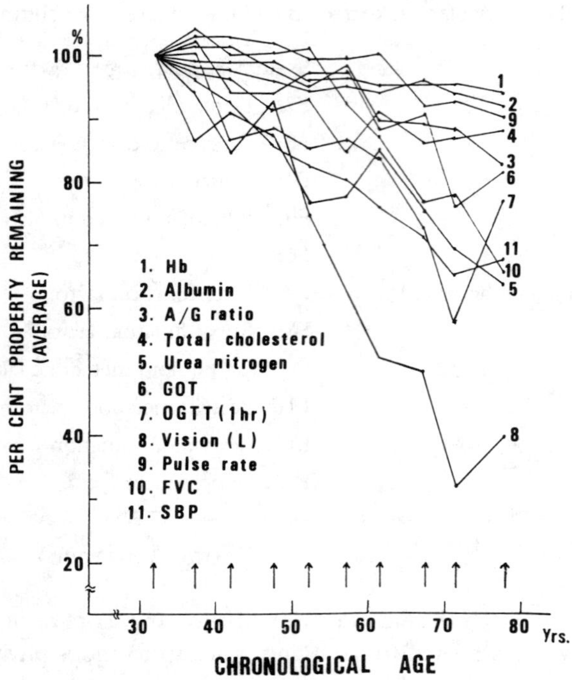

Figure 2 Declines in the selected 11 physiological variables with age. Values were adjusted so that the mean value of the 30 to 34 age group equaled 100%. As for the five variables urea nitrogen, GOT, OGTT (1 h), pulse rate, and systolic blood pressure, they were inversely plotted to allow direct comparison with other variables, which progressively decline with age.

Table 5 Principal components for the selected 11 physiological variables

	Factor loadings				
Test items	**F1**	**F2**	**F3**	**F4**	**Communality (h_j^2)**
Hb	−0.254	0.664	−0.152	−0.022	0.529
Albumin	−0.381	0.558	0.256	−0.198	0.561
A/G ratio	−0.639	0.154	0.317	0.081	0.539
Total cholesterol	0.183	0.479	0.540	−0.102	0.565
Urea nitrogen	0.215	−0.191	0.532	0.566	0.685
GOT	0.406	0.365	−0.465	0.138	0.534
OGTT (h)	0.435	0.433	−0.037	0.364	0.511
Vision (L)	−0.353	0.178	−0.347	0.584	0.617
Pulse	0.442	0.099	−0.113	−0.399	0.376
FVC	−0.641	0.027	−0.191	−0.061	0.452
SBP	0.659	0.192	0.084	−0.005	0.527
Eigenvalue	2.265	1.443	1.158	1.031	
Percentage of variance	20.6	13.1	10.5	9.4	

principal component score was used as a unitary index (biological score, BS) of age-related changes in physiological functions. To calculate individual BS, each score was first standardized and then summed across tests in a weighted manner using the coefficients of factor scores obtained from the principal component analysis. This procedure was complicated, so we reduced the equation so that individual BS was calculated directly by applying the raw scores of the 11 variables into the following equation:

$$\begin{aligned} BS = {} & 2.616 - 0.102\,(\text{Hb}) - 0.646\,(\text{albumin}) - 1.343\,(\text{A/G ratio}) \\ & + 0.002\,(\text{total cholesterol}) + 0.031\,(\text{urea nitrogen}) + 0.024\,(\text{GOT}) \\ & + 0.005\,(\text{OGTT (1 h)}) - 0.3\,(\text{vision (L)}) + 0.026\,(\text{pulse}) - 0.0005\,(\text{FVC}) \\ & + 0.018\,(\text{SBP}) \end{aligned}$$

where individual BSs are distributed with the mean of 0 and a standard deviation of 1.0.

At first glance, the evaluation of individual biological age based on the obtained BS lacks persuasive power when compared to the result of the multiple regression model, which can be expressed as years. To remove this disadvantage, individual BSs were transformed to years (biological age, BA) using the T-scale procedure (technique of transformation from standard score to T score).

$$BA = (BS \times 12.09) + 50.86$$

where 50.86 and 12.09 are the mean and standard deviation of the chronological age of our sample of 462 healthy men, respectively. This procedure assured that the mean biological age of all the subjects was equal to the mean chronological age and the pattern of the distribution of the biological age agreed with that of the scores of first principal component without changing the characteristics of the scores of first principal component.

Figure 3 shows the relationship between individual biological and chronological ages (Y) in 462 healthy men. The correlation between the estimated biological and chronological ages was 0.75 ($p < 0.01$). Individual biological ages were scattered relatively symmetrically above and below the identity line Y = BA. However, the agreement of the mean biological age with the mean chronological age for each group was not perfect. The differences for the age groups of 30 to 34, 35 to 54, 55 to 59, 60 to 64, and 75+ were significant at or beyond the 5% level.

D. EFFECTS OF PATHOLOGICAL CONDITION ON BIOLOGICAL AGE

The predictors of the maximum life span may have a high probability of being a valid equation of biological age.[6,21,26,27] Based on the hypothesis that individuals estimated to be biologically older will encounter more illness or premature death, some researchers reported that patients with symptoms such as diabetes, hypertension, and cardiovascular morbidity had higher "biological ages" than chronological ages when an equation standardized on healthy subjects was applied to data obtained from them.[4,15,43]

To examine whether some pathological conditions such as hypertension and diabetes affect biological age, the biological age of 62 hypertensive and 65 diabetic men were calculated using the healthy subject equation devised in this study. Because two tests of OGTT (1 h) and SBP were included in the equation, the biological age of hypertensive and diabetic men was logically expected to be higher than their chronological age when their raw data were used for calculating biological age. Therefore, the SBP of hypertensive men and OGTT (1 h) of diabetic men were replaced with the mean values of SBP and OGTT (1 h) of healthy men in the same age groups (10-year age interval), respectively (Figure 4). Most biological ages estimated on hypertensive and diabetic men

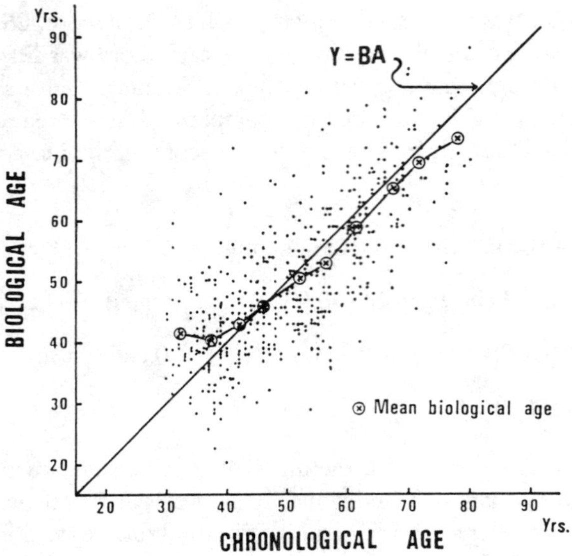

Figure 3 Relationship between biological ages (BA) and chronological ages (Y) in 462 healthy men. (Data from Nakamura, E., *Mech. Age. Dev.*, 46, 1, 1988. With permission.)

were scattered above the identity line Y = BA. The mean biological age of the hypertensive men was estimated as 57.25 years old and was higher by 4.17 years than their mean chronological age (53.08 years old). The mean biological age of the diabetic men was estimated as 55.57 years old, and was higher by 4.57 years than their mean chronological age (51.0 years old). The differences between the mean biological age and chronological age for both groups were statistically significant at the 1% level.

Figure 5 shows a radar chart for assessing one's biological condition based on a biological age and ten kinds of system-specific biological ages of an individual. As for the computation of the ten kinds of system-specific biological ages, the first, factor scores of F2, F3, F4, F5, F7, F8, F9, F10, F11, and F12 in Table 3 were calculated. Second, each of the ten kinds of factor scores was transformed to years (system-specific biological age) by using the same principle and methods as those for calculating the biological age of an individual. An overall "biological age" calculated by combining scores from different types of tests is shown as a thin circle in a radar chart. The chronological age as well as ten kinds of system-specific biological ages of an individual are shown with thick lines as a profile of 11 faces. From this diagram, we can easily understand that the biological age of this subject is higher by 4 years than his chronological age, and also the deteriorations of pulmonary function and lipid metabolism advance more than other functions. Furthermore, we can estimate that if this individual does not take any countermeasure for the prevention of hypertension and diabetes, he may have hypertensive and diabetic diseases.

V. DISCUSSION

Biological age can be viewed as an objective measure for the assessment of one's biological vigor which declines with advancing age.[9,12,20,22,37] A reliable and valid equation for measuring one's biological age can provide a tool for detecting age-related diseases and also for examining the effectiveness of such interventions as drug, diet, and exercise that may influence the rate of aging. However, the question arises as to how a concept such as biological vigor can be measured. At the present time, a standardized system for measuring biological age has not been developed because the nature of the primary aging process or processes is unknown.

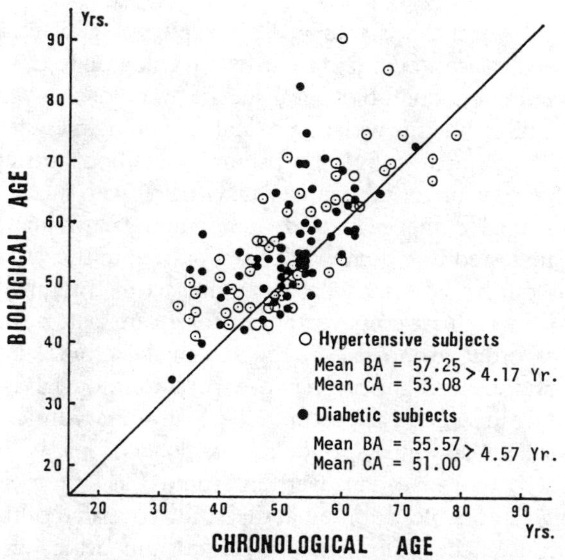

Figure 4 Relationship between biological ages (BA) and chronological ages (CA) in 62 hypertensive and 65 diabetic men. (Data from Nakamura, E., *Mech. Age. Dev.*, 46, 1, 1988. With permission.)

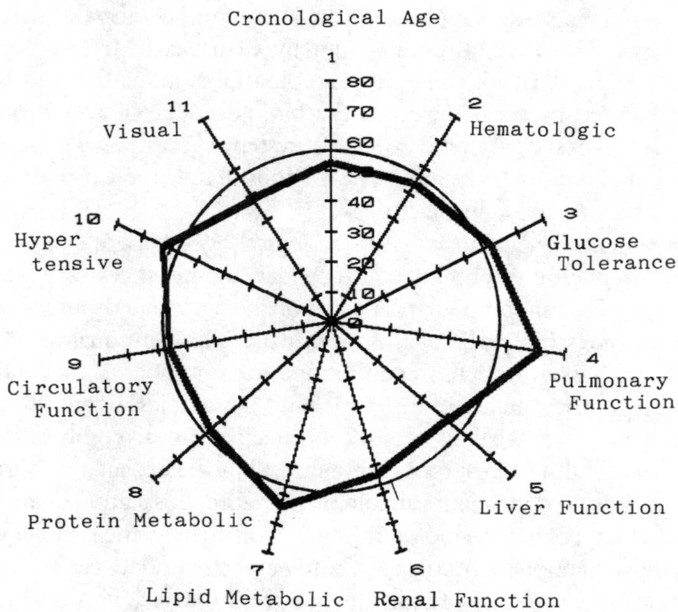

Figure 5 A radar chart for assessing an individual's biological vigor based on biological age and 10 kinds of system-specific biological ages of an individual. The chronological age as well as 10 kinds of system-specific biological ages are shown with thick lines, as a profile of 11 faces. The biological age is shown as a thin circle in the radar chart.

In this chapter, we hypothesized the existence of a unitary aging process that controlled the rate of aging in a number of different functions. However, Costa and McCrae[10] denied its existence because aging rate might be substantially different for different physiological systems and hence each system would have its own temporal pattern of age change. They also pointed out that if aging was a single process, factor analysis of change scores on different physiological tests administered to subjects of different ages should yield a factor common to many physiological tests. Of course, the researchers who are interested in determining one's biological age are aware of these pitfalls and recognize that it is difficult to assess one's biological age with only a single physiological system. Generally, the pattern of age changes is a linear decrement in function beginning at about the age of 30 and continuing throughout life; furthermore, many of the same changes occur with increasing age.[5,39]

Both results of principal component and hierarchical factor analyses of the age-related physiological variables suggested that there was a fixed pattern in the variations of the physiological variables employed in our studies. In other words, the factor structure of age parameters shows hierarchical group-factors, which are composed of major group factors, minor group factors, and specific factors. The first-order group factor, the so-called factor 1, loaded with most of the physiological variables and also highly correlated with chronological age, was interpreted as a single general aging factor in which each score reflects an unitary index underlying aging. The third-order group factors, the so-called specific factors, loaded only with a few variables related to a single physiological system or organ, were interpreted as system-specific secondary aging factors. All the physiological variables adopted in this study consisted of the tests for the diagnosis of conditions or functions such as properties of blood and urine, protein metabolism, lipid metabolism, renal function, liver function, glucose tolerance, visual acuity, and cardiorespiratory functions. These physiological variables were considered to represent vital organic functions, closely related to the maintenance of life. Therefore, the score of first-order group factor, the so-called factor 1, was fully expected to represent one's state of viability (the so-called biological age), and the scores of system-specific aging factors were expected to represent one's state of system-specific deteriorations. This study supports the basic assumption for the derivation of a single index of biological age. However, as pointed out by Costa and McCrae,[10] it is also true that different physiological ages exist for different physiological systems that can be measured. This problem could be resolved by breaking down the biological age of an individual into different biological ages of specific systems (the so-called system-specific ages). Therefore, it will be necessary to develop an aging measurement system considering the existence of a single general aging factor and system-specific aging factors.

From the above-mentioned point of view, biological age changes can be viewed as a time-dependent complex integration of primary and secondary aging processes. Thus, the first component obtained from a principal component analysis of the age-related physiological variables was employed to estimate one's biological age. A principal component analysis is generally a useful procedure whenever the task is to determine the minimum number of independent components needed to explain most of the variance in the original set of variables. Especially as the first principal component obtained from this analysis was the normalized linear combination with maximum variance, it becomes a useful statistical tool combining all of the explanatory variables into a single expression, in case there is no dependent variable.[18] Therefore, this statistical model can be used for determining a concept such as human biological vigor. Fortunately, the biological age estimated on the basis of the principal component model gave better agreement between the mean biological age and the chronological age in a group of individuals at the same age. This is a prerequisite to assess one's biological age because difference in aging rate is assessed on the basis of the difference between the predicted and actual ages. We can say that the biological age estimated by the principal component model is practically useful and theoretically valid.

One problem with the majority of aging measurement systems is that few have been validated in longitudinal studies.[4,14] The models have to be based on longitudinal data collected over at least 10 years of senescence. It is said that the validation of assessing biological age requires a correlation with mortality.[6,21,26,27] However, it is not easy to follow the life span of subjects until death and also correct the data longitudinally because the humans are a long-lived species. Because the life expectancy of hypertensive and diabetic persons is shorter than that of normotensives,[7,15,21,41] the biological age of hypertensive and diabetic men were compared with those of normotensives by using a biological age equation devised in this study. The estimated biological age of most hypertensive and diabetic men was higher by about 4.5 years than their chronological age. What the relationship is between disease and aging is not yet clear. However, a reasonable view taken by most gerontologists is that aging increases the probability of disease occurring and that some disease may even accelerate aging.[6] The individual biological age estimated by the principal component model shows the equation's high sensitivity in detecting abnormalities. This finding may indicate the adequacy of estimated biological age by showing that various pathological conditions deteriorate physiological functions and then advance the biological age. It is questionable, however, whether the estimated biological age can be used to estimate life expectancy.

ACKNOWLEDGMENTS

The author wishes to express his sincere gratitude to Dr. Donald K. Ingram, Molecular Physiology and Genetics Sections, Gerontology Research Center, National Institutes on Aging, for valuable advice and criticism. I would like to thank Dr. Arthur K. Balin, the past president of the American Aging Association, for his constructive comments.

REFERENCES

1. Benjamin, H., Biologic versus chronologic age, *J. Gerontol.*, 2, 217, 1947.
2. Bell, B., Significance of functional age for interdisciplinary and longitudinal research in aging, *Aging Hum. Dev.*, 3, 145, 1972.
3. Birren, J.E., Principles of research on aging, in *Handbook of Aging and the Individual*, Birren, J.E., Ed., University of Chicago Press, Chicago, 1959, 3.
4. Borkan, G.A. and Norris, A.H., Assessment of biological age using a profile of physical parameters, *J. Gerontol.*, 35, 177, 1980.
5. Bourliere, F., Ecology of human aging, in *The Physiology and Pathology of Human Aging*, Goldman, R. and Rockstein, M., Eds., Academic Press, New York, 1978, 9.
6. Brown, K.S. and Forbes, W.F., Concerning the estimation of biological age, *Gerontology*, 22, 428, 1976.
7. Caird, F.I. and Dall, J.L.C., The cardiovascular system, in *Textbook of Geriatric Medicine and Gerontology*, Brocklehurst, J.C., Ed., Churchill Livingstone, Edinburgh, 1978, 125.
8. Clark, J.W., The aging dimension: a factorial analysis of individual differences with age on psychological and physiological measurements, *J. Gerontol.*, 15, 183, 1960.
9. Comfort, A., Test-battery to measure ageing-rate in man, *Lancet*, 27, 1411, 1969.
10. Costa, P.T., Jr. and McCrae, R.R., Functional age: a conceptual and empirical critique, in *Epidemiology of Aging*, Haynes, S.G. and Feinleib, M., Eds., NIH Publ. No. 80-969, U.S. Government Printing Office, Washington, D.C., 1980, 23.
11. Damon, A., Predicting age from body measurements and observation, *Aging Hum. Dev.*, 3, 169, 1972.
12. Dean, W. and Morgan, R.F., In defense of the concept of biological aging measurement — current status, *Arch. Gerontol. Geriatr.*, 7, 191, 1988.
13. Dean, W., *Biological Aging Measurement*, The Center for Bio-Gerontology, Los Angeles, 1988.
14. Dubina, T.L., Dyundikova, V.A., and Zhuk, E.V., Biological age and its estimation. II. Assessment of biological age of albino rats by multiple regression analysis, *Exp. Gerontol.*, 18, 5, 1983.
15. Furukawa, T., Inoue, F., Kajiya, F., Inada, S., Takasugi, S., Fukui, S., Takeda, H., and Abe, H., Assessment of biological age by multiple regression analysis, *J. Gerontol.*, 30, 422, 1975.
16. Guttman, L., Some necessary conditions for common-factor analysis, *Psychometrika*, 19, 149, 1954.
17. Hayflick, L., Theories of biological aging, *Exp. Gerontol.*, 20, 145, 1985.

18. Harman, H.H., *Modern Factor Analysis,* 2nd ed., University of Chicago Press, Chicago, 1967.
19. Heikkinen, A., Kiiskinen, B., Käyhty, B., Rimpelä, M., and Vuori, I., Assessment of biological age. — Methodological study in two Finnish populations, *Gerontologia,* 20, 33, 1974.
20. Hofecker, G., Skalicky, M., Kment, A., and Niedermüller, H., Models of the biological age of the rat. I. A factor model of age parameters, *Mech. Age. Dev.,* 14, 345, 1980.
21. Hollingsworth, J.W., Hashizume, A., and Jablon, S., Correlations between tests of aging in Hiroshima subjects. — an attempt to define "physiological age", *Yale J. Bio. Med.,* 38, 11, 1965.
22. Ingram, D., Toward the behavioral assessment of biological aging in the laboratory mouse: concepts, terminology, and objectives, *Exp. Age. Res.,* 9, 225, 1983.
23. Ingram, D., Key questions in developing biomarkers of aging, *Exp. Gerontol.,* 23, 429, 1988.
24. Jalavisto, E. and Makkonen, T., On the assessment of biological age. I. A factor analysis of physiological measurements in old and young women, *Ann. Acad. Sci. Fenn. Med.,* 100, 5, 1963.
25. Jackson, R.A., Diabetes, in *Principles and Practice of Geriatric Medicine,* Pathy, M.S.J., Ed., John Wiley & Sons, London, 1985, 987.
26. Linn, B.S., Chronologic vs. biologic age in geriatric patients, in *The Physiology and Pathology of Human Aging,* Goldman, R. and Rockstein, M., Eds., Academic Press, New York, 1975, 9.
27. Masoro, E., Physiological system markers of aging, *Exp. Gerontol.,* 23, 391, 1988.
28. Nakamura, E., Kimura, M., Nagata, H., Miyao, K., and Ozeki, T., Evaluation of the progress of aging based on specific biological age as estimated by various physiological functions, *Jpn. J. Hyg.,* 36, 853, 1982 (in Japanese).
29. Nakamura, E., Development and Standardization of Theoretical Formulas for the Assessment of Physical Fitness Age as an Index of Aging, Summary Reports of Research, Japan Foundation for Health Sciences, 1985, 7. (in Japanese).
30. Nakamura, E., Assessment of biological age by principal component analysis, *Mech. Age. Dev.,* 46, 1, 1988.
31. Nakamura, E., A study on the basic nature of human biological aging processes based upon a hierarchical factor solution of the age-related physiological variables, *Mech. Age. Dev.,* 60, 153, 1991.
32. Nunnally, J.C., *Test and Measurement,* McGraw-Hill, New York, 1959.
33. Report of the Committee on Statistics of the Japan Diabetes Society, Standardization of oral glucose tolerance test, *Diabetes,* 18, 299, 1970.
34. Rockstein, M., Chesky, J.A., and Sussman, M.L., Comparative biology and evolution of aging, in *Handbook of the Biology of Aging,* Finch, C.E. and Hayflick, L., Eds., Van Nostrand Reinhold, New York, 1977, 3.
35. Schmid, J. and Leiman, J.M., The development of hierarchical factor solutions, *Psychometrika,* 22, 53, 1957.
36. Shock, N.W., Physiological aspects of aging in man, *Annu. Rev. Physiol.,* 23, 97, 1961.
37. Shock, N.W., Physical activity and the "rate of ageing", *Can. Med. Assoc. J.,* 96, 836, 1967.
38. Shock, N.W., System integration, in *Handbook of the Biology of Aging,* Finch, C.E. and Hayflick, L., Eds., Van Nostrand Reinhold, New York, 1977, 639.
39. Shock, N.W., Physiological and chronological age, in Aging — Its Chemistry, Dietz, A.A., Ed., The American Association for Clinical Chemistry, Washington, D.C., 1980, 3.
40. Strehler, B.L., *Time, Cell and Aging,* Academic Press, New York, 1977.
41. Veterans Administration Cooperative Study Group on Antihypertensive Agents, Effects of treatment on morbidity in hypertensive. II. Results in patients with diastolic blood pressure averaging 90 through 114 mm Hg, *JAMA,* 213, 1143, 1970.
42. Voitenko, V.P. and Tokar, A.V., The assessment of biological age and sex differences of human aging, *Exp. Age. Res.,* 9, 239, 1983.
43. Webster, I.W. and Logie, A.R., A relationship between functional age and health status in female subjects, *J. Gerontol.,* 31, 546, 1976.
44. World Health Organization, The Uses of Epidemiology in the Study of the Elderly, Rep. WHO Sci. Group on the Epidemiology of Aging, World Health Organization, Geneva, 1984.

CHAPTER 27
AGE DIFFERENCES IN BIOLOGICAL MARKERS OF MORTALITY

LARRY J. BRANT, JAMES L. FOZARD, AND E. JEFFREY METTER

TABLE OF CONTENTS

I. INTRODUCTION

Regardless of how chronological age is used in the determination of biological age, chronological age remains important as a point of reference or basis of comparison for any estimate of biological age. By knowing chronological age, which shall be referred to as "age" throughout this discussion, we can say whether an individual is young or old in relation to their estimated biological age. For example, Borkan et al.[3] compared a visual estimate of age made by an examining physician at first examination, who had no knowledge of the person's actual age, with the actual age. They then demonstrated that the difference in this simple estimate of age and actual age was significantly associated with a more sophisticated determination of biological age based on a number of physiological variables collected on each individual.

In practically every study of morbidity or mortality that has considered age as a factor associated with the study's outcome, age is found to have a significant association and is often the most significantly related variable. In the Seven Countries Study, Keys et al.[17] found age to be the most important risk factor associated with mortality from all causes in all of the geographic areas studied. Pinsky et al.,[20] in a study of predictors of good function for males and females in the Framingham Heart Study, showed that age had the strongest relationship with good function in a multiple logistic regression carried out separately for men and women. Using a longitudinal method of analysis for investigating hearing acuity in a study of normal aging, Brant and Fozard[6] found age to be strongly related to audiometric threshold levels in each of seven different 15-year age cohorts of males ranging from 20 to 80 years. Unlike studies of human longevity where one finds the effect of age to be positively associated with subsequent mortality, the degree of association between age and hearing acuity declines over the adult age span. This finding coincides with the interindividual differences in hearing acuity that become more striking with age.

The relationship of age with a morbid or mortal outcome is not always characterized by a simple increase or decrease in the predictive power of age over the adult age span. Halperin et al.,[13] in a study of coronary heart disease (CHD) incidence in the Framingham Heart Study, found age to be insignificant in the presence of several other well-known CHD risk factors for a 29- to 39-year-old cohort of males. However, in a similar analysis carried out for 40 to 49 year old males, age emerged as a highly significant risk factor. In a final analysis of 50 to 62 year olds, the level of significance for age declined in the presence of the same risk factors.

Age changes in biological markers and their subsequent effect on mortality will be examined using data collected by the periodic examination of voluntary participants in the Baltimore Longitudinal Study of Aging (BLSA). In addition to investigating the importance of various biological markers on mortality and how their effect changes with age, this chapter also examines where in the life cycle each marker manifests itself. These findings regarding the relationship of age to many of the important biological markers of aging should prove to be useful information in considering any method of estimating human biological age.

II. BIOLOGICAL MARKERS AND RISK ASSESSMENT

A. POPULATION

The BLSA is an ongoing multidisciplinary study begun in 1958 to study normal human aging.[22] The study is carried out at the Gerontology Research Center in Baltimore and is part of the intramural research program of the National Institute on Aging. The BLSA was initially an all-male study, with female participation beginning in 1978. Because of the short follow-up period and low number of female decedents, this report deals only with data collected on BLSA male participants. The male cohort represents a predominantly upper-middle class group of community-dwelling men. They are generally married (85%), predominantly white (95%), well educated (75% are college educated and 45% hold higher degrees), of sufficient economic means (82% consider themselves to be financially comfortable or better), consider themselves having above average health (93%), and most live in the Baltimore-Washington metropolitan area. In effect, the population represents a relatively homogeneous socioeconomic group. Such a population has proved to be useful in the study of changes that occur in normal humans as they age, and in various risk-factor studies in which the confounding effect of many socioeconomic factors on the interested outcome has been implicitly diminished.

To investigate age changes in biological markers of mortality, serial measurements of each marker on the same individual over the study period were compared with each individual's subsequent mortality or status in the study. These measurements were collected from each participant at regularly scheduled visits to the study center in Baltimore, usually 2 years apart. Data from these measurements were used to define two longitudinal study cohorts. The first cohort was younger adult males who were first examined at approximately 40 years of age and the second cohort was older adult males who were first examined at 60 years of age. The two cohorts were thus disjointed, with no one in both cohorts. Whenever possible, each individual was reexamined 10 and 20 years later.

Information from the BLSA sample on the two male cohorts used in this report is summarized in Table 1. There were 432 males in the 40-year-old cohort and 361 males in the 60-year-old cohort. Because the BLSA is in its 30th consecutive year of operation, individuals tested at 40 or 60 years of age could have a maximum follow-up of 30 years. The average length of follow-up was

Table 1 Years of follow-up, sample size, and number of decedents by age of testing for the 40-year-old and 60-year-old BLSA male cohorts

Age of testing	Years of follow-up Maximum	Years of follow-up Average	Sample size	No. deceased
		40-Year-old cohort		
40	30	14.3	432	29
50	20	10.1	261	18
60	10	5.0	153	10
		60-Year-old cohort		
60	30	14.1	361	134
70	20	7.7	257	88
80	10	3.2	101	31

14.3 years for the 40 year olds and 14.1 years for the 60 year olds. Attrition in the BLSA male population has been measured and discussed,[21] and in a recent paper, Brant and Greene[7] demonstrated no difference in the observed values of several important physiological variables with respect to age between active and dropout participants. Table 1 indicates that there were 29 total deaths in the 40-year-old cohort, of which 18 occurred after 10 years of follow-up and 10 after 20 years of follow-up. Similarly, there were 134 total deaths in the 60-year-old cohort with 88 and 31 occurring after 10 and 20 years, respectively.

B. BIOLOGICAL MARKERS

The biological markers examined in this report are risk factors that were found to be predictive of morbidity and mortality in other studies. Most of those considered here have been used by others who have investigated the concept of biological or functional age.[4,9] These markers include anthropometric, biochemical, physiological, and psychological variables. Table 2 gives the list of markers that were considered in this report. A description of how these markers are measured in the BLSA is given in Chapter IV, "Tests Administered", of the 1984 book by Shock et al.[22] Measurements on the biological markers were obtained on each individual at their different ages of testing. By considering the association of each of these markers with mortality at the different ages of measurement, we can determine the age at which these markers manifest themselves and examine the resulting age changes in the degree of association that each of these manifested variables has with mortality.

C. STATISTICAL MODEL

For each of the ages tested in both the 40- and 60-year-old cohorts, the relationships between each of the biological markers in Table 2 and mortality were examined using the proportional hazards model.[10,14] The model is given by

$$h\ (t \mid x) = h_0(t) \exp\ (\beta x)$$

where t represents the age of the individual at any time during his follow-up period, x is the biological marker or explanatory factor believed to affect mortality, $h_0(t)$ is the force of mortality independent of x, and β is the regression coefficient or parameter to be estimated from the data. The response variables being modeled are the age-specific mortality rates. Long-term mortality was measured through monitoring the vital status of all participants throughout the course of the study. When a person's death was reported, death certificate information was obtained in order to

Table 2 Biological markers used in the assessment of mortality at different ages for both age cohorts

Total serum cholesterol (mg/dl)	Body mass index (kg/m^2)
Serum triglycerides (mg/dl)	Visual acuity (Snellen decimal)[a]
White blood cell count ($10^3/mm^3$)	Auditory threshold at 500–2000 cps (dB)[b]
Hemoglobin (g/dl)	Auditory threshold at 8000 cps (dB)
Creatinine clearance (ml/24 h)	Simple reaction time (ms)
FEV-1 (liters)	Benton visual memory test (errors)
Systolic blood pressure (mmHg)	Wechsler adult intelligence scale
Diastolic blood pressure (mmHg)	Vocabulary test (number correct)
Cardiac diagnosis (0, 1, 2)[c]	

[a] *Visual acuity is a binocular measurement without correction and is expressed as the decimal representation of the Snellen ratio.*
[b] *Average auditory threshold at pure tones of 500, 1000, and 2000 cps.*
[c] *Cardiac diagnosis is based on patient history, resting ECG, exercise ECG, and thallium scan of heart. Based on these 4 elements, a score of 0 represents no evidence of cardiac disease, 1 represents possible evidence of disease, and 2 represents definite CHD.*

determine the exact date and cause of death. This information was confirmed, when possible, through family members, physician, and/or hospital records.

Estimates of $h_0(t)$ and the unknown parameter β along with an estimate of its standard error were obtained using a maximum likelihood analysis,[14] in which the likelihood function is based on the product of the conditional probabilities of dying at each time where a death was observed in each cohort of our male population. Tests of significance for each biological marker were obtained using the usual asymptotic properties of these estimates. For those biological markers found significant, the relative risk (RR) per unit of measurement change in the marker x was calculated by the formula

$$\mathrm{RR} = h(t \mid x + 1)/h(t \mid x) = \exp\,(((x + 1) - x)\,\beta) = \exp\,(\beta)$$

where β is replaced by its estimated value. Using the calculated value of RR along with the standard error of the estimate of β, 95% confidence intervals were obtained for each of the RR values. These values provide the basis of comparing age differences in the degrees of manifestation for each of the biological markers found to be significantly associated with mortality.

III. BIOLOGICAL MARKERS AND AGING

Each of the markers listed in Table 2 were considered in an analysis using the proportional hazards model. For each of the three ages in both age cohorts, the hazard function $h(t \mid x)$ was estimated, and tests of significance were performed on the resulting coefficients. Those markers found to be significantly associated with mortality at the $p < 0.05$, for at least one of the ages in one of the cohorts, are given in Table 3. The table also gives the mean values, standard deviations, and ranges for these variables at all different ages.

A. BIOCHEMICAL MARKERS

Figure 1 shows the results of the hazards function analysis for total serum cholesterol, serum triglycerides, white blood cell count, and hemoglobin. Each estimated relative risk per unit of

Table 3 Mean values, standard deviations (S.D.), and other characteristics by age for biological markers found to be significantly associated with mortality in 40-year-old and 60-year-old cohorts

Biological marker	Age 40	Age 50	Age 60	Age 60	Age 70	Age 80
Cholesterol						
Mean	214.4	211.1	193.7	237.9	221.0	182.9
S.D.	46.0	42.6	30.7	47.4	42.5	37.4
Range	115–476	126–368	140–268	97–483	125–356	84–328
Triglycerides						
Mean	145.3	154.2	154.9	131.8	134.0	131.1
S.D.	97.1	95.1	116.9	66.8	94.1	68.6
Range	40–640	34–500	44–733	39–439	43–727	49–392
White blood count						
Mean	7.04	6.75	6.60	6.93	6.88	7.15
S.D.	1.85	1.79	1.43	1.89	1.72	3.04
Range	3.6–15.3	3.1–15.2	3.6–11.6	3.2–17.1	2.5–18.7	3.5–30.4
Hemoglobin						
Mean	15.25	15.25	15.16	15.19	14.97	14.69
S.D.	1.03	1.00	1.00	1.08	1.18	1.26
Range	11.3–18.2	12.5–18.5	12.6–17.7	11.5–19.1	7.8–18.2	10.9–17.8
FEV-1						
Mean	4.01	3.67	3.19	3.29	2.89	2.71
S.D.	0.66	0.67	0.58	0.55	0.62	0.58
Range	1.9–6.0	1.3–5.5	1.7–4.8	1.5–4.7	1.1–4.3	0.7–3.6
Systolic pressure						
Mean	120.1	122.8	125.8	133.3	137.6	139.2
S.D.	13.9	15.3	18.2	20.7	21.5	25.1
Range	88–178	92–180	85–200	88–200	95–206	94–230
Diastolic pressure						
Mean	79.9	81.8	80.9	83.9	81.2	78.8
S.D.	10.5	10.5	10.8	11.5	11.0	11.1
Range	50–130	58–124	44–104	60–122	55–120	55–108
Cardiac diagnosis						
% Scores 0	—	88	66	75	55	37
1	—	9	21	13	20	32
2	—	3	13	12	25	31
Visual acuity						
Mean	0.683	0.513	0.451	0.460	0.338	0.248
S.D.	0.541	0.452	0.424	0.394	0.325	0.251
Range	0–1.54	0–1.54	0–1.54	0–1.54	0–1.33	0–1.11
Body mass index						
Mean	25.56	25.88	25.78	25.57	25.40	24.87
S.D.	3.27	3.40	3.05	2.92	3.08	3.18
Range	18.3–40.0	18.9–41.1	18.3–43.5	18.8–37.2	18.5–36.6	17.9–37.8

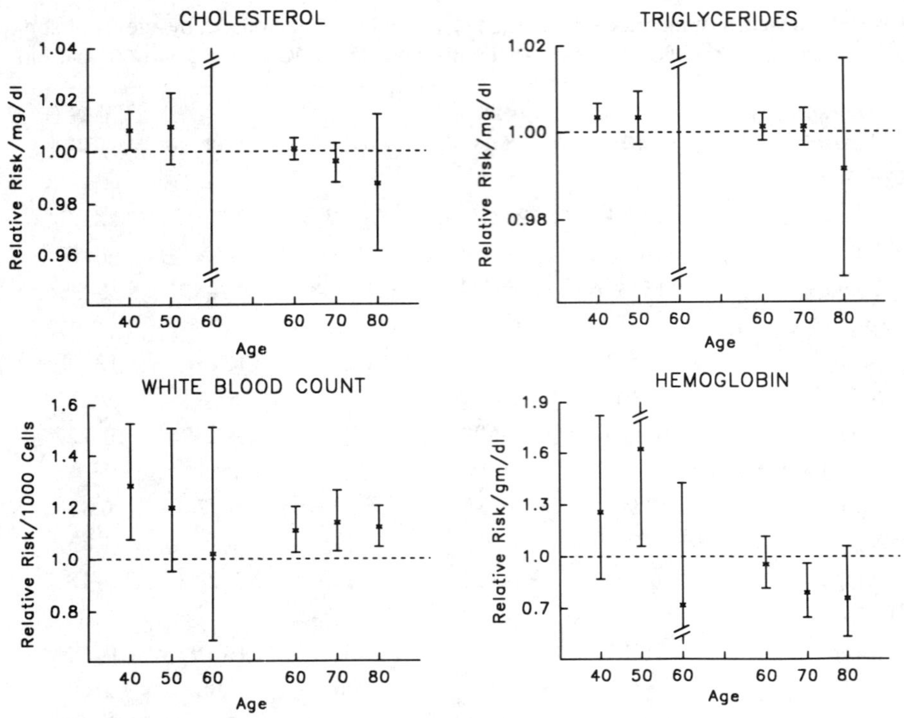

Figure 1 Relative risks (*) of mortality and 95% confidence intervals for the biochemical markers found to be significantly associated with mortality for at least one of the ages tested in the young (ages 40, 50, 60) and old (ages 60, 70, 80) adult male cohorts.

measurement change is denoted by an asterisk in the figure, and the vertical line passing through the asterisk is the corresponding 95% confidence interval for the relative risk. Confidence intervals lying totally above or below the value of 1 indicate a significant risk of mortality associated with the biological marker at that age. The relative risk per unit change for cholesterol was found to be 1.008/1 mg/dl change. Using the proportionality property of the model, this value can be used to find the estimated risk of mortality for any desired difference in cholesterol levels. For example, a total serum cholesterol value of 240 mg/dl relative to 200 mg/dl carries an estimated $(1.008)^{40} = 1.37$ greater risk of mortality for a given individual. As the 95% confidence intervals in the figure indicate, cholesterol shows a significant increase in the risk of mortality only at age 40. The estimated risk remains at approximately the same level for those who were reevaluated at age 50; however, the predictiveness of this marker has diminished somewhat because of the widened confidence interval. By age 60 for those still surviving in the 40-year-old cohort, there is no evidence present of cholesterol being associated with mortality. The very large width of the interval is indicative of the sample size of 153 males with only 10 deceased in the maximum possible follow-up of 10 years after measurement (Table 1). Neither is there any increase in risk in the 60-year-old cohort evaluated at age 60, as well as the older ages. Because of the larger sample size and larger number of deaths at age 60 in the older cohort, the 95% confidence interval here is quite narrow. Thus, by age 60 no evidence is present to suggest that the cholesterol levels occurring in this population are significantly related to mortality.

An examination of the mean values in Table 3 indicates the gradual reduction in cholesterol values for those remaining in the study from each cohort. In addition, the observed maximum values decreased from 476 to 268 mg/dl in the 40-year-old cohort and from 483 to 328 mg/dl in the 60-year-old cohort. The mean cholesterol values for those who died in the younger cohort were approximately 40 to 50 mg/dl higher than the population average at each age.

Thus, total serum cholesterol is a biological marker of mortality which was found to manifest itself at age 40. No evidence was present to conclude a significant increased risk at the other ages in the 40-year-old cohort. However, there tended to be a declining level of importance with respect to age in the 60-year-old cohort. This finding coincides with risk factor analyses of CHD carried out by the Framingham Study.[15] Kannel and Gordon[15] showed that the relationship to risk was strongest at the young ages and decreased with age. In fact, they showed that the predictive power of the most important CHD risk factors declines over the adult age span.

The relative risks for serum triglycerides followed essentially the same pattern with age as the results for total serum cholesterol. The only age at which triglycerides manifested themselves was at 40 years, with the relative risk of mortality per unit (mg/dl) change given by 1.0034. As with cholesterol, no significant risk in mortality is evident from our data at the older ages. This is not surprising because triglyceride and cholesterol are strongly related biological factors.

Because of the correlation between these variables, care must be taken in interpreting the results from any multivariate analysis that includes both these variables. Cambien et al[8] demonstrated this point in an examination of coronary death in "normocholesterolemic" subjects in the Paris Prospective Study. They found both cholesterol and triglyceride to be significant only in the presence of an interaction term. Our data shows evidence of this from examining the mean and maximum values given in Table 3. As we have seen, the cholesterol values are decreasing with age, while the triglyceride values tend to be nondecreasing.

White blood cell count showed an increased risk in mortality of 1.28 per unit change in the 40 year olds, where the count is given in units of 1000 cells per cubic millimeter. For those retested in this age cohort, no evidence of an increased risk in mortality was found. In addition, the mean values also declined with age. In the 60-year-old cohort, the relative risks of mortality at every age were all significantly greater than 1, while the mean values tended to increase with age.

Thus, white blood count manifested itself in young adulthood and diminished in importance to mortality for ages 50 and 60 in the younger cohort, perhaps because of the smaller sample sizes and number of deaths observed at these ages. These ages of repeated measurement bear further investigation, especially in light of the consistently high risk of mortality found for all ages in the older cohort.

The last set of relative risks in Figure 1 are for hemoglobin. For this biological marker of mortality, two different trends appear to be emerging. First, an increase in hemoglobin was found to carry an increase in the risk of mortality in the younger cohort. This risk was significant at age 50 with a value of 1.62 per unit change in gram per deciliter. Second, an increase in hemoglobin was found to be associated with a decrease in mortality in the older cohort. At age 70, the relative risk was 0.79. Thus, for example, an individual with a hemoglobin of 15 as compared to 11 would have a 61% lower risk of mortality.

Hemoglobin thus appears to manifest itself differently in the younger and older age groups. The increase in risk of mortality in the 40-year-old cohort perhaps reflects the greater proportion of smokers at the younger ages. Smoking has long been known to affect numerous biochemical markers, and it is a variable that merits special attention as a possible confounding variable in any analysis. The decrease in the risk of mortality associated with an increase in hemoglobin is indicative of decreases in hemoglobin that often have been associated with higher mortality at older ages. As people age, they develop a variety of diseases, many of which result in the reduction of hemoglobin levels.

B. PHYSIOLOGICAL MARKERS

Several different physiological markers were found to be significantly associated with mortality in one or both of the age cohorts. They were systolic and diastolic blood pressure, cardiac diagnosis, forced expiratory volume in 1 s (FEV-1), and visual acuity. Figure 2 shows the corresponding age-specific relative risks of mortality for both blood pressures, cardiac diagnosis, and FEV-1, and Figure 3 gives the results for visual acuity.

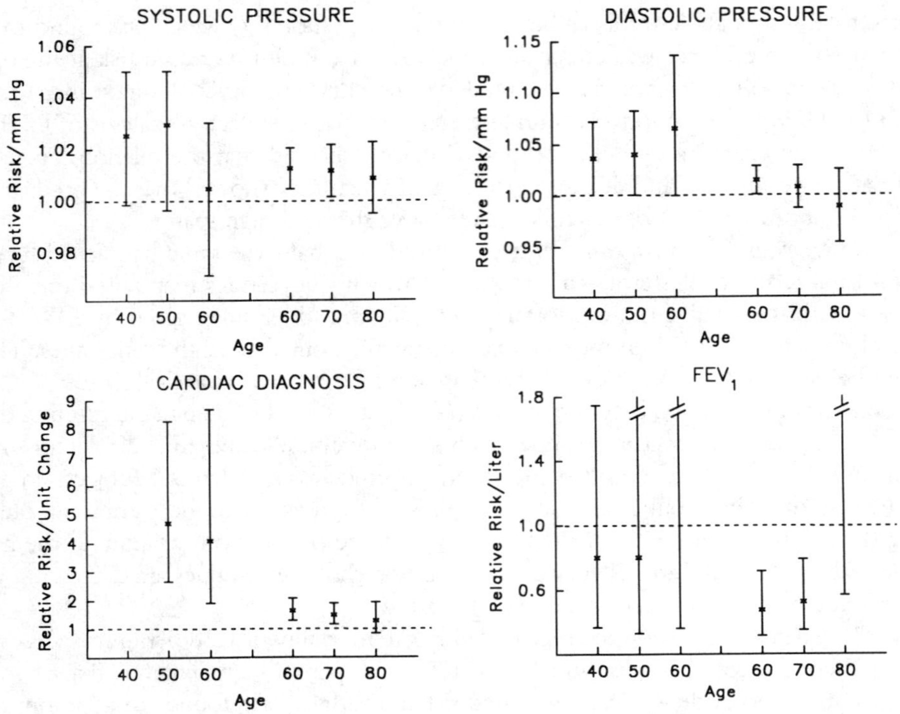

Figure 2 Relative risks (*) of mortality and 95% confidence intervals for physiological markers found to be significantly associated with mortality for at least one of the ages tested in the young (ages 40, 50, 60) and old (ages 60, 70, 80) adult male cohorts.

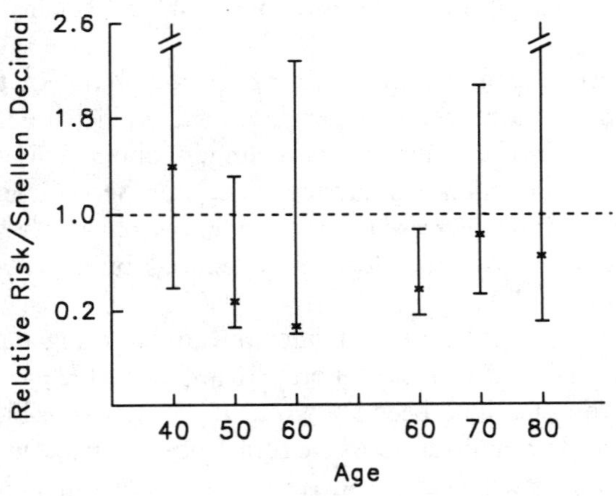

Figure 3 Relative risks (*) of mortality and 95% confidence intervals for visual acuity measurements taken in the young (ages 40, 50, 60) and old (ages 60, 70, 80) adult male cohorts.

Systolic blood pressure was found to manifest itself at only the ages of 60 and 70 in the older-age cohort. The estimated values of the relative risks of mortality were 1.012 and 1.011/1 mm Hg increase. Thus, a 60-year-old with a 20 mmHg increase in systolic pressure would have a $(1.012)^{20} = 1.27$ times greater risk of mortality. The relative risk at 80 years was estimated to have a similar value, though there was not enough evidence to find significance. No evidence of an increased risk of mortality for systolic blood pressure was found in the younger 40-year-old cohort.

The mean systolic values showed a gradual increase over all the ages studied. This coincides with the well-documented age-related increases found in both cross-sectional and longitudinal studies of systolic blood pressure. Data from the Framingham Study[15,16] has illustrated this very well. Based on our hazards analysis, systolic blood pressure was found to be significantly associated with mortality for blood pressure measurements taken at 60 and 70 years of age in the older-age cohort. Because death due to stroke accounts for a larger percentage of the deceased BLSA males at the older ages, this finding is consistent with the importance of systolic pressure reported in a recent study of predictors of stroke-associated mortality in an upper middle class population of community-dwelling elderly in Rancho Bernardo, CA.[18]

The results for diastolic blood pressure were different than those for systolic pressure. Diastolic pressure manifested itself at every age of observation in the younger cohort, but manifested itself at only age 60 in the older cohort. For the 40-year-old cohort, the relative risks of mortality were 1.037, 1.040, and 1.066/mmHg at ages 40, 50, and 60, respectively. At age 60 in the 60-year-old longitudinal cohort, the relative risk was 1.015, but as the small 95% confidence interval indicates, this estimate is quite reliable and within the range of the other 95% confidence intervals for the younger cohort. It should also be noted that the mean diastolic blood pressure values tended to increase up to age 60 in the older cohort, but started to decline sometime between the ages of 60 and 70. This compares with the findings of the Framingham Study[15,16] and with other studies as well.

Thus, diastolic pressure was found to manifest itself with regard to mortality at the younger adult ages of observation. A large proportion of the deaths in this younger group are due to coronary heart disease. This suggests that in this population, diastolic blood pressure might also be a good predictor of coronary heart disease-associated mortality. In any case, systolic and diastolic blood pressure manifested themselves at different ages, with mortality more strongly associated with systolic pressure in older males and with diastolic pressure in younger males.

The next physiological marker found to be significantly associated with mortality was cardiac diagnosis. As seen in Table 2, cardiac diagnosis was based upon a medical interview and history conducted by a physician, a resting electrocardiogram (ECG), an exercise stress ECG, and a thallium scan of the heart done during exercise. This information was reviewed by staff cardiologists and a score of 0, 1, or 2 was assigned representing no, some, or definite evidence of CHD. As might be expected, this marker was highly associated with mortality in the younger cohort. At age 50, the risk of mortality was approximately 22 times greater ($(4.69)^2$) in those males with a diagnostic score of 2 relative to a score of 0. A similar high relative risk was found at age 60. No analysis was available at age 40 because this marker was not collected in the earlier years of the study when many of the 40 year olds were first examined. In the older cohort, significant relative risks were found at age 60 (1.69) and age 70 (1.49). These values are considerably lower than the relative risks for the 40-year-old cohort; however, their level of significance is quite strong as evidenced by the narrow confidence interval. By age 80, the relative risk for cardiac diagnosis was no longer found to be statistically significant.

An examination of the percentage distribution of the cardiac diagnosis scores show an interesting pattern in the different ages. At age 80, the scores are essentially evenly distributed, with only 37% of the males having no evidence of CHD. At age 60 the corresponding percentage of disease-free males was 75% in the older cohort and 66% in the younger cohort. At age 50 in the younger cohort, 88% of the males showed no evidence of CHD.

In summary, cardiac diagnosis was found to be a biological marker of mortality that manifested itself at all the ages studied, except the most elderly. In younger adulthood, a nonzero score carries a very high increased risk of mortality. At age 80 the highest percentage of CHD was observed, but this did not show any significant increase in the risk of mortality at this age.

Pulmonary function as measured by FEV_1 showed a decreased risk in mortality for increased FEV-1 values only at the ages of 60 and 70 in the older cohort. The estimates of the relative risks per 1 l increase in FEV-1 were 0.47 and 0.52, respectively. If a 60-year-old BLSA male had a FEV-1

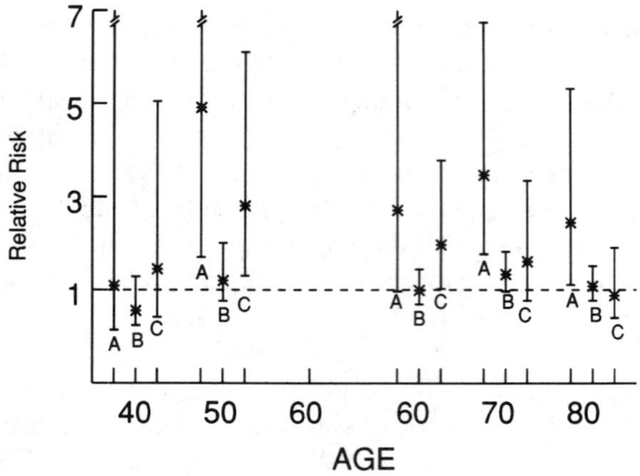

Figure 4 Relative risks (*) of mortality and 95% confidence intervals for BMI < 20 (A), 25 ≤ BMI < 30 (B) and BMI ≥ 30 (C) relative to 20 ≤ BMI < 25 for height and weight measurements taken in the young (ages 40,50,60) and old (ages 60,70,80) adult male cohorts.

value of 4 liters instead of 2 l, he would have a 78% lower risk of mortality ($(0.47)^2 = 0.22$). Again, because of the lack of data at age 60 in the younger longitudinal cohort, no evidence of any risk was found (RR = 1).

Other population-based studies have shown an association between poor pulmonary function and mortality.[2] Similar to those studies, the mean FEV-1 values for the BLSA males declined with age from a high of 4.01 l at age 40 to a low 2.71 l at age 80. The effect of this variable on mortality, however, did not manifest itself until the ages of 60 and 70, as seen in the older cohort. Thus, while higher FEV-1 values were suggestive of a lower risk of mortality at all ages studied, their importance based on our evidence was most profound in the older adult male group.

The final physiological marker found to be related to mortality was visual acuity, which was a binocular measurement without correction. The only age showing any significant degree of manifestation with mortality was at age 60 in the older cohort (Figure 3). At this age, the relative risk of mortality was estimated to be 0.37. The mean values of visual acuity decreased from 0.683 at age 40 to 0.248 at age 80 (Table 3). These values represent Snellen fractions of approximately 20/30 and 20/80, respectively. The best uncorrected visual acuity was 1.54 (20/13), which was observed in the younger cohort, while at age 80 in the older cohort the highest acuity observed was 1.11 (20/18). Thus, if a 60-year-old male's vision decreased from 20/30 to 20/80 his risk of mortality would increase by 52% as $RR = (0.37)^{0.25-0.67} = 1/(0.37)^{0.42} = 1.52$.

Gittings and Fozard,[12] in a recent examination of visual acuity in the BLSA, also showed that there were both significant longitudinal and cross-sectional age-related changes in acuity. In the present study, while the estimated RR of mortality tended to show a decrease in risk associated with higher measures of visual acuity, the only age to show a significant association between visual acuity and mortality was at age 60 in the older cohort.

C. ANTHROPOMETRIC MARKERS

Measurements of each person's height and body weight were used to obtain a value of relative body weight. The value calculated was body mass index (BMI) which is defined as weight in kilograms (kg) divided by the square of height in meters (m). Data collected in a number of studies has shown a correlation between BMI and mortality, and the data from many of these studies suggests that this association is characterized by a nonlinear U- or J-shaped relationship.[11,19,23] Because of these studies and a similar finding in a study of obesity and mortality in BLSA males,[5] BMI has been treated as

Table 4 Biological markers found to be significantly associated with mortality at the youngest, middle, and oldest (40, 60, 80) ages tested

	Age	
40	**60**	**80**
White blood count	White blood count	White blood count
Cardiac diagnosis	Cardiac diagnosis	
Diastolic pressure	Systolic pressure	
Total cholesterol		
Triglycerides		
	FEV-1	
	Visual acuity	
	BMI	BMI

a categorical variable in the hazard model analysis. The categories used were <20 (lean), 20 to 24.9 (normal), 25 to 29.9 (overweight), and ≥30 (obese) kg/m^2. Relative risks of mortality for BMI were calculated as relative to the normal range of $20 \leq BMI < 25$.

Figure 4 shows the results of the hazards analyses for the different ages in the two cohorts. No results are available for age 60 in the younger cohort because not enough deaths occurred to estimate RR in all three weight groups. The labels A, B, and C in the figure denote the RR results for the lean, overweight, and obese BMI groups, respectively, relative to the so-called normal BMI group. An examination of the figure shows no significant difference in the risk of mortality for BMI at age 40. However, there is an increased risk for obesity relative to a normal BMI at the ages of 50 and 60, but there is no evidence of such an increased risk in the older ages of 70 and 80. On the other hand, lean males showed an increased risk of mortality relative to the reference BMI normal range at the ages of 70 and 80, and the lean weight group also tended to have an increased risk at the ages of 50 and 60 as well. No increased risk of mortality was found for the overweight group at any of the ages studied.

These results are consistent with age-related differences in the impact of weight on mortality discussed by Andres et al.[1] in a reexamination of data from the 1979 Build Study. The relationship of RR with respect to their corresponding weight categories has a U- or J-shaped nature at each of the ages studied. The mean values of BMI in Table 3 tend to increase at the ages studied in the younger cohort, and they tend to decrease with age in the older cohort.

Thus, BMI is a biological marker that not only manifests itself at different ages, but the nature of the manifestation varies with the value of the marker in a manner in which the risk of mortality does not change in a proportional way. This has been demonstrated through the use of categorical variables in assessing the RR of mortality corresponding to BMI. Obese males were found to have a significantly greater risk of mortality over normal weight males only at the ages of 50 and 60. No such increased risk was found in the oldest males. Leanness, however, was found to be associated with an increased risk of mortality in the older males. This could be due to the fact that leanness results with the occurrence of disease in the elderly, or that lean males are less equipped for dealing with various medical conditions and illnesses that threaten life in the elderly.

IV. SUMMARY AND CONCLUSIONS

This report has examined the relationship between a number of different kinds of biological markers and mortality at several ages in two longitudinal cohorts of younger and older adult males. The markers examined represent variables that have been used in various investigations of the concept of biological and functional age. Table 4 summarizes our results. Of all the markers examined, only

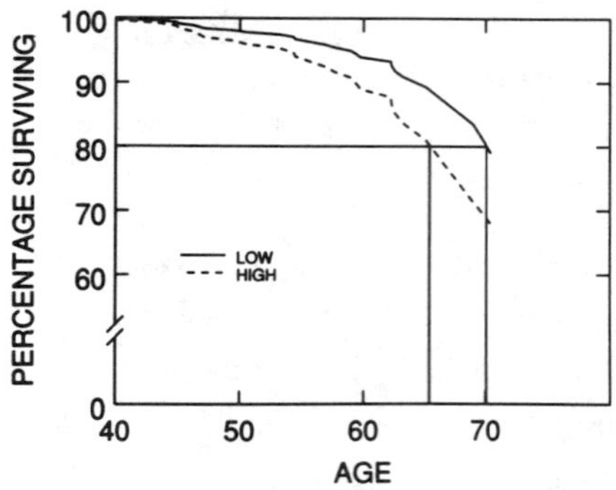

Figure 5 Estimated survival probabilities for BLSA males measured at age 40 with low (diastolic pressure = 75 mmHg, serum cholesterol = 200 mg/dl, serum triglycerides = 110 mg/dl), and high (diastolic pressure = 95 mmHg, serum cholesterol = 250 mg/dl, serum triglycerides = 140 mg/dl) levels of coronary risk factors. The vertical lines show the ages at which both the high and low risk groups have an estimated 80% chance of surviving the next year.

white blood cell count manifested itself in the youngest adult males (age 40), the middle-aged adult males (age 60), and the oldest adult males (age 80). The RR per unit change were all significantly greater than 1.0, with a slightly higher estimate of risk at age 40 than at the ages of 60 and 80. Cardiac diagnosis showed a significant importance at all the ages examined except for the most elderly. Furthermore, the estimated RR showed a reduction with age. Systolic and diastolic blood pressure appeared to perform differently with age. Diastolic pressure manifested itself more at age 40, while systolic manifested itself more at age 60. Neither showed any evidence of an association at age 80.

Other significant markers behaved differently with regard to age as well. Total serum cholesterol and serum triglycerides were found to manifest themselves only at age 40. Forced expiratory volume in 1s and visual acuity were associated with mortality only at age 60. The association of BMI with mortality differed not only by age, but the relative risks for changes in BMI varied in an unproportional manner. For example, obese levels of BMI showed a significantly greater risk of mortality over normal levels of BMI at age 60, but this association disappeared by age 80. Lean levels showed no significant change in risk relative to the normal level at age 60; however, at age 80 leanness was the only level to manifest itself.

The results from the study of these biological markers demonstrate that the relationship of a given marker to mortality can be quite different depending on the individual's age of measurement. This suggests that special care should be taken when using such age-specific measurements in any evaluation of biological age. This could take the form of stratifying the study population by the age of observation in some multivariate analysis of the entire study population, or by first stratifying the entire population into limited age ranges and then carrying out separate evaluations for each age group.

For example, in an analysis of a marker such as hemoglobin, which does not allow for a special treatment of the age of measurement but considers age in a continuous fashion, one could conclude that hemoglobin has no association with mortality. However, as seen from the results presented in this report (Figure 1), hemoglobin is a marker in which increases in the gram per deciliter level are associated with an increased risk of mortality in the younger adult cohort and a decreased risk in the older cohort. As mentioned earlier, often there are confounding variables, such as smoking, which can make the interpretation of results more difficult.

Finally, the potential impact that several of these markers can have together on an individual health status indicator such as biological age is illustrated in Figure 5. The figure shows the estimated ages at which there is an 80% probability of surviving the next year for a high and low risk group of BLSA males measured at age 40. The biological markers considered in the multivariate survival analysis using the proportional hazards model were diastolic blood pressure, total serum cholesterol, and serum triglycerides, all important CHD risk factors and all factors among the variables found to individually manifest themselves in the 40-year-old BLSA males. The high-risk group was defined as males with a diastolic pressure of 95 mmHg, a cholesterol of 250 mg/dl, and a triglyceride of 140 mg/dl. The low risk group was taken to be males with a diastolic pressure of 75 mmHg, a cholesterol of 200 mg/dl, and a triglyceride of 110 mg/dl. Figure 5 shows an approximate 5-year difference in the estimated ages at which there is an 80% yearly survival rate. These ages were found to occur near 70 and 65, respectively, for the low- and high-risk groups.

This chapter has demonstrated that in examining biological markers of mortality, the issue goes beyond whether a marker is important to where in the life cycle it manifests. The combined effect of these important markers has a definite impact on longevity which can change with the age at which the individual is measured. Thus, any formulation of biological age is much more complex than a group of markers which are highly correlated across the entire age span.

REFERENCES

1. Andres, R., Elahi, D., Tobin, J.D., Muller, D.C., and Brant, L., Impact of age on weight goals, *Ann. Intern. Med.,* 103, 1030, 1985.
2. Ashley, F., Kannel, W.B., Sorlie, P.D., and Masson, R., Pulmonary function: relation to aging, cigarette habit, and mortality, *Ann. Intern. Med.,* 82, 739, 1975.
3. Borkan, G.A., Bachman, S.S., and Norris, A.H., Comparison of visually estimated age with physiologically predicted age as indicators of rates of aging, *Soc. Sci. Med.,* 16, 197, 1982.
4. Borkan, G.A. and Norris, A.H., Assessment of biological age using a profile of physical parameters, *J. Gerontol.,* 35, 177, 1980.
5. Brant, L.J., Andres, R., and Tobin, J.D., A longitudinal examination of the association between obesity and mortality, in *Proc. Social Statistics Section of the American Statistical Association,* American Statistical Association, Washington, D.C., 1986, 222
6. Brant, L.J. and Fozard, J.L., Age changes in pure-tone hearing thresholds in a longitudinal study of normal human aging, *J. Acoust. Soc. Am,.* 88, 813, 1990.
7. Brant, L.J. and Greene, M.E., Cohort differences in a study of aging, in *Proc. Social Statistics Section of the American Statistical Association,* American Statistical Association, Washington, D.C., 1988, 412.
8. Cambien, F., Jacqueson, A., Richard, J.L., Warnet, J.M., Ducimetiere P., and Claude J.R., Is the level of serum triglyceride a significant predictor of coronary death in "normocholesterolemic" subjects?, *Am. J. Epidemiol.,* 124, 624, 1986.
9. Costa, P.T. Jr. and McCrae, R.R., Functional age: a conceptual and empirical critique, in *Second Conference on the Epidemiology of Aging,* Haynes, S.G. and Feinleib, M., Eds., NIH Publ. No. 80-969, U.S. Government Printing Office, Washington, D.C., 1980, 23
10. Cox, D.R., Regression models and life-tables, *J. R. Stat. Soc., Ser. A,* 34, 187, 1972.
11. Dyer, A.R., Stamler, J., Berkson, D.M., and Lindberg, H.A., Relationship of relative weight and body mass index to 14-year mortality in the Chicago Peoples Gas Company Study, *J. Chronic. Dis.,* 28, 109,
12. Gittings, N.S. and Fozard, J.L., Age related changes in visual acuity, *Exp. Gerontol.,* 21, 423, 1986.
13. Halperin, M., Blackwelder, W.C., and Verter, J.I., Estimation of the multivariate logistic risk function: a comparison of the discriminant function and maximum likelihood approaches, *J. Chronic. Dis.,* 24, 125, 1971.
14. Kalbfleisch, J.D. and Prentice, R.L., *The Statistical Analysis of Failure Time Data,* John Wiley & Sons, New York, 1980.
15. Kannel, W.B. and Gordon, T., *The Framingham Study. An Epidemiological Investigation of Cardiovascular Disease.,* DHEW Publ. No. 1740-0320, U.S. Government Printing Office, Washington, D.C., 1971.
16. Kannel, W.B. and Gordon, T., *The Framingham Study. An Epidemiological Investigation of Cardiovascular Disease,* DHEW Publ. No. (NIH) 74-478, U.S. Government Printing Office, Washington, D.C., 1973.

17. Keys, A., Menotti, A., Aravanis, C., Blackburn, H., Djordevic, B.S., Buzina, R., Dontas, A.S., Fidanza, F., Karvonen, M.J., Kimura, N., Mohacek, I., Nedeljkovic, S., Puddu, V., Punsar, S., Taylor, H.L., Conti, S., Kromhout, D., and Toshima, H., The Seven Countries Study: 2,289 deaths in 15 years, *Prev. Med.*, 13, 141, 1984.
18. Khaw, K., Barrett-Connor, E., Suarez, L., and Criqui, M.H., Predictors of stroke-associated mortality in the elderly, *Stroke,* 15, 244, 1984.
19. Metropolitan Life Insurance Company., *Build Study 1979*, Society of Actuaries and Association of Life Insurance Medical Directors of America, New York, 1980.
20. Pinsky, J.L., Leaverton, P.E., and Stokes, J., Predictors of good function: The Framingham Study, *J. Chronic. Dis.,* 40, 159S, 1987.
21. Sharma, S.K., Tobin, J.D., and Brant, L.J., Factors affecting attrition in the Baltimore Longitudinal Study of Aging, *Exp. Gerontol.,* 21, 329, 1986.
22. Shock, N.W., Greulich, R.C., Andres, R., Arenberg, D., Costa, P.T., Lakatta, E.G., and Tobin, J.D., *Normal Human Aging: The Baltimore Longitudinal Study of Aging*, NIH Publ. No. 84-2450, U.S. Government Printing Office, Washington, D.C., 1984.
23. Waaler, H.T., Height, weight and mortality: the Norwegian experience, *Acta Med. Scand. Suppl.,* 679, 1, 1984.

CHAPTER 28

ASSESSMENT OF THE ADEQUACY OF THE MULTIREGRESSION METHOD TO ESTIMATE BIOLOGICAL AGE

Toshiyuki Furukawa

TABLE OF CONTENTS

I. INTRODUCTION

The expression of an objective reference value of aging by an index such as a mathematical formula is considered to be important in facilitating the understanding of aging and the development of related research. Since 1967, the author along with colleagues has provided evidence demonstrating that adoption of a mathematical model using a multivariate regression analysis for estimating biological age is possible.[4,5,13]

In addition, a useful simulation model for age-dependent mortality rates based on a random Monte Carlo analysis by the authors,[6] as well as a mathematical model for an accurate understanding of the age-dependent mortality rate curve by adoption of the mixed Weibull distribution function, were proposed also by the authors.[8]

In this chapter, the concept of research on estimating human chronological age which could serve as a standard for determining the degree of senescence is briefly reviewed from the author's previous paper.[5] Then, the adequacy adopting this method to estimate biological aging based on certain biological parameters is evaluated by other multivariate analytical techniques such as principal

0-8493-0129-7/94/$0.00+$.50

component analysis, which has no external criterion. The part of the latter analysis was reported in a conference by the authors,[7] and quoted as an exercise case in a textbook of medical statistics.[9]

II. ESTIMATION OF CHRONOLOGICAL AGE BY MULTIPLE REGRESSION ANALYSIS

The most adequate means of expressing the degree of senescence is to use chronological age, because most of one's activities within society such as schooling, work, and retirement are generally determined based on age. Because chronological age stipulates the basic role in social life, the close association between this expression of age and daily decision making may show its superiority over other measures.

In addition, the physician often relates the health condition of subjects to the physical condition at a certain age. In the case of the elderly, for example, one can usually hear the following expression as "though 70 years old, he maintains the sprightliness of a man in the 50s". Therefore, an attempt to estimate chronological age by a multiple regression equation was started.

A. METHOD

Several physical laboratory examinations are known to exhibit clear age dependency; however, it is impossible to estimate age from the results of one or two examinations. Therefore, from the physical laboratory examinations exhibiting clear age dependency, a suitable combination of those physical examinations were empirically selected by trial and error in preparing multiple regression formulas to estimate chronological age. The ease of performing the examination was an important condition in the selection of these laboratory tests. Details of these many efforts are explained in previous reports by Furukawa et al.[4,5]

First, kidney functions such as renal blood flow, glomerular filtration rate, and urine concentration ability of the kidney were clearly demonstrated to be age dependent. In order to express kidney function, we utilized the PSP (phenolsulfophthalein) test whereby 15-min excretion rates of PSP are determined. This test is easy to handle and closely reflects renal blood flow. Because respiratory function is also known to exhibit age dependency, vital capacity (VCAP) was also selected. Age dependency in relation to systolic blood pressure (SBP) is represented by a formula for calculating blood pressure, [age + 90], and diastolic blood pressure (DBP) also showed a tendency to be elevated corresponding with an increase in age. Lowering of visual accommodation, which is experienced by the elderly during the progress of presbyopia (farsightedness) is also known to be age dependent, and this alternation in function was expressed as the range of visual accommodation (ACR, ACL). The velocity of nerve conductance is also reportedly reduced with increased age. Instead of directly measuring nerve conductance, the change in the threshold of vibratory sensation produced by 300 Hz applied to the tip of the index finger (VIBR, VIBL) was measured as a simple index of nerve sensitivity. Both the right and left side of the eye or the index finger were utilized for the measurement of visual accommodation, or vibration sensitivity, respectively. The suffixes R or L indicates right or left side. Although cardiac output is considered to show significant age-dependent change, the laboratory examination did not include a simple method for measurement of cardiac output and was subsequently eliminated from this study. Body height (HT) and weight (WT) were added to correct the effect of the body size on physical examination data.

A total of 111 healthy males, whose ages ranged from the 20s to the 80s, were subjects in this study. The numbers of subjects of each age class are 20s, 24; 30s, 38; 40s, 11; 50s, 12; 60s, 12; 70s, 9; 80s, 5.

The correlation between age and ten laboratory data is presented in Table 1. The parameters demonstrating a significant simple correlation with age were visual accommodation, vibratory sensing threshold, and vital capacity. The relationship between age and all of the measured

Table 1 Correlation coefficient matrix

	Age	HT	WT	SBP	DBP	VCAP	PSP	ACR	ACL	VIBR	VIBL
Age	1.000	–0.685	–0.556	0.634	0.542	–0.771	–0.637	–0.884	–0.886	0.30	0.821
HT		1.000	0.669	–0.477	–0.432	0.702	0.381	0.594	0.586	–0.510	–0.514
WT			1.000	–0.273	–0.242	0.528	0.336	0.455	0.460	–0.366	–0.385
SBP				1.000	0.709	–0.442	–0.544	–0.506	–0.524	0.492	0.492
DBP					1.000	–0.493	–0.468	–0.500	–0.524	0.420	0.370
VCAP						1.000	0.419	0.694	0.709	–0.648	–0.629
PSP							1.000	0.524	0.539	–0.488	–0.468
ACR								1.000	0.966	–0.777	–0.755
ACL									1.000	–0.778	–0.754
VIBR										1.000	0.951
VIBL											1.000

Note: Abbreviations—Age: chronological age; HT: *body height;* WT: *body weight;* SBP *and* DBP: *systolic and diastolic blood pressure;* VCAP: *vital capacity;* PSP: *phenolsulfophthalein excretion test;* ACR *and* ACL: *range of visual accommodation, right and left eye;* VIBR *and* VIBL: *threshold of vibratory sensation, right and left index fingertip.*

From Furukawa, T. et al., J. Gerontol., *30, 422, 1975. Copyright © The Gerontological Society of America. With permission.*

parameters yielded a high multiple correlation coefficient of $r = 0.957$. These results were expected to produce considerably accurate multiple regression analytical formulas.

B. RESULTS

The first-order multiple regression formula yielded the following results:

$$\begin{aligned} \text{Age} = {} & 95.232 \\ & - 0.138\ (\text{HT}) \\ & - 0.180\ (\text{WT}) \\ & + 0.142\ (\text{SBP}) \\ & - 0.072\ (\text{DBP}) \\ & - 0.003\ (\text{VCAP}) \\ & - 0.252\ (\text{PSP}) \\ & - 1.433\ (\text{ACR}) \\ & - 0.816\ (\text{ACL}) \\ & + 0.262\ (\text{VIBR}) \\ & + 0.315\ (\text{VIBL}) \end{aligned}$$

The scattergram between the chronological and estimated ages showed a fairly good correlation (Figure 1). The variance of error was 26.51.

However, it is very difficult to demonstrate whether age estimated by the formulas can be applied as a standard biological criterion in order to evaluate aging. If the age estimated by multiple regression analysis represents the correct individual variation of senescence after the classification of individuals according to estimated age, continuous observation of each group until death should enable us to observe the remaining life span based on an age estimation. However, because cohort analysis of this type is theoretically desirable, it is almost impossible to realize.

Then, in order to explore new ways of applying the formulas, the data obtained from hypertensive and atherosclerotic patients were fitted to multiple regression analysis using data from healthy male subjects (Figure 2). It is, of course, mathematically proper to apply another new

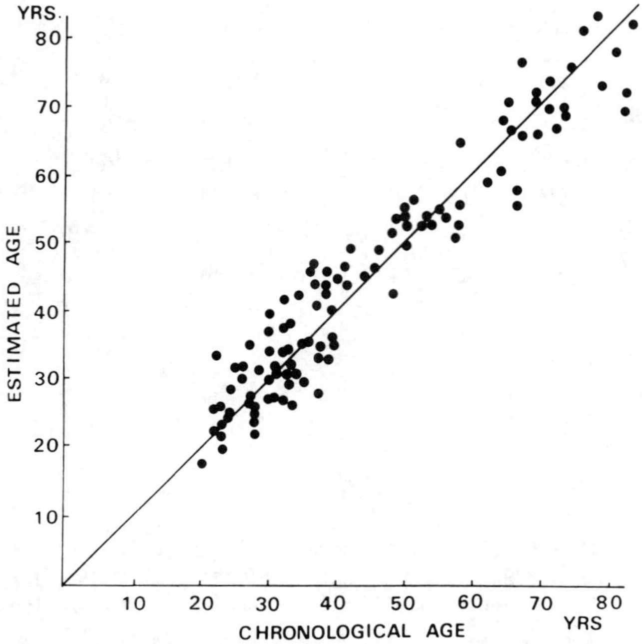

Figure 1 Comparison of chronological age and estimated age. (From Furukawa, T. et al., *J. Gerontol.*, 30, 422, 1975. Copyright © The Gerontological Society of America. With permission.)

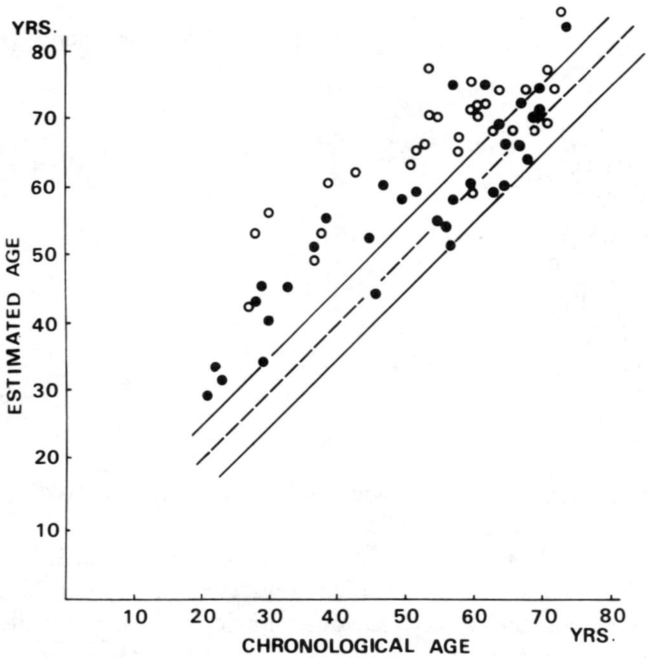

Figure 2 Estimated ages of hypertensives by the regression formula of healthy subjects. The upper and lower solid lines represent ±5 years limit (almost equal to ±1 S.D.) of healthy subjects. Dots and open circles correspond to males and females, respectively. (From Furukawa, T. et al., *J. Gerontol.*, 30, 422, 1975. Copyright © The Gerontological Society of America. With permission.)

regression equation obtained from healthy and hypertensive individuals, but only a rough prospect may be found.

The estimated biological age for each group of the patients was found to be significantly higher than the chronological age, and the distribution of most of the estimated values was higher than the maximum allowable variation of +5 years. In addition, a good correlation between the severity of illness and the degree of difference in estimated age as compared with chronological age was suggested. At first, when we represented the severity of disease based on arbitrary or empirical considerations, biological age estimated for the period of illness of the subject appeared probable as a newly devised objective reference value to indicate severity of the disease, i.e., the time lag until death. The new trend in etiological research related to aging was not retrievable in previous works, and therefore well-organized systemic confirmational studies are much needed.

III. ASSESSMENT OF ADEQUACY OF BIOLOGICAL AGE BY MULTIVARIATE ANALYSIS WITHOUT EXTERNAL REFERENCE

In order to get a better understanding of biological meaning of estimated age by multiple regression analysis, the study was conducted to insight of the main tendency with which the aging is reflected in the physiological examinations.[14]

A. METHOD

The analytical methods used were the multivariate statistical analysis without any external criterion, i.e., principal component analysis, factor analysis, and its varimax rotation. These methods are useful to reveal the important elements that may be a common factor underlying various phenomena. The details of these statistical procedures are provided in textbooks of multivariate statistical analysis. The data utilized for analysis were obtained from 111 healthy males as described in the previous section.

First, the relevance of data was analyzed by the principal component analysis. The purpose of this analysis is to summarize the meaning of various data and to propose an epitomized description of phenomena. The principal component analysis is to obtain major axes in the multidimensional data space so that they can explain the original data variation maximally. Moreover, each component has no relation, so it gives a result by what is designated as an "orthogonality". The relationships between those principal components and age or between each component were observed.

Factor analysis has almost a similar purpose as that of principal component analysis. For the application of factor analysis, the variables should be separated into two factors, *viz.*, common and specific factors, with no correlation assumed between the two factors. No correlation should exist between each factor which comprises the different variables. In this analysis, the variance of the common factor is exclusively analyzed to interpret the phenomena.

In addition, according to the varimax rotation of the results of factor analysis, the extraction of the smallest number of variables explains most of the variations observed. As a result, the simplest structure of the phenomena by using the most essential variables can be acquired.

B. RESULTS

The results of the analysis were remarkably successful, considering the simplicity of the analytical method. The following were the main outcomes of the analyses.

1. Analysis of Meaning of the First Principal Component

The first component expresses a general trend predicted by the sum of the results of ten physiological parameters. The eigenvalues (characteristic roots) and the variance ratios of principal components

Table 2 Eigenvalues and variance ratios of principal components

Principal component	Eigenvalue	Variance ratio	Cumulative ratio
1	5.99495	59.9	59.9
2	1.09277	10.9	70.9
3	0.97833	9.8	80.7
4	0.58866	5.9	86.5
5	0.43603	4.4	90.0
6	0.34417	3.4	94.3
7	0.27959	2.8	97.1
8	0.20810	2.1	99.2
9	0.04475	0.4	99.7
10	0.03262	0.3	100.0

Table 3 Factor loads of the principal components

Variables	1st Component	2nd Component	3rd Component	4th Component
HT	0.75401	0.26162	0.43237	–0.11365
WT	0.59378	0.45385	0.52400	0.20899
SBP	–0.69396	0.54894	–0.17394	0.07308
DBP	–0.65384	0.56653	–0.24175	0.27622
VCAP	0.81962	0.20287	0.12257	–0.20581
PSP	0.65698	–0.33787	0.04946	0.63715
ACR	0.89724	0.09103	–0.20439	–0.03153
ACL	0.90523	0.06713	–0.19398	–0.03069
VIBR	–0.85504	–0.09893	0.41011	0.01004
VIBL	–0.84011	–0.13484	0.40380	–0.00913

Note: See Table 1 for abbreviations.

are shown in Table 2. The factor loads of principal components to the physiological parameters are shown in Table 3.

As is evident from Table 2, the first principal component showed an extremely high contribution ratio of almost 60%. Moreover, in Table 3, the first principal component showed high relationships to each physiological parameter without exception.

To make the meaning of the first principal component more conspicuous, the relation between chronological age and overall scores calculated from the first principal component of individuals was plotted and revealed a fairly linear relationship (Figure 3).

In contrast, the effect of chronologic age should be eliminated by classification of the parameters according to the age of the subjects. The eigenvalue for the first principal component calculated after categorizing the data with age showed a marked classification. Also, the difference between the eigenvalues of the first principal component and successive ones became smaller (Table 4).

These results indicate that a major unrecognized factor governing variance is the alteration caused mainly in relation to chronological age. In the other expression, the major trend revealed by the principal component analysis was indirectly predicted to be the factor associated with the aging process, or the

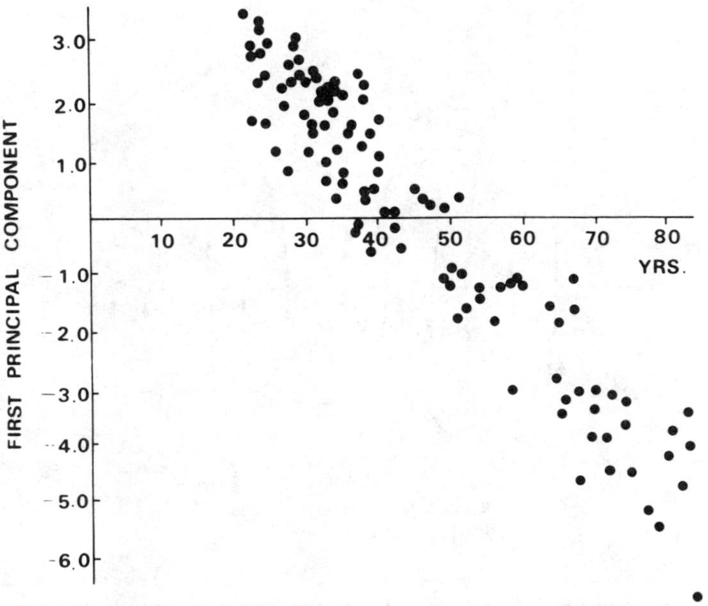

Figure 3 Comparison of chronological age and the first principal component.

Table 4 Difference of eigen values of principal components without and with classification of age group

Principal component	Without classification by age group	With classification by age group
1st	5.99	1.12
2nd	1.10	0.90
3rd	0.98	0.56
4th	0.59	0.46

duration of the individual existence after birth. Therefore, it is considered very reasonable to estimate chronological age from the measurement of the physiological items selected for study in this chapter.

2. Analysis of the Structure of Age-Related Changes of the Principal Components

About 80% of the total variance of the observed physiological parameters could be explained by the first to the third principal components as shown in Table 2. In order to inspect the characteristics of the data space composed of the three major principal components, the relation between the first and the second and the first and the third principal component vectors was calculated for individuals. The scores of the vectors were plotted on a section graph as the distribution of concentric ellipses. The center of the ellipse corresponds to the mean value of the principal component vector for each age group. The ellipse covers 64% of individual scores.

In the chart of concentric ellipses of the first and the second principal components, a linear progression with aging was observed along the first principal component axis, but no distinct progression was observed along the second component axis (Figure 4). However, regarding the first and third components chart, the distribution of the third component vectors showed a deflection for the age group of 40 years (Figure 5). This phenomenon is discussed later.

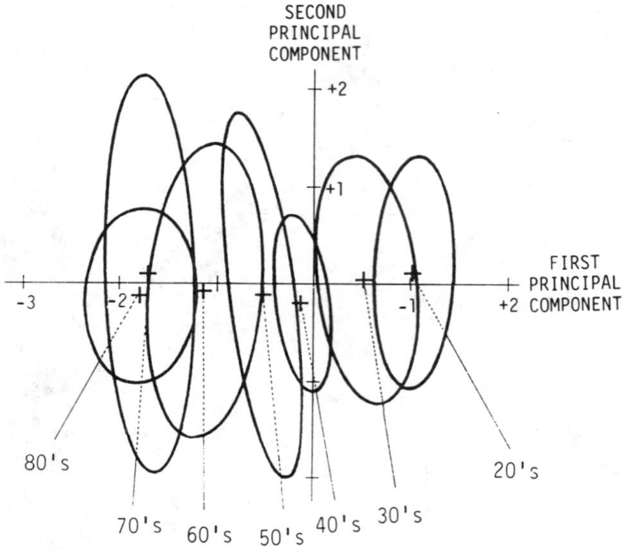

Figure 4 Comparison of the first and second principal component by the age groups.

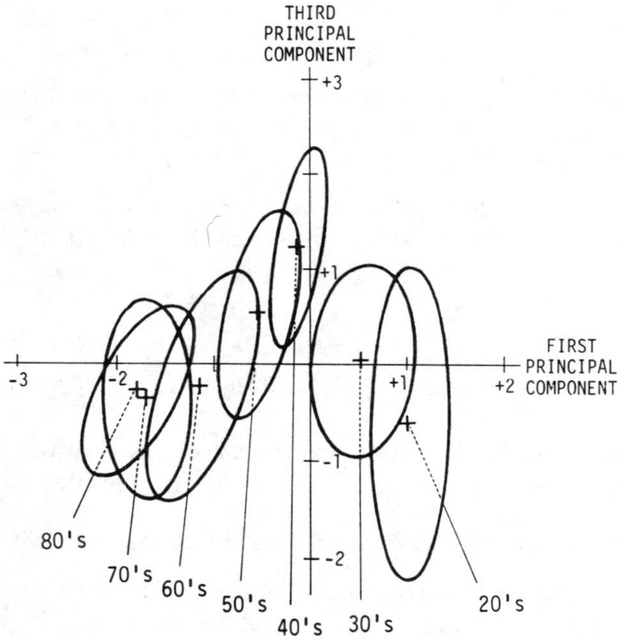

Figure 5 Comparison of the first and third principal component by the age groups.

3. Analysis of Meanings of Factor Analysis

The purpose of factor analysis is to extract the common factors from the total variation, and to try to reconstruct the factors by the smallest number of variables.

In the first step, the contribution ratio of the first factor was the highest, as with the first principal component. Then, by the varimax rotation, a more simple data structure was explored.

Table 5 Factor loading vectors after varimax rotation of factor analysis

Variables	Factor 1	Factor 2	Factor 3
HT	0.26754	–0.29091	0.80722
WT	0.20625	–0.11348	0.70541
SBP	–0.26353	0.79646	–0.17698
DBP	–0.19765	0.78246	–0.19417
VCAP	0.48957	–0.30629	0.57926
PSP	0.35872	–0.47847	0.22045
ACR	0.73346	–0.34871	0.39524
ACL	0.73137	–0.37411	0.39185
VIBR	–0.88995	0.25549	–0.21877
VIBL	–0.86074	0.22652	–0.24299

Note: See Table 1 for abbreviations.

As shown in the varimax rotated factor loading matrix (Table 5), factor 1 had a greater amount of factor load on visual accommodation of 0.73 and vibratory sensing threshold of 0.86 and 0.89. These results meant that factor 1 mainly contributed to the age change of sensory and nerve functions. Factor loading of the second varimax rotated factor found that the contribution of systolic and diastolic blood pressure was as high as 0.80 and 0.78, respectively. This factor seemed to indicate the involvement of the blood pressure regulation system in the aging process. The third varimax rotated factor had the highest contribution from body height (0.81) and weight (0.71) and vital capacity (0.58). These parameters are related to body dimensions and, therefore, possibly appeared to reflect the quantity of the functioning cells.

4. Analysis of the Structure of Age-Related Changes of the Factor Analysis

The results obtained by the factor analysis made the interpretation somewhat simple. Following the preceding analysis of the principal component analysis, the characteristics of the major three factors were investigated on a section graph as the distribution of concentric ellipses.

The charts of concentric ellipses distribution were drawn for factor 1 vs. 2, and 1 vs. 3. The calculated factor values of individuals were grouped in age ranges from the 20s to the 80s in concentric ellipses (Figures 6 and 7). The data show that the migration of ellipses along the factor 1 axis occurred from the 20s to the 40s, but there were almost no migrations along the factor 2 and 3 axes. By contrast, migration along the factor 2 and 3 axes were found after age 50.

According to physiological and medical knowledge, the irreversible hardening change of the human ocular lens begins just after birth. The factor analysis suggests that age associated changes in visual accommodation as well as in the threshold of vibratory sensation occur between the ages of 20 and 40. After age 40, a reduction in the number of functioning cells was estimated to occur.

IV. DISCUSSION

A decline in physiological function with an increase in age could be an easily understandable phenomena, if an organism is considered via a mechanical view. Because many physiological functions seem to decrease in a straight-line trend, we can use this to explain that age-associated exhaustion of physiological function may occur as a random process. Physiological functions that exhibited a straight-line degradation with age include:

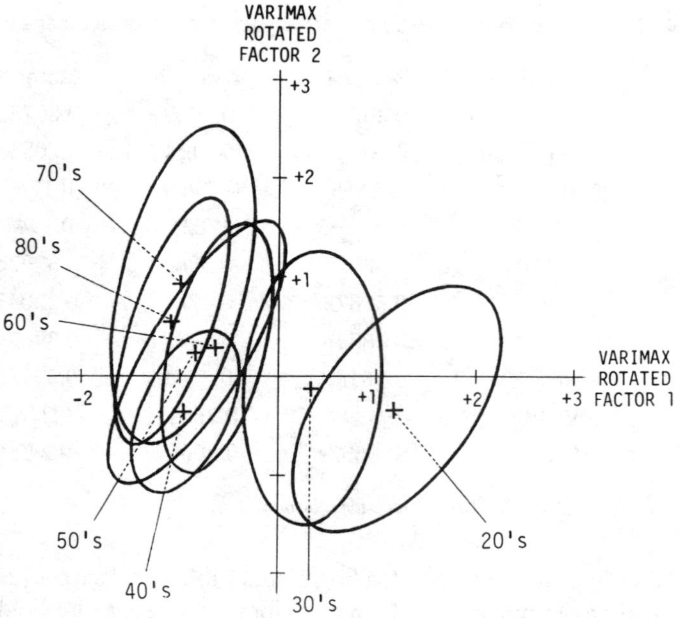

Figure 6 Comparison of the factor 1 and 2 after varimax rotation of factor analysis.

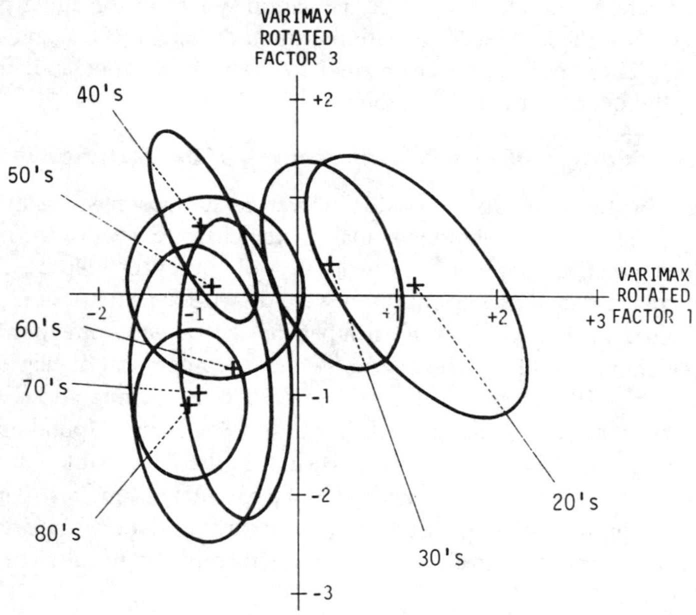

Figure 7 Comparison of the factor 1 and 3 after varimax rotation of factor analysis.

1. Functions reflecting the number of functioning cells such as brain weight, total body water, and basal metabolic rate
2. Neural functions such as the pulse conduction velocity rate, the capability of hearing, vision, visual accommodation, as well as the threshold of vibratory sensations
3. Several other organic functions such as cardiac output, renal blood flow, glomerular filtration rate, and vital capacity or maximum oxygen uptake

Functions of various organs after the period of growth decreased linearly with an increase in age. Generally, marked variations are recognizable during the growth period with regard to body size such as height; these are known to show variation governed by a Gaussian distribution curve as well as a growth rate curve. During the process of aging, those individual variations in various test values observed during the growth period were further exaggerated by the differences in the varied individual rates of aging. In addition, considerable natural variations in the rates of decline of functions were detected among individual organs. For that reason, the integration of various test values by multivariate statistical analysis is considered to be the only rational method to estimate an individual biological age. Furthermore, by using such a statistical treatment, it is possible to generate a reference value of aging or biological age.

The results presented here were the result of a series of investigations and were obtained by using multivariate statistical analysis of age-dependent physiological functions. By using multiple regression analysis, the chronological ages of healthy volunteers could be estimated from the results of ten tests of physiological function. This portion of the results is a summary of the reports already published in a Japanese article[13] and after that in the *Journal of Gerontology*.[5]

The applicability of multiple regression analysis to estimate chronological age was first examined in 1962 by Dirken.[3] In his research, Dirken used this method to estimate the functional age of factory workers. From the results of multiple regression analysis of data concerning maximum respiratory rate, maximum oxygen uptake, systolic blood pressure, maximum heart rate, hand steadiness, maximum load, and psychological capabilities such as picture recognition, semantic categorization test, concentration test, and four choice reaction times, the chronological age of factory workers was estimated. In this analysis, however, the estimated functional capacity of the elderly is shown to be less accurate, while in the younger population the analysis has a higher accuracy. Unfortunately, this report barely attracted the attention of specialists involved in aging research.

In 1975, we reported the accurate estimation of chronological age by using multiple regression analysis of data with exercise abilities. It is known in an empirical sense that there is a reduction in exercise abilities with an increase in age. Therefore, maximum momentary force, durability, maintenance of balance, and quick reflex movement were all found to decrease with an increase in age. Taking these results into consideration, a simple mobility test, which could be easily conducted in routine health examinations, was conducted on 110 subjects. Heavier exercise loads were given to an additional 33 subjects. In addition to basic data (such as body height and weight), SBP and DBP finger tapping rate in 30 s, hand-grip power, and the degree of body flexibility represented by degrees of bending forward, to the sides, and backward were used.

Furthermore, the recovery of heart rate after exercise was evaluated by measuring RR intervals from an ECG while resting, and at 30 s, 1 min, 1.5 min, 2 min, 3 min, and 4 min after exercise, respectively. The exercise loads were given by Master's double two-step test. Multiple correlations generated by regression analysis between age and the results of the test measurements were found to be very high, especially using Master's exercise test. After 70 up and down exercises, an unexpected high multiple correlation coefficient ($r = 0.939$) was obtained, while after 40 up and down exercises the multiple correlation coefficient was $r = 0.863$.

The multiple regression formula used to estimate chronological age under an exercise load of 70 steps up and down showed a variance of error as low as 15.60, indicating unexpectedly high reliability of the formula. If exercise load was 40 times, variance of error calculated from the adjusted formula for 40 times exercise load was higher than the former at 34.15. This appeared to indicate the difficulty in eliminating variables generated from factors other than the aging process after the lighter exercise load.

In addition, in order to investigate the hypothesis with regard to a correlation between the working environment and physical age, data from personnel involved in an outdoor, walking job in a sales promotion department were compared to data from personnel involved in clerical jobs, staying inside the company. Although the regression equation with a 40-step exercise test was used

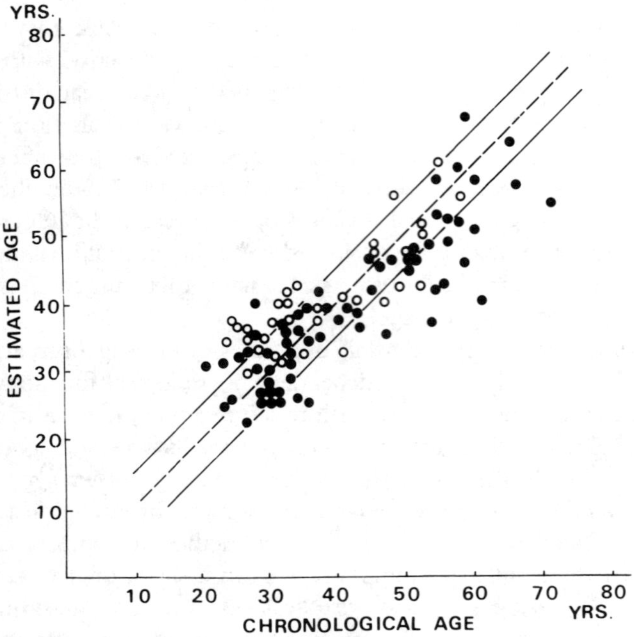

Figure 8 Comparison of chronological and estimated age using a multiple regression analysis consists of exercise abilities and according to the type of jobs. The upper and lower solid lines represent ±5 years limit (almost equal to ±1 S.D.) of total subjects. Dots and open circles correspond to the subjects working in clerical and sales promotion jobs, respectively.

and the difference was not statistically significant, estimated physical age generated from personnel involved in clerical jobs with less of a labor burden was slightly younger, indicating that the younger biological age tended to be generated in association with a lighter physical load (Figure 8). Although a detailed examination appeared to be required to evaluate these data, it seemed to generate some discussion. However, in this study, the principal component analysis of data was not carried out. This is because the extraction of the main components or main factors from the homologous exercise test, unlike the extraction of components from a variety of heterogeneous data as well as physiological examinations, is not considered to result in the detection of hidden factors.

Webster and Logie[15] reported the estimation of chronological age from data such as blood urea nitrogen, forced vital capacity, SBP, plasma alkaline phosphatase, plasma cholesterol concentration, and erythrocyte sedimentation rate. A 1974 study conducted by Heikkinen et al.[11] at Jyväskylä University, Jyväskylä, Finland used similar parameters as described in the work reported by Webster and Logie in 1976; however, the correlation was not as high ($r = 0.865$). The items studied such as audiometry and the hand grip dynamometer showed values almost identical to those reported by Dirken, supporting a reexamination of the study conducted previously. In a National Institute on Aging (NIA) report, Borkan and Norris[1] reported the estimation of biological age with data obtained from measurements of hemoglobin, forced expiratory volume, creatinine clearance, SBP, hand grip strength, and tapping test. A report presented by the Atomic Bomb Casualty Commission (ABCC) had some unique features. In order to evaluate the hypothesis that radioactivity exposure might accelerate the aging process, Hollingsworth and colleagues[12] adopted the measurement of the degree of skin elasticity, in addition to other tests such as hand grip strength, auditory acuity, the threshold of vibratory sensitivity, near vision, and light extinction time.

Dean's comprehensive book[2] gathers the methods applied to measure "biological" or "functional" age of humans. It describes the details of the methods proposed by specialists around the world to assess physiological changes in humans with age. Also, it covers the papers of many other scientists which were not referred to in the present report. However, the point common to all of the research cited here and in the above-mentioned book is the estimate of chronological age by combining the results of various biochemical and physiological tests, without any firm rationale with mortality functions. The principles of most of the tests were based on the differences in physical fitness levels, health conditions, and working conditions. In addition, none of the studies conducted could provide evidence as to whether the chronological ages estimated really reflected the biological ages.

This chapter, with the utilization of multivariate statistical analysis which does not require an external criterion, proved the adequacy of estimations conducted by multiple regression analysis. Namely, measurement of variables obtained from subjects ranging from young to old age appeared to reflect closely the duration of individual existence. Therefore, the estimate of age by multiple regression analysis of these multiple variables can be considered reasonable both empirically and theoretically.

In this study, the "deflection" was found not only on the distribution of principal component scores of individuals, but also in the factor analysis and its varimax rotation values. Moreover, the canonical analysis (multiple discriminant analysis) which was not mentioned in this chapter, a "deflection" of canonical scores was observed at the same age, 40.[7] The definitive mean of "deflection" found in these analyses was not clearly understood. However, it may reflect some difference in starting time of age changes of each of the biological functions. For example, the hardening of ocular lens begins earlier. On the other hand, the decrease in number of functioning cells starts later. In addition, there is additional supporting evidence. For example, the mortality rates for humans are known to increase remarkably after age 40, as proposed by Gompertz[10] using a simple exponential model. On the other hand, in a life table analysis by the Weibull distribution model done by the authors,[8] there was no change in the mode of mortality rate at age 40, but the component corresponding to the wear-and-tear failure mode of senescence death of the Weibull model had its location parameter at around 30 years. Nevertheless, because the effect of the wear-and-tear failure mode on the death rate appeared substantially around 40 years, the deflection may indicate the general alteration of physiological functions. Therefore, this fact, by referring to information previously obtained, suggests important points to be investigated in the future.

The basis of scientific research is to unmask important factors that might commonly underlie various phenomena. Conventional methods of medical research attempt to analyze and elucidate essential concepts hidden behind various phenomena. As precedents in the medical field, findings of pathogens, detection of diseases induced by deficiency or hyperproduction of hormones, and findings of degenerative lesions in specific organs or cells as causative factors of disease were the results of research based on the analytical method. However, in response to the increased amount of reliable information on particular research subjects, additional information is likely to be obtained from mathematical treatment of data.

REFERENCES

1. Borkan, G.A. and Norris, A.H., Assessment of biological age using a profile of physical parameters, *J. Gerontol.*, 35, 177, 1980.
2. Dean, W., *Biological Aging Measurement — Clinical Applications*, The Center for Bio-Gerontology, Los Angeles, 1988.
3. Dirken, J.M., The Development of A Measuring Device for Determining the Functional Age of Elderly Industrial Workers Doc. 22-6-1962, The Netherlands Institute for Preventive Medicine, Leiden, 1963.
4. Furukawa, T., Karita, M., Yoshikawa, H., Inada, H., Moriwaki, K., Abe, H., Miyazaki, M., Kajiya, F., and Miyawaki, K., Assessment of biological age by multiple variant analysis methods, *Korei-Igaku,* 6, 1, 1968 (in Japanese).
5. Furukawa, T., Inoue, K., Kajiya, F., Inada, H., Takasugi, S., Fukui, S., Takeda, H., and Abe, H., Assessment of biological age by multiple regression analysis, *J. Gerontol.*, 30, 422, 1975.

6. Furukawa, T., Takasugi, S., Hori, M., Takeda, H., Inada, H., Inoue, M., and Abe, H., Assessment of environment with application of stochastic model of mortality, in *Proceedings of the Second World Conference on Medical Informatics (Medinfo 77)*, Shires, D.B. and Wolf, H., Eds., North Holland, Amsterdam, 1977, 603.
7. Furukawa, T., Takasugi, S., Tanaka, H., and Yajima, K., Multivariate statistical analysis of biological data in the process of aging, in *Proceedings of the Fourth International Symposium on Medical Information Systems, (MEDIS '78)*, edited by the Organizing Committee, Kansai Institute of Information Systems, Osaka, Japan, 1978, 525.
8. Furukawa, T., Hara, S., and Hong, Y., A mathematical model of senescence and aging, *Byoutai-Seiri (Medicina Philosophica)*, 7, 199, 1988 (in Japanese).
9. Furukawa, T. and Tanaka, H., *Multivariate Statistical Analysis — How to Use the Program Package*, Igaku Shoin Publishing, Tokyo, 1983 (in Japanese).
10. Gompertz, B., On the Nature of the Function Expressive of the Law of Human Mortality and on a New Mode of Determining the Value of Life Contingencies, *Philos. Trans. R. Soc. London, Ser. A,* 115, 513, 1825.
11. Heikkinen, E., Kiiskinen, A., Katyhty, B., Rimpela, M., and Vouri, I., Assessment of biological age, *Gerontologia,* 20, 33, 1974.
12. Hollingsworth, J.W., Hashizume, A., and Jablon, S., Correlations between tests of aging in Hiroshima subjects — an attempt to define "physiologic age", *Yale J. Biol. Med.,* 38, 11, 1966.
13 Kajiya, F., Aso, Y., Inada, H., Kato, T., Itakura, N., Hayashi, R., Miki, K., Furukawa, T., and Abe, H., Medical Applications of Multivariate Statistical Analysis, Res. Rep. Med. Electr. Biol. Med., (MBE 67-15, 1967, 1.)
14 Takeuchi, K., Yanai, H., and Mukherjee, B.N., *The Foundations of Multivariate Analysis,* Willy Eastern Ltd., New Delhi, 1982.
15 Webster, I.W. and Logie, A.R., A relationship between functional age and health status in female subjects, *J. Gerontol.,* 31, 546, 1976.

CHAPTER 29
AN APPROACH TO BIOLOGIC AGE ASSESSMENT

Donald G. Lindsay and Stanley Kaplan

TABLE OF CONTENTS

I. INTRODUCTION

Many attempts have been made to develop a decisive indicator of biologic age (bioage). There is an intuitive notion, growing out of everyday experience, that a difference exists among individuals' aging bodies and their chronological age; some seem older, some seem younger. What might biomarkers tell us about the probable time of death, and with what certainty? What could we learn about the aging process? If there is some intrinsic biologic age, or if there are biomarkers, they may well be complex. The concept is poorly defined. If one could bring together all the information available about biologic age, and form this into a new kind of integrated, computerized, knowledge base, could we further develop this hypothesized biologic age? This chapter describes such an experimental method.

Life forms appear to proceed along some time course, encompassing embryonic development, growth, sexual maturity, involution, and senescence. With senescence comes a rapidly increasing death rate. We desire to fit an individual to a point on that biotrajectory at any given real time. Measuring group changes may have distorted our thinking. Many parameters decline with age when measured as a group. Individuals within that group may not decline at all, as longitudinal studies have shown. Some functions, renal function, for example, may improve.[1] People 80 and 90 years old show a great deal of individual variation.

What crucial parts of species knowledge must we know to understand and calibrate individual biologic age? It may be life span is a compromise, a balance between the potent directive growth factors and their mitogenic-oncogenic effects. Transforming growth factors-α and -β (TGF-α, TGF-β) are

0-8493-0129-7/94/$0.00+$.50

known to be second mitogens. Transforming growth factors are potent immunosuppressors. How do signals work to initiate proliferation, differentiation, and inhibition of proliferation? We know that calcium and cyclic adenosine monophosphate (cAMP) are essential signal transducers. What do we know about the specifics of these control mechanisms and the effects of time and entropy on this complexity? Matters of signal transduction, amplification, and redundancy are beginning to be elucidated. We find ourselves touching the edges of quantum mechanics with its counterintuitiveness. The complexity is staggering. We need more help from computers, for we know many disconnected things.

Self-repair of many systems diminishes with age. Changes in cytosine methylation occur as time since birth lengthens. We know many hormone levels diminish with age; yet we cannot rejuvenate by replacing those we have been able to replace. Must some unknown factors dictate a certain time for hormones to be effective? Perhaps what occurs is simply feedback inhibition with a shift in set point? Giving hormones (e.g., estrogen) to some older people increases their incidence of malignancy. Growth hormone given to older people firms muscle, but the muscles regress soon after treatment is stopped. Strangely, growth hormone treatment produces an increased incidence of carpal tunnel syndrome, among other things. We know of several instances in which changes in receptor populations or receptor affinity are responsible for inexplicable hormonal action. Some of these are genetic and inheritable. Now we have steroid receptor antagonists that directly block these receptors.[2,3] Our understanding of the changing reaction to drugs with age has been advanced by studies of drug receptors and studies of untoward drug effects mediated through calcium channels. Why are survivors survivors? Any point in a signal pathway is a place for an oncogene to arise. We could go on and on. Why recount this? The aim is to prepare the reader for what follows, to illustrate the many parameters that would lend themselves well to inclusion in the type of knowledge base we describe.

Perhaps the whole notion of bioage is illusory, the product of our hope, our need to simplify, and our need for certainty. However, given the hypothesis that biologic age exists, is measurable, and once measured is valuable, the next task is to develop a methodology, a tool to discern it, and perhaps define it, to at least find a biomarker or two. Perhaps we have a way to put it all together.

The methodology proposed can be built around a principle in probability theory known as Bayes theorem. The methodology is similar to that used by the authors to do computer-aided diagnoses in medicine (dermatology) and engineering (nuclear plants, diesel engines, and aviation navigation equipment). In this methodology the general human knowledge of the system or equipment of interest is encoded into the computer in what is called the knowledge base. This knowledge base is then used, along with symptoms or observations of the specific system at hand, to determine the disease, condition, or state of the system. Some prerequisite discussion is necessary.

II. DEALING WITH UNCERTAINTY AND COMPLEXITY

When we look at someone, it seems easy for us to guess that person's age with a fair degree of accuracy. When we seek to assess biological age precisely, we are confounded, rambling through an entangled thicket of data, conflicting motivation, concepts, and semantics. Why is that so? No prediction can be made with certainty. Is there some way to approach this problem? We are confounded by our need for simplicity, for certainty.

One must recognize the interdependent complexity and implicit uncertainty in such a process as the progression toward increased probability of death, and find a pragmatic way to cope with this fuzzy information thrust upon us by reality. Uncertainty is the very thing we are trying to avoid by seeking to establish a notion called biologic age or by seeking to find biomarkers of aging. How can we make uncertainty more certain? By dealing in probabilities, especially conditional probabilities, by thinking in terms of degrees of confidence and by quantifying this.

Consider this switch. When *X* equals 1, then *Y*. What if *X* would be better represented by equaling nearly 1, or somewhere around 1 to trigger *Y*? Suppose *X* is not a definite digital quantity or even an analogue expression, but rather an uncertain complex of the interplay and interdependence of numerous uncertain (nearly or almost) quantities, qualities, or events. What then? There may be a way to put this very complexity to work against itself to produce a workable definitiveness. Each aspect is assigned a probability. While any one probability may be a bit fuzzy or even an expert opinion, the sum of many of these hardens into a definitive quantity, which we can view with a quantifiable degree of confidence.

Consider the uncertainty implicit in the act of making a diagnosis. Does this patient with an acutely painful belly have appendicitis? The diagnostician is never certain. His situation at any point in time is best expressed as a probability. We say he has *X* degrees of confidence. As time progresses each new piece of evidence or lack of it can change this degree of confidence in a given diagnosis. The diagnostician's degree of confidence can be expressed as a number. That number brings together all the many bits of information and judgment calls made by the diagnostician and focuses them into a useful quantity. A similar number about biologic age is what we seek by this experiment. One has only to bring together the basis for this number, and as time progresses to upgrade it with new data, new discoveries, and even new speculations so long as their probable truth is expressed with reasonable accuracy. These new discoveries, new bits of evidence, or lack of them will move this number toward certainty. One of the virtues of the Bayesian approach is that it explicitly tells us, quantitatively, the degree of uncertainty present at each stage of the endeavor. It is helpful to learn a bit more about conditional probabilities and Bayes theorem.

III. CONDITIONAL PROBABILITIES AND BAYES THEOREM

Conditional probabilities are expressed as P(A/B), P(B/A). These are read the probability of A given B; or the probability of B given A. What is the probability of A given B? Suppose we are given the information that it is raining. What is the probability it is September? Now turn that around. It is September, what is the probability of rain? These express two entirely different things. P(A) simply says, what is the probability it is September? Thus, P(A) is 1 in 12, i.e., 0.083, if we have no other information, as the months offer us only 12 choices. The conditional probabilities are a bit more complex. They embody a condition and a probability given that condition. The relation between P(A/B) and P(B/A) is expressed by Bayes theorem:

$$P(A/B) = P(A)\frac{P(B/A)}{P(B)}$$

What do we have here? Return to the September analogy where A equals September and B equals Rain. What this equation says is the probability that it is September given rain (called the posterior probability) can be calculated as follows. Take the probability P(A) = 1/12 it is September (this is called the prior probability), and multiply it by the probability that if it is September it is also raining; then divide by the probability that it would be raining at a randomly chosen time of the year. Again, one thus calculates the posterior probability, i.e., the probability it would be September if it were raining. Those who find this rather nonmathematical way of expressing it distressing see References 4 to 6. For those who find this theorem rather counterintuitive, so have several generations since Bayes. Even knowing a bit about this relation helps for an understanding of what the authors will be developing. Another prerequisite follows.

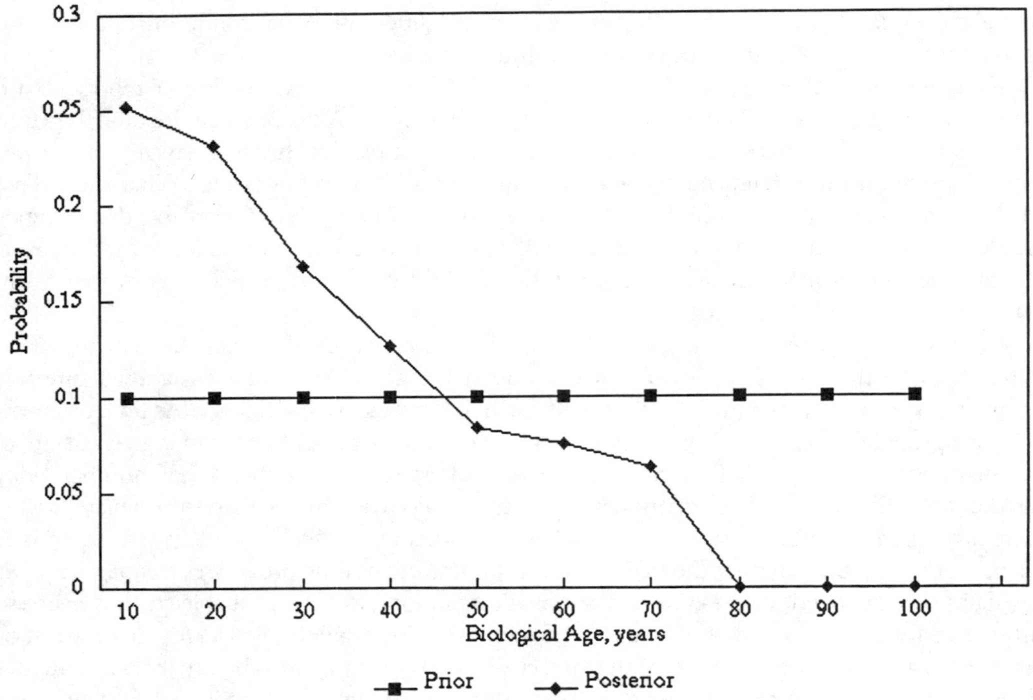

AGE	PRIOR	POSTERIOR	VARIABLE		VALUE	
10	0.10000	0.25209	Mitochondrial Por	V1	6.0	
20	0.10000	0.23108	DHEA male	V2		0
30	0.10000	0.16806	Estradiol	V3		0
40	0.10000	0.12604	Dermal estrogen	V4		0
50	0.10000	0.08403	Urinary hydroxy	V5		0
60	0.10000	0.07563	Acetylcholine rec	V6		0
70	0.10000	0.06302	Beta1 adrenergic	V7		0
80	0.10000	0.00002				
90	0.10000	0.00002				
100	0.10000	0.00002				
	1.00000	1.00000				

Figure 1 Probability distribution, one variable.

IV. THE SPREADSHEET

Picture a spreadsheet as long rows of columns and long columns of rows. Perhaps a matrix would be a better description of a spreadsheet. The information therein can be converted for use as a graph. Figures 1 through 8 illustrate computer-generated graphs of the spreadsheet material. Figures 9 and 10 show an excerpt from such a spreadsheet. Figure 9 shows a spreadsheet as we see it. Figure 10 shows a spreadsheet as the computer sees it. We will first describe in words our dermatology diagnosis spreadsheet. An illustration is not shown.

Down the left side, the title column, we list the names of the possible observable variables. These are the things a person looks at to make a diagnosis. The dermatology spreadsheet has 273 variables or observables listed down this first vertical or title column of the spreadsheet. Each one of these makes a row as it stretches across horizontally. Across the horizontal title bar at the top of the spreadsheet are arrayed the diseases. Each makes a column. This column, as it extends down vertically crossing the rows, creates cubicles. At the top, beneath the row of diagnostic titles, is a special row for the priors, a number that represents P(A). Prior here means the presumed probability of an event before the individual had any prior information. For example, a physician is driving to his office with a friend. The friend wants to know what would be the prior probability, the chance, the first patient the physician saw had hives. Knowing the conditions of his area and his practice,

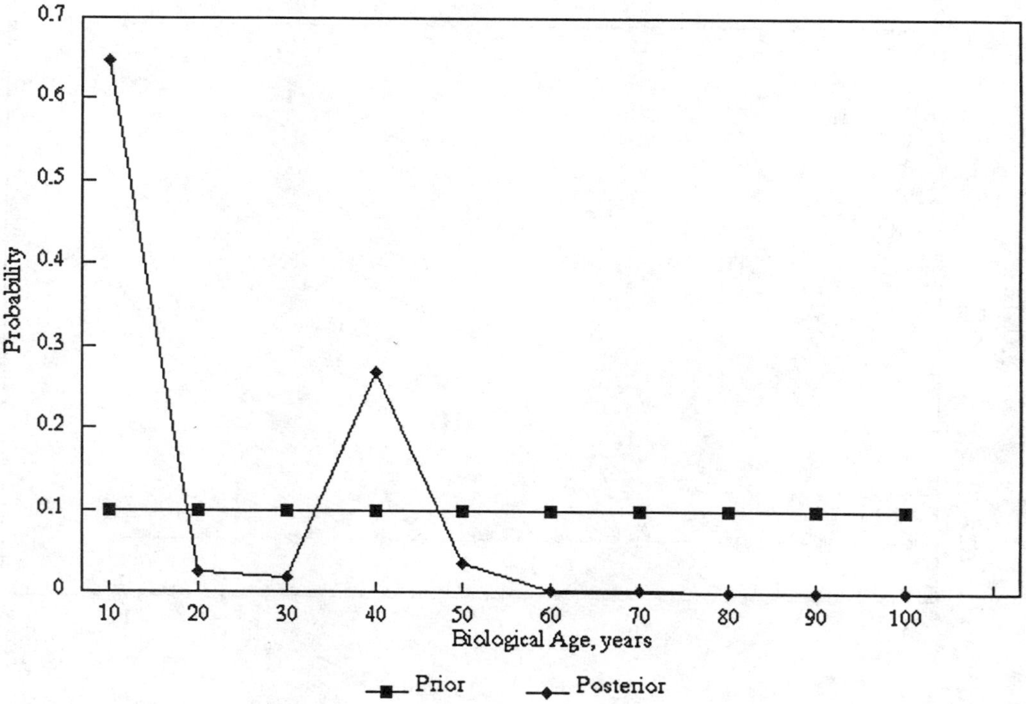

AGE	PRIOR	POSTERIOR	VARIABLE		VALUE
10	0.10000	0.64690	Mitochondrial Por	V1	6.0
20	0.10000	0.02372	DHEA male	V2	2.5
30	0.10000	0.01797	Estradiol	V3	0
40	0.10000	0.26954	Dermal estrogen	V4	0
50	0.10000	0.03594	Urinary hydroxy	V5	0
60	0.10000	0.00323	Acetylcholine rec	V6	0
70	0.10000	0.00270	Beta1 adrenergic	V7	0
80	0.10000	0.00000			
90	0.10000	0.00000			
100	0.10000	0.00000			
	1.00000	1.00000			

Figure 2 Probability distribution, second variable added.

the physician could arrive at an approximate answer. This is interchangeable practically with the question, what is the incidence of hives in your area for which people consult a physician?

Note the numbers seen in each cubicle represents an expert's opinion of the probability that this symptom or finding (observable) will appear in that disease. To create the expert system, the expert simply fills in each cubicle with a number, a decimal fraction that represents the conditional probability that a given symptom will occur in that disease. The number 0.0001 is a way of saying the observable very rarely occurs. Nevertheless, that small number is very important. It is important because a zero would give the very important information that the event never occurs. Each number represents the conditional probability that this symptom will occur given that disease. Visualize there are roughly 300 diseases listed across the top.

Consider a mole (dermal nevus). There would be a probability that it would be raised, and one that it would be brown, and one that it would be black, etc. To review, conditional probability here means given a dermal nevus, what is the probability it would be brown? To use this, the user simply inputs what he sees. For example, he sees a flat (macular), black lesion with irregular borders that bleeds easily. Then, with Bayes theorem and a few computer program macros it is a simple procedure to have the computer scan this roughly 90,000-cell spreadsheet, considering the conditional probabilities of all the user input observables over the range of diseases (diagnostic possibilities). It then arrives at three (if it is programmed that way) diagnostic possibilities expressed as a probability.

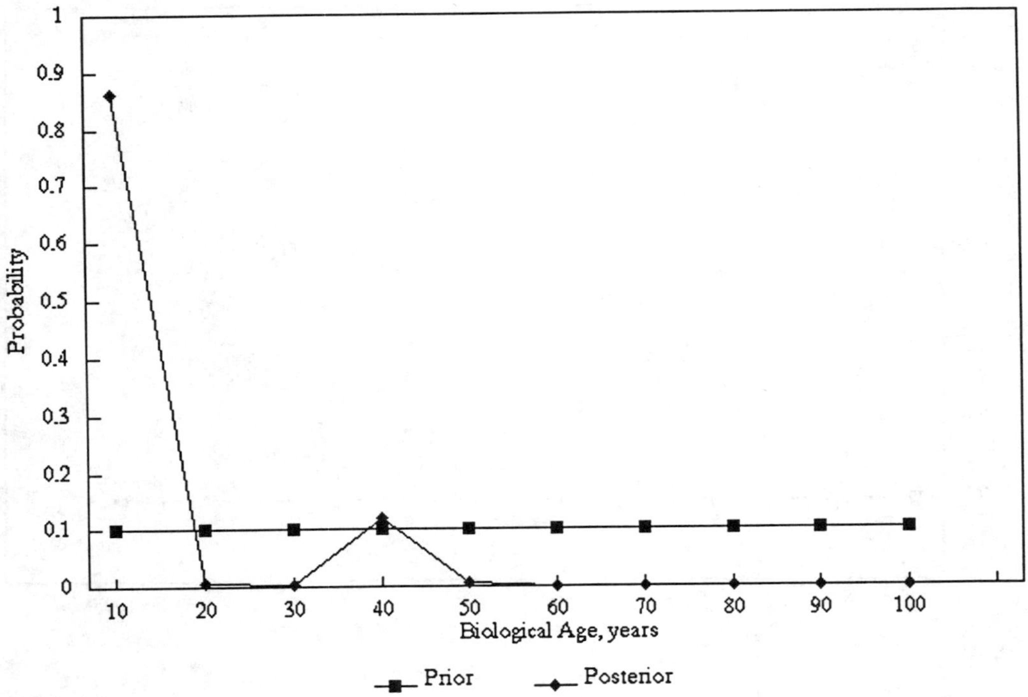

AGE	PRIOR	POSTERIOR	VARIABLE		VALUE	
10	0.10000	0.86202	Mitochondrial Por	V1	6.0	
20	0.10000	0.00527	DHEA male	V2	2.5	
30	0.10000	0.00399	Estradiol	V3		0
40	0.10000	0.11972	Dermal estrogen	V4	.01	
50	0.10000	0.00798	Urinary hydroxy	V5		0
60	0.10000	0.00072	Acetylcholine rec	V6		0
70	0.10000	0.00030	Beta1 adrenergic	V7		0
80	0.10000	0.00000				
90	0.10000	0.00000				
100	0.10000	0.00000				
	1.00000	1.00000				

Figure 3 Probability distribution, third variable added.

It might say melanoma, 0.90; pigmented basal cell carcinoma, 0.05; and something else, 0.05. This says the knowledge base is 90% confident the diagnosis is a melanoma, but there exists a 5% probability from the information given it that the diagnosis is a pigmented basal cell carcinoma, etc. If given different information, that is to say given different query input, the knowledge base might say melanoma, 0.38; irritated seborrheic keratosis, 0.30; dermal nevus, 0.42. This would mean the computer is indecisive and needs more data input. While it is a simple procedure for the computer to scan 90,000 cells, to put the conditional probabilities into 90,000 cells is a lot of work.

V. APPLICATION TO BIOLOGIC AGE

Diagnosis, the arriving at an uncertain conclusion from the synthesis of a set (the expert's knowledge), or stream (new findings) of information is indeed similar to the problem of determining biologic age. The reader perhaps has expert knowledge about an aspect of aging, and some knowledge about many other variables pertaining to the subject. How would one develop this into a workable knowledge base? How broad or how narrow does the reader want the consideration to be? Is help needed from other experts? One can construct an input sheet to send to other experts to facilitate their return of requested information in a form that could be easily added to the

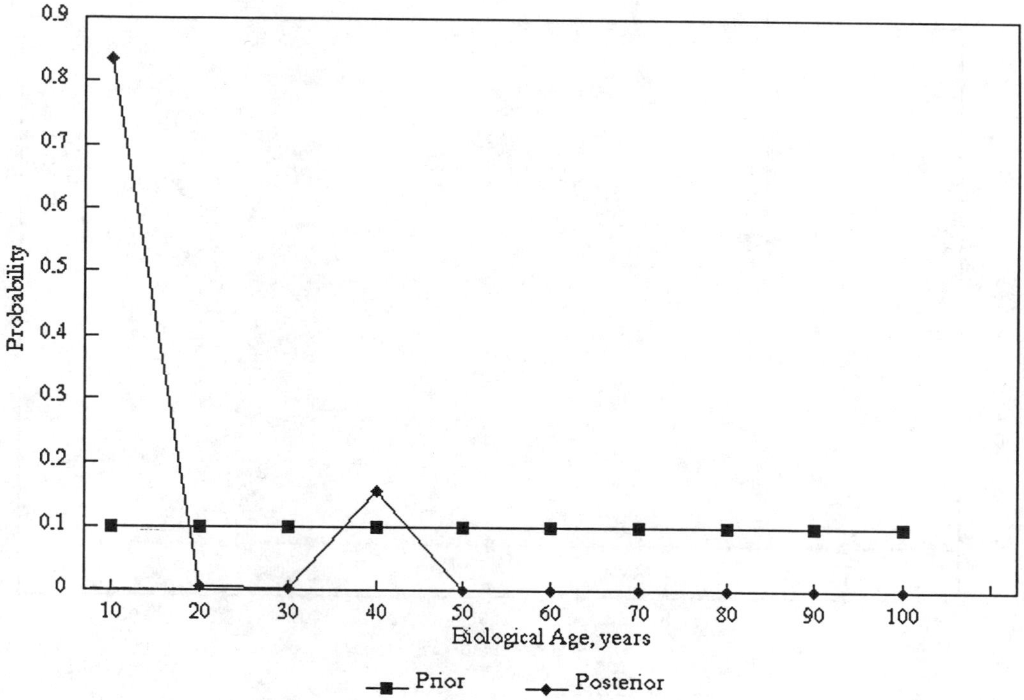

AGE	PRIOR	POSTERIOR	VARIABLE		VALUE
10	0.10000	0.83499	Mitochondrial Por	V1	6.0
20	0.10000	0.00510	DHEA male	V2	2.5
30	0.10000	0.00387	Estradiol	V3	0
40	0.10000	0.15463	Dermal estrogen	V4	.01
50	0.10000	0.00129	Urinary hydroxy	V5	20
60	0.10000	0.00009	Acetylcholine rec	V6	0
70	0.10000	0.00003	Beta1 adrenergic	V7	0
80	0.10000	0.00000			
90	0.10000	0.00000			
100	0.10000	0.00000			
	1.00000	1.00000			

Figure 4 Probability distribution, fourth variable added.

spreadsheet. From what viewpoint will one begin? For example, take a physician's view, an endocrine physiologist's viewpoint, a biochemist's view, a marine biologist's view, or a molecular geneticist's view. All of these modules can be put together to form a master knowledge base.

Whatever else one wants to define as pure biologic age variables can be set against time increments in years, months, or decades. Subsets of observables can be logically grouped so long as their combined possible probabilities add up exactly to the number 1, when these are put in by the expert. This will become clearer later. Subsets of observable variables are grouped until the list is exhaustive, or sufficiently definitive, for the category, so long as the members of the group are mutually exclusive. They add to one by definition. When each member of a group is given a numerical probability represented by a decimal fraction which is a part of one, the whole must be one.

In the case of dermatology, lesion color is one such group, consisting of brown, black, red, pink, orange, skin color, and other. The expert responds in the case of a common skin mole (dermal nevus), thus: brown, 0.6; black, 0.2; pink, 0.1; red, 0.05; other, 0.05. What color is a dermal nevus? It may be any of a number of colors. The previous statement of conditional probabilities answers this question more definitively. What factors comprise "pure bioage"? There could be a myriad of factors, many inextricably mixed with disease, and a host of other things known, unknown, or theorized. A knowledge base spreadsheet of the kind illustrated by this simple skin mole color example shows a way to a more definite answer about bioage.

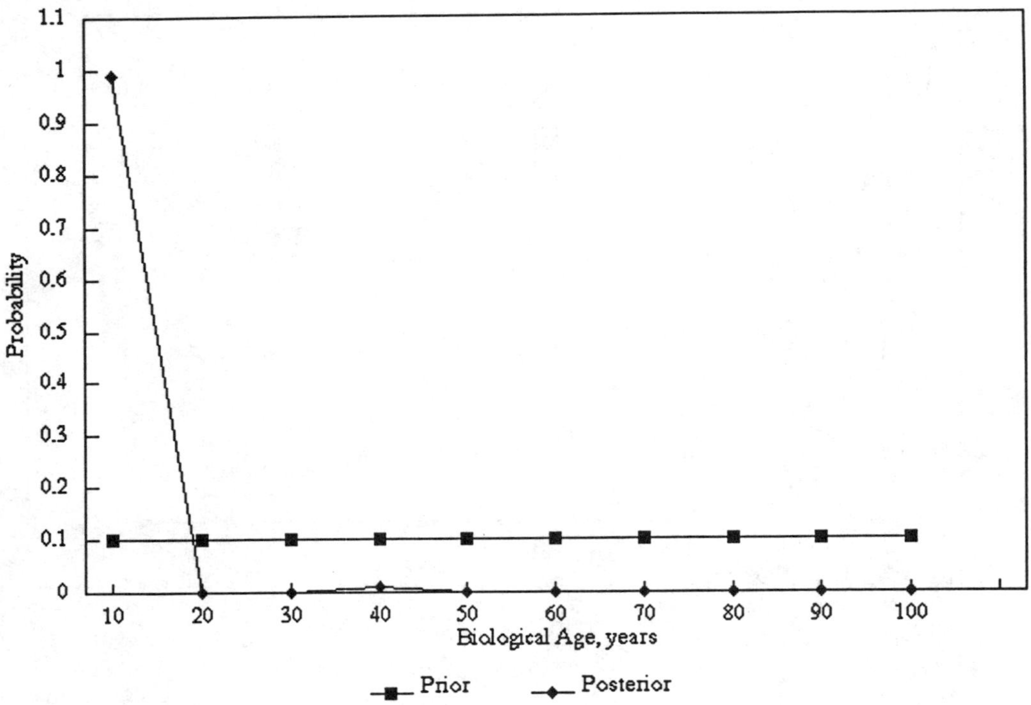

AGE	PRIOR	POSTERIOR	VARIABLE		VALUE	
10	0.10000	0.98910	Mitochondrial Por	V1	6.0	
20	0.10000	0.00121	DHEA male	V2	2.5	
30	0.10000	0.00046	Estradiol	V3	<50	
40	0.10000	0.00916	Dermal estrogen	V4	.01	
50	0.10000	0.00008	Urinary hydroxy	V5	20	
60	0.10000	0.00000	Acetylcholine rec	V6		0
70	0.10000	0.00000	Beta1 adrenergic	V7		0
80	0.10000	0.00000				
90	0.10000	0.00000				
100	0.10000	0.00000				
	1.00000	1.00000				

Figure 5 Probability distribution, fifth variable added.

Another spreadsheet can be constructed where the observables are diseases common to later life. Another can be about perceived overlap between what is seen as "pure biologic age" and disease. A similar spreadsheet could be about predisposing conditions, and so on. These can be combined and compared with cross-sectional or longitudinal study findings; this information in turn can be used to improve the knowledge base. Many possibilities would present as one becomes more familiar with this tool. This knowledge base can be quite large. It can focus on a great number of variables, and it compares each aspect of the query data against the entire range of this complexity.

VI. THE DYNAMIC KNOWLEDGE BASE

This is a method that can be used for storing large quantities of complex interrelated information in what might be termed a dynamic form, and testing against this another pattern of information called query data. It works for the management and utilization of a large body of complex interdependent, nondefinitive information and for putting the entire mass to use quickly, as if it were a single, responsive body. Thanks to the computer, the queries tested against this dynamic in effect give the data mass a focus. The computerized data mass can be thought of fancifully as being asked to bring its knowledge to bear on a question, on a set of observables posed to it.

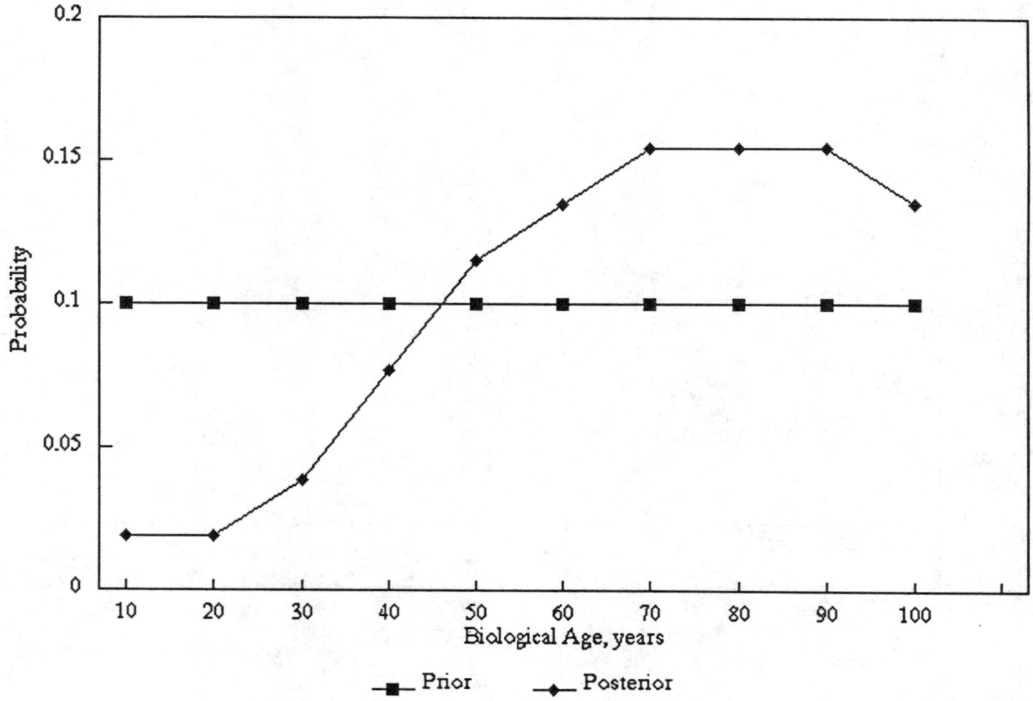

AGE	PRIOR	POSTERIOR	VARIABLE		VALUE
10	0.10000	0.01923	Mitochondrial Por	V1	2.4
20	0.10000	0.01923	DHEA male	V2	0
30	0.10000	0.03846	Estradiol	V3	0
40	0.10000	0.07692	Dermal estrogen	V4	0
50	0.10000	0.11538	Urinary hydroxy	V5	0
60	0.10000	0.13462	Acetylcholine rec	V6	0
70	0.10000	0.15385	Beta1 adrenergic	V7	0
80	0.10000	0.15385			
90	0.10000	0.15385			
100	0.10000	0.13462			
	1.00000	1.00000			

Figure 6 Probability distribution, one variable, age 50.

It requires thought and effort to compile, group, and understand the logic of this list of observables. It takes work and care to fill in the conditional probabilities. However, the reader should not be intimidated by the work, the use of expert opinions, or hard data. Judgments from experience are important.

To form an example, we have set down some fictitious arbitrary data points. We have arranged these into a small spreadsheet format. In the case of mitochondrial porphyrins illustrated in Figure 9, the points are 1.2, 2.4, 3.6, 4.8, and 6. nmol/ml. These could correspond with red, orange, brown, black, and skin color. Now we look at our hard data and ask ourselves, what is the probability a 10-year-old would have a mitochondrial porphyrin of 1.2 nmol/ml? Only. 0.5% of the time was this noted. In Figure 9, what has been done is to take data and give them a probability distribution. The reader must understand this converting hard data into the same information given as a conditional probability. It should be clear that much less quantitative data, even judgments, can be handled effectively in this way. They tend to summate with a surprising degree of robustness. This notion of converting numerical data into the same information expressed as a probability may not be clear at first. Examples to follow should clarify this essential maneuver.

We can arrange widely different forms of information in this uniform way. We can arrange a high school class of 100 around the data points A, B, C, D, and F. In the case of mitochondrial porphyrins, given a group of 100 10-year-olds, and arbitrarily choosing the five data points in the

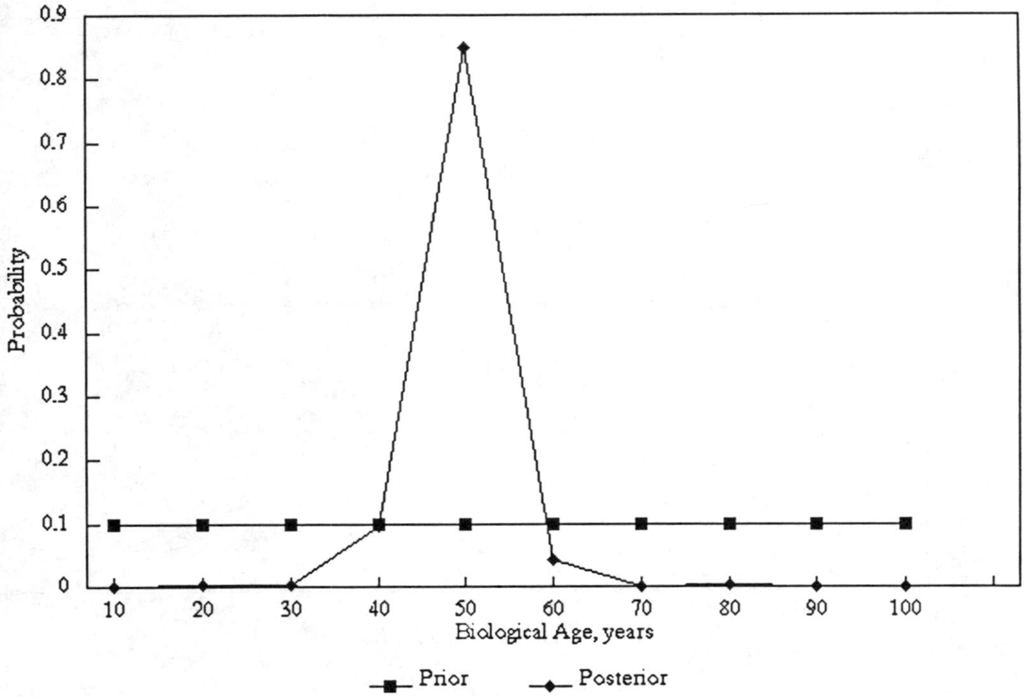

AGE	PRIOR	POSTERIOR	VARIABLE		VALUE	
10	0.10000	0.00000	Mitochondrial Por	V1	2.4	
20	0.10000	0.00242	DHEA male	V2	2.0	
30	0.10000	0.00279	Estradiol	V3	150	
40	0.10000	0.09692	Dermal estrogen	V4	1.0	
50	0.10000	0.84804	Urinary hydroxy	V5		0
60	0.10000	0.04240	Acetylcholine rec	V6		0
70	0.10000	0.00162	Beta1 adrenergic	V7		0
80	0.10000	0.00363				
90	0.10000	0.00162				
100	0.10000	0.00057				
	1.00000	1.00000				

Figure 7 Probability distribution, five variables, age 50.

paragraph above (again, refer to Figure 9), we would find that 0.05 would cluster around 1.2 and around 2.4 nmol/ml; but 0.6 would cluster around 6 nmol/ml mitochondrial porphyrins. Given that we have 100 10-year-olds, 5 would have a mitochondrial porphyrin of 1.2 nmol/ml, and 60 would have levels of 0.6. Had we 100 70-year-olds, 35 would have levels of only 1.2 nmol/ml (Figure 9).

Now if we have a means of collecting hundreds of different parameters, different aspects of aging that are definitive and arrange them in this way, we can develop on the computer this dynamic database we call a knowledge base. Some refer to this as a form of artificial intelligence or decision support. No matter what it is called, the computer once programmed to calculate Bayes formula at each point performs the miracle of scanning vast amounts of these data in seconds against a constellation of data put to it. In other words, once the correct probability is put in each cubical where an age column crosses an input row, and once this database is sufficiently complete and properly programmed, then the findings of a patient can be queried against this knowledge base and the computer would give that person's biological age. Further, the computer can be programmed to show by graphs how its opinion changes as more data are added (see Figures 1 through 8).

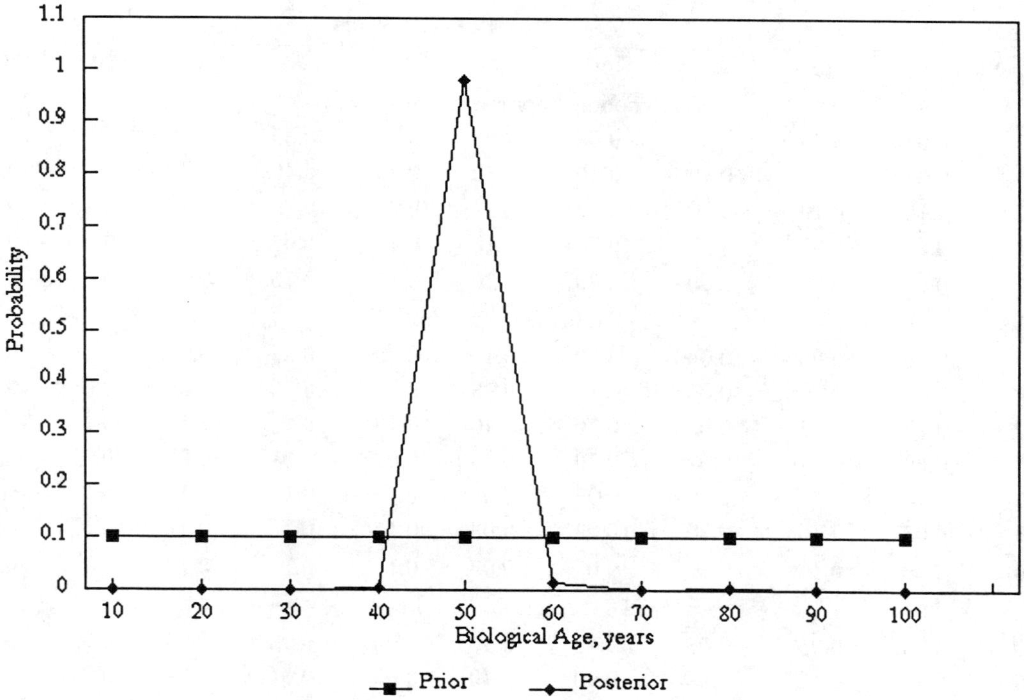

AGE	PRIOR	POSTERIOR	VARIABLE		VALUE
10	0.10000	0.00000	Mitochondrial Por	V1	2.4
20	0.10000	0.00004	DHEA male	V2	2.0
30	0.10000	0.00000	Estradiol	V3	150
40	0.10000	0.00310	Dermal estrogen	V4	1.0
50	0.10000	0.97760	Urinary hydroxy	V5	30
60	0.10000	0.01426	Acetylcholine rec	V6	.8
70	0.10000	0.00083	Beta1 adrenergic	V7	25
80	0.10000	0.00242			
90	0.10000	0.00124			
100	0.10000	0.00051			
	1.00000	1.00000			

Figure 8 Probability distribution, seven variables, age 50.

The output is usually written as follows. The biological age of this person is 50 years with a degree of certainty of 90%. It might, on the other hand, report this person is age 50 with a degree of certainty of 30%, age 55 with a probability of 50%, and age 45 with a probability of 20%. In such a case, insufficient information was input about the person being assessed, or the database was inadequate, or the computer was "confused".

Another exciting aspect emerges. The adequacy of the computer program itself can be checked against standards put to it. By observing a given graph following each data input, weak spots, indeed strong spots, can be located. These so-called strong spots may be the biomarkers we are seeking. By the slang term "strong spots" is meant that within a given constellation of input about a person, some certain input will at once push the age decisively to a certain age and it will tend to stay there. An example from dermatology is given. In the midst of putting what one sees about a pigmented tumor into the computer, the feature of asymmetry or the feature of bleeding when entered, will immediately swing the diagnosis to the consideration of malignancy and keep it there regardless of a myriad of other variables added.

It is assumed the data taken in about test subjects reflect both their chronological and biological age at the time taken. In the earlier ages the two are apt to coincide. How and over what time course

Prior variables	Biological age, years 10	20	30	40	50	60	70	80	90	100
				Mitochondrial porphyrins (nmol/ml)						
1.2	0.05	0.05	0.05	0.08	0.08	0.10	0.35	0.40	0.50	0.35
2.4	0.05	0.05	0.10	0.20	0.30	0.35	0.40	0.40	0.40	0.35
3.6	0.10	0.10	0.10	0.12	0.24	0.25	0.05	0.18	0.10	0.30
4.8	0.20	0.25	0.35	0.30	0.18	0.17	0.05	0.02	0	0
6.0	0.60	0.55	0.40	0.30	0.20	0.18	0.15	0	0	0
				DHEA male (mg/ml)						
1.0	0.001	0.000	0.000	0.00	0.1	0.36	0.85	0.90	0.85	0.80
1.5	0.01	0.000	0.001	0.19	0.35	0.50	0.10	0.05	0.05	0.10
2.0	0.25	0.024	0.023	0.20	0.40	0.10	0.1	0.1	0.1	0.1
2.5	0.60	0.024	0.025	0.50	0.10	0.01	0.01	0.01	0.01	0.01
3.0	0.10	0.10	0.199	0.05	0.04	0.1	0.1	0.1	0.1	0.1
3.5	0.03	0.40	0.50	0.04	0.03	0.1	0.1	0.1	0.1	0.1
4.0	0.009	0.45	0.25	0.01	0.03	0.1	0.1	0.1	0.1	0.1
				DHEA female (mg/ml)						
1.0	0.20	0.05	0.05	0.40	0.40	0.90	0.95	0.95	0.95	0.95
1.5	0.40	0.10	0.35	0.40	0.40	0.05	0.01	0.01	0.01	0.02
2.0	0.20	0.20	0.35	0.05	0.05	0.01	0.01	0.01	0.01	0.01
2.5	0.10	0.40	0.10	0.05	0.05	0.01	0.01	0.01	0.01	0.01
3.0	0.05	0.20	0.10	0.05	0.05	0.01	0.01	0.01	0.01	0.01
3.5	0.04	0.049	0.025	0.04	0.05	0.01	0.01	0.01	0.01	0.00
4.0	0.01	0.001	0.025	0.00	0.00	0.01	0.00	0.00	0.00	0.00

Figure 9 Simple sample spreadsheet.

do they separate? It is possible that not one, but some grouping of several parameters taken together are necessary to determine biologic age, or to develop a so-called biomarker.

Thus, as people age and the disparity between their biological and chronological age widens, to whatever extent this is true, important distinguishing data can be collected by converting it all to probabilities and treating it as suggested. The knowledge base then can be used in several other interesting ways that present themselves as one works with the computer. The knowledge base can be made to continually check over and update itself. In a fascinating variety of ways one can play with the data.

VII. AN EXAMPLE

The likelihood function which means the body of conditional probability numbers used in this example knowledge base, and the data from which they were derived are based on fictitious estimates rather than on a literature search. After all, the purpose of this chapter is to exemplify only the format and operation of the methodology. Even so, one cannot help being influenced by the literature[7-10] to develop a bit of science fiction. If the reader disagrees with the numbers, the reader should remember that they are contrived to serve as example data so that attention may be concentrated on the thesis.

Variable	value	10	20	30	40	50	60	70	80	90	100
		Biological age, years									
		Mitochondrial porphyrins (nmol/ml)									
V1	1.2	0.05000	0.05000	0.05000	0.08000	0.08000	0.10000	0.35000	0.40000	0.50000	0.35000
V1	2.4	0.05000	0.05000	0.10000	0.20000	0.30000	0.35000	0.40000	0.40000	0.40000	0.35000
V1	3.6	0.10000	0.10000	0.10000	0.12000	0.24000	0.25000	0.05000	0.18000	0.10000	0.30000
V1	4.8	0.20000	0.25000	0.35000	0.30000	0.18000	0.17000	0.05000	0.02000	0.00000	0.00000
V1	6.0	0.60000	0.55000	0.40000	0.30000	0.20000	0.18000	0.15000	0.00000	0.00000	0.00000
		DHEA (mg/ml)									
V2	1.0	0.00100	0.00000	0.00000	0.00000	0.10000	0.36000	0.85000	0.90000	0.92000	0.93000
V2	1.5	0.01000	0.00000	0.00100	0.19000	0.35000	0.50000	0.10000	0.05000	0.03000	0.02000
V2	2.0	0.25000	0.02400	0.02300	0.20000	0.40000	0.10000	0.01000	0.01000	0.01000	0.01000
V2	2.5	0.60000	0.02400	0.02500	0.50000	0.10000	0.01000	0.01000	0.01000	0.01000	0.01000
V2	3.0	0.10000	0.10000	0.19900	0.05000	0.04000	0.01000	0.01000	0.01000	0.01000	0.01000
V2	3.5	0.03000	0.40000	0.50000	0.04000	0.03000	0.01000	0.01000	0.01000	0.01000	0.01000
V2	4.0	0.00900	0.45000	0.25000	0.01000	0.03000	0.01000	0.01000	0.01000	0.01000	0.01000
		Estradiol (pmol/ml)									
V3	<50	1.00000	0.20000	0.10000	0.05000	0.05000	0.02000	0.01000	0.00500	0.00100	0.00100
V3	100	0.00000	0.50000	0.50000	0.40000	0.35000	0.20000	0.09000	0.03500	0.01000	0.00500
V3	150	0.00000	0.10000	0.20000	0.30000	0.35000	0.30000	0.10000	0.09000	0.05000	0.02000
V3	200	0.00000	0.10000	0.10000	0.15000	0.15000	0.30000	0.20000	0.20000	0.20000	0.17400
V3	250	0.00000	0.04900	0.04900	0.04900	0.04900	0.10000	0.20000	0.20000	0.25000	0.25000
V3	300	0.00000	0.04800	0.04800	0.04800	0.04800	0.05000	0.20000	0.20000	0.20900	0.22000
V3	350	0.00000	0.00100	0.00100	0.00100	0.00100	0.02000	0.10000	0.15000	0.15000	0.17000
V3	400	0.00000	0.00100	0.00100	0.00100	0.00100	0.00700	0.09000	0.10000	0.10000	0.12000
V3	450	0.00000	0.00100	0.00100	0.00100	0.00100	0.00300	0.01000	0.02000	0.03000	0.04000
		Dermal estrogen receptor (nmol/g)									
V4	0.01	0.60000	0.10000	0.10000	0.20000	0.10000	0.10000	0.05000	0.10000	0.25000	0.30000
V4	0.5	0.10000	0.20000	0.10000	0.40000	0.10000	0.10000	0.10000	0.20000	0.35000	0.39000
V4	1.0	0.10000	0.50000	0.15000	0.20000	0.50000	0.10000	0.10000	0.25000	0.20000	0.20000
V4	1.5	0.05000	0.10000	0.20000	0.05000	0.10000	0.20000	0.15000	0.15000	0.10000	0.05000
V4	2.0	0.05000	0.05000	0.40000	0.05000	0.05000	0.25000	0.20000	0.10000	0.05000	0.03000
V4	2.5	0.05000	0.02500	0.025000	0.02500	0.02500	0.15000	0.25000	0.10000	0.03000	0.02000
V4	3.0	0.05000	0.02500	0.025000	0.02500	0.02500	0.10000	0.15000	0.10000	0.02000	0.01000
		Urinary hydroxy proline (mg/24h)									
V5	10	0.30000	0.25000	0.200000	0.03800	0.02500	0.01000	0.01000	0.02000	0.05000	0.05000
V5	15	0.30000	0.25000	0.200000	0.20000	0.02500	0.01000	0.01000	0.03000	0.05000	0.05000
V5	20	0.30000	0.30000	0.300000	0.40000	0.05000	0.04000	0.03000	0.05000	0.05000	0.05000
V5	25	0.05200	0.17000	0.260000	0.25000	0.20000	0.04000	0.05000	0.07000	0.10000	0.05000
V5	30	0.02500	0.02700	0.019000	0.10000	0.40000	0.10000	0.10000	0.13000	0.15000	0.20000
V5	35	0.00100	0.00100	0.010000	0.01000	0.20000	0.30000	0.20000	0.25000	0.20000	0.20000
V5	40	0.00100	0.00100	0.001000	0.00100	0.07000	0.30000	0.30000	0.25000	0.20000	0.20000
V5	45	0.00100	0.00100	0.001000	0.00100	0.03000	0.20000	0.30000	0.20000	0.20000	0.20000

Figure 10 Example knowledge base spreadsheet for biological age (male).

		Acetylcholine receptor antibody (nmol/l)									
V6	.1	1.00000	0.15000	0.200000	0.10000	0.05000	0.05000	0.05000	0.01000	0.01000	0.01000
V6	.2	0.00000	0.20000	0.200000	0.10000	0.05000	0.05000	0.05000	0.01000	0.01000	0.01000
V6	.3	0.00000	0.20000	0.200000	0.10000	0.15000	0.10000	0.05000	0.02000	0.02000	0.01000
V6	.4	0.00000	0.15000	0.150000	0.10000	0.10000	0.10000	0.10000	0.06000	0.06000	0.02000
V6	.5	0.00000	0.10000	0.150000	0.15000	0.10000	0.10000	0.10000	0.10000	0.10000	0.05000
V6	.6	0.00000	0.10000	0.050000	0.15000	0.10000	0.10000	0.10000	0.15000	0.10000	0.10000
V6	.7	0.00000	0.04900	0.040000	0.10000	0.15000	0.15000	0.15000	0.15000	0.15000	0.15000
V6	.8	0.00000	0.04900	0.005000	0.10000	0.15000	0.15000	0.20000	0.20000	0.20000	0.20000
V6	.9	0.00000	0.00100	0.003000	0.05000	0.10000	0.15000	0.10000	0.15000	0.20000	0.25000
V6	1.0	0.00000	0.00100	0.002000	0.05000	0.05000	0.05000	0.10000	0.15000	0.20000	0.20000
		Beta 1 adrenergic receptor antibody (nmol/ml)									
V7	5	1.00000	0.05000	0.01000	0.01000	0.00500	0.00100	0.00100	0.00100	0.00100	0.00100
V7	10	0.00000	0.10000	0.05000	0.10000	0.07500	0.04900	0.03900	0.01900	0.01900	0.01900
V7	15	0.00000	0.30000	0.40000	0.35000	0.12000	0.10000	0.0600	0.03000	0.03000	0.03000
V7	20	0.00000	0.30000	0.40000	0.45000	0.30000	0.25000	0.20000	0.15000	0.10000	0.10000
V7	25	0.00000	0.20000	0.10000	0.05000	0.30000	0.35000	0.40000	0.40000	0.40000	0.35000
V7	30	0.00000	0.04900	0.03000	0.03000	0.10000	0.15000	0.20000	0.30000	0.30000	0.30000
V7	35	0.00000	0.00100	0.01000	0.01000	0.10000	0.10000	0.10000	0.10000	0.15000	0.20000

Figure 10 Example knowledge base spreadsheet for biological age (male) (continued).

To demonstrate this methodology, we have constructed a sample knowledge base for humans, making use of the following seven physiologic variables:

V1. Mitochondrial porphyrin 12 (nmol/ml)
V2. DHEA, in mg/ml plasma
V3. Estradiol, in pmol/ml plasma
V4. Dermal estrogen receptor, in fmol/g dermis
V5. Urinary hydroxyproline, in mg/24 h urine specimen
V6. Acetylcholine receptor binding antibody, in nmol/l
V7. Beta 1 adrenergic receptor antibody, in nmol/ml

In this sample knowledge base, we have discretized the possible values of bioage, allowing only even decade values from 10 to 100 years. A more realistic knowledge base could easily allow more detail, down to 1 year or less if desired. There are also ways to program for sexual differences. One need only put this information in the computer.

Notwithstanding the fiction, the numerical results worked out rather well. For example, Figure 1 shows the results of a calculation in which we took the prior distribution to be flat over the range 10 to 100 years of biological age. We then told the system that the mitochondrial porphyrins of the individual in question were 6 nmol/ml. That single piece of information is sufficient to tell us that the individual's biologic age is probably 10 to 20 years, and possibly in the mid-range of 30 to 40 years. It is quite unlikely to be in the range of 50 to 70, and essentially impossible that it is higher than that.

In Figure 2, we have added the information that the individual is male and that his dehydroepiandrosterone (DHEA) is 2.5 mg/ml. This information raises our confidence that the biologic age is in the neighborhood of 10 years with a secondary possibility, because of the cyclic pattern of the DHEA data, that the bioage is about 40 years.

Figure 3 adds the information that dermal estrogen receptor is 0.01 fmol/g. This confirms still further the confidence in a 10-year biologic age and reduces the probability of 40 years to about 10%.

In Figures 4 and 5, added information on estradiol and acetylcholine receptors produces essentially complete confidence in a biologic age of about 10 years.

Figures 6, 7, and 8 show another example in which the first piece of information suggests a 70 to 90 bioage, but as successive pieces of information are entered, the curve gradually narrows down to essentially complete confidence in a 50-year bioage.

Finally, remember the computer adage "garbage in, garbage out". A database is no better than the quality and pertinence of the input information. This knowledge base is unique, however, in that through proper manipulation it can derive better quality information which then can be readded to upgrade a master knowledge base.

VIII. MITOCHONDRIAL PORPHYRINS

Consider this example fictitious article, "Age differences in mitochondrial levels of porphyrin 12 as measured by benzodiazepine affinity studies" (idea from Snyder[10]). The levels ranged from 1.2 $nmol/cm^3$ to 6.0 $nmol/cm^3$ with no sex differences. Note the row on the spreadsheet example (Figure 9) entitled "mitochondria por." Unless the original experimental work showed natural break points, the observable variables section could be written: 1.2, 2.4, 3.6, 4.8, 6.0.

To help the reader have clearly in mind the different aspects of what we are trying to explain, we attempt here by this digression to review the parts of a database. There are three. First is a comprehensive, succinct list of the possible variables. This puts into some suitable form each bit of information against which each age will be considered. The second part, the likelihood function, results from the work of the expert who gives these possible variables meaning within a certain context by inserting into the spreadsheet cell a number that says: Given that age, this is the change that the variable is true. This may be expert opinion. It may be hard data. These numbers en masse are called the likelihood function. Third is a user with a question; one aspect of that query data being this point, this level of mitochondrial porphyrins. The user, for example, has a patient with (among other data) a reading of this patient's level of mitochondrial porphyrins. He wants to know this patient's biologic age. A tiny part of this biologic age determination would be the comparison against the mitochondrial porphyrin data shown in Figures 9 and 10. Through proper programming he is able to present the constellation of variables he has collected to the dynamic database.

When we created the mitochondria row of the spreadsheet (Figure 9), and the data beneath it about mitochondrial prophyrins, we were inputting only the first part, described in the preceding paragraph. The next step would be for the expert to come along and fill each cell along the row belonging to a reading about mitochondrial prophyrins for each age group. To do that, note the columns after each mitochondrial porphyrin level reading in Figures 9 and 10. Again, note that these numbers could be estimates by the expert who did the work, or they could be hard experimental data. A corresponding cell, reading down from above, beneath each age, has a decimal number entered. Notice that for the column called age ten, the probability that the mitochondrial porphyrin 12 level is 1.2 is only 0.05; that it is 2.4 is 0.05; that it is 3.6 is 0.1; that it is 4.8 is 0.2; that it is 6.0 is 0.6. Note that these add to the number 1. If the reader can grasp this way of presenting data and grasp the significance of it, there remains only the art of fitting the information into this format.

IX. DEHYDROEPIANDROSTERONE SULFATE

Nearly everyone is familiar with the measurement of some hormone, for example, estrogen or DHEA, measured in some group of subjects of different ages. The same kind of measurements could be done on the same individual over time. They could be done on many subjects in some longitudinal study. Could such studies tell anything about bioage? Consider DHEA sulfate plasma levels in males and females of different ages. These contrived example data are presented here as follows:

Age (years)	Male (mg/ml)	Female (mg/ml)
10	2.5	1.6
20	3.8	2.6
30	3.4	1.8
40	2.5	1.3
50	1.8	1.2
60	1.0	0.6
70	1.0	0.8
80	1.0	0.8
90	1.0	0.5
100	1.5	0.8

After viewing the data, go to Figures 9 or 10 to see how they are presented in "probability form". These data have the appearance of digital data. Such data are usually the average of many individual measurements taken from different subjects, not all of whom were exactly on their birthday when the blood was drawn. One can view this as many different data points compressed into an average.

Using conditional probabilities, the frequency of occurrence of each measurement can be expressed as a probability, preserving more of the information content. One must work within the constraints of the arbitrary subdivisions selected to go down the left side of the spreadsheet. In this case these are 1, 1.5, 2, 2.5, 3, 3.5, and 4. According to this spreadsheet (Figure 9), if DHEA plasma levels from 1000 10-year-old males were determined, 1 of them showed a DHEA level (all mg/ml) of 1.0, 10 showed a DHEA level of 1.5, 250 a level of 2, 600 a level of 2.5, 100 a level of 3, 30 a level of 3.5, and 9 a level of 4. These numbers refer to clustering around such values.

Consider again how to tease biologic age out of data based on chronological age. One could compare the query subjects' testosterone level against the database which contained information about this. What if there were about 50 carefully chosen parameters entered, against which to query the knowledge base? Suppose after gaining experience with the knowledge base and after inputting into that knowledge base experience, the operators became aware of the most significant 50 parameters to use? A patient would not come with just a testosterone level but also those 50 variables. Suppose there were more sophisticated measurements to begin with. What if all 50 of those measurements were taken simultaneously before and several times after different knowledgeable perturbations of the subject? The measurements could be then evaluated in mass by a large similarly sophisticated knowledge base.

Given a profusion of input variables from the query subject taken singly, in combination, and at various times. To more efficiently handle this profusion of data taken over a large complex database, Kaplan has incorporated the strategy of "homing in". Any scenario can be considered as a set of subscenarios. The subscenarios can be aggregated into a small number of large categories. The query input set is then considered over a limited set of large categories. Those large categories that have a high probability of being important in the final result are expanded. Those that have low probabilities remain coalesced into their large categories. The result is a new set of scenario categories that contain more detail in the region of interest. A new calculation is made over this new set of categories and the process is repeated until the desired level of detail is obtained. In this way the process "homes in" on the solution with far greater computational efficiency.

Another simple use of this knowledge base idea, perhaps of interest to insurance companies, would be risk analysis. A knowledge base could be constructed containing the known risk factors as to life span of a queried individual. It would offer a more sophisticated method perhaps than is presently used. For example, if a person were a smoker with a family history of emphysema, one could bring in pulmonary function studies and sophisticated cardiac studies if an insurance policy were expensive enough to merit it. Such a method would have special application in the high risk and/or large policy situation. The art would be in the development of the list of observables, and in grouping them into mutually exclusive categories.

Finally, whatever was done, no information would be wasted. Information gleaned anywhere could be used everywhere.

X. CONCLUSION

This chapter gives the reader a glimpse of a new type of computerized dynamic database called here a knowledge base. This was originally developed by the authors in an effort to make better artificial intelligence or decision support systems. We realized that a methodology built around such a knowledge base can be well adapted to the assessment of biologic age. The reader is given some notion of the suitability of such a knowledge base for the definition and utilization of bioage. The assessment is presented in the form of a probability curve over an axis representing possible values of biologic age. The probability curve format allows one to explicitly acknowledge the degree of uncertainty in such an assessment. This degree of uncertainty depends on the amount and pertinence of the available information. Our experience has shown that results calculated thus are quite accurate with respect to approximations and moderate inaccuracies in the large knowledge base. The methodology has the advantage that it can make use of all the measurements, judgments, and approximations on all the individuals being assessed. It thus seems to come closer to dealing with the inherent complexity of the concept of biologic age as we understand it.

REFERENCES

1. Segerberg, O., *Living to be 100,* Charles Schribner Sons, New York, 1982, 8.
2. Bauleau, E.E., Molecular mechanism of antisteroid hormones at the receptor level, *Kidney Int.,* 34(Suppl. 26), S2, 1988.
3. Snyder, S.H., Drug and neurotransmitter receptors, *JAMA,* 261(No. 21), 3126, 1989.
4. Sox, H.C., Blatt, M.A., Higgins, M.C., and Marton, K.I., Medical *Decision Making,* Butterworths, Boston, 1988, 27.
5. Kaplan, S., Frank, M.V., Bley, D.C., and Lindsay, D.G., Outline of COPILOT, an expert system for reactor operational assistance, using a Bayesian diagnostic module, *Reliability Eng. System Safety,* 22, 411, 1988.
6. Kaplan, S., Keter, A., Lindsay, D.G., Bley, D.C., Epstein, S.A., and Emerson, M.A., Expert Systems for Diagnosis and Decision Under Substantial Uncertainty, A Classical (Bayesian) Approach, presented to the Forum on Artificial Intelligence in Management, sponsored by the U.S. Department of Defense, 1990, 1.
7. Collins, S., Balanowski, M.A., Caron, M.G., and Lefkowitz, R.J., Genetic regulation of beta adrenergic receptors, 203, 1989.
8. Bakken, C.L., Ed., *Mayo Medical Laboratories Handbook,* Mayo Medical Laboratories, Rochester, MN, 1981.
9. Peter, J.B., *The Use and Interpretation of Tests in Clinical Immunology,* 6th and 7th eds., Interstate Press, Omaha, NE, 1989 and 1990.
10. Verma, A., Nye, J.S., and Snyder, S.H., Porphyrins are endogenous ligands for the mitochondrial (peripheral-type) benzodiazepine receptor, *Proc. Natl. Acad. Sci. U.S.A.,* 84: 2256, 1987.

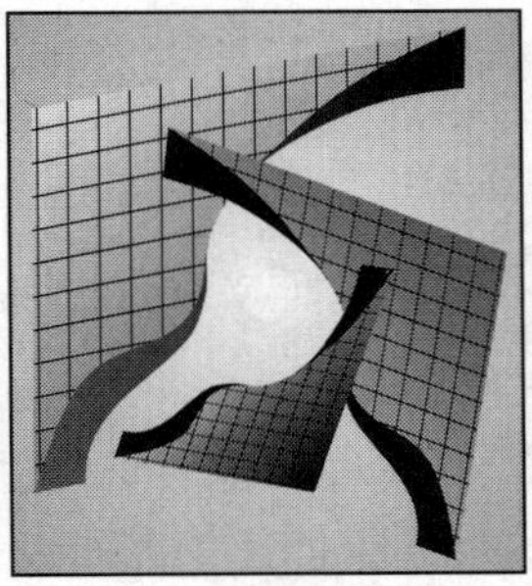

INDEX

INDEX

C

E

L

M

S

T

U

V